Date Due

OCT - 8 2001			
NOV 19 2001	DISCARDED		
DEC 1 6 2003			
OCT 0 3 2007			
NOV 2 6 2008			
DEC 0 6 2013			

BRODART, CO.　　　Cat. No. 23-233-003　　　Printed in U.S.A.

Tooth Wear and Sensitivity

The Council of Europe Group for Research on Colloidal Phenomena in the Oral Cavity was established under the auspices of the then Parliamentary Assembly of the Council of Europe Committee on Science and Technology in 1975. Since then the Group has met on a variety of occasions throughout Europe and has brought together clinical and basic scientists from around the world.

On a sad note, we must report the untimely passing away of one of our founder members, Professor Joop Arends from the Department of Biomedical Engineering, Groningen, The Netherlands. Joop Arends – a key member of our Group and a scientist renowned for his work on the physical aspects of tooth surface and structure considerations – will be sadly missed by all who knew him. Chapter 22 in this book is dedicated to his memory.

Tooth Wear and Sensitivity

Clinical advances in restorative dentistry

Edited by

Martin Addy BDS, MSc, PhD, FDSRCS
Professor of Restorative Dentistry (Periodontology)
Bristol Dental School and Hospital
Bristol BS1 2LY, UK

Graham Embery BSc, PhD, DSc
Professor of Dentistry
Head, Department of Basic Dental Science
Dental School
University of Wales College of Medicine
Heath Park
Cardiff CF4 4XY, UK

W Michael Edgar BSc, BDS, PhD, DSc, FDSRCS
Emeritus Professor of Dental Science
Department of Clinical Dental Sciences
School of Dentistry
University of Liverpool
Liverpool L69 3BX, UK

Robin Orchardson BSc, BDS, PhD
Senior Lecturer, Division of Neuroscience
Institute of Biomedical and Life Sciences
University of Glasgow
Glasgow G12 8QQ, UK

Published in association with the Council of Europe

MARTIN ■ DUNITZ

© Martin Dunitz Ltd 2000

First published in the United Kingdom in 2000 by
Martin Dunitz Ltd
The Livery House
7–9 Pratt Street
London NW1 0AE

Tel: +44 (0)20 7482 2202
Fax: +44 (0)20 7267 0159
E-mail: info@mdunitz.globalnet.co.uk
Website: http://www.dunitz.co.uk

A CIP catalogue record for this book is available from the British Library

ISBN 1–85317–826–8

Distributed in the United States by:
Blackwell Science Inc.
Commerce Place, 350 Main Street
Malden MA 02148, USA
Tel: 1 800 215 1000

Distributed in Canada by:
Login Brothers Book Company
324 Salteaux Crescent
Winnipeg, Manitoba R3J 3T2
Canada
Tel: 1 204 224 4068

Distributed in Brazil by:
Ernesto Reichmann Distribuidora de Livros, Ltda
Rua Coronel Marques 335
03440–000 São Paulo–SP
Brazil

Composition by Scribe Design, Gillingham, Kent, UK
Printed and bound in Singapore by Kyodo Pte Ltd

CONTENTS

† Deceased

CONTRIBUTORS

Martin Addy BDS, MSc, PhD, FDSRCS
Professor of Restorative Dentistry
(Periodontology), Bristol Dental School and
Hospital, Bristol BS1 2LY, UK

John I Alexander MB, BS, FRCA
Consultant in Anaesthesia and Pain
Management to the United Bristol Healthcare
Trust and Senior Clinical Lecturer to the
University of Bristol, Sir Humphry Davy
Department of Anaesthesia, Bristol Royal
Infirmary, Bristol BS2 8HW, UK

Bennett T Amaechi BSc, BDS, MSc, PhD
Research Associate in Cariology, Cariology
Research Group, Department of Clinical Dental
Sciences, School of Dentistry, University of
Liverpool, Liverpool L69 3BX, UK

David Andrew BDS, PhD
Research Fellow, Department of Physiology,
School of Medical Sciences, University of
Bristol, Bristol BS8 1TD, UK

†Joop Arends PhD
Professor of Materials Science, Department of
Biomedical Engineering, University of Groningen,
9712 KZ Groningen, The Netherlands

Lori A Bacca BS
Research Associate, Oral Care Product
Development, The Procter and Gamble Co.,
PO Box 8006, Mason, OH 45040, USA

David Bartlett BDS, PhD, MRD FDS(Rest.)RCS
Senior Lecturer in Conservative Dentistry,
Department of Conservative Dentistry, Guy's,
King's and St Thomas' Dental Institute, King's
College, London Bridge, London SE1 9RT, UK

Rolf Bos PhD
Department of Biomedical Engineering,
University of Groningen, 9712 KZ Groningen,
The Netherlands

Henk J Busscher PhD
Professor of Biomaterials, Department of
Biomedical Engineering, University of
Groningen, 9712 KZ Groningen, The
Netherlands

Jacob M ten Cate BSc, PhD
Professor of Preventive Dentistry, Department of
Cariology Endodontology Pedodontology, and
Associate Dean, Academic Center for Dentistry
Amsterdam (ACTA), 1066 EA Amsterdam, The
Netherlands

Edward R Cox BS
Senior Research Associate, The Procter and
Gamble Co., PO Box 8006, Mason, OH 45040,
USA

Frederick A Curro DMD, PhD
Vice-President and Director, Corporate Clinical
and Medical Affairs, Research and Technology,
Block Drug Company, Inc., Jersey City,
NJ 07302, USA

Monique M Danser DDS, PhD
Assistant Professor in Periodontology,
Department of Periodontology, Academic Centre
for Dentistry Amsterdam (ACTA), 1066 EA
Amsterdam, The Netherlands

Heinz Duschner Dr rer. nat. et med. dent. habil.
Professor, Applied Structure and Microanalysis,
Medical Faculty, University of Mainz, D-55101
Mainz, Germany

† Deceased

Toon Dykman MD PhD
Senior Researcher, Department of Biomedical
Engineering, University of Groningen, 9712 KZ
Groningen, The Netherlands

W Michael Edgar BSc, BDS, PhD, DSc, FDSRCS
Emeritus Professor of Dental Science,
Department of Clinical Dental Sciences, School
of Dentistry, University of Liverpool, Liverpool
L69 3BX, UK

Graham Embery BSc, PhD, DSc
Emeritus Professor of Dentistry and Head of
Department of Basic Dental Science, Dental
School, University of Wales College of Medicine,
Heath Park, Cardiff CF4 4XY, UK

Michael Friedman PhD
Director, Biostatistics and Data Management,
Block Drug Company, Inc., Jersey City,
NJ 07302, USA

Abdul Gaffar PhD
Vice-President Research and Development, Oral
Care Advanced Technology, Colgate–Palmolive
Co. Technology Center, PO Box 1343,
Piscataway, NJ 08855, USA

David G Gillam BA, BDS, MSc, DDS, FRSH
Senior Research Fellow and Lecturer,
Department of Periodontology, Eastman Dental
Institute for Oral Health Care Sciences,
University of London, London WC1X 8LD, UK

Wieke Goedhardt
Department of Biomedical Engineering,
University of Groningen, 9712 KZ Groningen,
The Netherlands

Hermann Götz Dipl. phys.
Applied Structure and Microanalysis, Medical
Faculty, University of Mainz, D-55101 Mainz,
Germany

Rachel C Hall BDS, PhD
Lecturer, Department of Basic Dental Science,
Dental School, University of Wales College of
Medicine, Cardiff CF4 4XY, UK

Matthias Hannig Dr med. dent.
Professor, Clinic of Operative Dentistry and
Periodontology, Christian-Albrechts-University
of Kiel, Germany

Susan M Higham BSc, PhD, CBiol., MIBiol.
Lecturer in Oral Biology, Cariology Research
Group, Department of Clinical Dental Sciences,
School of Dentistry, University of Liverpool,
Liverpool L69 3BX, UK

Margaret L Hunter BDS, MScD, FDS(Paed.)RCS
Department of Oral and Dental Science,
University of Bristol, Bristol BS1 2LY, UK

Robert J Jackson BSc, PhD
Honorary Senior Research Fellow and Deputy
Director – Clinical Research Centre, Eastman
Dental Institute for Oral Health Care Sciences,
University of London, London WC1X 8LD, UK

Klaus D Jandt Dipl. Phys., Dr rer. nat.
Senior Lecturer in Dental Materials Science and
Biomaterials, Department of Oral and Dental
Science, University of Bristol, Bristol BS1 2LY,
UK

Paul A King BDS, MSc, FDSRCS
Consultant in Restorative Dentistry, Bristol
Dental Hospital and School, University of
Bristol, Bristol BS1 2LY, UK

Vuokko Kontturi-Närhi DDS, PhD
Private practice, Kuopio, Finland; formerly
Professor and Head of Department of
Periodontology, Institute of Dentistry, University
of Turku, FIN-20520 Turku, Finland

Anthony C Lanzalaco PhD
Principal Research Scientist Beauty Care
Product Development, The Procter and Gamble
Co., Miami Valley Laboratories, Ross, OH 45061,
USA

Ronald S Leight PhD
Manager, Data Management, Block Drug
Company, Inc., Jersey City, NJ 07302, USA

Philip Lumley BDS, MDentSc, FDSRCPS, PhD
Senior Lecturer in Conservative Dentistry,
Department of Oral Biology, School of Dentistry,
University of Birmingham, Birmingham B4 6NN,
UK

Adrian Lussi Dr med. dent.
Professor, Department of Operative, Preventive
and Paediatric Dentistry, School of Dentistry,
University of Bern, Bern, Switzerland

Lawrence H Mair BDS, FDSRCS, FADM, PhD
Senior Lecturer in Restorative Dentistry,
Department of Clinical Dental Sciences,
Liverpool University Dental Hospital and School
of Dentistry, Liverpool L3 5PS, UK

Bruce Matthews BDS, PhD
Professor of Physiology, Department of
Physiology, School of Medical Sciences,
University of Bristol, Bristol BS8 1TD, UK

John B Matthews BSc, MSc, PhD
Senior Lecturer in Immunopathology,
Department of Oral Biology, School of Dentistry,
University of Birmingham, Birmingham B4 6NN,
UK

Henny C van der Mei PhD
Department of Biomedical Engineering,
University of Groningen, 9712 KZ Groningen,
The Netherlands

Jukka H Meurman MD, PhD, Dr odont.
Professor of Dentistry, Institute of Dentistry,
FIN-00014 University of Helsinki, PO Box 41,
Helsinki, Finland

William Moffat BS
Senior Research Technician, Colgate–Palmolive
Co. Technology Center, PO Box 1343,
Piscataway, NJ 08855, USA

Anthony Moskwa AS
Scientist, Colgate–Palmolive Co. Technology
Center, PO Box 1343, Piscataway, NJ 08855, USA

Peter E Murray BSc, PhD
Research Fellow in Oral Biology, Department of
Oral Biology, School of Dentistry, University of
Birmingham, Birmingham B4 6NN, UK

Matti VO Närhi DDS, PhD
Professor of Pain Physiology, Institute of
Dentistry, University of Turku, FIN-20520 Turku,
Finland

June H Nunn PhD, BDS, FDSRCS(Edin.),
DDPHRCS(Eng.)
Senior Lecturer and Honorary Consultant in
Paediatric Dentistry, Department of Child Dental
Health, School of Dentistry, University of
Newcastle, Newcastle upon Tyne NE2 4BW, UK

Robin Orchardson BSc, BDS, PhD
Senior Lecturer, Division of Neuroscience,
Institute of Biomedical and Life Sciences,
University of Glasgow, Glasgow G12 8QQ, UK

David H Pashley BSc, DMD, PhD
Regents' Professor of Oral Biology, Department
of Oral Biology, Medical College of Georgia,
Augusta, GA 30912, USA

Gunnar Rölla Dr odont.
Emeritus Professor, Department of Pedodontics
and Caries Prophylaxis, Faculty of Dentistry,
University of Oslo, PO Box 1109, Blindern,
N-0317 Oslo, Norway

Jan Ruben
Department of Dentistry, University of
Groningen, 9712 KZ Groningen, The Netherlands

Morten Rykke Dr odont.
Associate Professor, Department of Cariology,
Faculty of Dentistry, University of Oslo, PO Box
1109, Blindern, N-0317 Oslo, Norway

Jackie B Shaffer PhD
Section Head Health Care Research, The Procter
and Gamble Co., PO Box 8006, Mason,
OH 45040, USA

R Peter Shellis BSc, MSc, PhD
Research Fellow, Division of Restorative
Dentistry, Department of Oral and Dental
Science, Dental School, University of Bristol,
Bristol BS1 2LY, UK

Alastair J Sloan BSc, PhD
Lecturer in Oral Biology, Department of Oral
Biology, School of Dentistry, University of
Birmingham, Birmingham B4 6NN, UK

Anthony J Smith BSc, PhD
Professor of Oral Biology, Department of Oral
Biology, School of Dentistry, University of
Birmingham, Birmingham B4 6NN, UK

Bernard GN Smith BDS, MSc, PhD, MRD,
FDSRCS(Eng.), FDSRCS(Edin.)
Professor of Dentistry, Department of
Conservative Dentistry, Guy's, King's and St
Thomas' Dental Institute, King's College, London
Bridge, London SE1 9RT, UK

Torleif Sønju Dr odont.
Professor, Department of Cariology, Faculty of
Dentistry, University of Oslo, PO Box 1109,
Blindern, N-0317 Oslo, Norway

Anne Beate Sønju Clasen Dr odont.
Department of Cariology, Faculty of Dentistry,
University of Oslo, PO Box 1109, Blindern,
N-0317 Oslo, Norway

Rita Sorvari DDS, PhD
Lecturer, Department of Anatomy, University of
Kuopio, PO Box 1627, FIN-70211 Kuopio, Finland

Michael Stranick PhD
Senior Technical Associate, Colgate–Palmolive
Co. Technology Center, PO Box 1343,
Piscataway, NJ 08855, USA

Roger Walker
Dentist, Department of Operative Dentistry,
School of Dentistry, University of Bern, Bern,
Switzerland

Sitthichai Wanachantararak DDS
Research Fellow, Department of Physiology,
School of Medical Sciences, University of
Bristol, Bristol BS8 1TD, UK

Fridus Van der Weijden DDS, PhD
Associate Professor in Periodontology,
Department of Periodontology, Academic Center
for Dentistry (ACTA), 1066 EA Amsterdam,
The Netherlands

Nicola X West BDS, PhD, FDSRCS
Lecturer and Honorary Senior Registrar in
Restorative Dentistry (Periodontology),
Department of Oral and Dental Science,
University of Bristol, Bristol BS1 2LY, UK

Donald J White PhD
Research Fellow, Oral Care Product
Development, The Procter and Gamble Co.,
PO Box 8006, Mason, OH 45040, USA

David K Whittaker BDS, PhD, FRSA, FDSRCS, Dip.
forens. odont.
Reader in Oral Biology and Forensic Dentistry,
Department of Basic Dental Science, Dental
School, University of Wales College of Medicine,
Heath Park, Cardiff CF4 4XY, UK

Malcolm Williams PhD
Senior Technical Associate, Colgate–Palmolive
Co. Technology Center, PO Box 1343,
Piscataway, NJ 08855, USA

Alix R Young PhD
Department of Pedodontics and Caries
Prophylaxis, Faculty of Dentistry, University of
Oslo, PO Box 1109, Blindern, N-0317 Oslo,
Norway

Domenick T Zero DDS, MS
Professor and Chair, Department of Preventive
and Community Dentistry, and Director, Oral
Health Research Institute, Indiana University
School of Dentistry, Indiana University,
Indianapolis, IN 46202, USA

PREFACE

After caries and periodontal disease, tooth wear and dentine hypersensitivity must rank next as the most common conditions affecting human dentition. Tooth wear has implications for the aesthetics, function and longevity of the primary and secondary dentitions. On the other hand, dentine hypersensitivity is a painful condition of the permanent dentition, thereby affecting oral comfort and function rather than longevity. The two conditions have a commonality in respect of aetiology, and a consideration of aetiological and predisposing factors suggests that both are increasing in incidence and severity. The consequences of tooth wear and sensitivity are potentially enormous, not least in financial terms to the profession, health services and patients.

The aim of this book is to draw together, in a single volume, the most up-to-date information on tooth wear and dentine hypersensitivity. The two conditions are considered from basic science, laboratory and clinical research, and clinical viewpoints. To our knowledge, no other book is available at this time which deals with these two associated common clinical conditions in such a comprehensive fashion. Each chapter has been contributed by recognized leaders in the field today; contributors from Europe and North America have been drawn from the basic sciences, clinical academia, clinical practice and industry, and all are considered experts in their own particular field.

The topics associated with tooth wear include: the anatomy, physiology, biology and histology of the dental hard tissues and pulp; the historical and forensic aspects of tooth wear; the definition, classification, measurement and aetiology of tooth wear and the processes involved, together with the consequences to the patient and clinician. Dentine hypersensitivity is considered from a number of perspectives including prevalence, aetiology, pulpal response and evaluation, with a separate chapter devoted to the clinical and physiological aspects of pain. The management of dentine hypersensitivity is considered with individual chapters on preventional present and future home use and in-office treatments.

This book is aimed at a wide range of individuals interested in basic and clinical dental science and clinical practice. As a whole, this book will be of interest to those in academic dentistry and to scientists involved in academic and industrial research. Individual chapters, particularly those based on up-to-date literature and data reviews, will be of great value and a source of extensive pertinent information to dental undergraduate and postgraduate students and to general and specialist dental practitioners.

It is hoped that this book will form a basis from which to understand tooth wear and dentine hypersensitivity, whereby effective management protocols can be designed and, more importantly, preventive strategies can be developed.

ACKNOWLEDGEMENTS

This is the book of the 1998 workshop of the Council of Europe Research Group on Surface and Colloidal Phenomena in the Oral Cavity. The workshop was held in Bristol, UK, on 18–21 November 1998 and was opened by Professor Graham Embery, Secretary General of the Research Group Council.

The meeting was most generously sponsored by the following organizations: Block Drug Co. (USA); Braun (Germany); Coca-Cola (UK); Colgate–Palmolive (USA); Gaba (Switzerland); Mars (UK); Oral B (USA); Procter and Gamble (USA); SmithKline Beecham (UK); and Unilever (UK). The financial help from these companies is gratefully acknowledged by the editors.

The editors and Council also gratefully acknowledge and sincerely thank Mrs Marjorie Addy and Mrs Mary Hall of the Department of Oral and Dental Science, University of Bristol, for their tremendous efforts in the organization of all aspects of the meeting.

PART I

Tooth Structure

1

Biological and structural features of enamel and dentine: current concepts relevant to erosion and dentine hypersensitivity

Rachel C Hall, Graham Embery and R Peter Shellis

Introduction

The underlying theme throughout this book recognizes the susceptibility of tooth mineral, primarily enamel, to erosion in response to a variety of chemical and mechanical stimuli, and also that the dentine has distinct structural features which give the dentition a capacity to recognize and respond to stimuli. Therefore the purpose of this chapter is to give an account of the structural biology of enamel and dentine, where it pertains to such trauma, and this underpins subsequent treatises governing more clinically related aspects of these problems.

Much is known about the synthesis and formation of enamel and dentine, although the key molecular events governing the influence of specific matrix molecules on the process of amelogenesis and dentinogenesis have not yet been fully elucidated. However, it is not the objective of this chapter to describe the highly complex biology which is known to be involved and the reader is referred to excellent reviews on amelogenesis (Robinson *et al.* 1995, Chadwick and Cardew 1997) and dentinogenesis (Linde and Goldberg 1993, Goldberg *et al.* 1999).

Instead, this chapter will focus on the mineral elements of both enamel and dentine, as this is the phase that is at risk. The dentition is unique in terms of mineralized tissue biology, because calcium phosphate is exposed to the outer environment. It is at risk from foodstuffs and beverages that are themselves vital for the nutri-

tional status and health of the organism. The delicate balance between ingestion and structural risk to the dentition is recognized as an important issue in dental health in modern society. The following accounts of the structural features of enamel and dentine aim to lay a foundation for an understanding of the issues which have arisen and are of concern to dental public health specialists.

Enamel structure and physiology

Enamel is the most highly calcified and hardest tissue of the body. Unlike dentine, cementum and bone, it is produced by cells of ectodermal origin. In the human tooth, the enamel normally forms a covering layer for the whole of the crown, but varies considerably in thickness in different parts of the crown.

Histological variation

Mineral content and porosity have been examined by quantitative microradiography and density mapping and show significant variation within enamel (Wilson and Beynon 1989). The mineral content is lowest at the enamel–dentine junction (EDJ) and highest at the outer surface. The volume of enamel not occupied by mineral is 50–100% greater in the inner enamel compared with the outer enamel; in inner enamel both protein (Robinson *et al*. 1971) and water (Dibdin and Poole 1982) are more abundant.

Structure

The prism (or rod) is the fundamental structural unit of enamel; each prism extends from its site of origin at the EDJ to the outer enamel surface and is composed of millions of individual crystals of hydroxyapatite. All enamel, with few exceptions (e.g. very thin enamel), is made up of superassemblies of these structures, combined with varying amounts of interprismatic material. Changes in the orientation of the crystals, relative to each other, mark the boundaries of the prisms (Figs 1.1 and 1.2).

In human enamel, the boundary of the prism body is incomplete cervically. Here the prism is continuous with a wedge-shaped 'tail', which comparative studies (Boyde 1965) show to be interprismatic enamel. The combined shape of the prism body and tail is that of a keyhole. The body of the prism is approximately 5 µm wide and the prism plus tail keyhole is approximately 9 µm long. The apatite crystals are most closely packed in the prism bodies, which occupy 60–65% v/v of enamel (Shellis 1984). When considering the generally accepted model for the prismatic structure of human enamel (Poole and Brookes 1961, Boyde 1965), a number of levels of perfection of crystal packing associated with prism bodies, prism tails and prism junctions (Shellis 1984) must be considered.

The configuration of enamel crystals is related to the organization of the ameloblast and its Tomes' process. The forming surface of enamel consists of pits, each defined by a wall made up of newly formed interprismatic enamel. During active secretion, each of these walled pits is occupied by a Tomes' process. The interprismatic walls are formed slightly earlier than the prism enamel, which constitutes the floors of the pits, and are formed by secretion by sites at the ameloblast peripheries (Warshawsky *et al*. 1981). The presumptive prism boundary is defined by the position of the junction between the pit wall and the floor. In human enamel the pit is at its

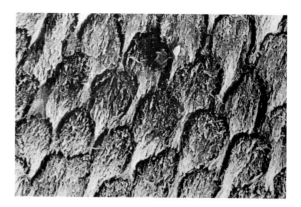

Figure 1.1

Enamel prisms in transverse section. The prisms in this section demonstrate the characteristic keyhole appearance of type 3 enamel, the tail of one prism lying between the body of two lower prisms. Differences in crystal orientation between the tail and body are apparent (etched section, SEM ×1900).

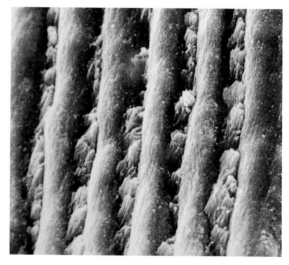

Figure 1.2

Longitudinal section of enamel prisms. SEM showing enamel prisms running parallel (SEM ×400).

deepest occlusally, and rises to become confluent with the wall cervically, thus eliminating the boundary in this region. Each wall (interprismatic region) is formed as a cooperative effort by adjacent secretory ameloblasts. Based on current knowledge of enamel formation, it is clear that each ameloblast is responsible for the formation of one prism at its central secretory site and a portion of the surrounding interprismatic region at its cooperative peripheral sites.

Interprismatic enamel contains more enamel protein than the prism bodies, because the crystals meet at different angles and thus cannot be packed as tightly together. The consistent arrangement of the interprismatic enamel, with its greater protein content, accounts for the fish-scale appearance observed in ground sections.

Enamel microporosity

Due to its ultrastructural organization, enamel – despite its hardness and density – has apprecia-ble porosity. The pore structure affects the mechanical and optical properties of enamel; the formation of carious lesions is strongly influ-enced by the pathways for diffusion and by electrochemical effects arising from the charge on the pore wall (Shellis and Dibdin 1998).

The prism junctions or boundaries, which are the sites where crystals of the tail region of one prism meet with those in the body of another, are sites where there is an abrupt change in crystal orientation. Consequently, prism junctions have enlarged pores, filled with matrix, and hence increased porosity (Hamilton et al. 1973, Orams et al. 1974, 1976, Shellis and Dibdin 1998). In human enamel the incomplete prism junctions form laminar pores with curved cross-section running from the EDJ to the outer surface (Shellis and Dibdin 1998). In outer enamel the prism junctions tend to be separate, and thus exist as independent channels, whilst those in inner enamel (especially in molars) interconnect to form a three-dimensional network of laminar pores (Boyde 1989, Shellis 1996).

Enamel mineral is composed of relatively small crystals, the arrangement of which results in internal pores that are small and variable in form, orientation and distribution. Chromium sulphate demineralization has been used to provide ultrastructural information on the distri-bution of matrix (Sundström and Zelander 1968). Silness et al. (1973) used this technique, and reported individual crystals with a coating of

matrix. Matrix is more apparent in the tail region than in the body region.

The material at prism junctions has a raised solubility (Shellis 1996), which may be due to the deposition of mineral with increased magnesium and carbonate content during amelogenesis, leading to the formation of sites with defective, more soluble apatite (Shellis 1996). The increased solubility at the prism junctions, combined with faster diffusion in this region, accounts for the demineralization pattern observed in advancing carious lesions (Shellis and Hallsworth 1987). At such lesion sites demineralization occurs preferentially via these prism junctions and then spreads laterally into the intraprismatic regions. While the largest pores in enamel are associated with the prism junctions, they only contribute in a small way to the total porosity, most of which is associated with prism bodies and tails (Shellis and Dibdin 1998). Here, the pores exist as very narrow gaps between closely packed crystals but some, while small, are elongated and tubule-like and may communicate with the prism-junction pores only through narrow intercrystalline pores.

Enamel tufts which are found in inner enamel adjacent to the EDJ are regions of high porosity, as they cut across the prism structure, in which crystals are small and dispersed (Orams et al. 1976) and protein abundant (Weatherell et al. 1968) (Figure 1.3). In addition, it has been reported that there is locally increased porosity at the incremental growth lines which constitute the striae of Retzius (Newman and Poole 1974). Striae of Retzius may form as a result of the temporary constriction of Tomes' process associ-ated with a corresponding increase in the secre-tory face forming the interprismatic enamel (Risnes 1990). As a result, enamel structure is altered along these lines and electron microscopy has revealed a possible decrease in the number of crystals in the striae. There is also increased porosity in cross striations (Boyde 1989), which are a pattern of periodic banding noted at 2–6 μm intervals along the length of the prisms, and which represent circadian variation in secretory activity of the ameloblast. Shellis (1996) produced methacrylate replicas of some cross striations in inner enamel, but was unable to do so in outer enamel, suggesting that the pores at most striations are very small or inaccessible.

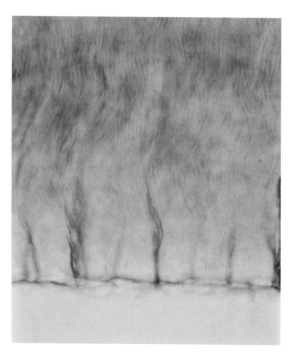

Figure 1.3

Enamel tufts. Seen in ground section, these branched wavy structures are seen in the inner one-third of enamel, originating at the enamel–dentine junction. These are regions of high porosity, as they run between the prism structure, in which crystals are small and dispersed and protein abundant (ground transverse section ×180).

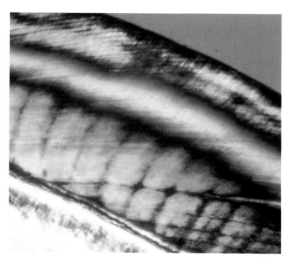

Figure 1.4

Hunter–Schreger bands. These bands can be observed when enamel is viewed in polarized light. The bands appear as alternating light and dark bands, and are observed in the inner one-third to one-half of enamel. They are the results of variation in the course of adjacent groups of prisms (×40).

Organic matrix seems to be present within all pores, and may alter pore size and modify diffusion in a number of ways (Shellis and Dibdin 1998). The effective pore size may be reduced; protein hydration may reduce water movement within the pores; and the diffusion of charged solutes may be altered by interaction with the negative charge of the protein. In addition, the lipid component may influence diffusion of solutes according to their hydrophobicity.

Prism orientation

The direction of movement of secretory ameloblasts dictates the orientation of the prisms observed in mature enamel.

In longitudinal section, the angle between the EDJ and the prisms is about 70° and increases to about 90° cervically, sometimes exceeding 90° in the most cervical region. In the inner one-half to two-thirds of the enamel, curvature of the prisms is responsible for the formation of Hunter–Schreger bands (Figure 1.4). Each band consists of 10–13 prisms which in alternate bands are sectioned approximately longitudinally or approximately transversely. However, the transition between alternate bands is gradual. The Hunter–Schreger bands are also manifested in transverse sections of the tooth. In cuspal enamel the prism curvature gives rise to a related but often apparently more complicated appearance of 'gnarled' enamel (Figure 1.5). Bands in which the prisms run parallel with the section plane reflect the light to a different degree compared with those in which the prisms are perpendicular to the section plane (Lester 1965, Osborn 1965, Silverstone 1982). Because of the deviations in prism orientation, inner enamel is relatively porous. It is thought that the relatively complicated prism arrangement within

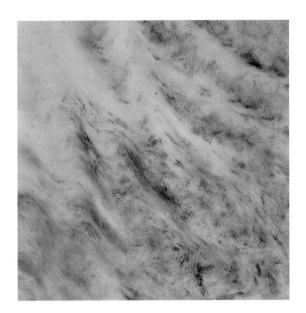

Figure 1.5

Gnarled enamel. Enamel in cuspal and incisal regions may demonstrate marked decussation of prisms. This altered arrangement of prisms gives rise to gnarled enamel (ground section ×250).

the Hunter–Schreger bands serves to reduce the propagation of fractures (Osborn 1968, Boyde 1989).

In the outer enamel, the prisms are straight and parallel in the cuspal and lateral regions, so do not show Hunter–Schreger banding. The angle at which prisms reach the surface varies with anatomical location on the tooth. At the cervical margin, the prisms follow an undulating course and approach the surface at very variable and sometimes acute angles (Boyde 1989). Occlusally, a different orientation is noted, with prisms on the lateral surface of the crown being angled at approximately 70°, whilst on the cuspal surface the angle returns to approximately 90°.

Prism shape and crystal orientation

The cross-sectional appearance of prisms is governed by the inter-relationship of prismatic and interprismatic enamel. Three classical prism patterns have been defined, termed 1–3 (Boyde 1965, 1978, 1989). Pattern 1 is characterized by prisms with complete boundaries, separated by well-defined interprismatic regions. In Pattern 2 enamel, the prisms have incomplete outlines and are arranged in rows. Within each row narrow bridges of interprismatic enamel separate the prisms, while more substantial sheets of interprismatic enamel separate the rows. Pattern 3 is the structure observed in human enamel, containing alternating prisms with horseshoe-shaped boundaries. Although Pattern 3 predominates in human enamel (Boyde 1978, 1989, Kodaka et al. 1990), the other patterns can be found in restricted areas. In particular, Pattern 1 enamel occurs close to the EDJ and also near the outer surface (Martin et al. 1988, Kodaka et al. 1990, 1991), i.e. in the enamel formed at the beginning and end of the ameloblast life-cycle. Comparative studies show that there is no correlation between prism pattern and incremental rate (Dumont 1995). In all three patterns, crystals in the interprismatic regions are orientated approximately perpendicular to the general forming surface (i.e. perpendicular to the plane of the Retzius lines), while the crystals within the prisms form perpendicular to the floor of the Tomes' process pit. In human enamel, this results in a gradual divergence of the crystals in the tail region from the parallel intraprismatic arrangement by angles of about 15–45° in the cervical direction (Poole and Brookes 1961). In Pattern 2 enamel, it results in a large angle between the intraprismatic crystals and those in the prism sheets. This distinction between Pattern 2 and Pattern 3 is important because of the widespread use of rodent and bovine enamel (Pattern 2) in dental research.

Crystal size and morphology

The crystals of mature enamel appear to grow and fill the bulk of the space available within the prism. The apatite crystals characteristically exhibit considerable irregularity of outline, but are roughly hexagonal in cross-section (Selvig and Halse 1972), with a mean width of 68.3 nm and mean thickness of 26.3 nm (Kérébel et al. 1979). Many of the crystals in mature enamel show evidence of crystallographic defects (Ichijo et al. 1993).

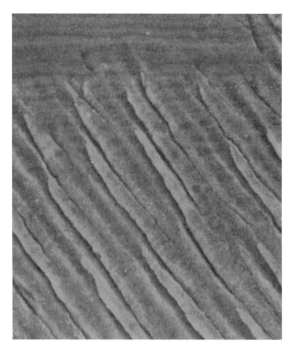

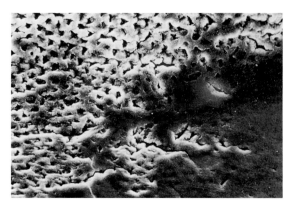

Figure 1.7

Aprismatic enamel – surface view. Aprismatic enamel may not cover the entire enamel surface, as seen in this SEM micrograph. Where aprismatic enamel is absent, the pit into which the Tomes' process would have projected is clearly present (SEM ×600).

Figure 1.6

Aprismatic enamel – transverse section. The surface enamel is often aprismatic with variable appearance and thickness. In prismatic enamel there are abrupt changes in crystal orientation at prism boundaries, whereas in aprismatic enamel the crystals are aligned parallel. Aprismatic enamel arises due to the loss of Tomes' process of the ameloblast, towards the end of enamel formation. A similar layer may also be present adjacent to the EDJ, which can be attributed to a poorly developed Tomes' process at the beginning of enamel formation (SEM ×70).

detectable in some areas (Kodaka *et al.* 1989). Because of the parallel alignment of crystals and the absence of prism boundaries, the surface layer is generally more highly mineralized than the subsurface enamel (Robinson *et al.* 1971). This relatively featureless layer is thought to result from the loss of the Tomes' process by the ameloblast; thus the structural feature which directs the deposition of crystal into prisms and interprismatic material is lost, altering enamel structure as a consequence (Figs 1.6 and 1.7).

Aprismatic enamel

Aprismatic enamel, up to 100 μm thick, has been reported to be present at the surface of both permanent and deciduous human enamel (Whittaker 1982, Boyde 1989, Kodaka *et al.* 1989). The thickness of aprismatic enamel varies both within and between tooth types (Whittaker 1982). Within aprismatic surface enamel, the crystals are arranged parallel to each other and perpendicular to the surface, although some deviation in crystal orientation, due to the presence of remnants of prism boundaries, may be

Dentine structure and physiology

Dentine can be defined as a porous biological composite composed of apatite crystal filler particles in a collagen matrix (Pashley 1996). The apatite crystallites are thought to provide strength (Burstein *et al.* 1975), whereas the collagen matrix provides toughness (Jepson *et al.* 1992).

Dentine contains micrometre-diameter dentinal tubules surrounded by highly mineralized (~95% volume mineral phase) intratubular dentine embedded within a partially mineralized (~30% volume mineral phase) collagen matrix (intertubular dentine) (Marshall 1993, Marshall *et al.* 1997).

The majority of tooth structure is composed of dentine, which is the vital component of the tooth. When compared with enamel (Knoop hardness number KHN 343), dentine is much softer (KHN 68) (Craig 1993), a characteristic which explains why dentine exhibits much faster wear. In addition, the modulus of elasticity of enamel is approximately 84 GPa (Craig 1993) compared with a value of 13–17 GPa reported for dentine (Smith and Cooper 1971, Sano *et al.* 1994). The more compliant nature of dentine compared with enamel allows dentine to function as a stress absorber for the overlying enamel. Dentine is composed of a calcium-deficient carbonate apatite whose crystallite size is smaller than that of enamel and larger than that of bone or cementum (LeGeros *et al.* 1970, LeGeros 1981, 1991).

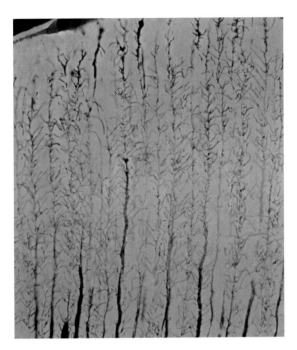

Figure 1.8

Branching of dentinal tubules. Marked terminal branching of dentinal tubules can be noted in outer dentine. It is apparent that tubule diameter increases in a pulpal direction (picrothionin ×300).

Developmental origins

It is well established that during tooth development, cells which originate from the neural crest migrate and interact with epithelial cells of the dental lamina, which eventually leads to the developmental stages termed bud, cap and bell. Newly differentiated odontoblasts (which are post-mitotic) polarize, and mineralized dentine is formed by odontoblasts which begin secreting collagen and other extracellular matrix proteins at the EDJ and then migrate centripetally whilst trailing their odontoblast processes. The deposition of predentine and its subsequent mineralization reduces the pulp area. The rate of dentine production is initially about 1.5 µm/day, increasing to 5–6 µm/day for the bulk of dentine formation, later slowing down (Dean and Scandrett 1995).

Dentine morphology

The foremost morphological characteristic of dentine is its tubular, branched structure connecting the pulp to the EDJ (Figure 1.8). Under normal conditions the tubules, which are largely filled with fluid, may be important in

hydraulically transferring and relieving stresses imparted to dentine through the supporting structures of the periodontium and enamel (Kafka and Jorova 1983, Pashley 1990). Indeed, this may explain why endodontically treated teeth are more brittle than vital teeth (Carter *et al.* 1983).

When isolated from the dentine, each individual dentinal tubule would have the appearance of an inverted cone, with the smallest dimension being recorded at the EDJ end and the largest dimension adjacent to the cell body in the pulp.

Intratubular dentine

Within each tubule is a collagen-deficient, hyper-mineralized layer of dentine which has been termed peritubular dentine, and which may be more accurately termed periluminal (Pashley 1996) or intratubular dentine (Linde and Goldberg 1993), which is calcium-deficient carbonate-rich hydroxyapatite. The small crystals present have a higher crystallinity and are five times harder than intertubular dentine (Kinney *et al.* 1996), with a KHN of 250 compared with a KHN of 52 for intertubular dentine (Kinney *et al.* 1996). The presence of this intratubular dentine narrows the lumen of the tubule from its original 3 μm to as little as 0.6–0.8 μm in superficial dentine near the EDJ (Frank and Nalbandian 1989). The width of intratubular dentine decreases in a pulpward direction, where there is a zone in which there is no intratubular dentine present and the tubule (luminal) diameter is approximately 3 μm (Garberoglio and Brannstrom 1976). There is little published information on the biological control of intratubular apposition, but it is known to be a slow process, slower than the incremental formation of secondary dentine in the pulp chamber.

The deposition of intratubular dentine, as a result of ageing or in response to attrition, results in a progressive reduction in the tubule lumen, and if continued, obliterates the tubule. If this occurs in several tubules in adjacent areas, the dentine assumes a glassy appearance (Figure 1.9). The term used to describe this progressive deposition and obliteration of the tubule is sclerosis, resulting in sclerotic dentine. This process begins in root dentine of 18-year-old premolars without any external influence. It can therefore be assumed that this is a physiological response and the occlusion of the tubules is achieved by continued intratubular deposition. The mechanisms by which intratubular dentine is formed are poorly understood and three possible mechanisms have been suggested (Torneck 1994). Firstly, it has been suggested that there may be a passive redistribution of mineral from intertubular dentine into the tubules around the pre-existing components of the tubule. Secondly, there may be an active response on the part of the odontoblast process, resulting in an organic matrix that is actively mineralized as a result of odontoblast activity. Finally, it has been suggested that the odontoblast may produce an organic matrix that becomes mineralized by redistribution of mineral from intertubular dentine, as in the first case. However it forms, the net result is that intratubular dentine is

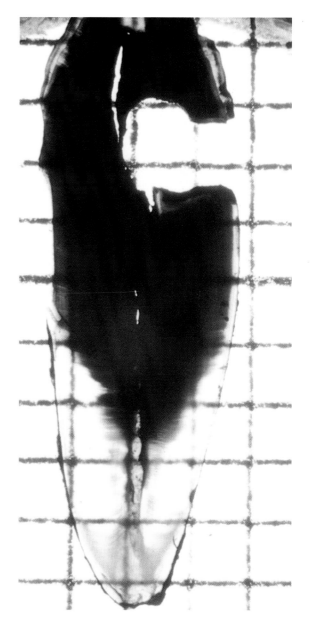

Figure 1.9

Translucent dentine. The appearance of translucent dentine, seen in the root, is associated with physiological ageing. The tubules become completely obliterated by mineral, by a process that is not completely understood, but is believed to be similar to intratubular dentine formation. In this section, occlusion of the tubules is demonstrated by the inability of dye placed in the pulp chamber to penetrate the dentinal tubule in the apical portion of the root, which thus appears translucent. The amount of translucent dentine increases linearly with age, and is not affected by function or external irritation (ground section ×5).

deposited at the expense of the odontoblast process, which is either retracted or shortened by the loss of its distal extremity. The amount of sclerosed dentine increases with age and is most frequently encountered in the apical third of the root. Sclerosis reduces the permeability of dentine, and thus may help prolong pulp vitality.

Although there is little evidence in the literature, it is thought that the processes which contribute to sclerotic dentine in the crown in response to attrition and caries may differ from the physiological deposition of sclerotic (translucent) dentine in the root, which is age-dependent and whose rate of deposition is not altered by attrition.

Extent of odontoblast processes

During tooth development, at the bell stage, odontoblast processes extend from the odontoblast cell body through predentine to the EDJ. As the thickness of dentine increases, the cellular processes must elongate. However, the true length of the processes in mature dentine, in the absence of blood vessels or supporting cells, is an issue that is open to debate. In human teeth, the thickness of dentine is about 3–3.5 mm, such that if an odontoblast process were to pass the entire distance from the pulpal border to the EDJ, then the volume of the cellular process would be four-fold larger than that of the cell body (Pashley 1996). This difference in volume between the cell body and the process is even greater if the situation with cuboidal or flattened odontoblasts is considered, as seen in the root towards the apex. It is generally agreed that the length of the process of most odontoblasts is between 0.1 and 1.0 mm (Holland 1976, Byers and Sugaya 1995).

The question of how far the odontoblast process penetrates dentine is of vital importance when considering dentine sensitivity. If odontoblasts were to participate directly in the sensitivity of dentine to surface stimuli, then the stimuli must interact directly with the process, which is unlikely to be the case.

Normally dentine is covered coronally with enamel and on the root surface by cementum. When these surface coverings are lost, dentine is subjected to a variety of stimuli, including mechanical, chemical, thermal and smaller mechanical stimuli to which intact teeth are responsive. When exposed, it is proposed that the fluid-filled tubules allow minute fluid shifts across the dentine when exposed to thermal, tactile, evaporative or osmotic stimuli. The effect of this is that mechanoreceptors in the pulp are stimulated (Pashley 1996). These fluid shifts can directly irritate odontoblasts, pulpal nerves and subodontoblastic blood vessels by applying large sheer forces on their surface as the fluid streams through narrow spaces. The effect of fluid shift on the release of neuropeptides has been assessed (Kimberly and Byers 1988, Byers et al. 1990, Byers 1996, Olgart 1996), and results in the release of calcitonin gene-related peptide (CGRP) or substance P (SP) from the pulpal nerves to generate a local neurogenic inflammatory condition.

Dentine characteristics change with depth

Both primary and secondary dentine contain tubules. The circumference of the dentine at the most peripheral part of the root or crown is much greater than that of the final circumference of the pulp chamber or root canal space. This results in the odontoblasts being much more crowded as they approach their final position, thus leading to the appearance of a columnar layer of odontoblasts, especially over the pulp horns (Couve 1986). The convergence of odontoblasts towards the pulp creates a unique structural organization, with functional consequences. The convergence has been estimated to be 4:1 (Walton et al. 1976) or 3:1 (Fosse et al. 1992).

The number of tubules per unit area and the radius of the tubules increases in the direction from the EDJ to the pulp, thus the area occupied by tubule lumina also increases (Mjor and Fejerskov 1979, Fosse et al. 1992, Olsson and Oilo 1993; Dourda et al. 1994). Pashley (1984) calculated the area occupied by tubule lumina at the EDJ to be approximately 1% of the total surface area of the EDJ and 22% at the pulp. As this area is occupied by dentinal fluid, which is 95% water (Pashley 1996), the surface area figures are also approximately equal to the tubule water content of these regions. Therefore, the water content or wetness of dentine increases 20-fold from superficial to deep dentine. This factor has clinical implications, in terms of dentine bonding of restorative materials to deep dentine; the water competes with resin monomers for surface collagen fibrils (Eick et al. 1997, Pashley and Carvalho 1997).

Fluid flow

In clinical conditions there is an outward fluid flow across exposed dentine in response to the low but positive pulpal tissue pressure (~14 cm H_2O: Ciucchi et al. 1995). The composition of this fluid is uncertain, but must have an ion product of calcium and phosphate which is above or near the solubility product constants for a number of forms of calcium phosphate (Pashley 1996). This would in turn lead to the formation of mineral deposits in dentinal tubules which have many forms (Mjor 1985), as the dentinal fluid moves outwards, larger amounts of mineral ions are presented to the walls of tubules than would occur in sealed tubules. Indeed, Shellis (1994) used this principle to reduce the depth of demineralization in vitro under simulated caries-forming conditions, by using a supersaturated surrogate dentinal fluid, which was perfused through the pulp chamber. When examined microscopically, translucent bands resembling sclerotic dentine were sometimes observed.

Clinically, patients who complain of dentine sensitivity report that a cold stimulus elicits a greater response than evaporative, tactile or osmotic stimulation (Orchardson and Collins 1987). Outward direct fluid movement (in response to cold) is far more effective at activating pulpal mechanoreceptors than is the inward movement of fluid (seen following a hot stimulus) (Matthews and Vongsavan 1994).

Permeability

The structure of dentine is tubular, as previously stated, and it is this characteristic that provides the channels for the permeation of solutes and solvents across dentine. The density of tubules per mm^2 varies from 15 000 at the EDJ to 65 000

at the pulp boundary (Garberoglio and Brannstrom 1976, Fosse et al. 1992, Dourda et al. 1994). The dentinal tubules are tapered structures measuring approximately 3.0 µm in diameter near the pulp, 1.2 µm in the mid-portion of the dentine and 900 nm near the EDJ. Because the diameter and density of tubules increases with the distance of the dentine from the EDJ, then it follows that the permeability of dentine is lowest at the EDJ and highest at the pulp. However, at any location within dentine the permeability in vitro is far below what would be predicted from tubule density and diameters (Koutsi et al. 1994), due to the presence of intratubular material such as collagen fibrils and mineralized constrictions of the tubules (Pashley 1996).

Dentine permeability can be subdivided into two broad categories (Pashley 1996): (1) trans-dentinal movements of substances through the entire thickness of dentine via dentinal tubules (such as fluid shifts in response to hydrodynamic stimuli) and (2) intradentinal movement of exogenous substances into intertubular dentine. The latter occurs during the infiltration of hydrophilic adhesive resins into demineralized dentine surfaces during resin bonding or demineralization of intertubular dentine by bacterially derived acids (Kinney et al. 1995), where the material enters the tubules but does not travel across the tubules. The presence of smear layers, smear plugs and/or intratubular deposits (i.e. sclerotic dentine) is thought to lower intratubular permeability to minimal values (Pashley et al. 1991).

Dentine permeability (transdentinal or intratubular) is not uniform across the tooth. Coronal dentine permeability is much higher than that of the root (Foegel et al. 1988). This can be attributed to the convergence of tubules towards the pulp chamber, the tubule density increases about four-fold in coronal dentine, but only two-fold in root dentine. Thus, within any location on the tooth peripheral dentine has a lower permeability than deeper dentine (Outhwaite et al. 1976, Reeder et al. 1978, Foegel et al. 1988, Koutsi et al. 1994). The permeability of intertubular dentine has never been quantified, but it must be very low and limited to patent lateral canals that branch off from tubules (Chappell et al. 1994, Mjor and Nordahl 1996).

Numerous methods have been used to assess dentine permeability (Pashley 1990). The easiest method of measuring transdentinal permeability is to quantify its hydraulic conductance. This measures the ease with which fluid can filter across a unit surface area of dentine in a unit time under a unit pressure gradient (Pashley 1990). It has been reported, in unobstructed dentine, that the hydraulic conductance increases as dentine thickness decreases (Fogel et al. 1988, Koutsi et al. 1994). However, the presence of intratubular material reduces the fluid conductance of dentine and hence lowers its permeability (Pashley 1996).

The structure of dentine means that it can be considered to be both a barrier and a permeable structure, depending on its thickness, age and other variables (Pashley and Pashley 1991). Dentine is very porous because of its tubular structure, and the minimum porosity of normal peripheral coronal dentine is about 15 000 tubules/mm^2. If the dentine is uncovered, then the tubules provide a diffusion channel from the surface to the pulp. The rate at which diffusional flux of exogenous material crosses dentine to the pulp is highly dependent on dentine thickness and upon the hydraulic conductance of dentine (Pashley 1985, 1990).

There is competition between the inward diffusional flux of materials and the rising action of outward convective fluid transport (Pashley and Matthews 1993). When dentine is exposed, the outward flow of fluid through the tubules is the first line of defence against inward diffusion of noxious substances, and thus may have a protective role in mitigating the inward flux of potentially irritating bacterial products into exposed sensitive dentine (Pashley 1996). Dentine permeability is not uniform, but varies widely – especially on occlusal surfaces, where only about 30% of the tubules are in free communication with the pulp (Pashley et al. 1987). Functional studies of fluid movement across occlusal dentine indicate that the tubules that communicate with the pulp are located over the pulp horns, with the central region being relatively impermeable (Pashley 1996).

Sclerotic dentine, formed in response to a number of stimuli, has a very low permeability (Tagami et al. 1992) because the tubules become filled with mineral deposits. The deposition of sclerotic dentine may have two effects; it may slow the ingress of bacteria and thus help protect the pulp, alternatively, sclerosis may aid the demineralization observed in advancing caries by reducing the supply of dentine tissue fluid. Although the exact composition of dentinal fluid is unknown, it is likely to be similar to serum ultrafiltrate, which is undersaturated with respect to brushite, slightly supersaturated with respect to octacalcium phosphate and moderately supersaturated with respect to hydroxyapatite (Shellis 1994). Thus a reduction in the supply of dentinal fluid due to tubule occlusion may aid caries progression.

The pulpo-dentinal complex

Dentine and pulp are embryologically, histologically and functionally united, and there is much evidence to support the concept of viewing the dentine and pulp as a functionally coupled unit which act as an integrated system. As soon as the tissues which normally cover dentine are lost, then the normal compartmentalization between the tissues is lost (Pashley 1996) and they become functionally continuous. The pulp responds to the stimuli generated by the loss of dentinal covering, in the short term by mounting an inflammatory response which produces an outward movement of fluid (Vongsavan and Matthews 1991, Matthews and Vongsavan 1994, Matthews 1996) and macromolecules (Byers 1996). The long-term response to this stimulus is the production of tertiary dentine, which is a biological response to reduce the permeability of the dentine–pulp complex (see Chapter 5).

Innervation of dentine and pulp

Nerves grow into the papilla in the bell stage of tooth development (Kollar and Lumsden 1979, Byers 1980, Mohamed and Atkinson 1983). Both afferent neurons and efferent autonomic nerves that innervate pulpal blood vessels are present. The number of myelinated axons in permanent teeth increases with age and/or tooth development, reaching a plateau value of about 500 myelinated axons per human premolar at age 15 (Johnson 1990), which remains constant up to 60 years. However, there are more unmyelinated axons (~1500 axons/premolar) and these appear to demonstrate a reduction in number with age (Fried and Hildebrand 1981, Byers 1984, Johnson 1990). Other age changes reported include a large reduction in axon number and CGRP, SP, neuropeptide Y and nerve growth factor receptor activity in the pulps of ageing cats (Fried 1992).

Histologically, nerves can be seen entering the apex as dental nerves in bundles. Less than 10% of nerves are given off in the root (Byers and Matthews 1981), whilst most continue to the coronal pulp where they diverge, branch and form the nerve plexus of Rashkow and innervate the blood vessels. From the plexus, some nerves pass peripherally to terminate in predentine and dentine, and a few pass >100 μm into the tubules (Byers 1984, Hildebrand et al. 1995). The percentage of dentinal tubules innervated by sensory nerves is >40% in the region of the coronal pulp horns, 4.1–8.3% in mid-crown, 0.2–1.0% at the CEJ and 0.02–0.2% in mid-root in humans (Byers 1984, 1990).

Sensory nerves are based into subgroups based on histological size, conduction velocity and function. Most of the myelinated fibres are classified as A-β or A-δ sensory fibres. These are relatively large, fast conducting fibres that respond to hydrodynamic stimuli such as tactile, evaporative, osmotic or thermal challenges (Närhi et al. 1996). Small C fibres that are unmyelinated have higher thresholds and slower conduction velocities than A fibres, and respond only to intense stimuli that reach the pulp, rather than to stimulation of dentine surfaces. It is now generally accepted that the great majority (>93%) (Nair et al. 1992) of apical myelinated axons of human teeth are A-δ fibres that show a unimodal distribution in fibre size. Only a small proportion (<7%) is in the A-β range, but they do not form a distinct group. The non-myelinated C fibres are much smaller and have an overall diameter of 0.5 μm (Nair and Schroeder 1995). All myelinated axons entering human teeth are considered to be sensory afferents, with their receptive field located in the pulp–dentine interface and the inner dentine (Nair 1995). The free endings of these nerve fibres located around the odontoblastic body and the inner dentine are probably activated by fluid movement within tubules from a variety of stimuli, according to the hydrodynamic mechanism (Brannstrom 1966). In physiological terms, it is thought that the A-δ fibres are associated with the sharp localized pain experienced when dentine is first exposed, whereas C fibres are associated with a dull and more diffuse pain. About 87% of all axons that enter human premolars are non-myelinated C fibres (Nair and Schroeder 1995). They are slow conductors, with their receptive field located in the pulp, the majority of which are believed to be sensory afferents.

The inner pulpal wall of dentine in human teeth has an estimated 50 000–80 000 tubules/mm² (Schellenberg et al. 1992). The dentine is innervated with the highest density believed to be around the pulp horns, where nearly 50% of the tubules are thought to contain neural elements (Byers and Dong 1983).

It is believed that coronal dentine is more densely innervated than the remaining dentine, in order to register external stimuli to which the crown is exposed after eruption (Nair 1995). Likewise, the root dentine, which is protected within a bony socket from external stimuli, is believed to be only sparsely innervated.

Acknowledgement

Thanks must be given to Dr David K Whittaker for the provision of the slides presented as Figures 1.1, 1.2 and 1.9.

References

Boyde A (1965) The structure of developing mammalian dental enamel. In: Stack MV, Fearnhead RW eds, *Tooth Enamel*, 163–7. Wright: Bristol.

Boyde A (1978) Development of the structure of the enamel in the incisor teeth in three classical subordinal groups in the Rodentia. In: Butler PM, Joysey KA, eds, *Development, Function and Evolution of Teeth*, 43–58. Academic Press: London.

Boyde A (1989) Enamel. In: Oksche A, Vollrath L, eds, *Handbook of Microscopic Anatomy*, Vol V/6 Teeth, 309–473. Springer-Verlag: Berlin.

Brannstrom M (1966) Sensitivity of dentine. *Oral Surg Oral Pathol Oral Med* **21**:517–26.

Burstein AH, Zika JM, Heiple KG, Klein A (1975) Contribution of collagen and mineral to the elastic properties of bone. *J Bone Joint Surg* **57**:956–61.

Byers MR (1980) The development of sensory innervation in dentine. *J Comp Neurol* **191**:413–28.

Byers MR (1984) Dental sensory receptors. *Int Rev Neurobiol* **25**:39–44.

Byers MR (1990) Neuroanatomical studies of dental innervation and pain. In: Spandberg L, ed, *Experimental Endodontics*, 77–113. CRC Press: Boca Raton, FL.

Byers MR (1996) Neuropeptide immunoreactivity in dental sensory nerves. Variations related to primary odontoblast function and survival. In: Shimono M, Takahashi K, eds, *Dentin/pulp Complex*, Quintessence: Tokyo.

Byers M, Dong WK (1983) Autoradiographic location of sensory nerve endings in dentin of monkey teeth. *Anat Rec* **205**:441–54.

Byers MR, Matthews B (1981) Autoradiographic demonstration of ipsilateral and contralateral sensory nerve ending in cat dentine, pulp and periodontium. *Anat Rec* **201**:249–60.

Byers MR, Sugaya A (1995) Odontoblast processes in dentine revealed by fluorescent DiI. *J Histochem Cytochem* **43**:159–68.

Byers MR, Taylor PE, Khayat BG, Kimberly CK (1990) Effects of injury and inflammation on pulpal and periapical nerves. *J Endodontics* **16**:78–84.

Carter JM, Sorenson SE, Johnson RR et al (1983) Punch shear testing of extracted vital and endodontically treated teeth. *J Biomech* **16**:841–8.

Chadwick D, Cardew G. eds. (1997) *Dental Enamel*. Ciba Foundation 205. Wiley: Chichester.

Chappell RP, Cobb CM, Spencer P, Eick JD (1994) Dentinal tubule anastomosis: a potential factor in adhesive bonding? *J Prosthet Dent* **72**:183–8.

Ciucchi B, Bouilleguet S, Holz J, Pashley DH (1995) Dentinal fluid mechanics in human teeth *in vivo*. *J Endodontics* **21**:191–4.

Couve E (1986) Ultrastructural changes during the life cycle of human odontoblasts. *Arch Oral Biol* **31**:643–51.

Craig RG (1993) *Restorative Dental Materials*, 9th edn, 64. CV Mosby: St Louis.

Dean MC, Scandrett AE (1995) Rates of dentine mineralization in permanent human teeth. *Int J Osteoarchaeol* **5**:349–58.

Dibdin GH, Poole DFG (1982) Surface area and pore size analysis for human enamel and dentine by water vapour sorption. *Arch Oral Biol* **27**:235–41.

Dourda AO, Moule AJ, Young WG (1994). A morphometric analysis of the cross-sectional area of dentine occupied by dentinal tubules in human third molar teeth. *Int Endodontic J* **27**:184–9.

Dumont E (1995) Mammalian enamel prism patterns and enamel deposition rates. *Scanning Microsc* **9**:429–42.

Eick JD, Gwinnett AJ, Pashley DH (1997) Current concepts on adhesion to dentine. *Crit Rev Oral Biol Med* **8**:306–35.

Fogel HM, Marshall FJ, Pashley DH (1988) Effects of distance from the pulp and thickness on the hydraulic conductance of human radicular dentin. *J Dent Res* **67**:1381–5.

Fosse G, Saele PK, Eide R (1992) Numerical density and distribution pattern of dentine tubules. *Acta Odontol Scand* **50**:201–10.

Frank RM, Nalbandian J (1989) Structure and ultrastructure of dentine. In: Berkovitz BKB, Boyde A, Frank RM et al, eds, *Teeth*, 212. Springer Verlag: New York.

Fried K (1992) Changes in pulp nerves with ageing. *Proc Finn Dent Soc* **88**: 517–28.

Fried K, Hildebrand C (1981) Pulpal axons in developing mature and ageing feline permanent incisors. A study by electron microscopy. *J Comp Neurol* **203**:23–36.

Garberoglio R, Brannstrom M (1976) Scanning electron microscopic investigations in human dentinal tubules. *Arch Oral Biol* **21**:355–62.

Goldberg M, Septier D, Torres-Quintana et al (1999) New insights on the dynamics of dentin formation. In: Goldberg M, Robinson C, Boskey A, eds, *Proceedings of the 6th International Conference on the Chemistry and Biology of Mineralized Tissue*. American Academy of Orthopedic Surgeons (in press).

Hamilton WJ, Judd G, Ansell GS (1973) Ultrastructure of human enamel specimens prepared by ion micromilling. *J Dent Res* **52**:703–10.

Hildebrand C, Fried K, Tuisk U, Johnson CS (1995) Teeth and tooth nerves. *Prog Neurobiol* **45**:165–222.

Holland GR (1976) The extent of the odontoblast process in the cat. *J Anat* **120**:133–49.

Ichijo T, Yamashita Y, Terashima T (1993) Observations on structural features and characteristics of biological apatite crystals 6: observations on lattice imperfection of human tooth and bone crystals I. *Bull Tokyo Med Dent Univ* **40**:147–53.

Jepson KJ, Mansours MK, Kuhn JL et al (1992) An *in vivo* assessment of the contribution of type I collagen to the mechanical properties of cortical bone (abst). *Trans Orthopaed Res* **17**:93.

Johnson DC (1990) Innervation of teeth: developmental aspects. In: Inoki R, Kuda T, Olgart L, eds, *Dynamic Aspects of Dental Pulp*, 13–28. Chapman and Hall: New York.

Kafka V, Jorova J (1983) A structural mathematical model for the viscoelastic anisotropic behavior of trabecular bone. *Biorheology* **20**:795–803.

Kérébel B, Daculsi G, Kérébel LM (1979) Ultrastructural studies of enamel crystallites. *J Dent Res* **58**:844–50.

Kimberly CL, Byers MR (1988) Response of nerve fibres containing calcitonin gene-related peptide to inflammation of rat molar pulp and periodontium. *Anat Rec* **222**:289–300.

Kinney JH, Balooch M, Haupt DL et al (1995) Mineral distribution and dimensional changes in human dentine during demineralization. *J Dent Res* **74**:1179–84.

Kinney JH, Balooch M, Marshall SJ et al (1996) Hardness and Young's modulus of peritubular and intertubular dentine. *Arch Oral Biol* **41**:9–13.

Kodaka T, Nakajima F, Higashi S (1989) Structure of the so-called 'prismless' enamel in human deciduous teeth. *Caries Res* **23**:290–5.

Kodaka T, Kuroiwa M, Abe M (1990) Fine structure of the inner enamel in human permanent teeth. *Scanning Microsc* **4**:975–99.

Kodaka T, Kuroiwa M, Higashi S (1991) Structural and distribution patterns of surface 'prismless' enamel in human permanent teeth. *Caries Res* **25**:7–12.

Kollar EJ, Lumsden AGS (1979) Tooth morphogenesis: the role of innervation during induction and pattern development. *J Biol Buccale* **7**:49–60.

Koutsi V, Noonan RG, Horner JA et al (1994) The effect of dentin depth on the permeability and ultrastructure of primary molars. *Pediatr Dent* **16**:9–35.

LeGeros RZ (1981) Calcium phosphates in oral biology and medicine. In: *Monographs in Oral Science, Vol 5,* 114–119. Karger: New York, NY.

LeGeros RZ (1991) Apatites in biological systems. *Prog Cryst Growth Charact* **4**:1–45.

LeGeros RZ, LeGeros JP, Trautz OR, Klein E (1970) Spectral properties of carbonate in carbonate containing apatites. *Dev Appl Spectrosc* **7**:3–12.

Lester KS (1965) The bands of Schreger, the role of flexion. *Arch Oral Biol* **10**:361–7.

Linde A, Goldberg M (1993) Dentinogenesis. *Crit Rev Oral Biol Med* **45**:679–728.

Marshall GW (1993) Dentine microstructure and characterisation. *Quintessence* **24**:606–17.

Marshall GW, Marshall SJ, Kinney JH, Balooch M (1997) The dentin substrate: structure and properties relating to bonding. *J Dent* **25**:441–58.

Martin LB, Boyde A, Grine FE (1988) Enamel structure in primates: a review of scanning electron microscope studies. *Scanning Microsc* **2**:1503–8.

Matthews B (1996) The functional properties of intradental nerves. In: Shimono M, Maeda T, Suda H, Takahashi K, eds, *Dentin/pulp Complex*, 146–53. Quintessence: Tokyo.

Matthews B, Vongsavan N (1994) Interactions between neural and hydrodynamic mechanisms in dentine and pulp. *Arch Oral Biol* **39**(Suppl):S87–S95.

Mjor IA (1985) Dentin-predentine complex and its permeability: pathology and treatment overview. *J Dent Res* **64**:621–7.

Mjor IA, Fejerskov O (1979) *Histology of the Human Tooth*, 2nd edn. Munksgaard: Copenhagen.

Mjor IA, Nordahl I (1996) The density and branching of dentinal tubules in human teeth. *Arch Oral Biol* **38**:541–6.

Mohamed SS, Atkinson ME (1983) A histological study of the innervation of developing mouse teeth. *J Anat* **136**:735–49.

Nair RPN (1995) Neural elements in dental pulp and dentin. *Oral Surg Oral Med Oral Pathol* **80**:710–19.

Nair RPN, Schroeder HE (1995) Number and size spectra of non-myelinated axons of human premolars. *Anat Embryol* **192**:35–41.

Nair RPN, Luder HU, Schroeder HE (1992) Number and size spectra of myelinated nerves in human premolars. *Anat Embryol* **92**:123–8.

Närhi M, Yamamoto H, Ngassapa D (1996) Function of intradental nociceptors in normal and inflamed teeth. In: Shimono M, Takahashi K, eds, *Dentin/pulp Complex*, 136–40. Quintessence: Tokyo.

Newman HN, Poole DFG (1974) Observations with scanning and transmission electron microscopy on the structure of human surface enamel. *Arch Oral Biol* **19**:1135–43.

Olgart L (1996) Neurogenic components of pulp inflammation. In: Shimono M, Takahashi K, eds, *Dentin/pulp Complex*, 169–75. Quintessence, Tokyo.

Olsson S, Oilo G (1993) The structure of dentin surfaces exposed for bond strength measurements. *Scand J Dent Res* **101**:180–4.

Orams HJ, Phakey PP, Rachinger WA, Zybert JJ (1974) Visualisation of micropore structure in human dental enamel. *Nature* **252**:584–5.

Orams HJ, Zybert JJ, Phakey PP, Rachinger WA (1976) Ultrastructural study of human dental enamel using selected-area argon-ion beam thinning. *Arch Oral Biol* **21**:663–75.

Orchardson R, Collins WJN (1987) Thresholds of hypersensitive teeth to two forms of controlled stimulation. *J Clin Periodontol* **14**:68–73.

Osborn JW (1965) The nature of Hunter-Schreger bands in enamel. *Arch Oral Biol* **10**:929–33.

Osborn JW (1968) Evaluation of previous assessments of prism directions in human enamel. *J Dent Res* **47**:217–22.

Outhwaite WC, Livingston MJ, Pashley DH (1976) Effects of change in surface area, thickness, temperature and post extraction time on human dentine permeability. *Arch Oral Biol* **21**:599–603.

Pashley DH (1984) Smear layer: physiologic consideration. *Operative Dentistry* **3**:13–29.

Pashley DH (1985) Dentin–predentin complex: physiological overview. *J Dent Res* **64**:613–20.

Pashley DH (1990) Dentin permeability: theory and practice. In: Spangberg L, ed, *Experimental Endodontics*, 19–49. CRC Press: Boca Raton, FL.

Pashley DH (1996) Dynamics of the pulpo-dentinal complex. *Crit Rev Oral Biol Med* **7**:104–33.

Pashley DH, Pashley EL (1991) Dentin permeability and restorative dentistry. *Am J Dent* **4**:5–9.

Pashley DH, Matthews WG (1993) The effects of outward forced convective flow on inward diffusion in human dentine, in vitro. *Arch Oral Biol* **38**:577–82.

Pashley DH, Carvalho RM (1997) Dentine permeability and adhesive bonding, *J Dent* **25**:355–72.

Pashley DH, Andringa HJ, Derkson GD et al (1987) Regional variability in dentine permeability. *Arch Oral Biol* **32**:519–23.

Pashley EL, Talman R, Horner JA, Pashley DH (1991) Permeability of normal versus carious dentin. *Endod Dent Traumatol* **7**:207–11.

Poole DFG, Brooks AW (1961) The arrangement of crystallites in enamel prisms. *Arch Oral Biol* **5**:14–26.

Reeder DE, Walton RE, Livingstone MJ, Pashley DH (1978) Dentine permeability: determinant of hydraulic conductance. *J Dent Res* **57**:187–93.

Risnes S (1990) Structural characteristics of staircase-type Retzius lines in human dental enamel analysed by scanning electron microscopy. *Anat Rec* **226**:135–46.

Robinson C, Weatherell JA, Hallsworth AS (1971) Variation in composition of dental enamel within thin ground tooth sections. *Caries Res* **5**:44–57.

Robinson C, Kirkham J, Shore R eds (1995) *Dental Enamel: Formation to Destruction*. CRC Press: Boca Raton, FL.

Sano H, Cuicchi B, Matthews WG, Pashley DH (1994) Tensile properties of mineralised and demineralised human and bovine dentin. *J Dent Res* **73**:1205–11.

Schellenberg U, Krey G, Boshardt D, Nair PNR (1992) Numerical density of dentinal tubules at the pulpal wall of permanent human premolars and third molars. *J Endodont* **18**:104–9.

Selvig KA, Halse A (1972) Crystal growth in rat incisor enamel. *Anat Rec* **173**:453–68.

Shellis RP (1984) Relationship between human enamel structure and the formation of caries-like lesions *in vitro*. *Arch Oral Biol* **29**:975–81.

Shellis RP (1994) Effects of supersaturated pulpal fluid on the formation of caries-like lesions on the roots of human teeth. *Caries Res* **28**:14–20.

Shellis RP (1996) A scanning electron-microscopic study of solubility variations in human enamel and dentine. *Arch Oral Biol* **41**:473–84.

Shellis RP, Hallsworth AS (1987) The use of scanning electron microscopy in studying enamel caries. *Scanning Microsc* **1**:1109–23.

Shellis RP, Dibdin GH (1998) Enamel microporosity and its functional implications. In: Teaford MF, Ferguson MJ, Smith MM, eds, *Teeth: Development, Evolution and Function*. Cambridge University Press: Cambridge (in press).

Silness J, Hegdahl T, Gustavsen F (1973) Area of the organic–inorganic interface of dental enamel. *Acta Odontol Scand* **31**:123–9.

Silverstone LM (1982) The structure and characteristics of human dental enamel. In: Smith DC, Williams DF, eds, *Biocompatibility of Dental Materials, Vol 1: Characteristics of Dental Tissues and Their Response to Dental Materials*, 39–74. CRC Press: Boca Raton.

Smith DC, Cooper WEG (1971) The determination of shear strength. A method using a micropunch apparatus. *Br Dent J* **130**:333–7.

Sundström B, Zelander T (1968) On the morphological organisation of the organic matrix of adult human enamel after decalcification by means of a basic chromium (III) sulphate solution. *Odont Rev* **19**:1–15.

Tagami J, Hosada H, Burrow MF, Nakajima M (1992) Effect of aging and caries on dentin permeability. *Proc Finn Dent Soc* **88**:149–54.

Torneck CD (1994) Dentin–pulp complex. In: Ten Cate AR, ed, *Oral Histology, Development, Structure and Function*, 169–217. Mosby: London.

Vongsavan N, Matthews B (1991) The permeability of cat dentine *in vivo* and *in vitro*. *Arch Oral Biol* **36**:641–6.

Walton RE, Outhwaite WC, Pashley DH (1976) Magnification, an interesting optical property of dentine. *J Dent Res* **55**:639–42.

Warshawsky H, Josephsen K, Thylstrup A, Fejerskov Ø (1981) The development of enamel structure in rat incisors as compared to the teeth of monkey and man. *Anat Rec* **200**:371–89.

Weatherell JA, Weidman SM, Eyre DR (1968) Histological appearance and chemical composition of enamel protein from mature human molars. *Caries Res* **2**:281–93.

Whittaker DK (1982) Structural variations in the surface zone of human tooth enamel observed by scanning electron microscopy. *Arch Oral Biol* **27**:383–9.

Wilson PR, Beynon AD (1989) Mineralization differences between human deciduous and permanent enamel measured by quantitative microradiography. *Arch Oral Biol* **34**:85–8.

2
Transport processes in enamel and dentine

R Peter Shellis

Introduction

The dental hard tissues are more or less porous materials and are therefore permeable, to different extents, to substances dissolved in the media bathing the surfaces of the teeth. Knowledge of the way in which substances are transported through the hard tissues is central to understanding the aetiology of disorders of the teeth and to delivery of therapeutic agents. Two kinds of transport need to be considered. The first is *diffusion*, which results from the random motion of solute molecules and is driven by concentration gradients. Transport through dental tissues is by diffusion in all situations where the solution filling the internal pores is static. The second mechanism is *convection*, which occurs where there is flow of the medium, caused by a pressure gradient. Where both concentration gradients and flow exist, both processes will operate, but the overall transport will depend on the relative magnitudes and directions of the respective driving forces.

Before discussing these mechanisms, it is useful to compare briefly the pore structures of the dental tissues, which are crucial to both transport mechanisms.

Pore structure of dental hard tissues

This subject has been reviewed recently with regard to enamel (Shellis and Dibdin 1999). In both enamel and dentine there is a set of relatively large pores which connect the outer and inner surfaces: the prism-junction pores and the dentinal tubules respectively. These may be referred to as 'through' pores. Although the prism-junction pores appear to interconnect in inner enamel and adjacent tubules in dentine are often connected by small lateral branches, the regular orientation of the prism junctions and tubules imposes a preferred direction on transport of substances. However, while dentinal tubules are 0.8–2.5 µm (mean 1.4 µm) in diameter and occupy 1–22% v/v (mean 6.5%) of dentine (Garberoglio and Brannstrom 1976), the prism-junction pores are only 1–30 nm wide (average 6 nm) and occupy only about 0.3% of enamel volume (Dibdin 1993, Shellis and Dibdin 1998). Consequently, dentine is much more permeable than enamel.

Separating the system of relatively large pores in both tissues is mineralized tissue containing a system of much smaller pores. In enamel, the intercrystalline pores show a high degree of orientation, parallel with the prism direction, because of the highly elongated crystal morphology, and many of these pores are themselves elongated (Orams *et al.* 1974). Although generally much smaller than the prism-junction pores, the intercrystalline pores together account for nearly all the porosity of enamel (about 6 % v/v) (Dibdin and Poole 1982). Whole dentine has a porosity of about 21% v/v (Dibdin and Poole 1982). From the data given above, it appears that the mineralized component of dentine has an average porosity of about 15% v/v, more than double that of enamel. Clearly the porosities of peritubular and intertubular dentine would be respectively lower and higher than this. The pore structure of intertubular dentine may be much less anisotropic than that of enamel, because the crystals are smaller and much less elongated.

Finally, it should be noted that tubular root dentine is covered not only by primary (acellular) cementum, but also by atubular dentine. These tissues probably have a pore structure very similar to that of intertubular dentine.

Diffusion

The solvent and solute molecules in a solution are all in constant, random motion. Where there is a gradient in solute concentration between two regions of a solution, the random movements of the solute molecules result in net transport from regions of high concentration to regions of lower concentration. The rate at which the net solute movement occurs is proportional to the concentration gradient and the constant of proportionality is the diffusion coefficient (D), which has the units of area/time, usually m^2/s or cm^2/s. In solution, D depends on molecular size, temperature and interactions between the solute and solvent molecules.

Diffusion through porous solids

Diffusion through a porous solid takes place in the solution filling the pores and is therefore controlled by the same factors as in free solution. However, in addition, the structure and composition of the solid now play an important role, as do interactions between the diffusing substance (diffusate) and the solid. These additional factors can be summarized as described below.

Porosity

This is the volume fraction of the material which is occupied by solution-filled pores. Clearly, the flux of diffusate (transport rate per unit area) through a material with a low porosity will be less than through a more porous sample of the same material, even where transport within the pores is unaltered.

Tortuosity

Unless the pores run straight between opposite faces of a sample, the diffusion pathway will be greater than the thickness. For instance, in a slice of enamel cut parallel to the outer surface, the linear pores at the prism junctions would run at about 70° to the section plane, so that the diffusion distance along the junctions would be 6% greater than the section thickness. More complex, and less predictable, tortuosity is found in materials with a 'grain' structure, in which particles, e.g. crystals, are packed together to form an irregular system of pores between the grains, as in intraprismatic enamel or intertubular dentine.

Molecular sieve effects

Diffusates may be excluded from some of the pores within a material because of their molecular size. This is referred to as *molecular sieve* behaviour and has been identified as a property of enamel (Poole *et al*. 1961). This may be due to the presence of ultramicroscopic pores (Dibdin and Poole 1982) or to the presence of pores which could themselves accommodate molecules of the substance but have constricted openings – so-called 'ink-bottle' pores (Poole and Stack 1965, Zahradnik and Moreno 1975).

Because, in narrow pores, the ratio between the surface area of solid and the volume of contained solution is higher than in wide pores, pore size will also affect diffusion by effects other than simple exclusion on the basis of size. First, the pore walls may impose structure on a layer of adjacent water molecules, in effect increasing the viscosity of the solution and hence retarding diffusion. In enamel and dentine, organic matrix within pores may also be associated with structured water. The narrower the pores, the larger will be the proportion of structured to free water molecules and hence the greater the effect on diffusion. Secondly, interactions between the diffusate and the solid, described below, will be increased.

Reactions between diffusate and the solid

The reactions of a diffusate migrating along pores within a material with the surrounding solid surfaces reduce the proportion of diffusate which is free to diffuse and thus slow down the rate of transport. The transport process is then one of *diffusion-with-reaction*.

Reactions may be reversible or irreversible. The principal reversible interaction to be considered here is electrostatic binding of ions to mineral or matrix. Both enamel and dentine are composites of an ionic mineral and protein matrix, so carry a fixed charge which influences diffusion of ionic substances by electrostatic attraction or repulsion. Several studies suggest that enamel has a low point of zero charge (pzc) – about pH 4 (Klein and Amberson 1929, Waters 1972, Kambara *et al.* 1978), so enamel is negatively charged at all pH values of interest. Dentine, like enamel, has a net negative charge under neutral, quasi-physiological conditions (Neiders *et al.* 1970), but its pzc has not been estimated. The actual charge density of the tissue will depend on the ionic composition of the solution, as the negative charge is increased by anions such as phosphate and decreased or reversed by cations such as calcium, through binding to the solid (van Dijk 1986).

An example of an irreversible reaction would be incorporation of calcium and phosphate into mineral if the solution bathing a specimen of enamel or dentine were supersaturated.

Measurement of diffusion in porous solids

Steady-state diffusion

Here, a sample of the material is placed between two chambers, each filled with solution, to form a 'diaphragm cell'. Such cells have been widely used to obtain diffusion coefficients for enamel, the sample consisting of a section with known surface area and thickness. The chambers are filled with solutions each containing the same concentration of diffusate (to eliminate osmotic gradients), but with the source chamber containing radiolabelled diffusate. After a lag phase, during which reactions between the diffusate and the solid reach a steady state, tracer accumulates in the receiver chamber at a rate determined by diffusion through the sample and a diffusion coefficient can be calculated.

Penetration and clearance methods

These methods measure the rate at which a 'front' of diffusate moves through the material. In penetration methods, a solution of radiolabelled diffusate is applied to the surface of a sample of material. Diffusion with time into the sample is then followed, by one of a variety of methods: total uptake by the sample (Braden *et al.* 1971); autoradiography of sections (Marthaler and Mühlemann 1960); serial grinding to obtain layers at successively greater depths (Flim and Arends 1977, de Rooij *et al.* 1980); or measurement of the buildup of diffusate in a solution on the opposite side of the sample (Merchant *et al.* 1977). In the clearance method, a sample is first equilibrated with solution containing radiolabelled diffusate at a high specific activity. The sample is then transferred to unlabelled solution and the accumulation of radioactivity in the solution is followed over time (Dibdin 1993).

Application of diffusion measurements

In some penetration experiments, the aim has been simply to determine qualitatively whether teeth or particular dental tissues were permeable to particular substances. Other experiments have been aimed at providing some quantitative information on how quickly a substance will penetrate a layer of the hard tissue and on the probable flux. This has been the case with many problems of dental interest, such as ascertaining the rate of penetration of therapeutic agents or potentially toxic substances through a layer of hard tissue. While these penetration experiments have provided invaluable information, the results can be extrapolated to other situations only to a limited extent. If more rigorous experimental procedures are applied, diffusion coefficients can be determined and these can in principle be applied to predictions about transport in situations other than those studied directly, by the use of mathematical models. This has been done most successfully in the case of enamel caries (van Dijk 1986). In such work, independent information about diffusion and reaction rates is required for the overall process to be evaluated in a valid fashion, but there are some difficulties in extracting the required information from diffusion experiments.

Following Dibdin (1993), the coefficient derived from steady-state diffusion experiments will be termed the *apparent diffusion coefficient* (D_a) and that derived from penetration or clearance experiments the *effective diffusion coefficient* (D_e). These coefficients provide different types of information.

In a diaphragm-cell experiment conducted as described above, there is a steady state with respect to any reactions between the diffusate and the material, so D_a is not influenced by these reactions. Neither is it influenced by diffusion along any blind pores connecting with the through pores. D_a is thus a kind of permeability coefficient, being influenced only by the molecular size of the diffusate, the porosity and tortuosity of the through pores and by the viscosity of the solution within the pores.

D_e, on the other hand, is influenced by any processes which alter the concentration of diffusate in the pores leading to the sample surface. Such processes include both reactions, such as electrostatic binding, and exchange with 'blind' pores.

Most systems of dental interest – for instance the inward diffusion of H^+ ions and outward diffusion of mineral ions in caries or erosion – are not at steady state, and many of the diffusates of dental interest are small ions which are not confined to the larger pores, so more appropriate information is provided by D_e. However, interpretation and measurement pose greater problems than for D_a. Reversible reactions can be allowed for if experiments are performed at different diffusate concentrations. Irreversible reactions can in principle be eliminated by thorough pre-equilibration, but present a potentially serious source of error in penetration experiments, leading to underestimation of D_e.

Permeability of dental hard tissues

Because the tubules are large in relation to molecular dimensions, dentine is permeable to macromolecules such as proteins and non-dialysable bacterial products (Bergenholtz 1977) as well as to ions and low molecular weight substances. Enamel has been shown to be permeable to ions, to low molecular weight substances such as dyes (Shellis and Dibdin 1999) and even to some quite large molecules. Thus, the porosity with respect to inulin (M_r ~5200) is about 1.3% v/v (Chatfield 1997). However, the pore sizes are such that sound enamel is probably effectively impermeable to macromolecules. Because the mineral associated with the prism junctions has a raised solubility, one of the earliest changes during enamel demineralization is likely to be increased diffusion along the junctions (Shellis 1996).

Apparent diffusion coefficients have been measured for a fairly wide range of low molecular weight substances and ions in enamel. Most values for D_a fall within the range of 10^{-9}–10^{-7} cm^2/s (see Table 2.2 in Shellis and Dibdin 1999). The small value of D_a compared with diffusion in aqueous solution (e.g. about 2×10^{-5} cm^2/s for water itself) is mainly due to the very low porosity and the tortuosity of the pores. Consideration of various pieces of evidence indicates that diffusion occurs essentially in free water within the prism-junction pores (Shellis and Dibdin 1999), although there is some hindrance to diffusion (Burke and Moreno 1975).

An additional effect of the small pore size in enamel is that the tissue acts as an imperfectly ion-selective material. Anions are hindered from entering the narrow pores by the electrostatic repulsion of the negatively charged pore walls, whereas cations enter more freely. Enamel is thus cation-selective. Brown (1974) suggested that this property of enamel might favour the development of undersaturated conditions during caries formation, since H^+ ions produced by plaque could in effect exchange for Ca^{2+} ions to reduce the internal pH of enamel; this effect was demonstrated by the use of ion-selective membranes *in vitro* (Chow and Brown 1984). However, van Dijk (1986) considered that under *in-vivo* conditions variations in the ion selectivity of enamel that could be produced by treatment with ionic substances would not be sufficient to alter the rate of caries formation.

Lindén *et al.* (1986) produced data suggesting that D_a is greater for enamel of deciduous teeth than for that of permanent teeth. This is consistent with the relative mineral contents (Wilson and Beynon 1989).

No D_a values have been reported for dentine. Because of its greater porosity, dentine is unlikely to be ion selective.

Penetration and effusion studies of hard tissues

In a series of studies, the penetration of fluorine, calcium and phosphate ions in enamel was studied by serial grinding to obtain depth profiles after allowing time for penetration (Flim and Arends 1977, Flim et al. 1977, de Rooij et al. 1980). The results were interpreted in terms of diffusion within two pore systems: the prism-junction pores and the intercrystalline pores in the intervening enamel. However, there are doubts about the analysis. The assumed pore dimensions are unrealistic (Shellis and Dibdin 1999). Also, the diffusion coefficients obtained, even for prism-junction diffusion, were very small and the extent of reaction between diffusate and solid may have been underestimated (van Dijk 1986, Shellis and Dibdin 1999). It was implicit in the analysis of these studies that diffusion occurs in parallel along the prism junctions and between the crystals and hence it was assumed that there is no connection between the two. Dibdin (1993) proposed an alternative model, based on clearance experiments with water. In this model, the prism junctions formed a through pore system, within which the diffusion coefficient was close to that of water. The intercrystalline pores formed an inner pore system, communicating with the prism junctions, and within which the diffusion coefficient was very much lower. This seems to accord well with knowledge of enamel ultrastructure. Electron microscopy shows that there are numerous connections between the intercrystalline pore system and the prism junctions, and hence diffusion away from the junctions would be significant even if each connection allowed access only to a limited volume of tissue.

Most diffusion studies of dentine have addressed practical problems of clinical interest, being concerned with the rate at which potentially cytotoxic substances such as bacterial products (Bergenholtz et al. 1993), components of restorative materials (Hume 1994, Gerzina and Hume 1994, 1996, Hamid and Hume 1997, Bouillaguet et al. 1998) or therapeutic agents (Wiebkin et al. 1996) penetrate the dentine. The cementum layer was shown to have diffusion-limiting properties (Wiebkin et al. 1996).

Recently, some limited data have been obtained for the effective diffusion coefficient of water in dentine (Chatfield 1997). At 37°C, D_e was 16.1×10^{-7} cm^2/s for diffusion parallel with the tubules and 11.5×10^{-7} cm^2/s for diffusion perpendicular to the tubules, compared with 4×10^{-7} cm^2/s for a similar thickness of enamel (Dibdin 1993). Clearly, diffusion occurs much more freely through dentine, even when the tubules are not orientated so as to act as through pores, and when the intertubular dentine must provide the main diffusion pathways.

Convective transport

It is well established that the hydrostatic pressure within the dental pulp is higher than atmospheric pressure, the difference being 13–42 cm water (Wynn et al. 1963, Pashley et al. 1981, Maita et al. 1991, Vongsavan and Matthews 1994, Jacobsen and Heyeraas 1997) and as a result there is a driving force for convective fluid movement through the dental tissues. However, such a flow has been demonstrated only through dentine, and only after the removal of the overlying enamel or cementum. This flow through exposed tubules has clinical implications. First, augmentation of the flow, e.g. by imposition of an osmotic gradient, may stimulate pulpal pain receptors, resulting in hypersensitivity (Addy and Pearce 1994). Secondly, leakage of dentine fluid, which is a solution of serum proteins in an electrolyte solution, on to the floor of a freshly cut cavity might interfere with bonding of restorative materials. Thirdly, it is important to establish the extent to which the outward flow opposes the inward diffusion of potentially harmful substances, including bacterial products and diffusible components of restorative materials. For these reasons, the flow of fluid through dentinal tubules has been studied extensively.

The outward flow of dentine fluid can be measured in vivo by collection from a cavity cut in the dentine. This allows comparison of treatments intended to block flow (Bergenholtz et al.

1993). With additional experimental manipulation, quantitative data on hydraulic conductance, pulpal pressure and other parameters can be obtained (Maita *et al.* 1991).

In-vitro experiments can be controlled more closely and thus allow quantitative investigation of such variables as site, dentine structure, tissue thickness and pressure gradients. In the main, 'classical' techniques have been used, but Macpherson *et al.* (1995) have successfully measured flow rates through individual tubules by scanning probe microscopy. Results are inevitably influenced by the fact that the tubules are often empty, or at least have altered contents – in particular they lack the odontoblast process which extends through the inner part of the tubule in vivo (Matthews and Hughes 1988). Nevertheless, much knowledge relevant to clinical practice has been obtained and some of the results are summarized below.

Smear layers

Flow is significantly impeded by the smear layer produced by cutting instruments during cavity preparation. Removal of the smear layer during placement of a restoration allows wetting of the cavity surface by dentine fluid and this can adversely affect bond strength (Mitchem *et al.* 1988, Tao and Pashley 1989).

Fluid flow and diffusion

When a pressure gradient acts in the same direction as a concentration gradient, total transport through dentine will naturally be greater than that produced by diffusion alone. Thus, Merchant *et al.* (1977) found that application of 240 cm H_2O pressure approximately doubled the penetration rate of ^{125}I compared with diffusion alone, with a smear layer present, and increased it 32-fold when the smear layer had been removed. Here, the pressure used was 6–16 times greater than that *in vivo* and it would be interesting to know the effect of physiological pressure gradients. Pashley and Matthews (1993) found that, when diffusion down an overall gradient of about 1 mmol/l/mm was

opposed by a pressure gradient of 15 cm H_2O/mm, transport of ^{125}I was reduced by 15–20% in the presence of a smear layer and by up to 60% after its removal. Stead *et al.* (1996) have developed a useful mathematical model to investigate the effects of interaction between inward diffusion and outward flow on delivery of K^+ ions to intradentinal nerve endings. The studies just discussed utilized a static pressure gradient. However, a recent study indicated that inward diffusion of NaCl might actually reach equilibrium more quickly with a pulsatile pressure (Camps *et al.* 1996).

Site-to-site variations

In specimens retaining the original pulpal surface of the dentine, the permeability, as measured by the hydraulic conductivity, varies according to the residual dentine thickness (Pashley *et al.* 1987). In part this is an effect of reduced resistance to flow along the shorter tubules, but is also due to the fact that tubule diameter and density increase from the outer to the pulpal surface of the dentine. Thus, any effects of fluid flow on bond strength of restorations will vary from site to site.

Differences in hydraulic conductivity also exist between different sites on the same tooth (e.g. between coronal and radicular dentine) (Fogel *et al.* 1988) and between species (Tagami *et al.* 1989). These are largely attributable to variations in tubule diameter and density.

Reduction in fluid flow

In vivo, the outward flow of dentine fluid decreases within a short time after cavity preparation (Pashley *et al.* 1984, Bergenholtz *et al.* 1993). This reduction appears to be due to occlusion of tubules by proteins of the dentine fluid and, in vivo, salivary proteins and even bacteria could also contribute to reducing permeability (Pashley *et al.* 1982). Fibrin precipitation may be particularly important in the reduction of permeability (Pashley *et al.* 1984). There is evidence that substances known to precipitate protein accelerate flow reduction (Bergenholtz *et al.* 1993).

Conclusions

The diffusion properties of enamel have been extensively investigated and the results have been applied with considerable success to modelling the formation of caries lesions. However, some uncertainty remains as to the most appropriate model of enamel structure to use in such modelling work. The model proposed by Dibdin (1993) seems the most realistic at present, but further work to establish its validity would be useful. An aspect of diffusion through enamel that deserves more attention is the possibility that the enamel of deciduous teeth is more permeable than that of permanent teeth.

Diffusion through dentine has been studied with the aim of answering definite clinical questions, and flow through dentine tubules has received considerable attention. However, the relative importance of these two processes has not been established. While the tubules provide pathways for very free diffusion, these occupy only a small proportion of the tissue and the limited data reported by Chatfield (1997) suggest that diffusion through intertubular dentine cannot be neglected. Because the tubules are separated by very small distances in relation to the tissue thickness, it seems that exchange between the tubules and intertubular dentine is likely to be significant, even though the peritubular dentine will provide a partial diffusion barrier. Fluid flow is an important component of transport only in dentine where the tubules have been exposed and diffusion will be the dominant mode of transport in unexposed dentine, or in exposed dentine where the tubules are occluded by protein or sclerosis. Although the rate of transport by diffusion will be low compared with that driven by fluid flow, it could be clinically important, for instance when pulpal circulation is impaired, so that exogenous substances are removed less efficiently. Diffusion will also play a central role in subsurface demineralization, as in caries formation and the advance of erosions. For these reasons, further quantitative studies of diffusion in this tissue seem well justified.

Acknowledgement

The author acknowledges with thanks the support of SmithKline Beecham.

References

Addy M, Pearce N (1994) Aetiological, predisposing and environmental factors in dentine hypersensitivity. *Arch Oral Biol* **39**(Suppl):S33-S38.

Bergenholtz G (1977) Effect of bacterial products on inflammatory reactions in the dental pulp. *Scand J Dent Res* **85**:122–9.

Bergenholtz G, Jontell M, Tuttle A, Knutsson G (1993) Inhibition of serum albumin flux across exposed dentine following conditioning with GLUMA, glutaraldehyde or potassium oxalates. *J Dent* **21**:220–7.

Bouillaguet S, Virgillito M, Wataha J et al (1998) The influence of dentine permeability on cytotoxicity of four dentine bonding systems *in vitro*. *J Oral Rehabil* **25**:45–51.

Braden M, Duckworth R, Joyston-Bechal S (1971) The uptake of ^{24}Na by human dental enamel. *Arch Oral Biol* **16**:367–74.

Brown WE (1974) Physicochemical mechanisms in dental caries. *J Dent Res* **53**:204–25.

Burke EJ, Moreno EC (1975) Diffusion fluxes of tritiated water across human enamel membranes. *Arch Oral Biol* **20**:327–32.

Camps J, Santin V, Rieu R et al, (1996) Effects of pulsatile versus non-pulsatile pulpal pressure simulations on diffusional transport across human dentine *in vitro*. *Arch Oral Biol* **41**:837–43.

Chatfield SR (1997) A study of the pore structure of human dental enamel using radiotracer techniques. PhD thesis, University of Bristol.

Chow LC, Brown WE (1984) A physicochemical bench-scale caries model. *J Dent Res* **63**:868–73.

De Rooij JF, Kolar Z, Arends J (1980) Phosphate diffusion in whole bovine enamel at pH 7. *Caries Res* **14**:393–402.

Dibdin GH (1993) The water in human dental enamel and its diffusional exchange measured by clearance of tritiated water from enamel slabs of varying thickness. *Caries Res* **27**:81–6.

Dibdin GH, Poole DFG (1982) Surface area and pore size analysis for human enamel and dentine by water vapour sorption. *Arch Oral Biol* **27**:235–41.

Flim GJ, Arends J (1977) Diffusion of ^{45}Ca in bovine enamel. *Calcif Tiss Res* **24**:59–64.

Flim GJ, Kolar Z, Arends J (1977) Diffusion of fluoride ions in dental enamel at pH 7: a theoretical model. *J Bioeng* **1**:209–13.

Fogel HM, Marshall FJ, Pashley DH (1988) Effects of distance from the pulp and thickness on the hydraulic conductance of human radicular dentin. *J Dent Res* **67**:1381–5.

Garberoglio R, Brannstrom M (1976) Scanning electron microscopic investigation of human dentinal tubules. *Arch Oral Biol* **21**:355–62.

Gerzina TM, Hume WR (1994) Effect of dentine on release of TEGDMA from resin composites *in vitro*. *J Oral Rehabil* **21**:463–8.

Gerzina TM, Hume WR (1996) Diffusion of monomers from bonding resin–resin composite combinations through dentine *in vitro*. *J Dent* **24**: 125–8.

Hamid A, Hume WR (1997) The effect of dentine thickness on diffusion of resin monomers *in vitro*. *J Oral Rehabil* **24**:20–5.

Hume WR (1994) Influence of dentine on the pulpward release of eugenol or acids from restorative materials. *J Oral Rehabil* **21**:469–73.

Jacobsen EB, Heyeraas KJ (1997) Pulp interstitial fluid pressure and blood flow after denervation and electrical tooth stimulation in the ferret. *Arch Oral Biol* **42**:407–15.

Kambara M, Asai T, Kumasaki M, Konishi K (1978) An electrochemical study on the human dental enamel with special reference to isoelectric point. *J Dent Res* **57**:306–12.

Klein H, Amberson WR (1929) A physico-chemical study of the structure of dental enamel. *J Dent Res* **9**:667–88.

Lindén L-A, Björkman W, Hattab F (1986) The diffusion *in vitro* of fluoride and chlorhexidine in the enamel of human deciduous and permanent teeth. *Arch Oral Biol* **31**:33–37.

Macpherson JV, Beeston MA, Unwin PR et al (1995) Scanning electrochemical microscopy as a probe of local fluid flow through porous solids. *J Chem Soc Faraday Trans* **91**:1407–10.

Maita E, Simpson MD, Tao L, Pashley DH (1991) Fluid and protein flux across the pulpodentinal complex in the dog. *Arch Oral Biol* **36**:103–10.

Marthaler TM, Mühlemann HR (1960) Das Eindringen von radioaktiv markiertem Schwefelharnstoff in den Schmelz nach Natrium- und Kalziumchloridvorbehandlung. *Schweiz Monatsschr Zahnheilk* **70**:10–17.

Matthews B, Hughes SHS (1988) The ultrastructure and receptor transduction mechanisms of dentine. In: Hamann W, Iggo A, eds, *Progress in Brain Research*, Vol 74, 69–76. Elsevier: Amsterdam.

Merchant VA, Livingston MJ, Pashley DH (1977) Dentin permeation: comparison of diffusion with filtration. *J Dent Res* **56**:1161–4.

Mitchem JC, Terkla LG, Gronas DG (1988) Bonding of resin dentin adhesives under simulated physiological conditions. *Dent Mater* **4**:351–3.

Neiders ME, Weiss L, Cudney TL (1970) An electrokinetic characterization of human tooth surfaces. *Arch Oral Biol* **15**:135–51.

Orams HJ, Phakey PP, Rachinger WA, Zybert JJ (1974) Visualisation of micropore structure in human dental enamel. *Nature* **252**:584–5.

Pashley DH, Matthews WG (1993) The effects of outward forced convective flow on inward diffusion in human dentine *in vitro*. *Arch Oral Biol* **38**:577–82.

Pashley DH, Nelson R, Pashley EL (1981) *In-vivo* fluid movement across dentine in the dog. *Arch Oral Biol* **26**:707–10.

Pashley DH, Nelson R, Kepler EE (1982) The effects of plasma and salivary constituents on dentin permeability. *J Dent Res* **61**:978–81.

Pashley DH, Galloway SE, Stewart F (1984) Effects of fibrinogen *in vivo* on dentin permeability in the dog. *Arch Oral Biol* **29**:725–8.

Pashley DH, Andringa HJ, Derkson GD et al (1987) Regional variability in the permeability of human dentine. *Arch Oral Biol* **32**:519–23.

Poole DFG, Stack MV (1965) The structure and physical properties of enamel. In: Stack MV, Fearnhead RW, eds, *Tooth Enamel*, 172–6. Wright: Bristol.

Poole DFG, Mortimer KV, Darling AI, Ollis WD (1961). Molecular sieve behaviour of dental enamel. *Nature* **189**:998–1000.

Shellis RP (1996) Solubility variations in human enamel and dentine: a scanning electron microscope study. *Arch Oral Biol* **41**:473–84.

Shellis RP, Dibdin GH (1999) Enamel microporosity and its functional implications. In: Teaford MF, Ferguson MJ, Smith MM, eds, *Teeth: Development, Evolution and Function*. Cambridge University Press: Cambridge (in press).

Stead WJ, Orchardson R, Warren PB (1996) A mathematical model of potassium ion diffusion in dentinal tubules. *Arch Oral Biol* **41**:679–87.

Tagami J, Tao L, Pashley DH, Horner JA (1989) The permeability of dentine from bovine incisors *in vitro*. *Arch Oral Biol* **34**:773–7.

Tao L, Pashley DH (1989) Dentin perfusion effects on the shear bond strengths of bonding agents to dentin. *Dent Mater* **5**:181–4.

Van Dijk JWE (1986) Caries mechanisms and the permeability of tooth enamel. In: Driessens FCM, Wöltgens JHM, eds, *Tooth Development and Caries*, Vol 2, 1–25. CRC Press: Boca Raton.

Vongsavan N, Matthews B (1994) Fluid flow through cat dentine *in vivo*. *Arch Oral Biol* **37**:175–85.

Waters NE (1972) Membrane potentials in teeth: the effect of pH. *Caries Res* **6**:346–54.

Wiebkin OW, Cardaci SC, Heithersay GS, Pierce AM (1996) Therapeutic delivery of calcitonin to inhibit external inflammatory root resorption I. Diffusion kinetics of calcitonin through the root. *Endodont Dent Traumatol* **12**:265–71.

Wilson PR, Beynon AD (1989) Mineralization differences between human deciduous and permanent enamel measured by quantitative microradiography. *Arch Oral Biol* **34**:85–8.

Wynn W, Haldi J, Hopf MA, John K (1963) Pressure within the pulp chamber of the dog's tooth relative to arterial blood pressure. *J Dent Res* **42**:1169–77.

Zahradnik RT, Moreno EC (1975) Structural features of human dental enamel as revealed by isothermal water vapour sorption. *Arch Oral Biol* **20**:317–25.

3

On the nature of the acquired enamel pellicle

Alix R Young, Morten Rykke and Gunnar Rölla

Introduction

The acquired enamel pellicle is a protective protein layer that forms rapidly on teeth after exposure to saliva in the oral environment. The pellicle protects the enamel against erosion by acid and is probably also involved in protection against hypersensitivity (Zahradnik et al. 1976; Rykke and Rölla 1992). The newly formed enamel pellicle has been seen to consist predominantly of globular structures (Lie 1977, Rölla and Rykke 1994, Hannig 1997), or to have an uneven, knotted appearance (Busscher et al. 1989), as observed by transmission and scanning electron microscopic morphological studies (Figure 3.1). Similar morphological structures have been shown in scanning electron microscopic studies of enamel exposed to milk or cream (Nyvad and Fejerskov 1984; Guggenheim et al. 1994). These structures have been shown to resemble the salivary micelle-like globules seen in human saliva using electron microscopic techniques (Caldwell and Shackleford 1967; Rölla and Rykke 1994; Rykke et al. 1995; Rykke et al. 1997a, 1997b) (Figure 3.2). Both types of globules are 200–300 nm in diameter and appear to consist of subunits. The salivary micelle-like globules are morphologically and chemically similar to the milk proteins that form structures termed casein micelles (Schmidt 1980; Rollema 1992; Rykke et al. 1997b). The casein micelles consist of four different casein molecules. These are largely amphiphilic phosphoproteins, exhibiting properties that allow the formation of very stable complexes with a relatively large amount of calcium phosphate (Swaisgood 1985, Holt 1992, Rollema 1992).

Preliminary data suggest that the amino acid profile of isolated salivary micelle-like structures is similar to that of the 2-h pellicle collected directly from human teeth in vivo (Rölla and Rykke 1994). Given that the salivary micelle-like globules are the predominant proteinaceous components of the 2-h pellicle, it would be of interest to determine how much of the total saliva protein exists in the form of these globules. This may give an indication of the relative importance of the salivary micelle-like globules. The aims of the study described in this chapter were therefore two-fold. The first aim was to test the hypothesis that the amino acid profile of the salivary micelle-like globules shows similarity to that of the 2-h pellicle based on more comprehensive material than in a previous study. If this can be established in a larger body of material this would support the observation that the 2-h pellicle consists mainly of salivary micelle-like globules. The second aim was to establish how much of the total salivary protein occurs in the form of salivary micelle-like globules.

Although time-consuming, amino acid analysis is considered to be the most suitable method for this type of investigation. Amino acid analyses have been widely used to compare salivas and enamel pellicles (Sönju and Rölla 1973, Mayhall 1977, Oste et al. 1981, Al-Hashimi and Levine 1989). The micro-Kjeldahl method for protein determination was also included because this method is extensively used in the analysis of milk protein and, as mentioned previously, milk contains casein micelles which are chemically closely related to the salivary micelle-like globules (Rölla and Rykke 1994; Rykke et al. 1996). One advantage of both methods is that they are independent of protein standards.

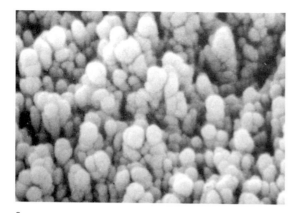

a

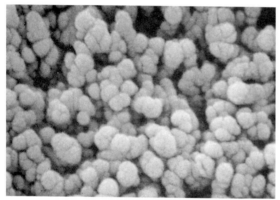
b

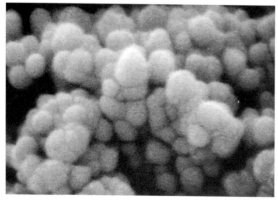
c

Figure 3.1

Scanning electron micrograph of pellicles formed on dental enamel carried in the mouth for 2 h (*b*, ×52,000 and *c*, ×80,000) or exposed to skimmed milk (*a*, ×52,000). Globules of similar size and structure are seen in both preparations (Rölla and Rykke 1994).

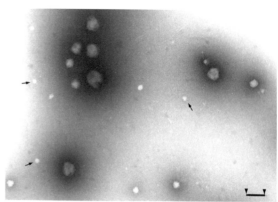

Figure 3.2

Transmission electron micrograph of freshly collected human parotid saliva, negatively stained with 2% ammonium molybdate for 1 min. The structures of about 90–180 nm diameter are multi-globular, consisting of subunits of 40–50 nm, also observed as single units in the micrograph (arrowed). Bar represents 200 nm.

Unclarified and clarified human whole saliva and human parotid saliva were included in the experiments. Clarified whole saliva and parotid saliva were tested because these fluids have been extensively used in studies relating to the physiology of human saliva, including studies on pellicle formation in vitro. Unclarified saliva was included because this fluid is the secretion encountered in the mouth and could thus be considered more relevant. The protein content of the isolated salivary micelle-like globules was compared with the total protein content of saliva, and the ratio was calculated.

Methodology

Saliva samples

Twelve-ml samples of paraffin wax-stimulated human whole saliva (HWS) and sweet/sour-stimulated human parotid saliva (HPS) were collected on ice from six healthy adult subjects (three male, three female, age range 32–70 years). Subjects were asked not to consume food or drink following their normal morning oral hygiene routine and saliva collected during the first minute was discarded. Three separate samples per subject of both HWS and HPS were collected on separate days between 9.00 and 11.00 am. The HPS samples were processed directly after collection at a flow rate of 0.9–2.3 ml/min, by means of Curby cups or individually fitted bilateral appliances made of Provil®-P impression material (BayerDental, Leverkusen, Germany) as described previously (Rykke et al. 1995). HWS samples were clarified immediately after collection at a flow rate of about 1.5–3 ml/min (approx. 1500 $\times$ g for 10 min). Three additional 6-ml HWS samples were collected from three of the subjects and not clarified (unclarified HWS). Aliquots (25 µl) of all HWS (unclarified and clarified) and HPS samples were transferred directly into hydrolysis tubes. After freezing the samples were freeze-dried in preparation for amino acid analyses. Six-ml aliquots of clarified HWS and HPS were immediately frozen until further analysis by the micro-Kjeldahl method. Following gentle water-bath warming of the remaining chilled saliva to room temperature, salivary micelle-like globules were isolated from 6-ml samples according to a procedure described previously, based on acidification of the saliva to the isoelectric point (Rölla and Rykke 1994; Rykke et al. 1996). The isolated salivary micelle-like globule pellets obtained were washed twice with de-ionized water and freeze-dried ready for amino acid analysis. The supernatants remaining after isolation and removal of salivary micelle-like globules were frozen until analysis by the micro-Kjeldahl method.

Amino acid analysis

Unclarified and clarified HWS, HPS and the respective isolated salivary micelle-like globule samples were subjected to quantitative amino acid analysis by standard procedures. The lyophilized samples were hydrolysed in 6 M HCl under pure nitrogen atmosphere for 24 h, at 108–110°C. The salivary micelle-like globule samples were transferred from the test tubes in which they were isolated to the hydrolysis tubes after the addition of acid. Some unavoidable loss of material occurred during the transfer, although precautions were taken to minimize these losses and all samples were treated similarly. Samples were then run on a Model 421

Amino Acid Analyser (Perkin Elmer, CA, USA), with phenyl isothiocyanate (PITC) as a detector reagent. The analysis is based on the Edman degradation and the use of high performance liquid chromatography (Stryer 1995). The results were obtained via connection to a Model 600 Data Module. Protein concentrations for the analysed samples were calculated by adding together the products (concentrations of the individual amino acid residues) $\times$ (molecular weight minus one water molecule per residue).

Micro-Kjeldahl method

HWS, HPS and the respective supernatants remaining after isolation and removal of the salivary micelle-like globules were analysed for their nitrogen content with a Kjeltec Auto Sampler System 1035 Analyser (Tecator, Höganös, Sweden). Triplicate 2-ml portions of the defrosted samples were digested in H_2SO_4 with added K_2SO_4 and selenium (Kjeltabs Auto, Thompson and Capper, Cheshire, UK). Recovery tests were carried out to ensure adequate yield using $(NH_4)_2SO_4$ and L-cysteine (Sigma Chemicals). Water blanks and skimmed milk control samples were employed. Calculation of the percentage of salivary micelle-like globules by the micro-Kjeldahl technique was based on the amount of protein remaining in the supernatant. It was assumed that the total salivary protein concentration minus the protein concentration of the supernatant after isolation and removal of salivary micelle-like globules was equivalent to the salivary micelle-like globule-related protein concentration. A Kjeldahl factor of 6.25 was used for all samples in the conversion of percentage nitrogen to percentage protein, as this has been employed previously in similar studies (Wolf and Taylor 1964; Dawes 1965).

Results

The amino acid profile of salivary micelle-like globules isolated from unclarified HWS is represented diagrammatically according to Robinson et al. (1975) (Figure 3.3) and showed resemblance to the previously determined amino acid

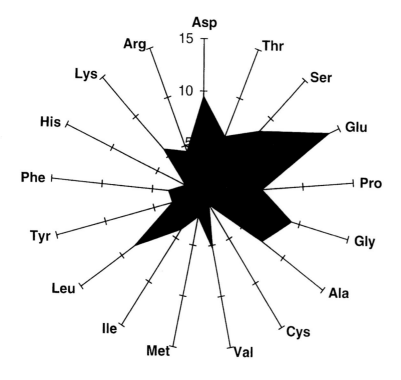

Figure 3.3

Amino acid profile of salivary micelle-like globules isolated from unclarified whole saliva based on the mean values for three subjects. The amounts of the different amino acids are calculated as mol/100 mol (Young *et al.* 1999). This profile shows a striking resemblance to the profile for 2-h pellicle (Figure 3.4) and differs significantly from the profile for unclarified whole saliva (Figure 3.5).

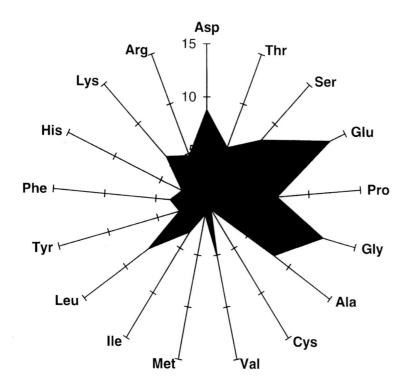

Figure 3.4

Amino acid profile of the 2-h acquired enamel pellicle (Rölla and Rykke 1994). The amounts of the different amino acids are calculated as mol/100 mol.

profile for the 2-h pellicle (Figure 3.4) (Rölla and Rykke 1994). These profiles were markedly different from the profile for unclarified HWS (Figure 3.5). Neutral and acidic amino acids accounted for on average 70–72% of the total for the salivary micelle-like globules and the 2-h pellicle. In comparison, these amino acids accounted for about 57–59 % of total salivary amino acids. The

amino acids to which the carbohydrate conjugate can be bound (ser, thr and asp) represented about 24–30% of the total amino acids for the salivary micelle-like globules compared with 14–18% for saliva.

The results for the protein quantification and calculation of the percentage of salivary micelle-like globules are shown in Table 3.1. The results

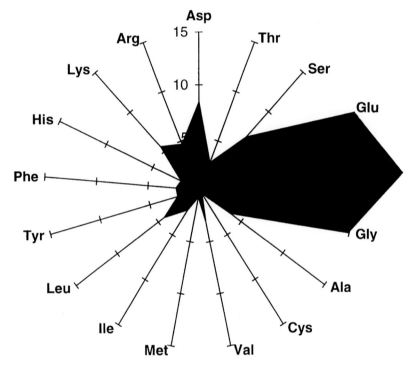

Figure 3.5

Amino acid profile of unclarified whole saliva based on the mean values from three subjects. The amounts of the different amino acids are calculated as mol/100 mol (Young *et al.* 1999). This profile differs markedly from the profile for salivary micelle-like globules isolated from unclarified whole saliva (Figure 3.3).

Table 3.1 Protein concentration (mg/ml) and ratio of salivary micelle-like globules (% SMGs), with mean and standard deviation (SD), as measured by amino acid analyses and micro-Kjeldahl determinations of unclarified and clarified whole saliva and parotid saliva (Young *et al.* 1999).

Protein content	Saliva (mg/ml) mean (SD)	SMGs (mg/ml) mean (SD)	% SMGs* mean (SD)
Amino acid analysis			
Clarified HWS[†]	1.543 (0.61)	0.072 (0.04)	4.7 (2)
Unclarified HWS[‡]	2.092 (0.77)	0.413 (0.13)	19.7 (13)
HPS[†]	2.224 (0.80)	Small amounts	
Micro-Kjeldahl method			
clarified HWS[§]	2.629 (0.91)	0.197 (0.11)**	7.5 (3)
HPS[†]	3.311 (0.98)	0.069 (0.05)**	2.1 (1)

HWS, human whole saliva; HPS, human parotid saliva.
*% SMGs calculated from the mean for saliva and SMGs.
[†]Data based on three samples from each of six subjects.
[‡]Data based on three samples from each of three subjects.
[§]Data based on three samples from each of five subjects.
**SMGs calculated from saliva minus supernatant.

for clarified HWS from one of the donors as determined by the micro-Kjeldahl method were excluded for technical reasons. Amino acid analysis gave 30–40% lower total protein measurements for the saliva compared with the micro-Kjeldahl method. Amino acid analyses indicated that the salivary micelle-like globules isolated from unclarified whole saliva contributed four times as much of the total protein in saliva compared with those isolated from clarified whole saliva. The average ratio of salivary micelle-like globules isolated from clarified HWS was similar with the two methods. HPS collected directly from the ducts contained only small (2.1% ± 1%, micro-Kjeldahl method) or very small amounts (amino acid analysis) of protein associated with the salivary micelle-like globules.

Discussion

The results of the study described above demonstrated that the amino acid profile of the salivary micelle-like globules was strikingly similar to that determined previously for the 2-h pellicle, which supports the concept that the globular micelle-like structures in saliva constitute the major part of the acquired enamel pellicle (Rölla and Rykke 1994). The results also showed that on average approximately one-fifth of the total amino acids in unclarified whole saliva were associated with salivary micelle-like globules, while HPS contained small or very small amounts of salivary micelle-like globules. However, the small amounts of micelle-like globules in human parotid saliva had been shown previously to be sufficient for electron microscopic and light scattering studies of these globules (Rykke *et al.* 1995; Rykke *et al.* 1996; Rykke *et al.* 1997a, 1997b). The present study was based on data from a total of 18 samples from six subjects, and confirmed the results of an earlier pilot study based on a sample from one subject. In the present study, unclarified whole saliva was considered to be of most interest. However, the relatively low levels of parotid salivary micelle-like globules compared with whole saliva could indicate that a major part of the formation of the salivary micelle-like globules occurs outside the ducts. A co-aggregation of salivary micelle-like

globules appears to occur after the individual secretions become mixed in the oral cavity, resulting in a larger salivary micelle-like globule fraction in whole saliva (Young 1999). Alternatively, salivary glands other than the parotid are the major source(s) of the salivary micelle-like globules in human whole saliva. Recent studies in our laboratory have indicated that salivary micelle-like structures are also present in human submandibular/sublingual saliva (Young 1999). Transmission electron microscopic and photon correlation spectroscopic studies demonstrated particulate aggregates in human submandibular/sublingual saliva that were 2–3-fold larger than the salivary micelle-like globules previously demonstrated in human parotid saliva (Rykke *et al.* 1995; Rykke *et al.* 1997a; Young 1999).

Previous studies have provided evidence suggesting a direct role for the salivary micelle-like globules in bacterial agglutination (Young *et al.* 1997). Amino acid analysis of a purified parotid saliva agglutinin indicated that it constituted about 0.4% of the total protein of the parotid saliva (Ericson and Rundegren 1983). This value is in the range between the small amounts measured by amino analysis and the average figure of about 2% based on the micro-Kjeldahl method for human parotid salivary micelle-like globules in the present study. The amino acids to which a carbohydrate conjugate can be bound (ser, thr and asp) represented 26.7% of the total parotid salivary micelle-like globule amino acids compared with 30.1% for the parotid agglutinin just mentioned.

Unclarified whole saliva is clearly the most relevant fluid of those examined and was considered of more interest than clarified whole saliva and parotid saliva. This oral fluid has an important role in such physiological functions as pellicle formation. However, clarified whole saliva has been used extensively in many salivary experiments, in most cases in order to minimize the possibility of contamination, and for convenience, and was therefore included in the present study. However, it appears likely that clarification removed not only any bacterial or cellular contamination, but also a proportion of the high-density fraction of salivary components, namely the largest salivary micelle-like globules. The fact that the amino acid profiles for unclarified and clarified human whole saliva were similar would support the choice of a lower level of centrifugation, as used in the present study. The ratio thus obtained for salivary micelle-like globules isolated from clarified whole saliva probably represents an underestimate. Conversely, the ratio of about 20% for salivary micelle-like globules isolated from unclarified whole saliva may represent a slight overestimate due to the likelihood of contamination with cells and bacteria. However, previous transmission and scanning electron microscopic studies of isolated salivary micelle-like globules have demonstrated minimal contamination and the amino acids commonly originating from bacteria were not observed in the present study (Rölla and Rykke, 1994). The isolation procedure is based on adjusting the saliva to the isoelectric point of the salivary micelle-like globules (pH 3.1), centrifugation to spin down the very high-density salivary micelle-like globules (the structures not repelling each other at this pH), followed by washing twice in de-ionized water (Rölla and Rykke 1994). This procedure is thus based on two properties, namely the low isoelectric point of the salivary micelle-like globules and their very high density. Initially, lipid-soluble dye was used in the isolation of salivary micelle-like globules in order to visualize their presence in the saliva (Rölla and Rykke 1994). The pellet formed during centrifugation and assumed to contain the salivary micelle-like globule fraction also contained all the staining from lipid-soluble dyes, except a layer on top of the supernatant that presumably represented the salivary lipids (Rölla and Rykke 1994). It has also been shown that > 90% of radioactive triclosan (which is lipid-soluble) added to human whole saliva was found in the pellet after the isolation process (Rölla et al. 1996). This indicated that the purification procedure resulted in sedimentation of almost all the salivary micelle-like globules.

It is widely agreed that the determination of salivary protein is difficult (Wolf and Taylor 1964, Söderling 1989). Many of the commonly used methods for protein determination are based on different characteristics of proteins. However, in biological fluids such as saliva, which contain mixtures of proteins, not all proteins have the same proportion of a given characteristic (Wolf and Taylor 1964). Furthermore, it has not been possible to find a suitable standard for establishing protein content of mixtures of proteins, as demonstrated in one study which showed that the choice of protein standard affected the results (Jenzano et al. 1986). The methods chosen for the calculation of protein content in the present study are independent of a protein standard. The average total protein content of human whole saliva and parotid saliva ranged from 0.9–4.3 mg/ml (with parotid saliva containing more protein than whole saliva), and was in accordance with previous studies (Wolf and Taylor 1964, Levine and Ellison 1973, Mandel 1974, Jenzano et al. 1986). The amino acid profile for human parotid saliva was in close agreement with previous studies (Levine and Ellison 1973, Mayhall 1977, Rykke et al. 1997a). Amino acid analysis of fractions isolated from human parotid saliva by gel chromatography (Rykke et al. 1997a) indicated much higher levels of proline in the peaks containing the salivary micelle-like structures compared with the parotid salivary micelle-like globules isolated in the present study. Differences may be due to the pretreatment of parotid saliva samples (filtration) and the large differences in the method of isolation (gel chromatography carried out over 10 h may allow for some partial destabilization of the globules).

However, both methods were associated with some problems, and the results indicated that the micro-Kjeldahl method measured higher protein concentrations than amino acid analyses for the same saliva samples. Amino acid hydrolysis is known to destroy tryptophan, and results in about 10% decomposition of serine and threonine. Asparagine and glutamine are transformed to the dicarboxylic amino acids with the loss of ammonia, whilst loss of the sulphur-containing amino acids, cysteine and methionine may occur due to oxidation processes when carbohydrates are present in the sample material (Savoy et al. 1975, Jakube 1977, Nair 1977, Stryer 1995). Furthermore, cysteine may be completely lost and methionine can only be traced as several oxidation products that are difficult to identify in the elution programmes. For this reason the values obtained for methionine and cysteine should not be regarded as absolute. However, the main cause of variation in the amino acid analyses of proteins is thought to be the hydrolysis with 6 M HCl, which may account for up to 10% variation (Savoy et al. 1975). Care was taken to ensure the exact measurement of HCl and use of the same batch of hydrolysing acid for all samples. In addition, although previous studies have indicated the presence of trace amounts of the amino sugars galactosamine and glucosamine (Levine and Ellison 1973, Rykke et al. 1990, Rölla and Rykke 1994), the analysis employed in the present study was not standardized to detect the hexosamines.

Despite these inadequacies, it has been stated previously that amino acid analysis is without doubt the most accurate procedure for calculating total protein, because the technique is independent of the composition of the proteins to be estimated (Levine and Ellison 1973). Although also independent of protein standards, the total protein results calculated after employing the micro-Kjeldahl method (that estimates the amount of protein nitrogen) are dependent on the empirical Kjeldahl factor. The Kjeldahl factor used in this study has been employed previously in similar studies and is derived from average nitrogen content for the amino acids of 16%. However, nitrogen content of individual proteins may vary from about 12 to 19%, dependent upon the varying amounts of carbohydrate in salivary proteins (Wolf and Taylor 1964, Dawes 1965). Therefore, the use of a Kjeldahl factor based on 16% protein nitrogen will yield only approximations. Researchers working with milk proteins have concluded that the only proper way of calculating the Kjeldahl factor for milk is from the amino acid sequences, or at least amino acid profiles (Karman and van Boekel 1986, van Boekel and Ribadeau-Dumas 1987). However, in the present study saliva and salivary supernatant samples had very similar amino acid profiles (results not shown), and based on this finding, the same Kjeldahl factor was used when converting percentage nitrogen to percentage protein for both saliva and supernatant samples.

Efforts were made to minimize the possible loss of salivary micelle-like globule-related protein during clarification of the whole saliva by avoiding excessive centrifugal forces in the isolation process. In the present study, whole saliva was clarified at about $1500 \times g$ for 15 min, compared with $10,000 \times g$ or higher as reported in previous studies (Hogg and Embery 1979, Jenzano et al. 1986). Despite this, the results of the present study indicate that about 25% of the total salivary protein was removed by clarification, thereby

adding strength to the above suggestion that the ratio for salivary micelle-like globules isolated from clarified whole saliva may represent an underestimate (see Table 3.1). The fact that the ratio for clarified whole salivary micelle-like globules in samples analysed by both amino acid analysis and micro-Kjeldahl was in the same order of magnitude would tend to strengthen the reliability of the results.

Many authors have shown that the acquired enamel pellicle contains many different proteins (Kraus et al. 1973, Rölla et al. 1983). This has posed a problem, because whereas it is known that certain proteins are selectively adsorbed to hydroxyapatite, it has not been understood how so many different proteins could be adsorbed to the tooth enamel at the same time. It was suggested in a previous study that acidic proteins adsorbed to the tooth mineral first, while other proteins were then adsorbed via protein–protein interactions (Rölla et al. 1982). However, the concept that the acquired enamel pellicle consists largely of salivary micelle-like globules (containing several different proteins), may explain the problem outlined above. The salivary micelle-like globules exhibit many exposed negatively charged protein terminals at their surfaces, as indicated by their low isoelectric point (Rykke et al. 1996), thus conferring a high affinity for the tooth enamel. This is a well known mechanism based on interaction between calcium ions in the hydration layer on the hydroxyapatite surface and negatively charged groups with high affinity for this cation (Rölla et al. 1982, Gorbunoff, 1984). The significance of this model is strongly supported by the observation that agents such as sodium lauryl sulphate and sodium pyrophosphate, which both exhibit high affinity for calcium, inhibit pellicle formation in vivo (Rykke et al. 1988, Rykke and Rölla 1990). As the salivary micelle-like globules at the same time consist of several proteins making up the complete structure, and have a surplus of negative charges on the surface, many proteins can become concentrated on the tooth surface by a single mechanism.

It appears reasonable to conclude that the salivary micelle-like globules represent at least 10% of the total protein of whole saliva. However, one of the donors had unclarified whole salivary micelle-like globules contributing up to 30% of the total salivary protein. Together with the confirmation that the amino acid profile for the salivary micelle-like globules is strikingly similar to that of the 2-h pellicle, the results suggest that the biological activities shown to be associated with the human whole salivary micelle-like globules are of physiological significance in the oral cavity. The amino acid profile of the salivary micelle-like globules was distinctly different to that of whole saliva, thus demonstrating that the selection of proteins for the formation of the salivary micelle-like globules is very specific in relation to salivary proteins as a whole. The results supported previous morphological studies which indicated that micelle-like globules represent a major component of the newly formed enamel pellicle (Lie 1977). This is also reasonable from a teleological point of view. The globules have high affinity for the tooth mineral, as discussed above, and their selective adsorption allows a rapid establishment of a thick protein layer. Such a layer may reduce the friction between the teeth, and between the teeth and the soft tissues of the oral tissues, and prevent or at least minimize erosion as the result of acid attack. The build-up of a similarly thick pellicle by selective adsorption of monolayers of single proteins would presumably be very time-consuming, supplying little protection during the long period of formation, and would scarcely provide for the selectivity and precision which are integrated in the process of pellicle formation (Rykke *et al.* 1990).

References

Al-Hashimi I, Levine MJ (1989) Characterization of in vivo salivary-derived enamel pellicle. *Arch Oral Biol* **34**: 289–95.

Busscher HJ, Uyen HMW, Stokroos I, Jongebloed WL (1989) A transmission electron microscopy study of the adsorption patterns of early developing artificial pellicles on human enamel. *Arch Oral Biol* **34**: 803–9.

Caldwell RC, Shackleford JM (1967) A chemical, immunological and electron-microscopic study of centrifuged human submaxillary saliva. *Arch Oral Biol* **12**: 333–40.

Dawes C (1965) Some characteristics of parotid and submandibular salivary protein. *Arch Oral Biol* **10**: 269–78.

Ericson T, Rundegren J (1983) Characterization of a salivary agglutinin reacting with a serotype c strain of *Streptococcus mutans*. *Eur J Biochem* **133**: 255–61.

Gorbunoff MJ (1984) The interaction of proteins with hydroxyapatite. II: Role of acidic and basic groups. *Anal Biochem* **136**: 433–9.

Guggenheim B, Nesser J, Golliard M, Schupbach P (1994) Salivary pellicle modified by milk components mediates caries protection. *Caries Res* **28**: 182 (ORCA abstracts).

Hannig M (1997) Transmission electron microscopic study of in vivo pellicle formation on dental restorative materials. *Eur J Oral Sci* **105**: 422–33.

Hogg SD, Embery G (1979) The isolation and partial characterization of a sulphated glycoprotein from human whole saliva which aggregates strains of *Streptococcus sanguis* but not *Streptococcus mutans*. *Arch Oral Biol* **24**: 791–7.

Holt C (1992) Structure and stability of bovine casein micelles. *Adv Protein Chem* **43**: 63–151.

Jakube H-D (1977) Analysis of amino acids. In: Jakube H-D, Jeschkeit H, eds, *Amino Acids, Peptides and Proteins: An Introduction*, 22–83. Macmillan Press: London.

Jenzano JW, Hogan SL, Noyes CM et al (1986) Comparison of five techniques for the determination of protein content in mixed human saliva. *Anal Biochem* **159**: 370–6.

Karman AH, van Boekel MAJS (1986) Evaluation of the Kjeldahl factor for conversion of nitrogen content of milk and milk products to protein content. *Netherlands Milk Dairy Journal* **40**: 315–36.

Kraus FW, Örstavik D, Hurts DC, Cook CH (1973) The acquired pellicle: variability and subject-dependence of specific protein. *J Oral Pathol* **2**: 165–73.

Levine MJ, Ellison SA (1973) Immuno-electrophoretic and chemical analyses of human parotid saliva. *Arch Oral Biol* **18**: 839–53.

Lie T (1977) Scanning and transmission electron microscope study of pellicle morphogenesis. *Scand J Dent Res* **85**: 217–31.

Mandel ID (1974) Relation of saliva and plaque to caries. *J Dent Res* **53** (Suppl): 246–66.

Mayhall CW (1977) Amino acid composition of experimental salivary pellicles. *J Periodontol* **48**: 78–91.

Nair BM (1977) Gas-chromatographic analysis of amino acids in food samples. *Journal of Agricultural Chemistry* **25**: 614–20.

Nyvad B, Fejerskov O (1984) Experimentally induced changes in ultrastructure of pellicle on enamel in vivo. In: ten Cate JM, Leach SA, Arends J, eds, *Bacterial Adhesion and Preventive Dentistry*, 143–51. IRL Press: Oxford.

Oste R, Rönström A, Birkhed D et al (1981) Gas-liquid chromatographic analysis of amino acids in pellicle formed on tooth surface and plastic film in vivo. *Arch Oral Biol* **26**: 635–41.

Robinson C, Lowe NR, Weatherell JA (1975) Amino acid composition, distribution and origin of "tuft" protein in human and bovine dental enamel. *Arch Oral Biol* **20**: 29–42.

Rölla G, Rykke M (1994) Evidence for the presence of micelle-like protein globules in human saliva. *Colloids and Surfaces B: Biointerfaces* **3**: 177–82.

Rölla G, Ciardi JE, Bowen WH (1982) Ionic exchange reactions on hydroxyapatite surfaces studied by the use of radioactive counterions (^{45}Ca and ^{32}PO$_4$). In: Frank RM, Leach SA, eds, *Surface and Colloid Phenomena in the Oral Cavity: Methodological Aspects*, 203–10: IRL Press: London.

Rölla G, Ciardi JE, Bowen WH (1983) Identification of IgA, IgG, lysozyme, albumin, α-amylase and glucosyltransferase in the protein layer adsorbed to hydroxyapatite from whole saliva. *Scand J Dent Res* **91**: 186–90.

Rölla G, Wåler SM, Kjærheim V, Rykke M (1996) The salivary micelle-like globules (SMGs) are the major retention site for Triclosan. *J Dent Res* **75**: 93 (IADR abstracts).

Rollema HS (1992) Casein association and micelle formation. In: Fox PF, ed, *Advanced Dairy Chemistry: Proteins*, Vol 1, 111–140. Elsevier Applied Science: London.

Rykke M, Rölla G (1990) Effect of sodium lauryl sulfate on protein adsorption to hydroxyapatite in vitro and on pellicle formation in vivo. *Scand J Dent Res* **98**: 135–43.

Rykke M, Rölla G (1992) Effects of sodium pyrophosphate and ethane-hydroxy-diphosphonate on albumin adsorption in vitro and pellicle formation in vivo. In: Embery G, Rölla G, eds, *Clinical and Biological Aspects of Dentrifrices*, 293–304. Oxford University Press: Oxford.

Rykke M, Rölla G, Sönju T (1988) Effect of pyrophosphate on protein adsorption to hydroxyapatite in vitro and on pellicle formation in vivo. *Scand J Dent Res* **96**: 517–22.

Rykke M, Sönju T, Rölla G (1990) Interindividual and longitudinal studies of amino acid composition of pellicle collected in vivo. *Scand J Dent Res* **98**: 129–34.

Rykke M, Smistad G, Rölla G, Karlsen J (1995) Micelle-like structures in human saliva. *Colloids and Surfaces B: Biointerfaces* **4**: 33–44.

Rykke M, Young A, Smistad G et al (1996) Zeta potentials of human salivary micelle-like particles. *Colloids and Surfaces B: Biointerfaces* **6**: 51–6.

Rykke M, Young A, Devold T et al (1997a) Fractionation of salivary micelle-like structures by gel chromatography. *Eur J Oral Sci* **105**: 495–501.

Rykke M, Young M, Rölla G et al (1997b) Transmission electron microscopy of human saliva. *Colloids and Surfaces B: Biointerfaces* **9**: 257–67.

Savoy CF, Heinis JL, Seals RG (1975) Improved methodology for rapid and reproducible acid hydrolysis of food and purified proteins. *Anal Biochem* **68**: 562–71.

Schmidt DG (1980) Colloidal aspects of casein. *Netherlands Milk Dairy Journal* **34**: 42–64.

Söderling E (1989) Practical aspects of salivary analyses. In: Tenovuo JO, ed, *Human Saliva: Clinical Chemistry and Microbiology*, Vol I, 1–19. CRC Press: Boca Raton, FL.

Sönju T, Rölla G (1973) Chemical analysis of the acquired pellicle formed in two hours on cleaned human teeth in vivo. Rate of formation and amino acid analyses. *Caries Res* **7**: 30–8.

Stryer L (1995) Protein structure and function. Exploring proteins. In: Stryer L, ed, *Biochemistry*, Vol IV, 22–70. WH Freeman: New York.

Swaisgood HE (1985) Characteristics of edible fluids of animal origin: milk. In: Fennema OR, ed, *Food Chemistry*, Vol 2, 791–828. Marcell Dekker: New York:

Van Boekel MAJS, Ribadeau-Dumas B (1987) Addendum to the evaluation of the Kjeldahl factor for conversion of the nitrogen content of milk and milk products to protein content. *Netherlands Milk Dairy Journal* **41**: 281–4.

Wolf RO, Taylor LL (1964) A comparative study of saliva protein analysis. *Arch Oral Biol* **9**: 135–40.

Young A (1999) Co-aggregation of micelle-like globules from human submandibular/sublingual and parotid saliva. *Colloids and Surfaces B: Biointerfaces* **13**: 241–9.

Young A, Rykke M, Smistad G, Rölla G (1997) On the role of human salivary micelle-like globules in bacterial agglutination. *Eur J Oral Sci* **105**: 485–94.

Young A, Rykke M, Rölla G (1999) Quantitative and qualitative analyses of human salivary micelle-like globules. *Acta Odontol Scan* **57**: 105–10.

Zahradnik RT, Moreno EC, Burke EJ (1976) Effect of salivary pellicle on enamel subsurface demineralization in vitro. *J Dent Res* **55**: 664–70.

4

Biology of the dental pulp with special reference to its vasculature and innervation

Bruce Matthews, David Andrew and Sitthichai Wanachantararak

Introduction

Dental pulp has a high resting blood flow. Resin casts of its microvasculature show arterioles and venules arranged axially with a high density of capillary loops extending out towards the dentine. Being surrounded by calcified dentine, pulp has a very low compliance that affects the properties of its circulation. Tissue fluid pressure is high and pulsatile, while arteriolar pressure is lower and the venular pressure is higher than in more compliant tissues. When dentine is exposed in vivo, fluid tends to flow out through the dentinal tubules, driven by the pulpal tissue fluid pressure. This flow slows down the diffusion of chemicals into dentine and pulp from the oral cavity.

Pulp is innervated by myelinated fibres (both A-β and A-δ) and non-myelinated C fibres. Most of these fibres are afferents, and all of these afferents are probably involved in pain and associated protective reflexes. Some of the A-δ and C fibre afferents produce vasodilatation by an axon reflex mechanism. Other C fibres are post-ganglionic, sympathetic, vasomotor fibres that produce vasoconstriction when activated.

Dentine has a limited innervation. Some pulpal fibres have terminals that extend ca. 100 μm into some dentinal tubules, particularly over the pulp cornu. Pulpal afferents in experimental animals respond to stimuli that also cause pain when applied to dentine or pulp in man. The larger myelinated fibres (A-β and some A-δ) respond to stimuli that cause displacement of the contents of dentinal tubules through a hydrodynamic mechanism. They are more sensitive to outward than inward flow. It is not known whether the movement of tubule contents excites the nerve endings directly (either in the inner ends of the tubules or in the superficial pulp) or whether the odontoblasts play a role in the transduction mechanism. The smaller fibres respond mainly to hot and chemical stimuli.

Dental pulp

Dental pulp is a highly vascular, richly innervated loose connective tissue that forms the soft tissue core of a tooth. In many respects the pulp of a fully formed tooth has physiological properties that are similar to those of loose connective tissue elsewhere in the body, but it is different in at least two important respects. First, it is exquisitely sensitive, so much so that just touching exposed pulp with a wisp of cotton wool can cause severe pain. Secondly, in a fully formed, intact tooth, it has a very low compliance, probably the lowest compliance of any tissue in the body. This low compliance is due to the surrounding calcified dentine, which prevents any significant volume change when the pressures within the tissue change. As a result of this low compliance, the equilibria between the various factors that affect blood flow and the circulation of tissue fluid in pulp are different from those in most other tissues.

The vasculature of dental pulp

Compliance

During tooth formation, the cells of the pulp (particularly the odontoblasts) are responsible for forming the dentine. The teeth of most mammals are of limited growth and once root formation is complete, the pulp is almost completely surrounded by calcified enamel and dentine. The only gap in this relatively impermeable barrier is at the tips of the roots where blood vessels and nerves pass into the pulp through one or more apical foramina. This arrangement means that the pulp of such teeth has an extremely low compliance, probably the lowest of any tissue in the body. As a consequence of this arrangement, there can be no change in the volume of one component of the pulp without a complementary change in the volume of another. For example, for a vessel to dilate to permit increased blood flow, there must be either constriction of another blood vessel, a reduction in the volume of lymph in the lymphatic vessels of the pulp, a reduction in tissue fluid volume, a reduction in intracellular fluid volume, or a combination of two or more of these changes. Such constraints do not apply in other, more compliant organs such as skin or mucous membrane, where an increase in blood flow can be accommodated by an overall increase in the volume of the tissue without such marked effects on other tissue elements. As a

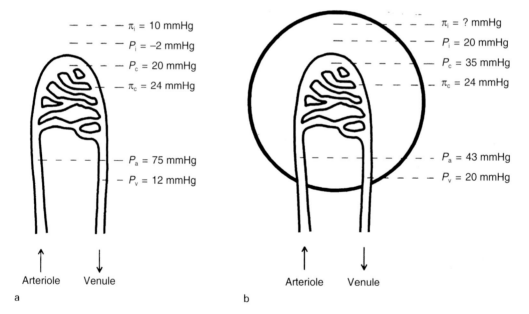

$\pi_i = 10$ mmHg
$P_i = -2$ mmHg
$P_c = 20$ mmHg
$\pi_c = 24$ mmHg

$P_a = 75$ mmHg
$P_v = 12$ mmHg

Arteriole   Venule

a

$\pi_i = ?$ mmHg
$P_i = 20$ mmHg
$P_c = 35$ mmHg
$\pi_c = 24$ mmHg

$P_a = 43$ mmHg
$P_v = 20$ mmHg

Arteriole   Venule

b

Figure 4.1

Hydrostatic pressures at the level of the heart in the arterioles (P_a), capillaries (P_c) venules (P_v) and tissue fluid (i.e. interstitial fluid) (P_i) in a typical compliant tissue such as skin, and in the non-compliant pulp of a fully-formed tooth of limited growth. The calcified dentine which encloses the pulp is represented by the circle. The oncotic pressures of plasma (π_c) and of the interstitial fluid (π_i) of skin are also shown. No estimates have been made of the corresponding value for the interstitial fluid of pulp. These figures are mean values and are based partly on data reviewed in the text and partly on values reported by Heyeraas (1985) and by Michel (1997). The differences in hydrostatic and oncotic pressure across the capillary wall will result in filtration or reabsorption of fluid between the blood and the interstitial fluid according to the following equation:

$$(J_v/A) = L_p((P_c - P_i) - \sigma(\pi_c - \pi_i))$$

where J_v/A is the flow per unit area of capillary wall, L_p is the hydraulic permeability of the capillary wall, and σ is the reflection coefficient of the capillary wall to protein (Michel 1997).

result of this low compliance, the pressures (Figure 4.1) and flow in the microvasculature and tissue fluid of dental pulp tend to be different from those in most other tissues.

In teeth with open root apices, such as the continuously growing incisors of rodents and partially formed teeth of limited growth, the pulp will have a lower compliance. It would be interesting to compare the haemodynamic properties of the pulp in these teeth with those in very low compliance pulp, but very little such information is available on teeth with open apices.

Pulpal blood vessels

The first detailed studies of the vascular architecture of pulp were made on human teeth by Kramer (1960). He used an elegant technique by which he was able to fill the blood vessels in the pulps of recently extracted teeth with India ink. He then examined the cleared specimens. He showed that venules tended to be in the peripheral part of the root pulp, whereas arterioles were more central. A capillary network extended over the surface of the pulp with loops extending up towards the odontoblast layer.

This pattern was described in greater detail in another very elegant study by Takahashi et al. (1982). They made resin casts of the pulpal vessels of cat teeth, digested away the surrounding tissues then examined the casts in a scanning electron microscope. Takahashi et al. confirmed that the main arterioles tended to run axially through the pulp with the main venules alongside. These were connected by capillary loops that extended up to the pulpal surface. They also described arteriovenous anastomoses, venous–venous anastomoses and U-turn arterioles. Such vessels are not generally found in loose connective tissue in other regions. It is not known what function they serve in the pulp: it may be that they have special functions related to the low compliance of the tissue.

Bishop (1987) studied the ultrastructure of pulpal capillaries in the cat and found that a high proportion of these were fenestrated, indicating a high permeability. Capillaries were present in the odontoblast layer in most parts of the tooth.

Pulp has a very high capillary density. Vongsavan and Matthews (1992b) estimated that, in the cat, the average capillary density was 1402/mm^2, which is comparable with that in tongue and the most vascular parts of the brain.

The flow of blood in individual vessels has been studied by observing the vessels in situ with a microscope by means of a window cut through the dentine (Kim et al. 1984a). A notable difference between the pulp (in this case the rat incisor) and many other tissues was that the velocity of the blood in the pulpal vessels was much slower. In capillaries the average flow velocity was 0.27 mm/s compared with 0.96 mm/s in rat mesentery (Zweifach and Lipowsky 1977, Driessen et al. 1979), indicating that the total cross-sectional area of the capillary bed is relatively large in the pulp. There was also a large difference between the mean velocity of the blood in the arterioles and that in the venules, indicating that the total cross-sectional area of the venules was much greater than that of the arterioles.

Pulpal blood flow

The blood flow through pulp is very difficult to measure accurately (see Meyer and Path 1979, Tønder 1980, Kim et al. 1983). The most reliable estimates are probably those obtained by injecting 15 μm diameter, radiolabelled microspheres into the general circulation of an animal then estimating the number that become lodged in the pulpal capillaries. The results obtained with this and other techniques indicate that pulpal blood flow in a normal, fully formed tooth is in the range 20–60 ml/min/100 g pulp (Meyer and Path 1979, Kim et al. 1980, Path and Meyer 1980, Kim et al. 1984b, 1986). The upper end of this range is comparable with the blood flow in the brain and much higher than would be expected for connective tissue with a low level of metabolic activity. The reason for this high blood flow is not known. Once dentine formation is complete, it seems unlikely that the metabolic rate of the pulp is high enough to require this level of blood perfusion. On the other hand, the high capillary density under the odontoblast cell layer suggests that these cells continue to have a high level of metabolic activity. It may be that the odontoblasts are actively transporting ions between the dentinal fluid and the pulpal tissue fluid to maintain a concentration gradient between the two tissues. Such a role is supported by recent evidence that the odonto-blast layer has a higher rate of oxygen consumption than the remainder of the pulp in rat incisors, of the order of 3 ml O_2/min/100 g tissue weight (Yu *et al.* 1999; Y. Yu, personal communication). An alternative explanation for the high pulpal blood flow is that it is an inevitable consequence of the tissue's low compliance, with a stable equilibrium between the several interacting factors that determine the distribution of water between the tissue compartments (see below) occurring under conditions in which there is a low resistance to flow through the pulpal vessels.

Pulpal blood flow is under neural control and the mechanisms of this control are similar to those in other tissues. Antidromic stimulation of pulpal afferent nerves supplying the teeth produces pulpal vasodilatation (Tønder and Næss 1978, Gazelius and Olgart 1980, Matthews and Vongsavan 1994), probably by an axon reflex mechanism involving both A-δ and C fibres. Nerve endings in the pulp and dentine contain neuropeptides (e.g. calcitonin gene-related peptide (CGRP) and substance P) (Olgart 1996, Jacobsen *et al.* 1998) and recent evidence suggests that a large part of the pulpal vasodilatation that results from antidromic stimulation is caused by CGRP (Berggren and Heyeraas 1998). Some of the nerve fibres that produce vasodilatation have been shown to respond to the application to dentine of stimuli that cause pain in man (Andrew and Matthews 1996).

Pulp is also innervated by sympathetic vasoconstrictor fibres (Matthews and Vongsavan 1994) and nerve endings close to pulpal vessels have been shown to contain noradrenaline (Olgart and Kerezoudis 1994).

Unlike some other oro-facial tissues, no evidence has been found for parasympathetic vasodilator fibres in dental pulp (Sasano *et al.* 1995, Matthews *et al.* 1996).

Intravascular and tissue pressures

One of the problems in studying the pulpal microcirculation is that gaining access to the tissue to make measurements may change significantly the variables under study. For example, when a cavity is cut in a tooth to expose the pulp so that the tip of a micropipette may be inserted into a vessel to measure the pressure within it (Heyeraas-Tønder and Næss 1979), the compliance of the pulp in the vicinity of the exposure inevitably increases and the local tissue fluid pressure is reduced to atmospheric. To minimize these effects, the exposure is kept as small as possible and the measurements are made from vessels below the exposed pulp surface.

Using this technique, Heyeraas-Tønder and Næss (1979) found that the average pressure in the arterioles (43, SD 6.2 mmHg) was lower, and the average venular pressure (19.8 ± 2.9 mmHg) higher than in most other tissues (Figure 4.1). Capillary pressure averaged 35 ± 0.8 mmHg. These values indicate that the resistance to flow through the pulpal microcirculation is less than in other vascular beds. They also indicate that there is an unusually high resistance to flow in the main arterioles and venules that link the pulpal circulation to the rest of the systemic circulation, either just outside the tooth or in the apical foramina (Heyeraas 1985).

The tissue fluid pressure in the dental pulp has been estimated with micropipettes inserted into exposed pulp, as described above. Measurements have also been made through exposed dentine by measuring the pressure that has to be applied to exposed dentine to stop the outward flow of dentinal fluid (Vongsavan and Matthews 1992a, Ciucchi *et al.* 1995). This latter technique has the advantage that the compliance of the pulp is nearer to normal, but it is still subject to some errors. For example, the pressure recorded will include any osmotic pressure gradient that exists across the odontoblast layer, which could be significant (Vongsavan and Matthews 1992a). The pressure required to stop flow is the net filtration pressure across the odontoblast layer. Also, the integrity of this barrier will depend upon how much damage was caused when the dentine was exposed (Turner *et al.* 1989). Whichever technique is used, the results show that the tissue fluid pressure in the pulp (11–30 mmHg) is much higher than in most other tissues (Figure 4.1) and is pulsatile (Brown and Beveridge 1966, Tønder and Kvinnsland 1983, Hartmann *et al.* 1996). This is also true of other low compliance tissues. Some of these measurements indicate that the hydrostatic pressure in the tissue fluid may be higher than that in the venules. If this is correct, there must be some form of external support, acting like 'guy ropes' that prevent these vessels from collapsing, as has been suggested in other tissues (MacPhee and Michel 1995).

Inflammation of the pulp is accompanied by vasodilatation of the pulpal arterioles and an increase in pulpal blood flow. It has been estimated that under these conditions pulpal tissue fluid pressure also increases by 8–10 mmHg (Tønder and Kvinnsland 1983). It may be that these changes result in an even larger hydrostatic pressure difference across the walls of the venules, tending to collapse them. If the venules were compressed, a point might be reached at which the stable equilibrium between the factors affecting blood and tissue fluid pressures (see below) would break down, leading to self-strangulation of the pulp (Kim 1985). However, Tønder (1983) and Tønder and Kvinnsland (1983) have argued that this probably does not happen. They presented evidence that an increase in tissue fluid pressure in an inflamed area of pulp would lead to an increase in tissue fluid uptake into the plasma in the capillaries in an adjacent area of normal pulp which, together with an increased lymph flow, would relieve the pressure on the venules. However, this might not be possible if the whole pulp was involved in the inflammatory process.

As in other tissues, the distribution of water between plasma, tissue fluid and intracellular fluid will depend upon the hydrostatic pressures in each of these compartments, as well as osmotic effects across the membranes separating them. The effective osmotic pressures will depend upon the composition of fluids and the reflection coefficients of the membranes to the solutes present (Brown et al. 1969, Heyeraas 1985, Michel 1997) (Figure 4.1). These factors interact and a steady-state is achieved in normal tissues.

Pulpal lymphatics

Small vessels (diameter 20–50 μm) with the typical structure of lymphatic vessels have been described in dental pulp (Bishop and Malhotra 1990). They were found in all regions of the pulp except in the odontoblast layer and in the pulp horns under cusps. They appear to be supported by 'guy ropes' of collagen that prevent them collapsing when the hydrostatic pressure in the tissue fluid is greater than that in the vessels, as with some blood vessels (see above).

Pulpal lymphatics provide a route back to the blood circulation for tissue fluid and plasma proteins that escape through the pulpal capillary membranes. Without such a route, both the protein content and the hydrostatic pressure of the pulpal tissue fluid would be the same as the plasma (Heyeraas 1985).

Fluid flow through dentine

When dentine is exposed in vivo, there is continuous outflow of fluid from the opened dentinal tubules (Vongsavan and Matthews 1992a, Ciucchi et al. 1995). This flow appears to be produced by the hydrostatic pressure of the pulpal tissue fluid, since it stops immediately when the blood supply to the pulp is cut off (Vongsavan and Matthews 1992a). In fact, under these conditions the outward flow is replaced by a very slow inward flow. This has been attributed to an osmotic effect due to protein in the pulpal tissue fluid, with the odontoblast layer forming a barrier to diffusion of the protein. Thus the normal outward flow of fluid through exposed dentine appears to result from a process of ultrafiltration from pulpal interstitial fluid.

The rate of outward flow increases when pulpal afferent nerves are stimulated antidromically (Matthews and Vongsavan 1994). This can be attributed to an increase in pulpal tissue fluid pressure that will accompany the vasodilatation that is produced by such stimulation (see above). Similarly, stimulation of the sympathetic supply to the pulp causes the flow to reverse into the pulp (Matthews and Vongsavan 1994) due to the vasoconstriction.

The normal outward flow can have a very significant effect in slowing the rate of diffusion of substances in solution from the cut dentine surface into the tubules towards the pulp. This was demonstrated in cats using the dye Evans' blue (Vongsavan and Matthews 1991). When the dye was applied to the cut dentine surface in recently extracted teeth, it diffused through to the pulp very easily (Figure 4.2a). However, when it was applied in the same way in vivo, no dye could be detected in the pulp after 30 minutes (Figure 4.2b). The opposite results were obtained when the dye was applied at a pressure of 20 cm H_2O above atmospheric in vivo, to stop or reverse the outward flow, or at a pressure of 20 cm H_2O below atmospheric in vitro, which was designed to produce outward flow through the tubules at approximately the same rate as that present in vivo.

The outward flow of fluid through exposed dentine may have functional importance in reducing the rate of inward diffusion of toxins from the mouth into the pulp. This effect will be enhanced when afferent nerves in teeth are stimulated, as is likely to occur when dentine is exposed, and vasodilatation is produced. Such a mechanism may therefore contribute to the neurogenic component of inflammation in the tooth and to the body's defences (Matthews and Vongsavan 1994).

It is difficult to predict how inward diffusion through the dentine will be affected by etching the exposed dentine surface. On the one hand, etching will increase the rate of outward flow through the tubules, which will reduce inward diffusion; but on the other hand, it will tend to facilitate diffusion by increasing the pore size of the exposed dentine surface. This is of importance clinically: is it better to etch exposed dentine or to leave it unetched to minimize the risk of toxic substances reaching the pulp from an exposed dentine surface? When this was investigated by estimating the rates at which lignocaine diffused through dentine in cat teeth (Amess and Matthews, unpublished observations), a surprising finding was that there was little difference in the effects of the lignocaine on the conduction of impulses in intradental nerves whether it was applied to etched or unetched dentine. For this relatively small molecule, it seems that the flux through the smear layer and near stationary tubular fluid was about the same as through a patent tubule in which there was an outward flow of fluid.

The outward flow of fluid through etched dentine will also affect the bonding of dental materials to the dentine surface, because the dentine cannot be dried and the flow of lining or filling materials into the tubules will be restricted.

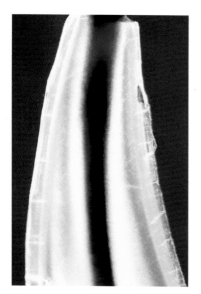

a

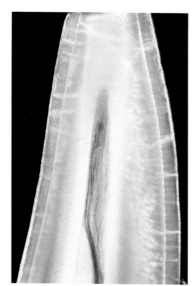

b

Figure 4.2

Photo-micrographs of ground longitudinal sections of the crowns of cat canine teeth. The sections were dehydrated and cleared in methyl salicylate. In both cases, a solution of Evans' blue was applied at atmospheric pressure for 30 minutes to the exposed dentine at the tip of the cusp immediately before the section was cut. In (a), the solution was applied to a recently extracted tooth; and in (b), it was applied before the tooth was extracted. Original magnification: ×35. (Colour originals of data published in Vongsavan and Matthews 1991)

The innervation of pulp and dentine

The pulps of the teeth are innervated by branches of the trigeminal nerve which include both afferent and post-ganglionic sympathetic axons (Matthews and Robinson 1980, Robinson 1980, Hildebrand *et al.* 1995). The trigeminal neurones have their cell bodies in the trigeminal ganglion and are primarily sensory in function, although some produce vasodilatation when stimulated (see above). The sympathetic fibres are vasomotor (see above). Their associated cell bodies are in the superior cervical ganglion, from which the axons pass via the trigeminal ganglion to the teeth in branches of the trigeminal nerve (Matthews and Robinson 1980, Robinson 1980). There is no conclusive evidence for a parasympathetic innervation of pulp (Sasano *et al.* 1995, Matthews *et al.* 1996).

Types of nerves

The pulps of teeth of limited growth in mammals (i.e. excluding those such as the continuously erupting incisors of rats which appear to have a very different type of innervation) contain large numbers of small myelinated and unmyelinated nerve endings (Beaseley and Holland 1978). The diameters of these axons in the pulp correspond with those of A-δ and C fibres in peripheral nerves. However, such data give a misleading impression of the numbers and types of neurone that innervate the tissue. There are several reasons for this: the terminal parts of the axons will be smaller in diameter than the parent axons more centrally, axons that are myelinated in the nerve trunk outside the tooth may have unmyelinated terminals in the pulp, and a single neurone may have several terminal branches.

The neurones that innervate pulp have conduction velocities outside the tooth ranging from >60 m/s to <1 m/s. The most accurate measurements have been made on the nerves that innervate the canine teeth of cats and dogs (Cadden *et al.* 1982, Närhi *et al.* 1982, Cadden *et al.* 1983). These data indicate that about half the myelinated A fibres have conduction velocities in the A-β range (>35 m/s), with the remainder being A-δ fibres. The number of neurones innervating pulp that have non-myelinated axons outside the tooth (i.e. true C fibres) is difficult to determine, because electrophysiological sampling techniques are very biased towards the larger, myelinated fibres. Their number appears to be small since they are very difficult to detect in compound action potential recordings from the nerve trunks or from the pulp (Carter and Matthews 1989). Some of these C fibres will be the non-myelinated axons of sympathetic neurones.

Thus, dental pulp is innervated by A-β, A-δ and C fibres, not by just A-δ and C fibres as is frequently stated.

The innervation of dentine and the contents of dentinal tubules

The dentinal tubules of mammalian teeth of limited growth taper from a diameter of about 2 μm at their pulpal ends to 0.5 μm or less peripherally (Forssell-Ahlberg *et al.* 1975, Garberoglio and Brännström 1976, Holland 1976a, Matthews and Hughes 1988). Dentine contains no blood vessels and, despite its apparently high sensitivity, has a very sparse innervation.

The most detailed quantitative data on the contents of the dentinal tubules have been obtained from studies on cat dentine. Each tubule contains the process of an odontoblast whose cell body is situated at the pulpal end of the tubule (Holland 1985). The cell bodies of the odontoblasts form a continuous layer that separates the pulp from the dentine. In the crown of a fully formed cat canine tooth, the odontoblast processes extend no more than half the length of the tubules (Holland 1976a) and under the tip of the cusp they are much shorter than this (Matthews and Hughes 1988). Here the length of the tubules is 1.5–2 mm and the odontoblast processes, no more than 300 μm. Beyond the ends of the odontoblast processes there is no evidence of other vital cellular elements, although in transmission electron-micrographs the luminal contents have a granular appearance (Matthews and Hughes 1988), indicating that they contain something in addition to simple extracellular fluid.

Some dentinal tubules also contain one or more fine, non-myelinated nerve terminals (diameter *ca*. 0.1 µm) (Byers 1984, Johnsen 1985). Again, quantitative data have been obtained mainly from the permanent canine teeth of cats (Holland *et al*. 1987, Matthews and Hughes 1988). In these teeth, the nerve terminals penetrate up to 100 µm into the dentinal tubules and the highest density of innervation – in terms of the proportion of tubules with at least one nerve terminal – is under the tip of the cusp, where it is almost 100%. The density falls off rapidly below this level: 3 mm below the pulp horn it averages 6.5% and lower down it is around 1%.

There are no axons with myelin sheaths in the odontoblast cell layer and it is not known whether the nerve endings there and in the dentinal tubules are the non-myelinated terminals of myelinated or of non-myelinated pulpal axons. Some of these nerve endings contain neuropeptides, including substance P and CGRP (Byers 1994).

Sensory mechanisms of dentine

It is not known how the different types of stimulus that cause pain from dentine in man excite intradental nerves (for reviews see Anderson *et al*. 1970, Matthews 1985). Such stimuli include hot, cold, mechanical, drying, large changes in hydrostatic pressure and solutions of high osmotic pressure. With the exception of the thermal stimuli, these must be applied to an exposed dentine surface to produce pain and they are most effective when the ends of the dentinal tubules are patent. Under these conditions, dentine is sensitive throughout its thickness. There is no conclusive evidence that any of these stimuli produce a sensation other than pain.

Despite the lack of vital cellular elements in the outer ends of the dentinal tubules, this area of the dentine is sensitive to stimulation and even very gentle mechanical probing of the enamel–dentine junction will evoke a discharge of impulses in intradental nerves if the smear layer left by drilling has been removed. So where are the receptors that respond to the pain-producing stimuli and how are they excited?

From simple physical principles it would be expected that all the different forms of stimulus that are capable of causing pain from dentine are capable of producing some movement of the contents of the underlying dentinal tubules, and this has been confirmed experimentally in extracted teeth (Brännström 1968, Horiuchi and Matthews 1973, Vongsavan and Matthews 1992c). These observations, together with the histological and clinical findings mentioned above, indicate that the dentinal tubules may act as passive hydraulic links between the site of stimulation and nerve endings located more deeply, either at the pulpal ends of the tubules or in the underlying pulp.

Such a mechanism was under discussion in the 1850s (Rosenthal 1990) and was discussed by Tomes (1856) in the paper in which he describes the process or fibre that came to be named after him. Similar mechanisms have been described by others such as Gysi (1900), but Brännström (1963) was the first to provide experimental evidence to support what has come to be known as the hydrodynamic hypothesis of dentine sensitivity. Kramer (1955) appears to have been the first person to use the term 'hydrodynamic' in this context. Incidentally, it seems likely that the fibre that Tomes described was the tube of lamina limitans that has confused later investigators (Thomas 1984, Thomas and Carella 1984).

There is much evidence to support the hydrodynamic hypothesis. This includes the finding that the latencies of sensory responses to cold stimuli in man (Naylor 1963) and of neural responses in the cat (Kollmann and Matthews 1982) are too short to be accounted for by a mechanism that involves nerves being excited by a temperature change at the pulp–dentine interface. In an intact cat canine, this may be of the order of 150 ms. Movement of fluid in the dentinal tubules would begin at the moment the stimulus was applied and a temperature gradient was set up in the tooth. Further support is provided by the observation that removing the smear layer from exposed dentine increases the neural response evoked by non-thermal stimuli such as probing, drying and changes in hydrostatic pressure; but probably the most conclusive evidence is the demonstration that single pulpal afferents each respond to many of the different stimuli that cause pain (Matthews 1985, Närhi 1985).

The relationship between fluid flow through dentine and the discharge evoked in pulpal afferents has been investigated during the application of hydrostatic pressure stimuli to exposed dentine (Matthews *et al.* 1996). A rather surprising finding was that the sensory receptors were very much more sensitive to outward than inward flow. Not all intradental afferents are excited by such a hydrodynamic mechanism; pulpal C fibres and some of the slowest A-δ fibres appear to respond directly to heating and to chemical stimuli (Matthews 1985, Närhi 1985).

Transduction mechanism

With those stimuli that appear to act through a hydrodynamic mechanism, it is not known how the displacement of tubule contents generates impulses in nerve endings in the dentinal tubules or in the adjacent pulp.

There might be pressure- or stretch-sensitive ion channels in the cell membranes of the nerve terminals (Matthews and Hughes 1988) that produce depolarization of the terminal axon when the membrane is subjected to mechanical deformation, with the result that impulses would be generated in the adjacent axon. Or the nerve endings might be depolarized non-specifically as a result of damage produced by the displacement of the tubule contents (Brännström 1963, Vongsavan and Matthews 1994, Matthews *et al.* 1996). The shear forces around nerve endings in the dentinal tubules that result from dentine stimulation may well be sufficient to damage the nerve membranes. Damage to the odontoblasts and the release of intracellular fluid would increase the concentration of potassium ions and ATP locally (Matthews *et al.* 1997), both of which could contribute to the impulse generation process. Consistent with such non-specific mechanisms, the neural response evoked by a cold (Kollmann and Matthews 1982) or negative hydrostatic pressure stimulus (both of which cause outward flow in the tubules) tends to decrease quite rapidly with repeated application of the stimulus.

An alternative explanation is that the odontoblasts function as the receptors. Such a mechanism would require that the odontoblasts were sensitive to the displacement of the tubule contents and were coupled to nerves, either electrically through gap junctions or through chemical synapses.

There is some evidence for gap junctions between nerves and odontoblasts, but this is not conclusive. Köling *et al.* (Köling *et al.* 1981, Köling and Rask-Andersen 1984a, 1984b) used freeze-fracture techniques and obtained evidence of gap junctions between odontoblasts and nerve-like fibres passing between the odontoblast cell bodies and into the dentinal tubules. Holland (1975, 1976b, 1977) has also obtained conventional TEM evidence of similar structures. With neither approach, however, has it been possible to prove conclusively that the fibres making contact with the odontoblasts are nerves. It has not been possible to prove that they are nerves because the nerve terminals in this region have no structural features uniquely associated with nerves. Other studies have failed to reveal evidence of specialized contacts between nerves and odontoblasts (Holland 1980, Tsukada 1987). It is known that there are many gap junctions between odontoblasts (Köling and Rask-Andersen 1984a, Ushiyama 1989, Fried *et al.* 1996) and it is possible the processes thought to be nerves may have been small processes of odontoblasts. Most recently, Fried *et al.* (1996) used double labelling of sections of rat molars with antibodies to the connexins that form the gap junctions and antibodies to the neuropeptide CGRP and found occasional sites at which the two were in close apposition. The labelling of connexins was not significantly reduced following denervation of the teeth.

The demonstration of gap junctions between odontoblasts and nerves would not prove that the odontoblasts are involved in sensory transduction; the gap junctions might be responsible for passing chemical messages between the cells, e.g. in the regulation of odontoblast function or the growth of nerve terminals.

Several attempts have been made to record intracellularly from odontoblasts in order to assess their possible role in sensory transduction. Recordings have been made either from mature teeth in situ (Winter *et al.* 1963) or isolated tooth germs (Magloire *et al.* 1979), or from cultured cells isolated from the pulps of teeth (Kroeger *et al.* 1961, Davidson 1993, 1994). Davidson (1993) obtained evidence from patch-clamp recordings for stretch-sensitive potassium channels in cultured pulp cells from human teeth, but otherwise these experiments have provided little support for the suggestion that the odontoblasts might function as sensory receptors. One limitation of all these experiments is that no evidence was obtained that the recordings were made from odontoblasts rather than other types of pulpal cell.

Finally, there is some evidence that the receptor may be more centrally located in the pulp. This idea is based on evidence that the odontoblast layer can be severely disrupted without destroying the sensitivity of the overlying dentine (Brännström and Åström 1964). If the receptors are located beneath the odontoblast cell layer, as these observations suggest, they must be exquisitely sensitive in order to be able to detect the local pressure changes set up by the displacement of the contents of just a few tubules in the overlying dentine. What is more, these pressure changes will have to be detected against a background of a fluctuating interstitial fluid pressure with a mean value of 20–30 mmHg (see above). Just touching exposed dentine very gently with the tip of a fine glass probe, with a diameter of <0.5 mm, is capable of generating a rapid discharge of impulses in an intradental nerve fibre. It may be that the histological evidence of disruption of the odontoblasts should be re-examined; a few surviving nerves may have been missed or delay in fixation could have led to deterioration in the structure of the tissue post-mortem.

References

Anderson DJ, Hannam AG, Matthews B (1970) Sensory mechanisms in mammalian teeth and their supporting tissues. *Physiol Rev* **50**:171–95.

Andrew D, Matthews B (1996) Some properties of vasodilator nerves innervating tooth pulp in the cat. In: Shimono M, Maeda T, Suda H, Takahashi H, eds, *Dentin/Pulp Complex*, 254–5. Quintessence: Tokyo.

Beaseley WL, Holland GR (1978) A quantitative analysis of the innervation of the pulp of the cat's canine tooth. *J Comp Neurol* **178**:487–94.

Berggren E, Heyeraas KJ (1998) Effect of CGRP on pulpal blood flow and tissue pressure in ferrets. *J Dent Res* **77** (Special issue):651.

Bishop MA (1987) An investigation of pulp capillaries and tight junctions between odontoblasts in cats. *Anat Embryol (Berl)* **177**:131–8.

Bishop MA, Malhotra M (1990) An investigation of lymphatic vessels in the feline dental pulp. *Am J Anat* **187**:247–53.

Brännström M (1963) A hydrodynamic mechanism in the transmission of pain-producing stimuli through the dentine. In: Anderson DJ, ed, *Sensory Mechanisms in Dentine*, 73–9. Pergamon: Oxford.

Brännström M (1968) Physio-pathological aspects of dentinal and pulpal response to irritants. In: Symons NBB, ed, *Dentine and Pulp: Their Structure and Reactions*, 231–46. University of Dundee: Dundee.

Brännström M, Åström A (1964) A study of the mechanism of pain elicited from the dentin. *J Dent Res* **43**:619–25.

Brown AC, Beveridge EE (1966) The relation between tooth pulp pressure and systemic arterial pressure. *Arch Oral Biol* **11**:1181–93.

Brown AC, Barrow BL, Gadd GN, Van Hassel HJ (1969) Tooth pulp transcapillary osmotic pressure in the dog. *Arch Oral Biol* **14**:491–502.

Byers MR (1984) Dental sensory receptors. *Int Rev Neurobiol* **25**:39–94.

Byers MR (1994) Dynamic plasticity of dental sensory nerve structure and cytochemistry. *Arch Oral Biol* **39**:13S-21S.

Cadden SW, Lisney SJW, Matthews B (1982) Aβ fibre innervation of tooth-pulp in the cat, with a discussion of the functions of nerves supplying tooth-pulp. In: Matthews B, Hill RG, eds, *Anatomical, Physiological and Pharmacological Aspects of Trigeminal Pain*, 41–9. Excerpta Medica: Amsterdam.

Cadden SW, Lisney SJW, Matthews B (1983) Thresholds to electrical stimulation of nerves in cat canine tooth-pulp with Aβ, Aδ and C-fibre conduction velocities. *Brain Res* **261**:31–41.

Carter GM, Matthews B (1989) Responses of jaw muscles to electrical stimulation of tooth-pulp in rat, cat and man. In: van Steenberghe D, De Laat A, eds, *Electromyography of Jaw Reflexes in Man*, 1st edn, 205–36. Leuven University Press: Leuven.

Ciucchi B, Bouillaguet S, Holz J, Pashley D (1995) Dentinal fluid dynamics in human teeth, in vivo. *J Endodontics* **21**:191–4.

Davidson RM (1993) Potassium currents in cells derived from human dental pulp. *Arch Oral Biol* **38**:803–11.

Davidson RM (1994) Neural form of voltage-dependent sodium current in human cultured dental pulp cells. *Arch Oral Biol* **39**:613–20.

Driessen GK, Heidtmann H, Schmid-Schönbein H (1979) Effect of hemodilution and hemoconcentration on red cell flow velocity in the capillaries of the rat mesentery. *Pflugers Arch* **380**:1–6.

Forssell-Ahlberg K. Brännström M, Edwall L (1975) The diameter and number of dentinal tubules in rat, cat, dog and monkey. *Acta Odontol Scand* **33**:243–50.

Fried K, Mitsiadis TA, Guerrier A, Haegerstrand A, Meister B (1996) Combinatorial expression patterns of the connexins 26, 32, and 43 during development, homeostasis, and regeneration of rat teeth. *Int J Dev Biol* **40**:985–995.

Garberoglio R, Brännström M (1976) Scanning electron microscopic investigation of human dentinal tubules. *Arch Oral Biol* **21**:355–62.

Gazelius B, Olgart L (1980) Vasodilatation in the dental pulp produced by electrical stimulation of the inferior alveolar nerve in the cat. *Acta Physiol Scand* **108**:181–6.

Gysi A (1900) An attempt to explain the sensitiveness of dentine. *Br J Dent Sci* **43**:865–8.

Hartmann A, Azerad J, Boucher Y (1996) Environmental effects on laser Doppler pulpal blood-flow measurements in man. *Arch Oral Biol* **41**:333–9.

Heyeraas KJ (1985) Pulpal, microvascular, and tissue pressure. *J Dent Res* **643** (Sp. iss.):585–9.

Heyeraas-Tønder KJ, Næss G (1979) Microvascular pressure in the dental pulp and gingiva in cats. *Acta Odontol Scand* **37**:161–8.

Hildebrand C, Fried K, Tuisku F, Johansson CS (1995) Teeth and tooth nerves. *Prog Neurobiol* **45**:165–222.

Holland GR (1975) Membrane junctions on cat odontoblasts. *Arch Oral Biol* **20**:551–2.

Holland GR (1976a) An ultrastructural survey of cat dentinal tubules. *J Anat* **122**:1–13.

Holland GR (1976b) Lanthanum hydroxide labelling of gap junctions in the odontoblast layer. *Anat Rec* **186**:121–6.

Holland GR (1977) Structural relationships in the odontoblast layer. In: Anderson DJ, Matthews B, eds, *Pain in the Trigeminal Region*, 25–35. Elsevier: Amsterdam.

Holland GR (1980) Non-myelinated nerve fibres and their terminals in the sub-odontoblastic plexus of the feline dental pulp. *J Anat* **130**:457–67.

Holland GR (1985) The odontoblast process: form and function. *J Dent Res* **64** (Special issue):499–514.

Holland GR, Matthews B, Robinson PP (1987) An electrophysiological and morphological study of the innervation and reinnervation of cat dentine. *J Physiol (Lond)* **386**:31–43.

Horiuchi H, Matthews B (1973) In-vitro observations on fluid flow through human dentine caused by pain-producing stimuli. *Arch Oral Biol* **18**:275–94.

Jacobsen EB, Fristad I, Heyeraas KJ (1998) Nerve fibers immunoreactive to calcitonin gene-related peptide, substance P, neuropeptide Y, and dopamine beta-hydroxylase in innervated and denervated oral tissues in ferrets. *Acta Odontol Scand* **56**:220–8.

Johnsen DC (1985) Innervation of teeth: qualitative, quantitative, and developmental assessment. *J Dent Res* **64** (Special issue):555–63.

Kim S (1985) Regulation of pulpal blood flow. *J Dent Res* **64** (Special issue):590–6.

Kim S, Fan F, Chen RYZ, Simchon S et al (1980) Effects of changes in systemic hemodynamic parameters on pulpal hemodynamics. *J Endodontics* **6**:394–9.

Kim S, Schuessler G, Chien S (1983) Measurement of blood flow in the dental pulp of dogs with the ^{131}xenon washout method. *Arch Oral Biol* **28**:501–5.

Kim S, Edwall L, Trowbridge H, Chien S (1984a) Effects of local anesthetics on pulpal blood flow in dogs. *J Dent Res* **63**:650–2.

Kim S. Lipowsky HH, Usami S, Chien S (1984b) Arteriovenous distribution of hemodynamic parameters in the rat dental pulp. *Microvasc Res* **27**:28–38.

Kim S, Trowbridge H, Dörscher-Kim J.(1986) The infuence of 5–hydroxytryptamine (serotonin) on blood flow in the dog pulp. *J Dent Res* **65**:682–5.

Köling A, Rask-Andersen H (1984a) Membrane junctions between odontoblasts and associated cells. *Acta Odontol Scand* **42**:13–22.

Köling A, Rask-Andersen H (1984b) Membrane structures in the pulp–dentin border zone. A freeze–fracture study of demineralised human teeth. *Acta Odontol Scand* **42**:73–84.

Köling A, Rask-Andersen H, Bagger-Sjöbäck D (1981) Membrane junctions on odontoblasts. *Acta Odontol Scand* **39**:355–60.

Kollmann W, Matthews B (1982) Responses of intradental nerves to thermal stimulation of teeth in the cat. In: Matthews B, Hill RG, eds, *Anatomical, Physiological and Pharmacological Aspects of Trigeminal Pain*, 51–65. Excerpta Medica: Amsterdam.

Kramer IRH (1955) The relationship between dentine sensitivity and movements in the contents of the dentinal tubules. *Br Dent J* **98**:391–2.

Kramer IRH (1960) The vascular architecture of the human dental pulp. *Arch Oral Biol* **2**:177–89.

Kroeger DC, Gonzales F, Krivoy W (1961) Transmembrane potentials of cultured mouse dentinal pulp cells. *Proc Soc Exp Biol Med* **108**:134–6.

MacPhee P, Michel CC (1995) Subatmospheric closing pressures in individual microvessels of rats and frogs. *J Physiol (Lond)* **484**:183–7.

Magloire H, Vinard H, Joffre A (1979) Electrophysiological properties of human dental pulp cells. *J Biol Buccale* **7**:251–62.

Matthews B (1985) Peripheral and central aspects of trigeminal nociceptive systems. *Philos Trans R Soc Lond [Biol]* **308**:313–24.

Matthews B, Hughes SHS (1988) The ultrastructure and receptor transduction mechanisms of dentine. In: Hamman W, Iggo A, eds, *Progress in Brain Research*, Vol. 74, 69–76. Elsevier: Amsterdam.

Matthews B, Robinson PP (1980) The course of post-ganglionic sympathetic fibres distributed within the trigeminal nerve in the cat. *J Physiol (Lond)* **303**:391–401.

Matthews B, Vongsavan N (1994) Interactions between neural and hydrodynamic mechanisms in dentine and pulp. *Arch Oral Biol* **39**:87S–95S.

Matthews B, Andrew D, Amess TR et al (1996) The functional properties of intradental nerves. In: Shimono M, Maeda T, Suda H, Takahashi H, eds, *Dentin/Pulp Complex*, 146–53. Quintessence: Tokyo.

Matthews B, Li F, Khakh BS et al (1997) Evidence on the possible function of P2X3 receptors in dental pulp. *Soc Neurosci Abst* **23**:1528.

Meyer MW, Path MG (1979) Blood flow in the dental pulp of dogs determined by hydrogen polarography and radioactive microsphere methods. *Arch Oral Biol* **24**:601–5.

Michel CC (1997) Starling: the formulation of his hypothesis of microvascular fluid exchange and its significance over 100 years. *Exp Physiol* **82**:1–30.

Närhi MVO (1985) The characteristics of intradental sensory units and their responses to stimulation. *J Dent Res* **64** (Special issue):564–71.

Närhi M, Virtanen A, Huopaniemi T, Hirvonen T (1982) Conduction velocities of single pulp nerve units in the cat. *Acta Physiol Scand* **116**:209–13.

Naylor MN (1963) Studies on the mechanism of sensation to cold stimulation of human dentine. In: Anderson DJ, ed, *Sensory Mechanisms in Dentine*, 80–7. Pergamon: Oxford.

Olgart L (1996) Neural control of pulpal blood flow. *Crit Rev Oral Biol Med* **7**:159–71.

Olgart L, Kerezoudis NP (1994) Nerve–pulp interactions. *Arch Oral Biol* **39**:47S–54S.

Path MG, Meyer MW (1980) Heterogeneity of blood flow in the canine tooth in the dog. *Arch Oral Biol* **25**:83–6.

Robinson PP (1980) An electrophysiological study of the pathways of pulpal nerves from mandibular teeth in the cat. *Arch Oral Biol* **25**:825–9.

Rosenthal MW (1990) Historic review of the management of tooth hypersensitivity. *Dent Clin North Am* **34**:403–27.

Sasano T, Shoji N, Kuriwada S et al (1995) Absence of parasympathetic vasodilatation in cat dental pulp. *J Dent Res* **74**:1665–70.

Takahashi K, Kishi Y, Kim S (1982) A scanning electron microscope study of blood vessels of the pulp using corrosion resin casts. *J Endodontics* **8**:131–5.

Thomas HF (1984) The lamina limitans of human dentinal tubules. *J Dent Res* **63**:1064–6.

Thomas HF, Carella P (1984) Correlation of scanning and transmission electron microscopy of human dentinal tubules. *Arch Oral Biol* **29**:641–6.

Tønder KJH (1980) Blood flow and vascular pressure in the dental pulp. *Acta Odontol Scand* **38**:135–44.

Tønder KJH (1983) Vascular reactions in the dental pulp during inflammation. *Acta Odontol Scand* **41**:247–56.

Tønder KJH, Kvinnsland I (1983) Micropuncture measurements of interstitial fluid pressure in normal and inflamed dental pulp in cats. *J Endodontics* **9**:105–9.

Tønder KJH, Næss G (1978) Nervous control of blood flow in the dental pulp of dogs. *Acta Physiol Scand* **104**:13–23.

Tomes J (1856) On the presence of fibrils of soft tissue in the dentinal tubes. *Philos Trans R Soc Lond [B]* **146**:515–22.

Tsukada K (1987) Ultrastructure of the relationship between odontoblast processes and nerve fibres in dentinal tubules of rat molar teeth. *Arch Oral Biol* **32**:87–92.

Turner DF, Marfurt CF, Sattelberg C (1989) Demonstration of physiological barrier between pulpal odontoblasts and its perturbation following routine restorative procedures: a horseradish peroxidase tracing study in the rat. *J Dent Res* **68**:1262–8.

Ushiyama J (1989) Gap junctions between odontoblasts revealed by transjunctional flux of fluorescent tracers. *Cell Tissue Res* **258**:611–16.

Vongsavan N, Matthews B (1991) The permeability of cat dentine *in vivo* and *in vitro*. *Arch Oral Biol* **36**:641–6.

Vongsavan N, Matthews B (1992a) Fluid flow through cat dentine *in vivo*. *Arch Oral Biol* **37**:175–85.

Vongsavan N, Matthews B (1992b) The vascularity of dental pulp in cats. *J Dent Res* **71**:1913–15.

Vongsavan N, Matthews B (1992c) Hydrodynamic effects in human dentine *in vitro*. *J Dent Res* **71** (Special issue):742.

Vongsavan N, Matthews B (1994) The relationship between fluid flow through dentine and the discharge of intradental nerves. *Arch Oral Biol* **39**:140S.

Winter HF, Bishop JG, Dorman HL (1963) Transmembrane potentials of odontoblasts. *J Dent Res* **42**:594–8.

Yu Y, Boyd N, Cringle S et al (1999) Intrapulpal oxygen distribution and vascular regulation in rat incisor pulp. *J Dent Res* **78** (Special issue):141.

Zweifach BW, Lipowsky HH (1977) Quantitative studies of microcirculatory structure and function. III. Microvascular hemodynamics of cat mesentery and rabbit omentum. *Circ Res* **41**:380–90.

5
Reparative processes in dentine and pulp

Anthony J Smith, Alastair J Sloan, John B Matthews, Peter E Murray and Philip Lumley

Introduction

The dentine–pulp complex represents a unique organ capable of responding in a variety of ways to environmental stimuli. Whilst the prime function of the pulp is to produce dentine, it also has a responsive sensory function which can influence the secretory behaviour of the cells present. Because of the nature of the environment in which the tooth functions, it can sometimes be difficult to distinguish between physiological and pathological responses to stimuli within the pulp. Tooth wear (attrition, abrasion and erosion) can invoke a response within the pulp and in its milder forms, might be considered a feature of the physiological life of a tooth. More extensive wear and dental caries, however, undoubtedly result in substantial tissue injury. Nevertheless, the dentinogenic response to all these stimuli tends to be focal, only occurring at the site of injury.

Tissue responses to injury

Nomenclature for the dentine laid down after primary dentinogenesis has long been confused, but increasingly the term physiological secondary dentine is being used to describe the slow and continuing apposition throughout life of circumpulpal dentine after completion of root formation. The dentine laid down at specific foci in the tooth in response to various stimuli is consequently referred to as tertiary dentine. However, within this group of responses, a broad spectrum can be observed and it is worthwhile to categorize these responses on the basis of the cellular behaviour

seen in the pulp. The most important cell in this respect is the odontoblast, which can either survive the injury and go on to participate in the tissue response, or if the injury is sufficiently severe it may die. In the latter case, the subsequent tissue fate is determined by the ability of progenitor cells within the pulp to give rise to a new generation of odontoblast-like cells that can participate in a reparative response. Thus, the terms reactionary and reparative dentinogenesis have arisen as subdivisions of the tertiary dentinogenic response (Smith *et al.* 1995a) (Figure 5.1). These are defined as follows. *Reactionary dentinogenesis* is a tertiary dentine matrix secreted by surviving post-mitotic odontoblast cells in response to an appropriate stimulus. *Reparative dentinogenesis* is a tertiary dentine matrix secreted by a new generation of odontoblast-like cells in response to an appropriate stimulus, after the death of the original post-mitotic odontoblasts responsible for primary and physiological secondary dentine secretion.

Even within each of these categories of dentinogenic response, a broad spectrum of tissue activities can be observed. These can give rise to considerable heterogeneity in tissue structure – from dentine matrix which shows virtually the same regularity of tubule structure as primary dentine to a very dysplastic dentine matrix with atubular structure (Mjor 1983). Such variations in tubule structure will obviously have an influence on dentine permeability and are likely to be considerations in terms of the sensitivity of the tissue. Incorporation of cells within the tertiary dentine matrix is also not an uncommon feature, although little is known of the factors influencing formation of such osteodentine matrices.

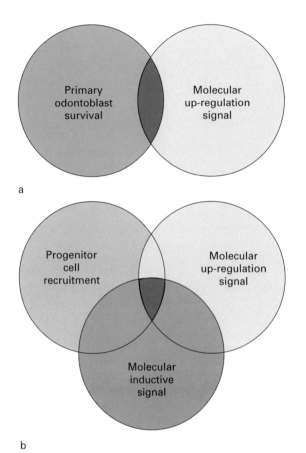

a

b

Figure 5.1

Schematic diagram of the interplay of factors determining dentinogenic responses. *a* Reactionary dentinigenesis. *b* Reparative dentinogenesis.

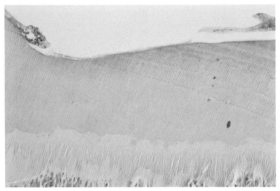

Figure 5.2

Secretion of a reactionary dentine matrix at the pulp–dentine interface beneath a cavity prepared in a ferret canine tooth after implantation of isolated dentine matrix components in the cavity base. The paler staining of the reactionary dentine matrix with haematoxylin and eosin compared to the matrix of the primary dentine is indicative of compositional differences and suggests some differential up-regulation of odontoblast synthetic activity (×120).

Pulpal inflammation after injury contributes to the tissue defence mechanisms and resolution of the inflammation can facilitate the reparative response. However, necrosis of the pulp can result if the inflammatory reaction is unresolved. The rather variable nature and intensity of the inflammatory reaction may well contribute to the heterogeneity of the reparative response observed. The vascular changes that occur during pulpal inflammation, subsequent neo-vascularization and production of inflammatory molecular mediators and cytokines will be important aspects of the overall tissue response.

Reactionary dentinogenesis

The tissue activities giving rise to these various dentinogenic responses reflect a complex sequence of molecular and cellular processes and it is important to distinguish between those processes involved in reactionary and reparative responses. Under physiological conditions, after completion of primary dentinogenesis the synthetic and secretory activities of the odontoblast cell are markedly decreased. This is reflected in the ultrastructural appearance of the odontoblast (Takuma and Nagai 1971, Couve 1986, Romagnoli *et al.* 1990), which shows a reduction in size and a decrease in cellular organelles. With appropriate stimulation, however, the largely quiescent odontoblast can be triggered to upregulate its synthesis and secretion of matrix components, giving rise to a reactionary dentine matrix (Figure 5.2). Magloire *et al.* (1992) described an acceleration of metabolic activities under the initial carious lesion, particularly focused on an increase in collagen synthesis (Karjalainen and Soderling 1980, 1984).

Growth factors and regulation of odontoblast activity

Whilst it has long been recognized that various non-specific stimuli (including tooth wear, caries, surgical procedures and dental restorative materials) can trigger a dentinogenic response in the mature tooth (Frank 1968, Harris and Griffin 1969, Bergenholtz 1981, Stanley 1981, Trowbridge 1981, Larmas 1986, Langeland 1987), attempts are now being made to understand the molecular basis of this stimulation of odontoblasts leading to reactionary dentinogenesis. Very little is known about the control of odontoblast matrix synthesis and secretion, but the involvement of growth factors in upregulating the synthesis of matrix proteins in various cells has been reported. Growth factors are peptides with potent bioactive properties, many of which regulate cell growth and function. Whilst it is beyond the scope of this paper to detail all the interactions of these molecules, members of the transforming growth factor-beta (TGF-β) super-family of growth factors have been implicated in the modulation of collagen (Ignotz and Massague 1986, Takuwa et al. 1991, Yu et al. 1991) and proteoglycan (Rapraeger 1989, Yu et al. 1991) synthesis. These growth factors are also involved in wound healing (Frank et al. 1996), where differential influences of the TGF-β isoforms on extracellular matrix biosynthesis have been observed (Shah et al. 1992, O'Kane and Ferguson 1997). However, the effects of TGF-βs can be anabolic or catabolic depending on concentration (Tashijian et al. 1985, Hock et al. 1990).

Many of the effects of TGF-βs in the body are under paracrine control; however, autocrine production of these growth factors allows a local level of regulation of cellular behaviour in the tissue. During tooth development, newly differentiated odontoblasts express both transcripts and the protein TGF-β1 (Cam et al. 1990, 1997, Inage and Toda 1996) and in mature human teeth, TGF-β isoforms 1, 2 and 3 have been detected immunohistochemically (Sloan, Matthews and Smith, unpublished observations). Secretion of TGF-βs and other growth factors by odontoblasts can lead to their sequestration within dentine matrix. The presence of TGF-β bioactivity, together with insulin-like growth factors I and II (IGF-I and -II), in dentine matrix was reported by Finkelman et al. (1990) and more recently, the amounts of TGF-β isoforms have been quantified for dentine in the continuously growing rabbit incisor and mature human teeth (Cassidy et al. 1997). This latter study indicated that TGF-β1 was the most prevalent isoform in dentine and the only one detected in mature human dentine. TGF-β2 and TGF-β3 were detected in smaller amounts in rabbit dentine, implying that these isoforms fulfil a more developmental role. The presence of these growth factors in dentine matrix provides an explanation for the bioactive properties of matrix fractions in the in-vivo stimulation of reactionary dentinogenesis (Smith et al. 1994, 1995a). Few studies have reported the experimental stimulation of reactionary dentinogenesis as information on the chronology of tissue events is essential for the identification of a reactionary response. This precludes categorical identification of reactionary dentinogenesis in the majority of human studies, because of the lack of such information.

Experimental stimulation of reactionary dentinogenesis

There have been numerous reports in the literature of reactionary-like responses to less severe injurious stimuli (particularly tooth wear and restorative materials) resulting in the secretion of what has been described variously as 'reaction, irritation, etc. dentine'. These reports are valuable in establishing such responses as a common feature of pulpo-dentinal wound healing, but provide little mechanistic information. Such information has come largely from experimental approaches to the study of reactionary dentinogenesis. Smith et al. (1994) implanted EDTA-soluble dentine matrix fractions in the base of unexposed cavities prepared under carefully controlled conditions in ferret canine teeth. Within 14 days, there was significant deposition of reactionary dentine by the odontoblasts beneath the cavities and there was no evidence of odontoblast death in the intervening period. In a subsequent study, the same dentine fractions were purified to enrich their content of TGF-βs and were found to stimulate deposition of significant amounts of reactionary dentine (Smith et al. 1995a). It was suggested that the

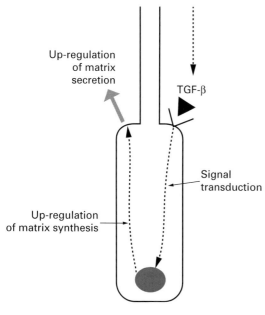

Figure 5.3

Schematic diagram of up-regulation of odontoblast synthetic and secretory activity by TGF-β during reactionary dentinogenesis.

reactionary dentinogenic events observed in these studies were the result of the diffusion of bioactive molecules down the dentinal tubules to the odontoblasts, leading to an up-regulation of synthetic and secretory activity (Figure 5.3). Trans-dentinal stimulation of odontoblasts by bone morphogenetic protein-7 (BMP-7/OP1), another member of the TGF-β superfamily, has also been reported (Rutherford 1995).

Direct evidence of the stimulatory effects of TGF-βs on odontoblasts has recently come from in-vitro studies using a rodent tooth slice organ culture approach (Sloan et al. 1999). Agarose beads were soaked in TGF-βs and applied over the odontoblast layer of the tooth slices. After culture, local stimulation of reactionary dentinogenesis was observed at the site of application with TGF-β1 and 3, but not TGF-β2 (Sloan and Smith 1999). A similar, but less intense, stimulation of reactionary dentinogenesis was also observed after application of BMP-7 under similar conditions (Sloan, Rutherford and Smith, unpublished observations). Interestingly, molar

teeth of TGF-β1 knock-out mice show marked attrition and it was suggested that this is the result of loss of TGF-β1 affecting primary and secondary dentinogenesis (D'Souza et al. 1998). Thus, the importance of TGF-βs in both physiological and pathological dentinogenesis is established, but there is still much to learn about the individual activities and interplay between members of the TGF-β superfamily of growth factors.

Restorative procedures and reactionary dentinogenesis

Such molecular triggers to odontoblast stimulation may also arise during normal dental restorative procedures. The tooth slice organ culture model of Sloan et al. (1998) has been used to examine the effects of various parameters involved with restorative procedures on the pulp–dentine complex. Cavities were prepared in rat tooth slices under carefully controlled conditions and the stimulation of reactionary dentinogenesis during subsequent culture of the slices was examined. The intensity of the reactionary dentinogenic response was observed to be related to the thickness of the residual dentine beneath the cavity and the conditioning of the cavity with EDTA (Murray et al. 1998) (Figure 5.4). In the rat incisor tooth model used, a residual dentine thickness of < 50 μ appeared to be critical for stimulation of reactionary dentinogenesis, suggesting that diffusion of solubilized bioactive molecules to the odontoblast may be a limiting factor. Treatment with EDTA for 60 s was optimal for the reactionary dentinogenic response, which was minimal in the absence of EDTA treatment. It would appear that EDTA used as a cavity conditioning agent has the capacity to solubilize bioactive molecules from the dentine matrix in situ, which can then go on to stimulate reactionary dentinogenesis in this culture model. Interestingly, the time course of this reactionary dentinogenic response indicated that most secretion occurred within the first 24 h after cavity treatment. This may reflect (a) the short half-life of TGF-βs, (b) limited solubilization of the growth factor by the cavity conditioning agent, (c) other factors modulating the bioactivity of the growth factor in the extracellular environment.

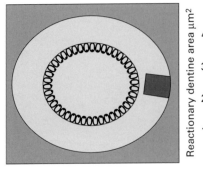 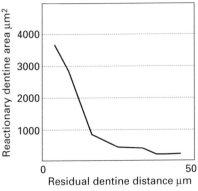

Figure 5.4

Stimulation of reactionary dentinogenesis in a rat incisor tooth slice
organ culture model and the
relationship with residual dentine
depth. The diagram on the left
shows a tooth slice in which a
cavity has been prepared under
carefully controlled conditions and
subsequently treated with EDTA
prior to culture. The graph on the
right shows the relationship
between the amount of reactionary
dentine formed during culture and
the residual dentine depth beneath
the cavity. Reactionary dentine
formation was observed with residual dentine depths of <50 μm.

Regulation of growth factor activity in pulpo-dentinal tissues

Regulation of growth factor activity in the pulpo-
dentinal tissues is important to avoid uncon-
trolled cellular behaviour. This could lead to
possible obliteration of the pulp chamber by
secretion of mineralized matrix in situations of
tissue repair. A number of factors are known to
modulate TGF-β bioactivity and Smith et al.
(1997) demonstrated that the TGF-β1 in dentine
matrix was partially associated with its latency-
associated peptide (TGF-β-LAP), beta-glycan and
decorin. Beta-glycan can sequester TGF-βs and
help in their presentation to cell surface receptors (Andres et al. 1989), whilst decorin can bind
TGF-βs and inhibit their activity (Yamaguchi et al.
1990). In this study, approximately half of the
TGF-β1 was found to be in an active form within
the dentine matrix and these other modulating
factors will almost certainly influence the growth
factor's availability and activity.

However, as well as a suitable signal for stimulation of reactionary dentinogenesis, the odontoblasts must also possess appropriate receptors to
the signalling molecules for signal transduction.
For TGF-βs, two cell surface receptors (TGF-β-RI
and -RII) are required for signal transduction and
the presence of both these receptors has been
demonstrated in rodent (Smith et al. 1997) and
human teeth (Sloan et al. 1999). In the case of
human teeth, the expression of these receptors

on odontoblasts does not appear to be affected
by caries, although the pulpal inflammatory infiltrate frequently seen during caries also expressed
these receptors. This highlights the complexity of
tissue events during caries and the possible interactions that could occur.

The foregoing discussion has emphasized the
possible importance of members of the TGF-β
family of growth factors in the reactionary
dentinogenic response, but it must be appreci-
ated that dentine matrix probably contains quite
a mixture of growth factors, many of which may
be able to influence odontoblast behaviour.
Finkelman et al. (1990) demonstrated the
presence of IGF-I and IGF-II in dentine matrix and
several workers have reported bone morphogenetic protein-like activity in dentine (Urist
1971, Bang 1973, Inoue et al. 1981). Recent
studies on angiogenesis during pulpal wound
healing have implicated a number of angiogenic
growth factors as constituents of dentine matrix
(Roberts-Clark and Smith 1999) and it is probable that other growth factor molecules will be
detected within the matrix in time. However, it is
important to consider how such growth factor
molecules are associated with the dentine
matrix. TGF-βs were found to be associated with
both the soluble and insoluble tissue compartments of dentine (Cassidy et al. 1997) and their
solubilization from the matrix and presentation
to cells will depend on the conditions that prevail
within the tissue.

Odontoblast synthetic and secretory processes

Whilst the possible stimulation of odontoblasts by TGF-βs, including those derived from the dentine matrix, has become apparent, there is still only limited understanding of the effects of such growth factors on the various synthetic pathways and secretory routes within the odontoblast cell. The morphological changes in the matrix during tertiary dentinogenesis imply compositional changes therein, but only very limited analytical data are available. Perry and Smith (1994) performed micro-analysis of the amounts of collagen and soluble non-collagenous proteins and glycosaminoglycans in human tertiary dentine samples. Whilst the samples probably represented a mixture of reactionary or reparative dentinogenic responses, they did show differential increases in the composition of some of the soluble matrix components. This suggests that the synthetic pathways for the various matrix components may be under differential control, whether it be at the cellular or genomic level. Much is still to be elucidated about the molecular control of gene transcription in the odontoblast and how it may be exploited to achieve optimal tissue repair.

In terms of odontoblast secretory processes, it seems probable that matrix components pass to the Golgi apparatus for packaging in secretory vesicles after synthesis and then pass from the cell by exocytosis. Linde (1984) has proposed that there may be two levels of secretion from the odontoblast, which could help to explain various aspects of tissue development and structure for dentine as well as reparative processes (Figure 5.5). In his model, Linde proposes that a major route of secretion is from the proximal end of the odontoblast cell body, giving rise to many of the structural components of the tissue, and then a more distal point of secretion of a number of tissue-specific components at the mineralization front. Such a model would help to explain the possible continuing apposition of peritubular dentine even when the secretion of matrix at the pulp–dentine surface slows right down. However, it also raises the question as to whether reactionary dentinogenesis involves secretion at the pulp–dentine interface alone, or also intratubularly. The dentinal sclerosis often seen as an early response to caries may well represent an increase in peritubular dentine

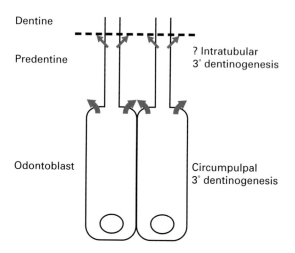

Figure 5.5

Schematic diagram of possible sites of matrix secretion from the odontoblast during reactionary and reparative dentinogenesis. Secretion from the proximal area of the cell would give rise to tertiary matrix deposition at the pulp–dentine interface contributing to a focal increase in circum-pulpal dentinogenesis. If secretion from the distal area of the odontoblast can occur during tertiary dentinogenesis, this would lead to intra-tubular matrix deposition which might represent the sclerosis often seen at sites of dentine injury.

formation (Magloire *et al.* 1992). A number of studies on reactionary dentinogenesis have used species such as the rat and ferret in which peritubular dentine is not seen. It is important to examine experimentally the processes of reactionary dentinogenesis in a species secreting peritubular dentine, as it could be critical to the understanding and management of dentine injury and hypersensitivity.

Reparative dentinogenesis

With more severe injury such as stronger carious challenge or other stimuli, odontoblast death frequently occurs at the site of injury and a response of reparative dentinogenesis is seen if the conditions in the pulp are conducive (Figure 5.6). However, the pulpo-dentinal tissues are often subject to the effects of injury and inflammation for prolonged periods and the sequence

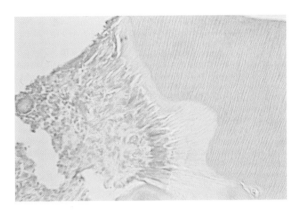

Figure 5.6

Reparative dentinogenic response after mechanical exposure in a ferret canine tooth and implantation of isolated dentine matrix components in the cavity base. The cavity at the top of the picture has been mechanically exposed on the left and cell migration from the pulp to the exposure site has been followed by induction of odonto-blast-like cell differentiation and tubular reparative dentine deposition on the exposure wall. Note the different orientation of the tubules in the new reparative dentine matrix compared to the residual dentine matrix underlying the cavity (haematoxylin and eosin; ×200).

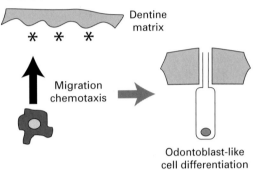

Figure 5.7

Schematic diagram of the role of the dentine matrix in immobilizing and presenting bioactive molecules to progenitor cells during the tissue events leading up to differentiation of a new generation of odontoblast-like cells and reparative dentinogenesis.

of events will depend on the influence of these other processes.

Initiation of reparative dentinogenesis involves a more complex sequence of events in the tissue than reactionary dentinogenesis, as a new generation of odontoblast-like cells must be recruited and induced to differentiate prior to matrix secretion. Therefore, a typical sequence of events might include progenitor cell recruitment (involving chemotaxis and migration), induction of cyto-differentiation and the up-regulation of dentinogenic activity (Figure 5.7) apart from any 'mopping-up' reactions to remove cellular debris from the injury process.

Progenitor cells for reparative dentinogenesis

Use of the term 'odontoblast-like cell' for those involved in reparative dentinogenesis is appropriate in view of the rather variable phenotype of these cells, reflected in the considerable heterogeneity observed in tissue structure. The derivation of the cells giving rise to the odonto-blast-like cell population is still unclear. The undifferentiated mesenchymal cells in the cell-rich zone of Hohl would be appropriate progenitor cells (Cotton 1968, Takuma and Nagai 1971, Slavkin 1974, Torneck and Wagner 1980). Many of these cells would have experienced the same history as the primary odontoblasts in terms of number of cell cycles and mainly differ in not having being exposed to the same epithelially derived epigenetic signal for initiation of odontoblast cyto-differentiation during tooth development. However, other pulpal cells including undifferentiated mesenchymal cells, fibroblasts, perivascular cells, etc. have also been implicated as progenitors for the odonto-blast-like cell (Sveen and Hawes 1968, Feit *et al.* 1970, Yamamura *et al.* 1980, Yamamura 1985, Fitzgerald *et al.* 1990).

Little is known of the processes involved in progenitor cell recruitment for reparative dentinogenesis. Many extracellular matrix molecules have been shown to have chemotactic properties in vitro, although their ability to display these properties in vivo remains unproven. It might be expected that intra-pulpal cell migration to the site of repair might not pose a significant problem. Certainly in terms of the neural crest-derived undifferentiated mesenchymal cells, the distance of migration might be regarded as insignificant in comparison with their early embryological migratory patterns. Molecular control of odontogenic patterning during embryogenesis appears to be determined by homeobox genes (Thomas and Sharpe 1998, Thomas *et al.* 1998, Weiss *et al.* 1998). Subsequently, early tooth morphogenesis might involve molecular control by growth factors such as the BMPs (Tureckova *et al.* 1995; Vaahtokari *et al.* 1996) and various transcription factors (Mackenzie *et al.* 1992, Mark *et al.* 1992, Weiss *et al.* 1994, Tureckova *et al.* 1995, Chen *et al.* 1996). During wound healing, TGF-β1 is chemotactic for fibroblasts, macrophages, neutrophils and monocytes (Pierce *et al.* 1989, Massague 1990) and in vivo, promotes cell influx into sites of wound healing and stimulation of extracellular matrix biosynthesis (Pierce *et al.* 1993, Sporn and Roberts 1993).

Odontoblast phenotype and progenitor cells during repair

In view of the rather specialized neural crest origin of the ecto-mesenchymal cells giving rise to the primary odontoblasts, it might be expected that progenitor cells of differing origin would not all be able to develop the true odontoblast phenotype. This may well contribute to the rather variable nature of the reparative dentinogenic response with quite differing cell morphologies and tissue structures. The pulpal environment is unique and the conditions therein tend to favour deposition of mineralized matrices. However, the specificity of those matrices in relation to true ortho-dentine may often be in question. For instance, it is not uncommon to observe secretion of a fibro-dentine matrix after injury, which subsequently has a more tubular ortho-dentine matrix laid down on its surface (Atkinson 1976, Senzaki 1980).

It is tempting to speculate that the fibro-dentine response may be a relatively non-specific one, and the presence of this matrix provides a suitable insoluble substratum on which inductive molecules might be immobilized, to trigger differentiation of more specific odontoblast-like cells – much as the role served by the basement membrane during tooth development. However, the possibility that the change from an atubular fibro-dentine matrix to a true tubular dentine matrix simply represents a change in the environmental conditions to which the cell has been exposed cannot be excluded. Nevertheless, this latter possibility implies a change in cell phenotype in developing a single cytoplasmic process, which becomes embedded within the dentine matrix. The importance of the pulpal environment which leads to the expression of the true odontoblast phenotype must not be underestimated. Transplantation of pulpal tissue can lead to loss of dentinogenic phenotype and result in the development of osteotypic characteristics (Hoffman 1966, Zussman 1966, Yamamura *et al.* 1980, Ishizeki *et al.* 1990). Maintenance of the odontoblast-like phenotype appears to be dependent on a pulpal environment (Takei *et al.* 1988).

Growth factors as signals for dental cyto-differentiation during repair

Recent progress in understanding the cellular and molecular processes that occur during physiological tooth development (Ruch *et al.* 1995) has provided considerable insight into the possible nature of the inductive process for odontoblast-like cell differentiation during reparative dentinogenesis. Many parallels exist between the induction of differentiation of a new generation of odontoblast-like cells during repair and embryonic tooth development, although a major difference is the absence of dental epithelium and its associated basement membrane in reparative situations. Terminal differentiation of odontoblasts during tooth development is under the control of the inner dental epithelium and a stage- and space-specific basement membrane, the latter of which may be important in the presentation of a functional network of bioactive molecules for induction of odontoblast differentiation (Ruch *et al.* 1995). The importance of growth factor molecules in signalling various cellular events (including odontoblast differentiation) during tooth development highlights the potential role that these molecules could play in reparative dentinogenesis. Several growth factors, including the TGF-βs and BMPs (Begue-Kirn et al. 1992, 1994), have been shown to mimic the role of the enamel organ and its associated basement membrane in the initiation of odontoblast cyto-differentiation in cultured dental papillae. Interestingly, each growth factor showed rather different characteristic effects on the dental papillae, and only TGF-β gave rise to gradients of cytological and functional differentiation of odontoblasts as seen during physiological tooth development.

When added alone, these growth factors were not capable of inducing odontoblast differentiation and required the presence of potentiating extracellular matrix molecules. The role played by these potentiating molecules is still unclear. It may be simply immobilization of the growth factor or may involve more complex potentiating reactions. Crude preparations of isolated dentine matrix fractions were very effective in stimulating initiation of odontoblast cyto-differentiation in cultured embryonic dental papillae and their effects could be blocked with neutralizing anti-TGF-β antibodies (Begue-Kirn et al. 1992). Similar preparations of dentine matrix fractions were also able to induce in-vivo reparative dentinogenesis within exposed cavities prepared in ferret canine teeth (Smith et al. 1990). These isolated matrix fractions gave rise to differentiation of odontoblast-like cells at the pulpal exposure site and deposition of a new tubular dentine matrix. Such findings provide an explanation for the formation of reparative dentine in association with dentinal chips displaced into the pulp during mechanical exposure (Seltzer and Bender 1984, Stanley 1989) and induction of dentine bridge formation in exposed pulps by demineralized dentine (Anneroth and Bang 1972, Nakashima 1989, Robson and Katz 1992). Clearly, dentine matrix contains bioactive components which are capable of initiating the induction of odontoblast differentiation.

Implantation of bone morphogenetic proteins in pulp-capping situations (Nakashima, 1990, 1994a, 1994b; Rutherford et al. 1993, 1994) has been shown to lead to in-vivo reparative dentinogenesis in several animal models. However, reparative events proceeded via a fibrodentine-like matrix and the amount of tubular dentine matrix produced was rather restricted in some cases. Whilst the effects of recombinant TGF-β1 were less convincing in a pulp-capping situation (Nakashima, 1994b), Tziafas et al. (1998) have reported induction of reparative dentinogenesis with tubular dentine formation when this growth factor was implanted at central pulpal sites. Similar results were observed previously when Millipore filters soaked in isolated dentine matrix fractions (rich in TGF-βs) were implanted at these central pulpal sites (Tziafas et al. 1995). The ability of these related but distinct growth factors to induce odontoblast-like cell differentiation requires further investigation to understand the nature and control of the molecular processes involved if they are to be exploited effectively in a clinical context. Importantly, a better understanding of the distinct biological activities of these growth factors in the pulpo-dentinal tissues is required.

The presence of other molecules in the extracellular matrix capable of modulating growth factor activity (Smith et al. 1997) highlights the potential role of various factors in regulating growth factor-induced dentinogenesis. The paracrine or autocrine nature of production of the growth factor, and its availability to the cells of the pulp, are also important factors. Endothelial cell production of TGF-βs might also be pertinent in view of the increased vascularity at sites of reparative dentinogenesis. An increase in the autocrine production of TGF-βs by odontoblasts during tertiary dentinogenesis is suggested from the raised levels found sequestered in dentine matrix (Perry and Smith 1997) and may be important in controlling cellular events.

New treatment modalities

It is probable that if new treatment modalities are to be developed based on the use of growth factors to stimulate local tertiary dentinogenesis at sites of dental injury, the mode of their delivery will be critical to the success of such treatment. If exogenous growth factors are to be applied to the tissues, it will be important to consider: (a) delivery vehicles, (b) dose responses and control of the extent of reparative responses, (c) growth factor half-life and local tissue factors which may modulate growth factor activity. The tissue events occurring after injury to the tooth and the reparative responses are very complex, involving a variety of cells, which show temporal and spatial differences in their activities within the tissues. Thus, as in any clinical situation of caries treatment, careful judgement of the relative importance of all these activities will be required. This implies that the rate of release of the growth factor from its delivery vehicle and maintenance of its bioactivity within the tissues will be important considerations. Whilst a variety of biomaterials could potentially be used to deliver recombinant growth factors at sites of dental tissue injury, control of growth factor release and bioactivity may be more problematical.

However, the endogenous tissue pools of TGF-βs and other growth factors in the dentine matrix (Finkelman *et al.* 1990, Cassidy *et al.* 1997) may provide a ready-made source of the growth factors which are necessary for pulpo-dentinal reparative processes to proceed. The release of these growth factors from dentine matrix to the site of tooth injury (Figure 5.8), may be augmented by some of the traditional restorative procedures commonly used in clinical dentistry. Calcium hydroxide is the most commonly used pulp-capping agent (Yoshiba and Iwaku 1994), and it has been used widely in the successful treatment of extensive dentinal caries and other pathological conditions. At least three major therapeutic actions have been ascribed to calcium hydroxide. These include: (a) its antibacterial activity (Fisher and McCabe 1978, Brannstrom *et al.* 1979), (b) its capacity for dissolving necrotic or injured tissue (Schroder and Granath 1971, Schroder 1985, Hasselgren *et al.* 1988) and (c) its ability to create localized alkaline conditions, which assist in dentine bridge formation (Tagger and Tagger 1985). The cellular events that occur following pulp-capping with calcium hydroxide have been described (Baume 1980, Schroder 1985, Yamamura 1985) and ultimately they can lead to differentiation of odontoblast-like cells and secretion of reparative dentine. Schroder (1985) has proposed that the necrotic material irritated the pulpal cells and stimulated odontoblast-like cell differentiation. However, the demonstration of solubilization of TGF-βs from dentine matrix by calcium hydroxide (Smith *et al.* 1995b) provides a more rational explanation for the inductive effect of calcium hydroxide on odontoblast-like cell

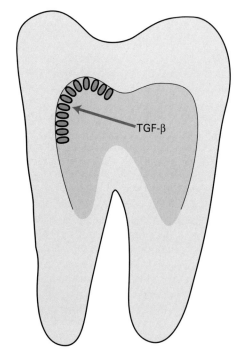

Figure 5.8

Schematic diagram of endogenous pools of TGF-βs sequestered in dentine matrix, which may be released after injury to the dentine–pulp complex and following use of clinical restorative procedures.

differentiation. This would also account for the lack of inductive effect of calcium hydroxide when implanted at central pulpal sites (Tziafas *et al.* 1996). The clinical success of calcium hydroxide would appear to rely on its ability to eliminate bacteria, and secondly to solubilize bioactive molecules at the site of injury where they are most needed to initiate the pulpal reparative processes. The solubilization of growth factors from the dentine matrix with the use of cavity conditioning agents (Smith and Smith 1998), including EDTA as discussed above, provides a further method of locally directing the bioactive molecules to the site of pulpo-dentinal injury.

These data provide an insight into how traditional dental restorative procedures may have encouraged reparative responses in caries management and also offer the opportunity to exploit our more recent understanding of the molecular and cellular processes taking place after tissue injury in the tooth. It is now important to extend our understanding of the presentation of growth factor and other bioactive molecules at sites of tissue injury in the dentine–pulp complex, and the signal transduction mechanisms that lead to the initiation of reparative processes.

Summary

The dentine–pulp complex shows a broad spectrum of reparative responses to injury. The nature of the response is determined, in part, by the type of cells involved. With survival of the primary odontoblasts, these cells can secrete a reactionary dentine matrix. After more severe injury, odontoblast death can often be succeeded by a differentiation of a new generation of odontoblast-like cells secreting a reparative dentine matrix. The factors controlling both differentiation of odontoblasts and regulation of their synthetic and secretory activity during repair show many parallels to developmental processes. Growth factors, particularly of the TGF-β superfamily, are able to initiate odontoblast differentiation and subsequently to up-regulate the activity of these cells to produce tertiary dentine matrices. Interaction of these molecules with others in the extracellular matrix appears to be important in both potentiating and modulating the activities of the growth factors. Odontoblast expression of growth factors and their sequestration within dentine matrix provides endogenous tissue pools of these molecules, which may be released after injury. These bioactive molecules offer exciting opportunities for the development of novel and innovative biological approaches to tissue repair in dentine and pulp.

Acknowledgement

Part of the work described in this paper was funded by a Sir Henry Wellcome Commemorative Award for Innovative Research from the Wellcome Trust; grant number 050834.

References

Andres JL, Stanley K, Chiefetz S, Massague J (1989) Membrane-anchored and soluble forms of betaglycan, a polymorphic proteoglycan that binds transforming growth factor-β. *J Cell Biol* **109**:3137–45.

Anneroth G, Bang G (1972) The effect of allogenic demineralised dentin as a pulp capping agent in Java monkeys. *Odontologisk Revy* **23**:315–28.

Atkinson ME (1976) The role of host tissue in repair of transplanted mouse molar teeth: a reappraisal of induction of odontoblasts during tooth development and repair. *Arch Oral Biol* **21**:91–3.

Bang G (1973) Induction of heterotopic bone formation by demineralised dentin: an experimental model in guinea pigs. *Scand J Dent Res* **81**:240–50.

Baume LJ (1980) *The Biology of the Pulp and Dentine, Monographs in Oral Science* **8**, 159–82. S Karger: Basel.

Begue-Kirn C, Smith AJ, Ruch JV et al (1992) Effects of dentin proteins, transforming growth factor β1 (TGF-β1) and bone morphogenetic protein 2 (BMP2) on the differentiation of odontoblasts in vitro. *Int J Dev Biol* **36**:491–503.

Begue-Kirn C, Smith AJ, Loriot M et al (1994) Comparative analysis of TGFβs, BMPs, IGFs, msxs, fibronectin, osteonectin and bone sialoprotein gene expressions during normal and in vitro induced odontoblast differentiation. *Int J Dev Biol* **38**:405–20.

Bergenholtz G (1981) Inflammatory response of the dental pulp to bacterial irritation. *J Endodontics* **7**:100–4.

Brannstrom M, Vojinovic O, Nordenvall KJ (1979) Bacteria and pulpal reactions under silicate cement restorations. *J Prosthet Dent* **41**:290–5.

Cam Y, Newmann MR, Ruch JV (1990) Immunolocalization of transforming growth factor β1 and epidermal growth factor receptor epitopes in mouse incisors and molars with a demonstration of in vitro production of transforming activity. *Arch Oral Biol* **35**:813–22.

Cam Y, Lesot H, Colosetti P, Ruch JV (1997) Distribution of transforming growth factor β1-binding proteins and low-affinity receptors during odontoblast differentiation in the mouse. *Arch Oral Biol* **42**:385–91.

Cassidy N, Fahey M, Prime SS, Smith AJ (1997) Comparative analysis of transforming growth factor-beta isoforms 1–3 in human and rabbit dentine matrices. *Arch Oral Biol* **42**:219–23.

Chen Y, Bei M, Woo I et al (1996) Msx-1 controls inductive signalling in mammalian tooth morphogenesis. *Development* **122**:3035–44.

Cotton WR (1968) Pulp response to cavity preparation as studied by the method of thymidine ³H autoradiography. In: Finn SB, ed, *Biology of the Dental Pulp Organ*, 69–101. University of Alabama Press: Tuscaloosa, Alabama.

Couve E (1986) Ultrastructural changes during the life cycle of human odontoblasts. *Arch Oral Biol* **31**:643–51.

D'Souza RN, Cavender A, Dickinson D et al (1998) TGF-β1 is essential for the homeostasis of the dentin–pulp complex. *Eur J Oral Sci* **106**(Suppl 1):185–91.

Feit J, Metelova M, Sindelka Z (1970) Incorporation of ³H-thymidine into damaged pulp. *J Dent Res* **49**:783–6.

Finkelman RD, Mohan S, Jennings JC et al (1990) Quantitation of growth factors IGF-1, SGF/IGF-11 and TGF-β in human dentin. *J Bone Miner Res* **5**:717–23.

Fisher FJ, McCabe JF (1978) Calcium hydroxide base materials; an investigation into the relationship between chemical structure and antibacterial properties. *Br Dent J* **144**:341–4.

Fitzgerald M, Chiego JD, Heys R (1990) Autoradiographic analysis of odontoblast replacement following pulp exposure in primate teeth. *Arch Oral Biol* **35**:707–15.

Frank RM (1968) Ultrastructural relationship between the odontoblast, its process and the nerve fibre. In: Symons NBB, ed, *Dentine and Pulp: Their Structure and Reaction*, 115–15. Churchill Livingstone: Edinburgh.

Frank S, Madlener M, Werner S (1996) Transforming growth factors β1, β2 and β3 and their receptors are differentially regulated during normal and impaired wound healing. *J Biol Chem* **271**:10189–93.

Harris R, Griffin CL (1969) The fine structure of the odontoblasts and cell rich zone of the human dental pulp. *Aust Dent J* **14**:168–77.

Hasselgren G, Olsson B, Cvek M (1988) Effects of calcium hydroxide and sodium hypochlorite on the dissolution of necrotic porcine muscle. *J Endodontics* **14**:125–7.

Hock JM, Canalis E, Centrella M (1990) Transforming growth factor-β stimulates bone matrix apposition and bone cell replication in cultured fetal rat calvariae. *Endocrinology* **126**:421–6.

Hoffman RL (1966) Tissue alterations in intramuscularly transplanted developing molars. *Arch Oral Biol* **12**:713–20.

Inage T, Toda Y (1996) Gene expression of TGF-β1 and elaboration of extracellular matrix using in situ hybridization and EM radioautography during dentinogenesis. *Anat Rec* **245**:250–66.

Ignotz RA, Massague J (1986) Transforming growth factor-β stimulates the expression of fibronectin and collagen and their incorporation into the extracellular matrix. *J Biol Chem* **261**:4337–45.

Inoue T, Sasaki A, Shimono M, Yamamura T (1981) Bone morphogenesis induced by implantation of dentine and cortical bone matrices. *Bull Tokyo Dent Coll* **22**:213–21.

Ishizeki K, Nawa T, Sugawara M (1990) Calcification capacity of dental papilla mesenchymal cells transplanted in the isogenic mouse spleen. *Anat Rec* **226**:279–87.

Karjalainen S, Soderling E (1980) The autoradiographic pattern of the in vitro uptake of proline by the coronal areas of intact and carious human teeth. *Arch Oral Biol* **24**:909–15.

Karjalainen S, Soderling E (1984) Dentino-pulpal collagen and the incorporation of ³H-proline by sound and carious human teeth in vitro. *J Biol Buccale* **12**:309–16.

Langeland K (1987) Tissue response to dental caries. *Endodont Dent Traumatol* **3**:149–71.

Larmas M (1986) Response of the pulpo-dentinal complex to caries attack. *Proc Finn Dent Soc* **82**:298–304.

Linde A (1984) Noncollagenous proteins and proteoglycans in dentinogenesis. In: Linde A, ed, *Dentin and Dentinogenesis*, Vol II, 55–92. CRC Press: Boca Raton FL.

Mackenzie A, Ferguson MWJ, Sharpe PT (1992) Expression patterns of the homeobox gene, Hox-8, in the mouse embryo suggest a role in specifying tooth initiation and shape. *Development* **115**:403–20.

Magloire H, Bouvier M, Joffre A (1992) Odontoblast response under carious lesions. *Proc Finn Dent Soc* **88**(Suppl 1): 257–74.

Mark M, Bloch-Zupan A, Ruch JV (1992) Effects of retinoids on tooth morphogenesis and cytodifferentiation in vitro. *Int J Dev Biol* **36**:517–26.

Massague J (1990) The transforming growth factor-β family. *Ann Rev Cell Biol* **6**:597–641.

Mjor I (1983) Dentin and pulp. In: Mjor IA, ed, *Reaction Patterns in Human Teeth*, 63–156. CRC Press: Boca Raton, FL.

Murray PE, Lumley PJ, Smith AJ (1998) Organ culture to assess pulpal responses to dental restorative materials. *J Dent Res* **77**:1035 (abstract 3226).

Nakashima M (1989) Dentin induction by implants of autolysed antigen-extracted allogenic (AAA) dentin on amputated pulps of dogs. *Endodont Dent Traumatol* **5**:279–86.

Nakashima M (1990) The induction of reparative dentine in the amputated dental pulp of the dog by bone morphogenetic protein. *Arch Oral Biol* **35**:493–7.

Nakashima M (1994a) Induction of dentin formation on canine amputated pulp by recombinant human bone morphogenetic proteins (BMP)-2 and -4. *J Dent Res* **73**:1515–22.

Nakashima M (1994b) Induction of dentine in amputated pulp of dogs by recombinant human bone morphogenetic proteins-2 and -4 with collagen matrix. *Arch Oral Biol* **39**:1085–9.

O'Kane S, Ferguson MWJ (1997) Transforming growth factor βs and wound healing. *Int J Biochem Cell Biol* **29**:63–78.

Perry H, Smith AJ (1994) Odontoblast expression of extracellular matrix components during tertiary dentinogenesis. *J Dent Res* **73**:838 (abstract 416).

Perry H, Smith AJ (1997) Transforming growth factor β1 in primary and tertiary human dentines. *J Dent Res* **76**:294 (abstract 2243).

Pierce GF, Mustoe TA, Lingelblach J et al (1989) Platelet-derived growth factor and transforming growth factor beta enhance tissue repair activities by unique mechanisms. *J Cell Biol* **109**:429–40.

Pierce GF, Tarpley J, Yanagihara D et al (1993) Platelet-derived growth factor (BB homodimer), transforming growth factor-beta and basic fibroblast growth factor in dermal wound healing. *Am J Pathol* **140**:1375–88.

Rapraeger A (1989) Transforming growth factor (type β) promotes the addition of chondroitin sulfate chains to the cell surface proteoglycan (syndecan) of mouse mammary epithelia. *J Cell Biol* **109**:2509–18.

Roberts-Clark D, Smith AJ (1999) Angiogenic growth factors in dentine matrix. *J Dent Res* **78**: 143 (abstract 299).

Robson WC, Katz RW (1992) Preliminary studies on pulp capping with demineralized dentin. *Proc Finn Dent Soc* **88**(Suppl 1):279–83.

Romagnoli P, Mancini G, Galeotti F et al (1990) The crown odontoblasts of rat molars from primary dentinogenesis to complete eruption. *J Dent Res* **69**:1857–62.

Ruch JV, Lesot H, Begue-Kirn C (1995) Odontoblast differentiation. *Int J Dev Biol* **39**:51–68.

Rutherford B (1995) Transdentinal stimulation of reparative dentine formation by osteogenic protein-1 in monkeys. *Arch Oral Biol* **40**:681–3.

Rutherford RB, Wahle J, Tucker M et al (1993) Induction of reparative dentine formation in monkeys by recombinant human osteogenic protein-1. *Arch Oral Biol* **38**:571–6.

Rutherford RB, Spanberg L, Tucker M et al (1994) The time-course of the induction of reparative dentine formation in monkeys by recombinant human osteogenic protein-1. *Arch Oral Biol* **39**:833–8.

Schroder U (1985) Effects of calcium hydroxide-containing pulp-capping agents on pulp cell migration, proliferation and differentiation. *J Dent Res* **64**:541–8.

Schroder U, Granath LE (1971) Early reaction of inert human teeth to calcium hydroxide following experimental pulpotomy and its significance to the development of the hard tissue barrier. *Odontologisk Revy* **22**:379–95.

Seltzer S, Bender IB (1984) *The Dental Pulp,* 3rd edn. JB Lippincott: Philadelphia.

Senzaki H (1980) A histological study of reparative dentinogenesis in the rat incisor after colchicine administration. *Arch Oral Biol* **25**:737–43.

Shah M, Foreman DM, Ferguson MWJ (1992) Control of scarring in adult wounds by neutralising antibodies to the growth factors TGF-βs and PDGF. *Lancet* **339**:213–14.

Slavkin HC (1974) Tooth formation: a tool in developmental biology. *Oral Sci Rev* **4**:1–136.

Sloan AJ, Smith AJ (1999) Stimulation of the dentine–pulp complex of rat incisor teeth by TGF-β isoforms 1–3 in vitro. *Arch Oral Biol* **44**: 149–56.

Sloan AJ, Shelton RM, Hann AC et al (1998) An in vitro approach for the study of dentinogenesis by organ culture of the dentine–pulp complex from rat incisor teeth. *Arch Oral Biol* **43**:421–430.

Sloan AJ, Matthews JB, Smith AJ (1999) TGF-β receptor expression in human odontoblasts and pulpal cells. *Histochem J* (in press).

Smith AJ, Smith G (1998) Solubilisation of TGF-β1 by dentine conditioning agents. *J Dent Res* **77**:1034 (abstract 3224).

Smith AJ, Tobias RS, Plant CG et al (1990) In vivo morphogenetic activity of dentine matrix proteins. *J Biol Buccale* **18**:123–9.

Smith AJ, Tobias RS, Cassidy N et al (1994) Odontoblast stimulation in ferrets by dentine matrix components. *Arch Oral Biol* **39**:13–22.

Smith AJ, Cassidy N, Perry H et al (1995a) Reactionary dentinogenesis. *Int J Dev Biol* **39**:273–280.

Smith AJ, Garde C, Cassidy N et al (1995b) Solubilisation of dentine extracellular matrix by calcium hydroxide. *J Dent Res* **74**:829 (abstract 59)

Smith AJ, Matthews JB, Hall RC (1997) Transforming growth factor-β1 (TGF-β1) in dentine matrix: ligand activation and receptor expression. *Eur J Oral Sci* **106**(Suppl 1):179–84.

Sporn MB, Roberts AB (1993) A major advance in the use of growth factors to enhance wound healing. *J Clin Invest* **92**:2565–6.

Stanley HR (1981) *Human Pulp Response to Restorative Dental Procedures*. Storte: Gainesville, FL.

Stanley HR (1989) Pulp capping: conserving the dental pulp – Can it be done? Is it worth it? *Oral Surg Oral Med Oral Pathol* **68**:628–39.

Sveen OB, Hawes RR (1968) Differentiation of new odontoblasts and dentine bridge formation on rat molar teeth after tooth grinding. *Arch Oral Biol* **13**:1399–412.

Tagger M, Tagger E (1985) Pulp-capping in monkeys with Realite and Life, two calcium hydroxide bases with different pH. *J Endodontics* **11**:394–400.

Takei K, Inoue T, Shimono M, Yamamura T (1988) An experimental study of dentinogenesis in autografted dental pulp in rats. *Bull Tokyo Univ Dent Coll* **29**:9–19.

Takuma S, Nagai N (1971) Ultrastructure of rat odontoblasts in various stages of their development and maturation. *Arch Oral Biol* **16**:993–1011.

Takuwa Y, Ohse C, Wang EA et al (1991) Bone morphogenetic protein-2 stimulates alkaline phosphatase activity and collagen synthesis in cultured osteoblastic cells MC3T3. *Biochem Biophy Res Comm* **174**:96–101.

Tashijan AH, Voelkel EF, Lazzaro M et al (1985) α and β human transforming growth factors stimulate prostaglandin production and bone resorption in cultured mouse calvaria. *Proc Natl Acad Sci USA* **82**:4535–8.

Thomas BL, Sharpe PT (1998) Patterning of the murine dentition by homeobox genes. *Eur J Oral Sci* **106**(Suppl 1):48–54.

Thomas BL, Tucker AS, Ferguson C et al (1998) Molecular control of odontogenic patterning: positional dependent initiation and morphogenesis. *Eur J Oral Sci* **106**(Suppl 1):44–7.

Torneck CD, Wagner D (1980) The effect of a calcium hydroxide cavity liner on early cell division in the pulp subsequent to cavity preparation and restoration. *J Endodontics* **6**:719–23.

Trowbridge HO (1981) Pathogenesis of pulpitis resulting from dental caries. *J Endodontics* **7**:52–60.

Tureckova J, Sahlberg C, Aberg T et al (1995) Comparison of the expression of the msx-1, msx-2, BMP-2 and BMP-4 genes in the mouse upper diastemal and molar tooth primordia. *Int J Dev Biol* **39**:459–68.

Tziafas D, Alvanou A, Panagiotakopoulos N et al (1995) Induction of odontoblast-like cell differentiation in dog dental pulp by in vivo implantation of dentine matrix components. *Arch Oral Biol* **40**:883–93.

Tziafas D, Veis A, Alvanou A (1996) Inability of calcium hydroxide to induce reparative dentinogenesis at non-peripheral sites of dog dental pulp. *Eur J Oral Sci* **104**:623–6.

Tziafas D, Alvanou A, Papadimitriou S et al (1998) Effects of recombinant fibroblast growth factor, insulin-like growth factor-II and transforming growth factor-β1 on dog dental pulp cells in vivo. *Arch Oral Biol* **43**:431–44.

Urist MR (1971) Bone histiogenesis and morphogenesis in implants of demineralised enamel and dentin. *J Oral Surg* **29**:88–102.

Vaahtokari A, Aberg T, Thesleff I. (1996) Apoptosis in the developing tooth: association with an embryonic signaling centre and suppression by EGF and FGF-4. *Development* **122**:121–9.

Weiss KM, Bollekens J, Ruddle FH, Takashita K (1994) Distal-less and other homeobox genes in the development of the dentition. *J Exp Zool* **270**:273–84.

Weiss K, Stock D, Zhao Z et al (1998) Perspectives on genetic aspects of dental patterning. *Eur J Oral Sci* **106**(Suppl 1):55–63.

Yamaguchi Y, Mann DM, Ruoslahti E (1990) Negative regulation of transforming growth factor β by the proteoglycan decorin. *Nature* **346**:281–4.

Yamamura T (1985) Differentiation of pulpal cells and inductive influences of various matrices with reference to pulpal wound healing. *J Dent Res* **64**:530–40.

Yamamura T, Shimono M, Koike H, Terao M (1980) Differentiation and induction of undifferentiated mesenchymal cells in tooth and periodontal tissue during wound healing and regeneration. *Bull Tokyo Univ Dent Coll* **21**:181–221.

Yoshiba N, Iwaku M (1994) Histological observations of hard tissue barrier formation in amputated dental pulp capped with tricalcium phosphate containing calcium hydroxide. *Endodont Dent Traumatol* **10**:113–20.

Yu YM, Becvar R, Yamada Y, Reddi AH (1991) Changes in the gene expression of collagens, fibronectin, integrin and proteoglycans during matrix-induced bone morphogenesis. *Biochem Biophy Res Comm* **177**:427–32.

Zussman W (1966) Osteogenic activity of odontoblasts in transplanted tooth pulps. *J Dent Res* **45**:144–51.

6

Erosion of dental enamel visualized by confocal laser scanning microscopy

Heinz Duschner, Hermann Götz, Roger Walker and Adrian Lussi

Introduction

Following a workshop held in 1995 in Limelette, Belgium on the state of the art in 'Etiology, Mechanisms and Implications of Dental Erosion' (published in a special issue of the *European Journal of Oral Sciences* in 1996), Grenby (1996) contributed a review on methods of assessing erosion and the erosive potential of beverages to this special publication. In addition to the well-known standard techniques for measuring the effect of erosive beverages on dental hard tissue he also mentioned a 'number of other innovative and sophisticated techniques, that should be capable of measuring erosive potential', namely 3-D tomography, laser scanning, nuclear magnetic resonance and micro-radiography. As far as we know, the potential of laser scanning, e.g. as confocal laser scanning microscopy (CLSM), has not yet been exploited for studying the erosive capacity of acidic beverages. This chapter describes the potential of CLSM for investigating the early processes of erosion in dental enamel.

Materials and methods

Preparation of enamel specimens

Enamel specimens were prepared as described previously by Lussi *et al.* (1993). Caries-free premolars with no cracks on the buccal site were selected from a pool of extracted teeth. The buccal sites were ground flat to obtain slabs of about 2.5 mm thickness, which were divided into the four test specimens. These were placed into 200-μm thick metal rings (fixed on a microscope glass) and embedded in resin. The specimens were polished down to the height of the metal rings with silicon paper disks of 30-, 18- and 6-μm grain and then with 3-μm and 1-μm diamond abrasive. Between the individual polishing processes the samples were rinsed with water, brushed and sonicated for 2 min in de-ionized water containing a detergent. One of the slabs was used without a pellicle; on the others (3-h in situ, 3 days in vitro or 7 days in vitro respectively) pellicles were grown as described below.

Pellicle formation

The in-situ pellicle was obtained by attaching one of the specimens to the rear denture of a panellist for 3 h. The in-vitro pellicles were obtained according to the method described by Meurman and Frank (1991). Stimulated saliva collected from one donor was centrifuged. Enamel slabs then were immersed in the clarified supernatant for 3 days or 7 days respectively. Saliva was changed daily. After pellicle formation slabs were washed with a buffered (0.1 M phosphate) sodium chloride solution and used directly for the erosion experiments.

Erosion experiments

Erosion experiments were carried out with 10 sets of teeth. The individual slabs prepared as described above were agitated slightly for 15 min at 37°C in a carbonated cola (Table 6.1). Then the specimens were rinsed with water and the slabs were removed from the embedding material. The pellicle was removed by carefully polishing the surfaces with a 3-µm diamond abrasive on a polishing cloth. Subsequently, the surfaces were dried with a soft paper towel. Prior to the hardness and CLSM experiments all specimens were stored in a saturated mineral solution (1.5 mmol/l $CaCl_2$, 1.0 mmol/l KH_2PO_4, 50 mmol/l NaCl, pH 7.0).

Table 6.1 Chemical characterization of a carbonated cola and the amount of NaOH required to achieve pH 5.5 or pH 7.0 respectively.

	pH	Amount 1N NaOH required to achieve pH 5.5	Amount of 1N NaOH required to achieve pH 7.0
Carbonated cola	2.4	0.3 ml	0.7 ml

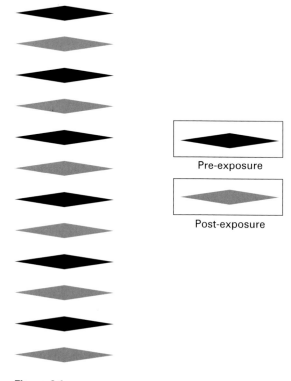

Pre-exposure

Post-exposure

Figure 6.1

Set-up of the hardness measurements.

Hardness measurements

The hardness measurements were carried out in an almost identical manner to those in a previous study by Lussi *et al.* (1995). Six pre-exposure baseline indentations (black) and six post-exposure final indentations (grey) were measured on each enamel specimen (Figure 6.1). The distance between two adjacent indentations was 50 µm. The mean values of the ratios between post- and pre-exposure indentation lengths were used for all further interpretations.

Confocal laser scanning microscopy

Confocal microscopy is a non-destructive, 3-dimensional microscopic tomography technique. The confocal principle is based on the elimination of stray light from out-of-focus planes by confocal apertures. Images are obtained by scanning over the sample with a spot-size laser beam (diameter ≈1 µm) and recording the light reflected from the in-focus plane. In-depth imaging (tomography) is possible by recording series of consecutive images either in the optical x–y plane (optical section parallel to the surface) or x–z plane (optical section perpendicular to the surface).

A Leica CLSM-DIAPLAN equipped with a variable energy mixed gas krypton/argon laser (up to 40 mW) was operated at 488 nm. The maximum lateral and axial resolution of the confocal microscope theoretically is a function of the wavelength of the laser light and the numerical aperture of the objective. Under the study conditions used (oil immersion objectives: ×40; numerical apertures 1.3; refractory index of the oil n = 1.518) the maximum resolution is about 200 nm laterally and about 300 nm axially.

Experimental details have been described earlier (Duschner *et al.* 1996).

An optical section perpendicular to the surface and optical sections parallel to the surface at 0, 10, 20, 30, 40, 50 and 60 µm depth were recorded for each specimen.

Results

Confocal laser scanning microscopy

Figure 6.2 shows non-destructive optical sections perpendicular as well as parallel to the surface of a polished piece of sound dental enamel from a surgically extracted fully impacted third molar. In this pseudo-colour visualization light red

colours stand for intense reflection of the laser light (interprismatic enamel), dark colours represent areas translucent to the laser light (enamel prisms). The perpendicular image was characterized by a regular band-like structure. The consecutive bands were directed to the surface at a relatively steep angle. The actual angle versus the surface varied with the different locations of the tooth crown. The image parallel to the surface appeared as the well-known honeycomb-like structure with relatively sharp contours.

The treatment of a polished enamel surface with the carbonated cola drastically affected the light remittance from surface and subsurface areas. In the perpendicular image there was almost no evidence for the band-like structure of enamel. The image was characterized by diffuse reflection of scattered light down to about 50 µm (Figure 6.3). As a consequence of the intensive

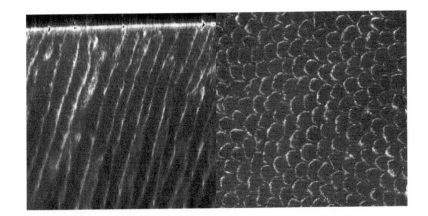

Figure 6.2

Optical section perpendicular to the surface of a polished slab of sound enamel.

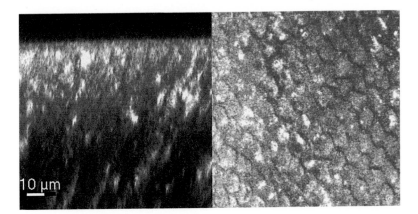

10 µm

Figure 6.3

Enamel without a pellicle after treatment with a carbonated cola for 15 min.

light scattering near the surface, the incoming laser light did not illuminate deeper areas of the enamel slab, so that these areas appeared dark and practically could not be observed. The image parallel to the surface (at a depth of 10 µm) gave only faint evidence of the initial honeycomb-like structure of enamel. Additionally, after erosion the reflection pattern reversed, so that the prism areas seemed to reflect and to scatter the light more intensively than the interprismatic enamel.

The presence of a 3-h in-situ pellicle on top of the enamel slabs had a drastic effect on the interactions of the carbonated cola with the microstructure on the enamel surface (Figure 6.4). In the image perpendicular to the surface the band-like structure of enamel could be identified, although with much more diffuse light scattering than in sound enamel. However, compared with the enamel slab with the 3-h in-situ pellicle, the

light scattering was reduced so that the laser illuminated an area down to about 100 µm. In particular, the interprismatic areas seemed to be affected most severely. Here the light was scattered most intensively, whereas the remaining prismatic areas still appeared dark and consequently were translucent to the laser light. This observation was also reflected by the CLSM images parallel to the surface (at a depth of 10 µm). Here the interprismatic enamel partly appeared as sharp edges and was partly characterized by spots of diffuse light scattering and by small areas with a breakdown of the honeycomb-like structure of enamel.

After the erosion experiment with enamel slabs coated with a 3-day in-vitro pellicle, the diffuse light scattering typical of the enamel slabs without pellicle was reduced again (Figure 6.5). The area illuminated by the laser extended

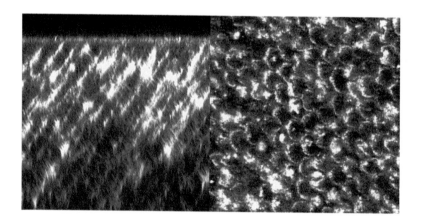

Figure 6.4

Enamel coated with a 3-h in-situ pellicle then treated with a carbonated cola for 15 min.

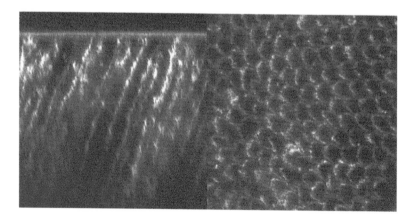

Figure 6.5

Enamel coated with a 3-day in-vitro pellicle then treated with a carbonated cola for 15 min.

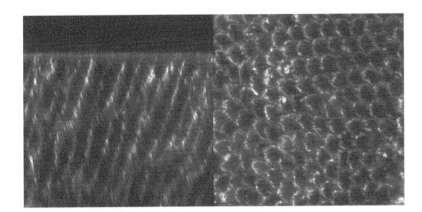

Figure 6.6

Enamel coated with a 7-day in-vitro pellicle then treated with a carbonated cola for 15 min.

down to about 80 µm. Nevertheless the band-like structure of the interprismatic enamel was still diffuse. Parallel to the surface, a well-organized honeycomb-like structure was typical for the carbonated cola-treated enamel, although the interprismatic areas are not nearly so sharp as in Figure 6.2.

There were only minute differences between the extent of light scattering by the enamel slabs that were coated during treatment with the carbonated cola with a 3-day or a 7-day pellicle (Figure 6.6). Nevertheless it is obvious from the above images that the bands of interprismatic enamel were sharper and not so broad as with the 3-day pellicle. Similar to the standard sound enamel in Figure 6.2 the laser light illuminated the piece of enamel down to about 100 µm. The image parallel to the surface almost showed the regular structure of sound impacted enamel, except for a few spot-like areas of increased light scattering.

Hardness measurements

The ratios between the post-erosion and pre-erosion indentation lengths are a relative measure of the softening of enamel due to the erosive capacity of the beverage. These ratios were as follows: 1.28 ± 0.07 for the enamel slabs without pellicle; 1.27 ± 0.07 for the enamel slabs with a 3-h in-situ pellicle; 1.14 ± 0.05 for the enamel slabs with a 3-day in-vitro pellicle; 1.10 ± 0.05 for the enamel slabs with a 7-day in-vitro pellicle.

The specimens without a pellicle and with a 3-h in-situ pellicle showed relatively high post-erosion/pre-erosion ratios and seemed to be markedly softened by the action of the carbonated cola. Although the value of the 3-h pellicle experiment was slightly lower than that without a pellicle, the difference between both values was not significant. However, there was a statistically significant difference ($P < 0.05$) in surface softening with respect to the experiments with the 3-day and 7-day pellicles. Here the surface softening was much less severe than before. The value with the 7-day pellicle was distinctly lower than that with the 3-day pellicle ($P < 0.1$).

Discussion

Confocal laser scanning microscopy provides indirect information on the micro-structure of dental hard tissue. This is mainly due to the fact that individual structures do not only reflect the incoming laser beam, but generate scattered light or fluorescence. Light scattering is due to organic material and to small particulate apatite mineral with anisotropic orientation. Under these conditions, the regularly aligned apatite micro-crystallites in prismatic enamel appeared dark because they were translucent to the laser light (Figure 6.2). Interprismatic enamel, with organic components and anisotronically aligned apatite crystallites, reflects and scatters light. The micro-structure of the non-erupted tooth (Figure 6.2) showed sharp contours and light scattering seemed to be restricted to the outermost surface layer. This may be due to a smear layer which could not be removed by the procedure of sample preparation used. When a tooth erupts into the oral cavity this ideal structure slowly changes, especially in the outermost subsurface layers of enamel, e.g. by the formation of an aprismatic surface area. Because these effects of maturing vary widely from one individual to another, non-erupted enamel was used as a standard for investigating the action of acidic beverages.

A clean polished enamel surface without a pellicle – according to the CLSM images – seemed to be relatively vulnerable to an acidic beverage such as the carbonated cola. Diffuse light reflection and light scattering could be observed down to about 40–50 μm (Figure 6.3). Deeper subsurface areas could not be observed because the intensive light scattering prevented the laser beam from illuminating deeper subsurface regions of the enamel slab. The image parallel to the surface was characterized by the reversal of light reflection/scattering. Prismatic enamel appeared in light colours, interprismatic enamel in dark ones. This might be due to the partial dissolution of the interprismatic mineral as observed by Meurman and ten Cate (1996) by scanning electron microscopy. The dissolution process breaks down the size and the order of the mineral particles of the apatite matrix; therefore light scattering is enhanced. Although the images obtained by confocal microscopy and by scanning electron microscopy were distinctly different, the interpretation was similar. In CLSM, however, this information was obtained non-destructively from natural wet specimens; in addition subsurface histo-tomographies could also be recorded. Thus some information on the in-depth migration of the acidic beverage could be obtained. The degradation of the enamel matrix visible by CLSM correlates with the relative decrease of micro-hardness compared with the pre-erosion measurements. The mean value of the ratios between post-erosion and pre-erosion indentation lengths was 1.28, with the relatively high standard deviation of ±0.07. In CLSM the post-erosion enamel appeared very inhomogeneous, with a widely varying degree and depth of degradation, locally and from specimen to specimen. It has to be taken into account that the vulnerability of natural samples to acid attack cannot be standardized; therefore the high standard deviations came as no surprise.

A 3-h in-situ pellicle obviously prevented the acidic beverage from degrading the enamel micro-structure as severely as that observed on enamel without a pellicle (Figure 6.4). In the image perpendicular to the surface the band-like structure was visible, though with much less sharp contours than the non-erupted standard enamel. Intense light scattering was evidence for the beginning of degradation of the interprismatic enamel. Obviously, components of the beverage migrated into deeper subsurface areas of the enamel slab along interprismatic enamel and then spread into the prismatic enamel. The image parallel to the surface showed that only individual parts of the interprismatic enamel were affected by the action of the acidic components of the carbonated cola. Despite these morphological differences, the pre-erosion/post-erosion hardness ratios were only slightly different (not statistically significant). It may be that this discrepancy cannot be readily explained with the present set of data. It might be speculated whether the observed enamel degradation did not affect the hardness of enamel or if the standard deviations were too high to differentiate between minor changes in hardness.

The 3-day in-vitro pellicle undoubtedly had a protective effect with respect to acid degradation. Although the light scattering in the interprismatic enamel was still visible, the micro-structure of this eroded tooth slab was near to that of the non-erupted standard (Figure 6.5). The pattern of reflected/scattered laser light in the image perpendicular to the surface was only slightly less sharp than before. The image parallel to the surface had only very few spots of more extended light scattering. Accordingly, the relative hardness values of the enamel slabs coated with the 3-day pellicle of 1.14 were distinctly lower than those without a pellicle or with the 3-h pellicle.

The 7-day in-vitro pellicle seemed to provide a very good protection against the action of the acidic components of the carbonated cola. The CLSM images – both perpendicular and parallel to the surface – were similar to those of the non-erupted standard. It is hard to say whether these differences were due to the maturation of enamel or to the action of the beverage. The problem is that the micro-structure of sound erupted enamel as seen in CLSM varies widely, laterally as well as individually. Even studies with enamel slabs partly coated or windowed with nail varnish are not an optimum solution, because the nail varnish may penetrate into interprismatic enamel. In consequence the coated parts of a tooth show similar histo-morphological effects to the uncoated but treated ones (Arends *et al.* 1997). The mean relative hardness value of this experiment was 1.10 and near to statistical significance below that of the 3-day pellicle.

Although the histo-tomographic observations in this study were in fairly good agreement with the hardness measurements, there was an obvious problem in comparing these data. The hardness measurements provided mean values of a series of studies on different locations of several tooth specimens. The statistical implications of confocal images in such an experiment must be interpreted with caution. The selection of representative images from hundreds of records taken during the experiments cannot fulfil strict objective criteria. However, when individual indentation spots were examined by CLSM the respective images clearly reflected the measured hardness values. Currently modified techniques of image processing to measure the amount of light scattering are being developed. It is hoped that the degree of degradation can not only be visualized but also quantified by such a technique.

The relevance of the present data for the in-vivo situation in the human mouth can only be speculated upon. The hardness measurements require polished specimens. Although confocal images can also be recorded with natural tooth surfaces, the extension of the aprismatic enamel may affect the illumination of deeper areas of the tooth by the laser beam. In addition to the experimental problems the biochemical situation in the mouth is totally different from that in the test tube. Nevertheless, the studies described above seem to provide some evidence for the protective action of a pellicle.

References

Arends J, Duschner H, Ruben JL (1997) Penetration of varnishes into demineralized root dentin in vitro. *Caries Res* **31**:201–5.

Duschner H, Sønju-Clasen B, Øgaard B (1996) Detection of early caries by confocal laser scanning microscopy. In: Stookey G, ed, *Early Detection of Dental Caries*, 145–56. Indiana University Press: Indianapolis, Indiana.

Grenby TH (1996) Methods of assessing erosion and erosive potential. *Eur J Oral Sci* **104**:207–14.

Lussi A, Jaeggi T, Schärer S (1993) The influence of different factors on in vitro enamel erosion. *Caries Res* **27**:387–93.

Lussi A, Jaeggi T, Jaeggi-Schärer S (1995) Prediction of the erosive potential of some beverages. *Caries Res* **29**:349–54.

Meurman JH, Frank RM (1991) Scanning electron microscopic study of the effect of salivary pellicle on enamel erosion. *Caries Res* **25**:1–6.

Meurman JH, ten Cate JM (1996) Pathogenesis and modifying factors of dental erosion. *Eur J Oral Sci* **104**:199–206.

PART II

Tooth Wear

7

Historical and forensic aspects of tooth wear

David K Whittaker

Introduction

Tooth wear, either natural or artificial, has proved a fascination to mankind since the dawn of history. The principal reason is that other parts of the animal or human body repair themselves to a degree and therefore the influences of life's events are eliminated as the individual gets older. Not so in the case of the teeth, which biologically speaking are almost inert, and certainly in a gross sense are incapable of repair as we know it in relation to the healing process. For this reason any life events affecting either the development or the permanent structure of the teeth will be recorded within the dentition and will theoretically be capable of analysis and interpretation. This feature has been used over countless generations to attempt, for example, to age the horse; hence the phrase 'never look a gift horse in the mouth' (Muylle *et al*. 1997).

Historical aspects

Patterns of wear in teeth are capable of providing information in relation to evolutionary phenomena and it seems clear that had the anatomists of the day been more informed in these matters the scandal of the Piltdown skull hoax might well have come to light much more rapidly than was the case. It was eventually demonstrated that part of an orang-utan jaw had been used in the preparation of the hoax material and occlusal wear and approximal wear patterns on this mandible would or should have indicated that its humanoid origins were in doubt. In a negative sense, lack of wear faceting

on the canine associated with this hoax should have raised awareness as to its origins – which were those of a deciduous orang-utan tooth rather than an adult humanoid canine.

Attrition in ancient material can be excessive due not only to massive muscle attachments, but also to the unrefined nature of the diet. This latter has resulted in studies on micro-wear patterns on the enamel surface of teeth – usually by scanning electron microscope – and it has been claimed that the patterns can be identified and related to particular food constituents, so that dietary habits in ancient populations may be determined. Wear patterns are usually due to silica phytoliths and recently it has been suggested that these can be classified and related to individual plant stems (Lalveza Fox *et al*. 1996). Although work in the past has usually associated these with the surface enamel of ancient teeth, we have recently demonstrated phytoliths in ancient calculus

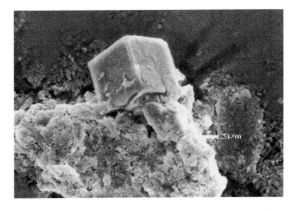

Figure 7.1

A silica phytolith in calculus from a neolithic skull.

deposits (Figure 7.1) and these are obviously more clearly attributable to the lifestyle of the individual than are surface phytoliths, which may be contaminants.

Preliminary studies of this nature are restricted to very small sample sizes, as are numerous reports in the archaeological literature relating to artificial tooth wear. Perhaps some of the more striking examples originated in the African continent in relation to tooth avulsion and filing practices. These have been related to individual tribal practices and a study of ancient skulls in the new world has utilized this phenomenon in order to study migration patterns either in ancient times or during, for example, slave practices in the 18th century.

There are numerous examples of wear patterns throughout the world which can be related not to therapeutic techniques but to cultural practices (Fastlicht 1948). For example, in the Mayan and Inca civilizations bow drills were used to modify teeth using carborundum as a means of abrasion, and inlays of various materials were structured to fit these abrasion cavities. Incidentally, in at least one case there is evidence of replantation of teeth following apicectomy in connection with these practices.

In Japan in the last century a common practice was to acid-etch the teeth followed by the application of lacquers and this was thought to markedly enhance the appearance of young females.

Population studies

Anthropologists working on human skeletal material in large populations have a major interest in determining age at death so that the demography of the population may be ascertained.

It is generally accepted that wear on the occlusal surfaces of teeth is to some extent a measure of the age of the individual, but in a given population it has to be presumed that dietary wear is similar in all members of that population. Even if nothing is known of the real diet, occlusal wear studies should still enable individual specimens to be ranked in order of age, rather than to reliably indicate what those age groups might be.

Scholarly contributions have been made by Brothwell (1981), who developed a simplified method of age grouping based on patterns of occlusal wear and assessment of islands of dentine and enamel on the occlusal surfaces of molar teeth. This method was refined by Miles (1962) who used juveniles from the population to determine relative wear in first, second and third molars and then to apply this information to wear patterns in the adult section of the population. The assumption has to be made that the diet will remain constant throughout life, but in spite of this limitation, at the present time there is no better way of estimating age at death in skeletal material without destroying some of the material.

Temporomandibular joint

Studies of wear patterns on the occlusal and proximal surfaces of historical populations have enabled these to be compared with changes in the temporomandibular joint, both in the condylar and glenoid fossa components (Figure 7.2). It has been shown that condylar shape and form vary markedly between different ethnic populations in Europe (Oberg et al. 1971) and also that pathological changes, particularly in the condyles, appear to be related more to loss of teeth than to attrition patterns (Whittaker et al. 1985a). It is difficult to disentangle the relationship of these processes to the ageing process in these studies, but there is evidence that early loss of teeth with consequent changes in masticatory patterns may be an important factor in the development of degenerative changes in the bony surfaces of the joint (Granados 1979). There is still controversy regarding the effect of occlusal attrition on the curves of Monson and Spee and their subsequent effect upon functional activity in the joints (Granados 1979). Recent work by Singleton on medieval archaeological material suggests that occlusal wear patterns do not accentuate the so-called curves of Monson and Spee (Hitchcock 1983) and the helicoid nature of wear in the molar teeth was described many years ago on Romano-British material in which it was shown that although the occlusal surfaces of the molar teeth may initially be arranged in the form of a portion of a sphere,

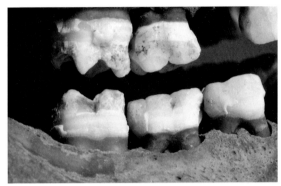

Figure 7.3

Cervical margin to alveolar crestal measurements were once used to indicate the extent of chronic infective periodontal disease in ancient skulls.

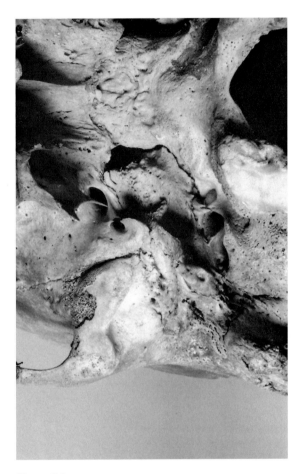

Figure 7.2

Remodelling in the glenoid fossa of an 18th century Londoner.

increasing wear results in bucco-lingual slope on the first molar, horizontal wear on the second molar and lingual-buccal slope on the third molar, resulting in a helicoid type of wear pattern (Brown *et al.* 1977). The significance of this in relation to temporomandibular joint activity is still unknown. It has been suggested that occlusal wear coupled with proximal wear may influence the incidence of impaction of third molars and that modern civilizations with minimal attrition may therefore have a higher incidence of impaction. Recent work (Sengupta, pers. comm.) has failed to show correlation between wear patterns and subsequent mal-eruption of the third molars.

Continuing eruption

Studies of chronic infective periodontal disease using skeletal material from ancient populations have commonly assumed that measurements from the cervical margin of the teeth to the alveolar crest give an indication of the extent of alveolar crestal bone loss and therefore some indication of the extent of chronic infective periodontal disease (Figure 7.3). This philosophy was based on earlier findings (Manson 1976) that horizontal alveolar crestal bone loss may occur slowly to some extent throughout life, resulting in exposure of the roots of the teeth, getting long in the tooth as epithelial migration occurred to compensate for this injury. This would seem to be a reasonable assumption, providing that it could be shown that the teeth remain in a static position throughout life in relation to fixed points in their bony support. However, it has been suggested (Murphy 1959) that teeth may continue to erupt beyond their normal occlusal position in the adult occlusion.

It has long been recognized that attrition may occur on the surfaces of teeth even in modern populations. Picton (1957) drew attention to the fact that if teeth continued to erupt in response to this wear then measurements from the neck of the tooth to the bone margin would not be the measure of a disease process. Darling and Levers (1975) showed strong evidence that the upper border of the alveolar canal was a fixed point and was static throughout life. They based this work on standardized radiographs in which deciduous teeth had become ankylosed and 'submerged'. Once this had been established it was possible to take standardized radiographs of skeletal material and to measure the position of the teeth in different age groups using the inferior alveolar canal as a fixed point. Newman and Levers (1979) applied this technique to radiographs of Anglo-Saxon skulls and measured from the inferior alveolar canal to the occlusal surfaces of the teeth. In that Anglo-Saxon population continuing eruption occurred throughout life and more or less exactly compensated for wear due to attrition. Their data appeared to show that there was surprisingly little bone loss, indicating that chronic infective periodontal disease was of minor significance. We have applied their method to a large series of Romano-British skulls (Whittaker *et al.* 1985b) which were grouped into ascending ages by a modification of the Miles method and we showed that a similar situation obtains in a large population of this nature (Figure 7.4).

Inaccuracies of ageing can either mask or accentuate studies on disease processes of this nature so that conclusions need to be interpreted with caution. However, over a period ranging from late teenage to late middle age, the apices of the molar teeth can be seen to move away from the inferior alveolar canal by a distance of about 2 mm and the occlusal surfaces remain at the same distance from the canal. The cervical margins of the teeth also move away from the inferior alveolar canal. It is interesting to note that bone appears to be added to the lower border of the mandible as age progresses. This presumably results in a slight increase in facial height in older members of a population.

A population exhumed from the crypt of Christchurch, Spitalfields, (London, UK) (Whittaker *et al.* 1990) has provided a sample of unique interest, as the age at death was accurately known in many of the cases from either burial records or coffin plates. This was an 18th century population, subject to little or no attrition because of refined diets and so it is of interest to determine whether continuing eruption occurs in modern day populations in the same way that it does to compensate for occlusal attrition. Standard radiographs were

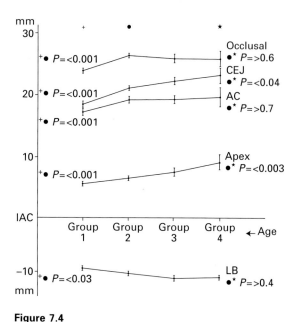

Figure 7.4

Continuing eruption of lower molar in Romano-British population. IAC, inferior alveolar canal; LB, lower border mandible; AC, alveolar crest; CEJ, cement–enamel junction.

used as described above, measurements being made from the inferior alveolar canal to specific points on each molar tooth and the results indicated that surprisingly the teeth were continuing to erupt at about the same rate as in more primitive populations, where occlusal attrition was manifest (Figure 7.5). As yet there is no evidence from the maxillary dentition, as no one has identified a fixed point in the maxilla from which to measure. However, it may be assumed that the maxillary teeth continue to erupt in the same manner. In the Spitalfields material, continuing eruption occurred for a distance of about 7 mm in maxilla and mandible together. Therefore in the absence of occlusal attrition it seems reasonable to suggest that providing a normal freeway space is maintained, then the facial height of these individuals should have increased over about 7 mm plus any bone added to the lower border of the mandible over their lifetime. As was found in other populations,

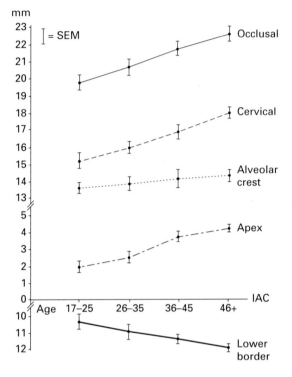

Figure 7.5

Continuing eruption in posterior teeth of 18th century Londoners. There is no occlusal wear, but apex and cervical margin move away from inferior alveolar canal (IAC) as age progresses.

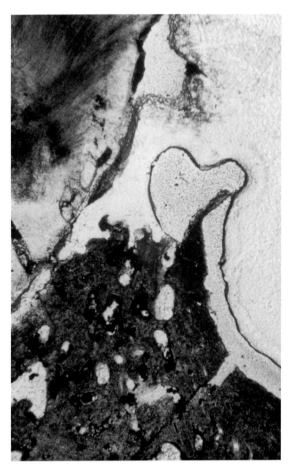

Figure 7.6

Remodelling of alveolar crestal bone in response to chronic infective periodontal disease (Romano-British specimen).

there seemed to be very little change in the level of alveolar bone when averaged in a horizontal fashion. Thus, it seems probable that chronic infective periodontal disease was not a major problem in the Spitalfields population, although there was vertical loss of bone around some of the teeth. Another interpretation is that bone is lost because of chronic periodontal disease, but that the continuing eruption stimulates bone growth and this more or less compensates for loss from infective processes. There is some histological evidence that bone is added in this way (Figure 7.6) and it has been shown (Anneroth and Ericsson 1967) that bone deposition may be stimulated by continuing eruption of teeth.

Localized periodontal bone loss is not measurable by these methods, but Kerr (1994) has developed a method which he has applied to the Spitalfields population and this is dependent upon microscopic examination of inter-dental bone. Proximal wear is considerable in populations of this nature and this might change the relationship of the occlusal surfaces of the teeth to the inferior alveolar canal due to mesial drift. This factor needs to be taken into consideration when considering apparent continuing eruption of molar teeth.

Tooth wear in forensic cases

Unlike the historical perspective, forensic cases are almost always of an individual nature rather than a study of populations. For this reason the statistical techniques applying to large population samples cannot be applied in the crime situation. However, there are a number of examples where the use of tooth wear helped to produce a dossier of information, e.g. about an unknown body, and there are also examples of bite mark analysis where tooth wear may be of importance.

Occupational tooth wear

There are a number of examples in the literature relating various occupations to changes in the teeth, although modern legislation regarding safety at work has fortunately made these extremely rare. Workers in acid battery factories have been reported to suffer from chemical erosion of the teeth and cobblers working in the Lancashire shoe factories were said to hold small nails or 'tingles' in the mouth and spit them out to catch them and hammer them into the welt of a shoe. This resulted in grooving of the incisal edges of the anterior teeth. Most changes to the dentition in the late 1900s are related to hobbies or pastimes, so that grooving of an incisal edge may be seen in a seamstress or a carpenter, the former holding or running cotton through the mouth prior to needle threading and the latter holding nails in a particular part of the occlusion. At least one example appears in the literature of excessive attrition on the anterior teeth related to playing the bagpipes.

Tooth wear in dentures

Artificial teeth, especially those manufactured from acrylic rather than porcelain, may be extremely prone to wear. The body of an elderly male was found in the basement of an empty unused property. There were no indications of identity except that he was wearing an unusual full denture with very severe wear patterns on the upper central incisors – which were acrylic –

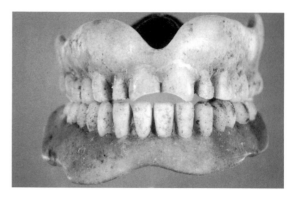

Figure 7.7

Anterior wear cause by pipe smoking. There has been a crude repair to the upper central incisors.

and none on the lower incisors, which were porcelain. There was evidence of the upper teeth having been detached from the baseplate and re-attached in an amateurish fashion, and it was possible to suggest that this individual smoked a pipe held in the front teeth and occasionally it had levered off his incisors and he had replaced them himself (Figure 7.7). Some 6 months later an elderly lady reported to a police station on the other side of the country that her husband had been missing for the previous 12 months, and some pipe stems were recovered from her household. Contour patterning on the pipe stems was compared to contour wear faceting on the denture and the individual was identified by means of this analysis.

In another case the body of a young female was found battered and decomposing in woodland and it was obvious from the oral condition that a partial denture had probably been worn. This was eventually found at some distance in the undergrowth and consisted of an unremarkable plastic Every type denture. Graphite enhancement and ultraviolet photographic techniques were used to identify a prescription number on the baseplate and a putative identification was made on the basis of this information. It became essential for the murder trial to determine that this denture had in fact been worn by the individual concerned and this was done by examination of small facets on the palatal surfaces of the upper anterior denture teeth. These facets were shown to relate to wear from the natural standing lower incisor teeth. In addition, a fitting of the denture around a small exostosis in the maxilla confirmed the relationship of the denture to the individual.

Tooth wear in reconstruction

Skeletal material in forensic cases is often fragmented and before identification procedures can be commenced it is necessary to reconstruct the facial bones. As the teeth developmentally precede the development of maxilla and mandibular bone the occlusion should be reconstructed as accurately as possible and the facial bones will to some extent take care of themselves. Small facets on the labial occlusal and palatal surfaces of teeth should be examined in detail and the teeth can then be mounted in correct relationship to each other with a high degree of accuracy. Once the facial skeleton has been reconstructed it may be possible to identify the individual by means of dental records, but these are frequently unavailable. Facial reconstruction of some type is therefore necessary and this can be carried out by artistic design (Pragg and Neave 1997), a procedure which is dependent upon average tissue thicknesses. This procedure may also be carried out by a computer, but neither of these techniques produces an accurate likeness. Photographic superimposition, if such photographs are available, is the most accurate method of determining identity and this was first employed in the case of the Ruxton murders in Lancaster in the 1930s (Brash and Glaister 1937). A major difficulty is that photographs are two-dimensional distortions of a three-dimensional object and therefore it is necessary to image the skull electronically and distort that image to the same extent as the photograph with which one is comparing identity. This procedure was used in the majority of remains in the Frederick and Rosemary West case (Whittaker et al. 1998) and resulted in positive identification acceptable to the courts in all the cases examined (Figure 7.8). Not only does facial superimposition allow positive identification to be made, but in the case of young individuals it may allow an opinion to be given as to the time elapsed between the photograph being taken and death occurring, by studying facial growth in the intervening period.

Tooth wear in bite marks

Bite mark analysis requires decisions to be made concerning whether the injury is indeed a bite mark. Then it must be determined whether it is a human bite mark and whether there is sufficient information within the mark to allow a positive identification to be made of the assailant. The more individuality there is relating to the assailant's dentition, the more likely an identification will be (Whittaker 1995). Wear patterns on the incisal edges of the anterior teeth may often be reproduced in the dimensions of a bite mark and if these wear patterns are unusual then it may be claimed with some degree of reliability that a specific individual caused the injury. The unusual incisal wear shown in Figure 7.9 has resulted in a mesial incisal edge of the upper left central incisor having a protruding portion of enamel and the laceration caused by the protruding edge is visible in the bruised and lacerated area above the nipple of the victim. Lower incisors frequently produce clear incised injuries to skin because of their small incisal surface area and rather sharp edges, but severe attrition of the lower incisors may result in very characteristic images in a bite mark. In this particular case, not only is marked incisal attrition obvious, but there is clearly a diastema between the lower central incisors. This was subsequently shown to be present in a suspect arrested in association with this murder case.

Future developments

It is now possible to image both soft and hard tissues in three dimensions using technology such as computerized axial tomography, where radiographic imaging in parallel planes from the vertex of the head to the neck region is digitalized, computer stored and recovered as three-dimensional data. Using this technology it is possible to scan an unopened sarcophagus of mummified Egyptian material to reconstruct the information within the sarcophagus and then –

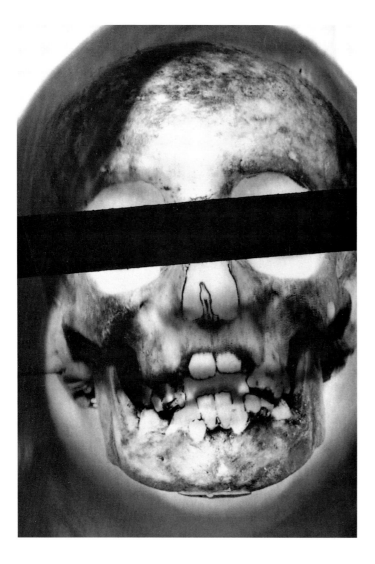

Figure 7.8

Superimposition of 'corrected' skull image and facial photograph shows exact match in teeth and facial bone structures.

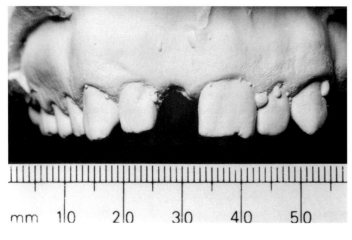

Figure 7.9

A missing tooth and unusual incisor wear matched this dentition to an unusual bite mark in a case of murder.

by measuring the absorbance radiographically speaking of the material of the coffin and mummified tissues within it from a similar opened specimen – to eliminate these data from the computer databank (Baldock *et al*. 1994). This results in the loss of imaging of the sarcophagus, the mummy wrappings and the mummified soft tissues and therefore enables the operator to study a three-dimensional image of the bones of the skull (and if necessary the details of individual teeth), without the requirement of opening the sarcophagus. These techniques are expensive and rarely used in individual forensic investigations but allow sufficient detail to be obtained for the study of wear patterns in both historical and forensic cases without invasion or destruction of any of the material.

References

Anneroth G, Ericsson SG (1967) An experimental histological study of monkey teeth without antagonists. *Odont Revy* **18**:345–59.

Baldock C, Hughes SW, Whittaker DK et al (1994) 3-D reconstruction of an ancient Egyptian mummy using x-ray computer tomography. *J R Soc Med* **87**:806–8.

Brash JC, Glaister J (1937) *Medico-legal Aspects of the Ruxton Case*. E and S Livingstone: Edinburgh.

Brothwell DR (1981) *Digging Up Bones*. Trustees of the British Museum: London.

Brown WAB, Whittaker DK, Fenwick J, Jones DS (1977) Quantitative evidence for the helicoid relationship between the maxillary and mandibular occlusal surfaces. *J Oral Rehabil* **4**:91–6.

Darling AI, Levers BGH (1975) The pattern of eruption of some human teeth. *Arch Oral Biol* **20**:89–96.

Fastlicht S (1948) Tooth mutilations in pre-Columbian Mexico. *J Am Dent Assoc* **36**:315–20.

Granados JI (1979) The influence of the loss of teeth and attrition on the articular eminence. *J Prosthet Dent* **42**:78–85.

Hitchcock HP (1983) The curve of Spee in Stone Age Man. *Am J Orthod* **84**:248–53.

Kerr NW (1994) Prevalence and natural history of periodontal disease in a London, Spitalfields population (1645–1852 AD). *Arch Oral Biol* **39**:581–8.

Lalveza Fox C, Juan J, Albert RM (1996) Phytolith analysis on dental calculus, enamel surface and burial soil: information about diet and paleoenvironment. *Am J Phys Anthropol* **101**:101–13.

Manson JD (1976) Bone morphology and bone loss in periodontal disease. *J Clin Periodontol* **3**:14–22.

Miles AEW (1962) Assessment of the ages of a population of Anglo-Saxons from their dentitions. *Proc R Soc Med* **55**:881–6.

Murphy TR (1959) Compensatory mechanisms in facial height adjustment to functional tooth attrition. *Aust Dent J* **4**:312–23.

Muylle S, Simoens P, Lauwers H, Van Loon G (1997) Ageing draft and trotter horses by their dentition. *Vet Rec* **141**:17–20.

Oberg T, Carlsson GE, Fajers CM (1971) The temporomandibular joint. A morphological study on human autopsy material. *Acta Odontol Scand* **29**:349–62.

Newman HN, Levers BGH (1979) Tooth eruption and function in an early Anglo-Saxon population. *J R Soc Med* **72**:341–50.

Picton DCA (1957) Calculus, wear and alveolar bone loss in the jaws of sixth century Jutes. *Practitioner* **7**:301–3.

Pragg J, Neave R (1997) *Making Faces*. British Museum Press: London.

Sengupta A, Whittaker DK, Barber G et al (1998) The effects of dental wear on third molar eruption and on the curve of Spee in human archaeological dentitions (personal communication).

Whittaker DK (1995) Forensic dentistry in the identification of victims and assailants. *J Clin Forens Med* **2**:145–51.

Whittaker DK, Davies G, Brown M (1985a) Tooth loss, attrition and temporomandibular joint changes in a Romano-British population. *J Oral Rehabil* **12**:407–19.

Whittaker DK, Molleson T, Daniel AT et al (1985b) Quantitative assessment of tooth wear, alveolar crest height and continuing eruption in a Romano-British population. *Arch Oral Biol* **30**:493–501.

Whittaker DK, Griffiths S, Robson A et al (1990) Continuing tooth eruption and alveolar crest height in an eighteenth century population from Spitalfields, East London. *Arch Oral Biol* **35**:81–5.

Whittaker DK, Richards BH, Jones ML (1998) Orthodontic reconstruction in a victim of murder. *Br J Orthod* **25**:11–14.

8

Definition, classification and clinical assessment of attrition, erosion and abrasion of enamel and dentine

David Bartlett and Bernard GN Smith

Introduction

Tooth wear is a common problem, estimates of its prevalence indicate that up to 97% of the population are affected, with about 7% exhibiting pathological degrees of wear that may require treatment (Smith and Robb 1996). The term tooth wear is used to describe the processes of erosion, attrition and abrasion, although the effect of one factor – most notably erosion – is often dominant (Smith and Knight 1984). Erosion is defined as the chemical dissolution of teeth by acids, attrition is the wear of tooth against tooth, abrasion is the wear of teeth by physical means other than teeth.

Erosion

The most important sources of acids are those found in the diet and from the stomach, although industrial sources have been described in the past. Current evidence suggests that erosion is the most important cause of tooth wear and if it occurs in combination with abrasion or attrition the damage will be greater than if these processes occurred independently (Smith and Knight 1984, Jarvinen et al. 1991). The palatal surface of the upper anterior teeth appears to be the most common site for erosion and is usually associated with acid originating from the stomach (O'Brien 1993), although some researchers have implicated that dietary acids could be important in this region (Milosevic et al. 1997). The most destructive source of acid is regurgitated gastric juice, which has a pH of about 1–2, whilst most dietary acids only reach a pH of around 3 (Bartlett and Smith 1995, Bartlett et al. 1998).

Gastric acid

It is now firmly established that regurgitated gastric juice causes dental erosion (Smith and Knight 1984, Jarvinen et al. 1991, Bartlett et al 1996). Stomach juice can enter the mouth passively, such as in patients with gastro-oesophageal reflux disease (Bartlett et al. 1996), and forcibly in patients with anorexia and bulimia nervosa (Bartlett and Smith 1995). Patients with chronic alcoholism may suffer from either passive regurgitation or chronic vomiting (Robb and Smith 1990). In all these examples the destruction caused by frequent exposure to gastric acid is catastrophic and may lead to the complete obliteration of the teeth. It is likely that gastric acid containing hydrochloric acid produced by the parietal cells in the stomach is associated with the more severe cases of erosion, whilst dietary acids may be related to the less severe forms.

Dietary acids

Dietary acids are commonly found in the Western diet. The dominance of the carbonated drinks market has resulted in this source of acid frequently being cited as the major cause of erosion, although there is little scientific evidence to support this assumption. The carbonation of a drink is probably not as potentially erosive as its underlying acidity, because the titratable acidity of carbonic acid is low and is probably not particularly erosive (Milosevic 1998). As it is relatively easy for most patients to describe their diet in detail, acidic drinks receive considerable research interest and in most circumstances admitting to a high intake of acidic drink and foods causes little psychological damage. On the other hand, admitting to frequent gastric regurgitation or vomiting is associated with a certain degree of stigma in modern life and is much more difficult to investigate. Consequently, acidic foods and drinks have been labelled as the most important cause of dental erosion by some authorities.

Acidic working environments have been associated with dental erosion, most commonly on the buccal or facial surfaces of the upper anterior teeth, but improvements in health and safety at work have made this type of erosion uncommon in the Western world (Skogedal et al. 1977, Petersen and Gormsen 1991).

Appearance of erosion

Early enamel erosion appears smooth and rounded, and the surface contour is lost. Once the less mineralized and more soluble dentine is exposed the damage to teeth increases (Davis and Winter 1977). The palatal surface of the upper incisor teeth represents a good example of the pathogenesis of erosion. In the early stages the cingulum and surface characteristics are eroded, later as the erosion progresses dentine is exposed which is less resistant to acids and consequently the rate increases. Enamel along the palatal gingival margin often is preserved, producing an appearance not dissimilar to a veneer preparation sometimes used on anterior teeth. This 'lip' of enamel along the gingival margin is a useful means of gaining sufficient retention when using adhesive materials to restore the worn tooth surface.

Eventually, the damage can result in the complete loss of palatal enamel and dentine

which undermines the incisal edge and so slowly breaks away, leaving an uneven surface. The appearance of a worn incisal edge may incite a patient to seek advice for an otherwise symptomless process. Severe erosion may expose the pulps of the teeth or leave a very thin shell of dentine protecting the vital tissue. The pulps often maintain their vitality despite the extent of the damage, but in extreme cases the pulps die. Surprisingly, sensitivity is rare even in the most extreme cases whilst the pulp remains vital (but see Chapter 27).

Early enamel erosion on the labial or facial surfaces of upper anterior teeth is characterized by loss of surface definition and appears to be common, especially in children and young adolescents (O'Brien 1993). If the erosion progresses depressions may develop on the labial surfaces of the anterior teeth which are concave and may expose the yellower underlying dentine. In more severe cases of erosion other tooth surfaces, most notably the palatal surfaces of the upper anterior teeth, also become involved. Eventually the incisal edge is weakened and undermined and crumbles, shortening the height of the clinical crown. In some extreme cases the clinical crown is lost completely, exposing the root of the tooth.

Erosion on the occlusal surface of molars follows a similar course to incisors in that early erosion causes minor surface changes. However, as the erosion continues discrete, rounded hollows appear on the cusps of the teeth. The aetiology of these lesions can be ascribed to acids, but whether the source is dietary or gastric is unclear. As the erosion progresses these areas coalesce, increasing the area of destruction and eventually destroying the surface topography of the teeth. In severe cases the whole occlusal morphology of the tooth is lost, resulting in a surface flush with the gingival margin. In such cases the vitality of the tooth is usually lost.

Most restorative materials used in the mouth are insoluble in acids, apart from glass ionomers. Acid attacks the mineralized component of the tooth, leaving the restoration intact and resulting in what appears to be unsupported restoration (Figure 8.1). Glass ionomers are soluble in acids and their surface quickly deteriorates, especially in the first few weeks after placement, so these

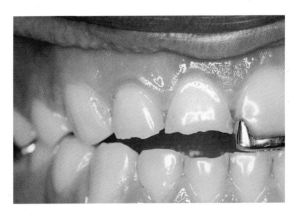

Figure 8.1

The incisal edge gold restoration was originally placed level with the adjacent teeth. Over time, acid from the stomach has eroded the unrestored central and lateral incisors, but the vertical dimension has remained unchanged, as the gold is resistant to the acid. The presence of restorations which are resistant to acids is a useful indicator of the activity of erosion.

materials are not normally used in patients with dental erosion.

The eating disorders and regurgitation erosion caused by gastro-oesophageal reflux are most commonly associated with erosion on the palatal surfaces of the upper anterior teeth (Hellstrom 1977, White *et al.* 1978, Robb and Smith 1990, Gilmour and Beckett 1994). The presence of stain on eroded surfaces can provide an indication of the activity of the erosion. Active erosions are usually seen as smooth and unstained, and tend not to be sensitive to hot or cold stimuli (Smith and Knight 1984). Inactive erosions become stained by dietary foods (such as tannin in tea and coffee) and nicotine if the patient smokes. This is important, because if the wear is progressing rapidly, treatment may be offered to restore the dentition, protecting the teeth from further damage.

Traditionally, dietary acids have been associated with erosion on the labial, facial or buccal surfaces of the upper incisors (Smith and Knight 1984). The labial surface was thought to be particularly prone to dietary acids, as this is the first tooth surface that acids contact on entering the mouth. The tooth surface appears smooth and somewhat dull, but as the erosion continues a 'saucer-shaped' lesion develops and the underlying yellow dentine begins to appear. Recently, the theory associating labial erosion with dietary acids has been challenged (Millward *et al.* 1994). Some patients are known to drink acidic beverages and then hold or 'swill' them in the palatal vault before swallowing. With this habit erosion is thought to occur on the palatal surfaces of teeth, which until recently has been associated with regurgitation erosion

Attrition

Wear caused by tooth-to-tooth contact without the influence of any other factor is called attrition. The amount of time that teeth are in contact during normal function is minute and is unlikely to compromise the longevity of a tooth. Contact of teeth for reasons other than eating can be termed bruxism and is the main cause of attrition seen in humans. The cause of bruxism remains unclear, but two possibilities have been suggested. Firstly, occlusal interferences may trigger bruxism and secondly the action may act as a form of stress relief used by the body overnight. Certainly, occlusal interferences are present in patients with severe attrition, but it is difficult to prove whether they were formed as a consequence of the wear or whether they stimulated it.

Appearance of attrition

In the early stages of attrition wear facets are formed on the occlusal surfaces of molar teeth and the incisal edges of anterior teeth become worn (Molnar *et al.* 1983). The surface of the wear facet is flat and flush with the opposing tooth on contact. Pure attrition is probably rare; however, when it does occur the teeth are seen to interdigitate accurately and there is equal wear on both arches (Figure 8.2). If the opposing surfaces do not contact evenly or there is a difference in the amount of wear in the opposite jaw the cause is probably multifactorial with erosion playing a major part.

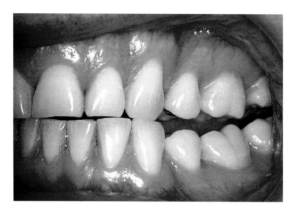

Figure 8.2

Pure attrition should have equal wear on both arches, as seen in this photograph. The facets should interdigitate accurately, but if they do not and it appears that wear is greater in one arch than the other, another aetiology of wear is active – usually erosion.

Abrasion

Abrasion has most commonly been associated with the cervical lesion or class V cavity. It is not clear why this surface is particularly prone to wear producing an angular lesion that is horizontal to the dentine margin and acute at the enamel margin. It is usually, but not exclusively, found on the buccal/facial surfaces of the upper canines and premolars, although it can be identified on the lingual surfaces of upper and lower molars. The cause of the cervical lesion remains unclear, but erosion, abrasion and attrition have all been implicated. Abfraction has also been suggested as a cause, although much of the evidence for the existence of this phenomenon remains theoretical (Lee and Eakle 1984, Grippo 1995). It has been suggested that abfraction weakens the tooth by forming stress concentrations near to the gingival margin and increasing the susceptibility to erosion and abrasion.

Symptoms associated with cervical lesions are common on this surface, whilst they are rare on the palatal surfaces of the upper anterior teeth, despite the latter sometimes involving near pulpal exposure. Why this occurs remains unclear and cannot be a reflection of the extent of the tooth wear, as early dentine exposure in palatal erosion is also not sensitive. Unusual patterns of wear caused by abrasion have been described, but are comparatively rare (Djemal *et al.* 1998).

Extra-oral appearance of tooth wear

When teeth wear they generally maintain contact with the opposing dentition by a process of alveolar compensation and the vertical dimension is conserved (Berry and Poole 1976, Dahl and Krogstad 1982). If the rate of wear is very rapid the teeth become shorter without the alveolar compensatory mechanism and a reduction in vertical dimension occurs, but this is rare. Clinically alveolar compensation is seen as a lowering of the gingival margin towards the incisal edge of adjacent teeth (Figure 8.3). If the wear is relatively localized margins of worn teeth do not appear flush with margins of the adjacent unworn teeth. The result is short clinical crowns at the original vertical dimension complicating their restoration, as more space is needed for tooth preparation.

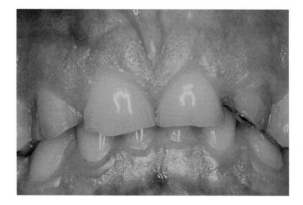

Figure 8.3

Wear on the palatal surface of the upper teeth has resulted in compensatory eruption of the lower incisors to maintain contact. The gingival margins of the lower incisors appear uneven, as the central incisors have erupted into the space created by the erosion on the palatal surfaces of the upper incisors. This process is called alveolar compensation.

Clinical assessment

Clinically tooth wear appears to progress relatively slowly, sometimes no obvious changes are seen on the teeth for many years. In most circumstances clinical assessment of tooth wear is achieved by comparing dated study casts taken at regular intervals to determine if the wear has progressed. The height from a restoration to a worn tooth surface can also make a convenient reference point to assess the rate of wear, as can the change in height of a clinical crown measured with dividers. None of these techniques can be considered accurate, as the surface characteristics of eroded teeth continually change, removing stable reference points. To complicate matters, tooth wear is probably episodic and therefore long-term review of patients with wear is necessary to identify the changes.

The main problem in measuring dental erosion, which has defeated previous workers, is the establishment of reproducible reference points which are themselves not affected by wear, particularly erosion (Bartlett *et al.* 1997). There have been some reports in the literature of using metal discs as reference points attached to the tooth surface or digital recordings, but to date these have only been used as research tools (Bartlett *et al.* 1997, Chadwick *et al.* 1997). Future research should concentrate on developing techniques to measure very small changes in the tooth surface so that preventive regimes can be scientifically and quantitatively assessed.

Conclusion

Tooth wear is an almost universal condition, with most people affected during their lives. In most cases the wear does not require treatment, but on occasion restorations are needed to preserve the longevity of the tooth. Erosion appears to be the most important factor in tooth wear and is either caused by the diet or stomach juice. The appearance of the eroded surface of teeth can provide some indication of the aetiology, but is by no means definitive.

References

Bartlett DW, Smith BGN (1995) The dental impact of eating disorders. *Dent Update* **21**:404–7.

Bartlett DW, Evans DF, Anggiansah A, Smith BGN (1996) A study of the association between gastro-oesophageal reflux and palatal dental erosion. *Br Dent J* **181**:125–32.

Bartlett DW, Blunt L, Smith BGN (1997) Measurement of tooth wear in patient with palatal erosion. *Br Dent J* **182**:179–84.

Bartlett DW, Coward PY, Nikkah C, Wilson RF (1998) The prevalence of tooth wear in a cluster sample of adolescent schoolchildren and its relationship with potential explanatory factors. *Br Dent J* **184**:125–9.

Berry DC, Poole DFG (1976) Attrition: possible mechanisms of compensation. *J Oral Rehabil* **3**:201–6.

Chadwick RG, Mitchell HL, Cameron I et al (1997) Development of a novel system for assessing tooth and restorations wear. *J Dent* **25**:41–7.

Dahl BL, Krogstad O (1982) The effect of partial bite raising splint on the occlusal face height. An X-ray cephalometric study in human adults. *Acta Odontol Scand* **40**:17–24.

Davis WB, Winter PJ (1997) Dietary erosion of adult dentine and enamel. *Br Dent J* **143**:116–19.

Djemal S, Darbar UR, Hemmings KW (1998) Case report: tooth wear associated with an unusual habit. *Eur J Prosthodont Rest Dent* **6**:29–32.

Gilmour AG, Beckett HA (1994) The voluntary reflux phenomenon. *Br Dent J* **175**:368–72.

Grippo JO (1995) Dental 'erosion' revisited. *J Am Dent Assoc* **126**:619–30.

Hellstrom I (1977) Oral complications in anorexia nervosa. *Scand J Dent Res* **85**:71–86.

Jarvinen V, Rytomaa II, Heinonen OP (1991) Risk factors in dental erosion. *J Dent Res* **70**:942–7.

Lee WC, Eakle WS (1984) Possible role of tensile stress in the aetiology of cervical erosive lesions of teeth. *J Prosthet Dent* **52**:374–9.

Millward A, Shaw L, Smith AJ et al (1994) The distribution and severity of tooth wear and the relationship between erosion and dietary constituents in a group of children. *Int J Paed Dent* **4**:151–7.

Milosevic A (1998) Toothwear: aetiology and presentation. *Dent Update* **25**:6–11.

Milosevic A, Lennon MA, Fear SC (1997) Risk factors associated with tooth wear in teenagers: a case control study. *Community Dent Health* **14**:143–7.

Molnar S, McKee JK, Molnar IM, Przybeck TR (1983) Tooth wear rates among contemporary Australian aborigines. *J Dent Res* **62**:562–5.

O'Brien M (1993) *Children's Dental Health in the United Kingdom*, 1–130. OPCS: London.

Petersen PE, Gormsen C (1991) Oral conditions among German battery factory workers. *Community Dent Oral Epidemiol* **19**:104–6.

Robb ND, Smith BGN (1990) Prevalence of pathological tooth wear in patients with chronic alcoholism. *Br Dent J* **169**:367–9.

Skogedal O, Silness J, Tangerud T et al (1977) Pilot study on dental erosion in a Norwegian zinc factory. *Community Dent Oral Epidemiol* **5**:248–51.

Smith BGN, Knight JK (1984) A comparison of patterns of tooth wear with aetiological factors. *Br Dent J* **157**:16–19.

Smith BGN, Robb ND (1996) The prevalence of tooth-wear in 1007 dental patients. *J Oral Rehabil* **23**:232–9.

White DK, Hayes RC, Benjamin RN (1978) Loss of tooth structure associated with chronic regurgitation and vomiting. *J Am Dent Assoc* **97**:833–5.

9
Prevalence and distribution of tooth wear

June H Nunn

Introduction

'There is no new thing under the Sun' (Ecclesiastes 9). Whilst many assume that tooth wear, and more specifically dental erosion, is a new phenomenon, that is not so. The earliest case reports of tooth wear go back to the last century (Royston 1808) and since then there have been many reports of such tooth tissue loss. It is important to distinguish between the different types of tooth wear, although in practice two or more types may be present in any one person, particularly with increasing age-related changes in the dentition. In earlier papers, there is confusion over this (Xhonga-Oja and Valdmanis 1986).

Attrition is usually found on incisal edges, occlusal surfaces, the palatal surfaces of upper anterior teeth or on the labial surfaces of lower anterior teeth. The affected teeth have flat-faceted areas that can be related to functional movements of the teeth together (Figure 9.1). In contrast, abrasion is characterized by rounded or V-shaped notching in the cervical area of the buccal surfaces of teeth in either jaw (Figure 9.2).

The appearance of erosion alone is quite different: the normal developmental lines are missing, giving the affected surface a smooth, glazed appearance. Initially, erosion will produce a 'frosted' surface but the additive effect of abrasion from soft tissues or a toothbrush, for example, will produce the smooth, glazed appearance. On smooth surfaces this usually occupies an area greater in width than depth. On anterior teeth, enamel may be thinned sufficiently for the edges to appear translucent and with further tissue loss there is chipping of the

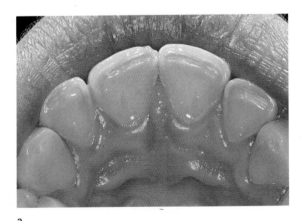

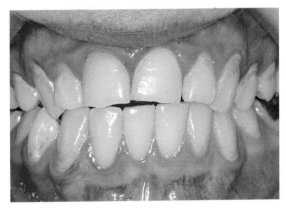

a   b

Figure 9.1

a and *b* Flattening of the incisal edges of permanent maxillary incisor teeth as a feature of the occlusion evidence of both attrition and erosion..

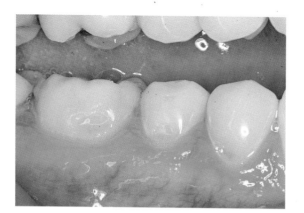

Figure 9.2

Abrasion lesions of the buccal cervical surfaces of teeth nos. 43 and 44.

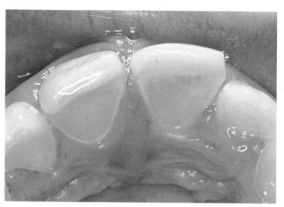

Figure 9.4

Wear into dentine on the palatal surfaces of these permanent maxillary incisor teeth. Note the 'shoulder-like' preparation adjacent to the margins of the teeth.

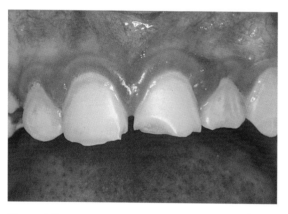

Figure 9.3

Thinned and chipped incisal edges in a young person with wear into dentine on the labial surfaces of his permanent maxillary incisor teeth.

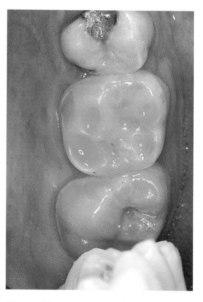

Figure 9.5

Erosion producing 'cupping' of the occlusal and palatal surfaces of this upper first permanent molar.

incisal edges (Figure 9.3). Palatally, loss of enamel may leave an appearance not dissimilar to a 'shoulder' preparation (well-defined margin) parallel to the margins of the gum, principally in the cervical area (Figure 9.4).

There may be evidence of 'cupping' on the occlusal surfaces of posterior teeth (Figure 9.5) and where there are restorations, their margins may be raised above the level of the surrounding tooth surface (Figure 9.6). Incisal edges may exhibit 'grooving', although it is important to distinguish

between this and the anatomical feature of a narrow line where the lingual and labial plates join at the incisal edge (see Figure 9.1a)

The clinical impression is that tooth wear is increasing, particularly in younger people. The assumption is that, from the presumed aetiolo-

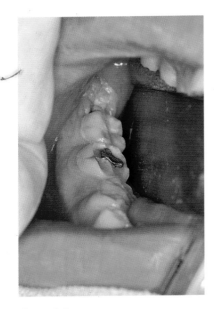

Figure 9.6

The amalgam restoration on this permanent mandibular molar 'standing proud' of the adjacent enamel surface.

gies, tooth wear is likely to persist as an issue for the dental profession. This is as much because the aetiological factors are unlikely to change very significantly, and because teeth are being retained for longer and patients' expectations are higher. Related to this is the greater significance of erosion in the process, linked in part to changes to healthier ways of eating (Bishop *et al.* 1997).

Almost without exception, the dental literature contains epidemiological evidence of tooth wear from case reports, in-vitro and in-vivo studies, cohort studies and some cross-sectional prevalence studies. The more significant of these different types of evidence, as they relate to prevalence of tooth wear but more specifically erosion, will now be considered.

Case reports

Although often dealing with only small numbers of subjects, case reports were the means whereby the dental profession became alerted

to the existence of excessive wear, more specifically erosion, in the dental literature. Levine (1973) warned against the use of excessive fruit and juice consumption in two cases of dental erosion in young females attending a dental hospital. The first subject drank fresh orange juice three times a day, each glass containing the juice of six oranges. The second subject, who was dieting, consumed the juice of 10 oranges and two whole oranges or apples per day, as well as a kilo of stewed rhubarb per week. Later papers have looked specifically at the drinking habits of younger children. Smith and Shaw (1987) highlighted the potential erosive effects of baby juices when given for prolonged periods of time in some form of comforter or bottle, used at night time. The authors cautioned against prolonged exposure and mentioned that in the case they reported, the juice had been given in a reservoir feeder for prolonged periods. In this case, that of a 2-year-old child, it was the palatal surfaces of the maxillary incisors that were worst affected, with pulpal exposure on one tooth. Asher and Read (1987) examined 12 patients aged between 9 and 15 years attending a dental hospital for their care. The children in this study were reported by parents to have drunk between one and three 725-ml bottles of fruit-flavoured drinks per week (equivalent to between 22 and 66 drinks if properly diluted, per week). It was obvious to the authors that many children drank the juice in a more concentrated form. The conclusions of that study were that erosion was directly related to the excessive consumption of low pH soft drinks. The study by Millward *et al.* (1994a) also involved a referred dental hospital population of children aged between 4 and 16.5 years. Of the 101 children, 49 were girls and 52 were boys. Using a modification of the Smith and Knight index of tooth wear (1984), they found that 21 children had 'mild' erosion, 45 'moderate' erosion and 35 'severe' erosion. Differences between the groups were highly statistically significant in relation to drinking habits. For example, of the children who had fruit-based drinks at bedtime, 60% had evidence of severe erosion compared with those with mild erosion of whom only 14% had such a bedtime drink. Many of these reports highlight the dangers of misuse of products, particularly drinks, which have frequently not been used in accordance with the manufacturer's instructions on dilution and often drunk in excessive amounts.

In a study involving adults referred to a dental hospital because of erosion (Eccles and Jenkins 1974), 26 subjects completed a dietary questionnaire. Although many of the subjects consumed large quantities of fruit and fruit-based drinks, the authors concluded that they were unable to relate the severity of the lesions to the quantity, frequency or period of consumption of the drinks involved.

Other reports of tooth surface loss in young adults have focused on some of the other causes of erosion rather than on purely dietary sources of acids. Eccles and Jenkins (1974), one of the first groups to propose an index for the measurement of erosion, recorded details of 19 patients, aged between 11 and 21 years, with erosion. In five of the patients, no cause could be elicited for the tooth tissue loss, in four patients a dietary cause alone was the reason, but in the remaining 11 subjects the most likely aetiology was some form of regurgitation, with or without an associated acid challenge from the diet.

Taylor et al. (1992) reported a case of asymptomatic gastro-oesophageal reflux in an 8-year-old child presenting initially as dental erosion. Appropriate drug therapy resolved the reflux phenomenon after thorough investigation. A case of voluntary reflux has been reported in the British literature and reference made to other, similar cases (Gilmour and Beckett 1993). This phenomenon may have serious psychiatric implications, but may only be detected by the dental team, because of its unusual presentation.

Bartlett and co-workers (1994) investigated 26 subjects presenting with occasional reflux symptoms and palatal dental erosion using two pH electrodes in the oesophagus, as well as an oral pH monitor, over a period of 18 h. Eighteen patients were diagnosed as having pathological gastro-oesophageal reflux on the basis of the proportion of time the oesophageal pH registered below a value of 4.

In Finland the problem of dental erosion was studied the other way around, with a dental examination of patients presenting with upper gastro-intestinal symptoms (Järvinen et al. 1988). Forty-four patients had pathology associated with increased acid output and of these, seven patients aged from 51 to 59 years had dental erosion as classified by the criteria of Eccles and Jenkins

(1974). Three of the patients also had markedly reduced salivary secretion rates and one of these patients also reported using acidic drinks. Another Finnish study reported prevalence data on erosion (Aine et al. 1993), but this time in children aged between 22 months and 16 years attending an outpatient clinic for gastro-oesophageal disease. Only two of the children had presented at the clinic because of dental symptoms, 10 had chronic respiratory problems and only two had overt gastro-intestinal symptoms. None of the children had consumed acid beverages or fruit juices daily. Erosive lesions were found in 13 of the 15 children (87%). Reflux during sleep or frequent daytime episodes of reflux appeared to produce the most severe erosion.

Case-control (cohort) studies

Järvinen et al. (1991) reported a case-control (cohort) study investigating factors that were thought to influence dental erosion. The study involved 106 subjects aged between 13 and 73 years with dental erosion selected from general dental practices in Helsinki. These patients were matched with a control group. Because five erosion cases were detected (according to strictly defined criteria) among 100 controls in the random sample from the source population (the patients of Helsinki dentists), the prevalence of erosion (with 95% confidence limits) was estimated from this sample. In only one of the study cases was it not possible to elicit a cause. For the remainder, dietary factors were isolated in 32 cases, gastric regurgitation in 27 cases and a combination of factors for 46 patients. Citrus fruits and soft drinks were identified as being the main causative agents for dental erosion in this Finnish population, being consumed by between one-third and one-half of the subjects. Gastric symptoms, reported at least weekly by the subjects, varied between vomiting in 11 cases to a sour taste in 32 subjects. A logistic multivariate model applied to these data gave the relative importance of the associations between erosion and the variables identified. Despite some possible deficiencies in the way the data were analysed, the study was an important one because it further highlighted the need to investigate salivary flow as a factor in the aetiology of erosion.

Lussi (1996) reported data on the change in tooth wear over time in a 6-year longitudinal study in Switzerland, indicating that erosion progresses. Explanatory factors such as dietary habits, gastric disturbances, drug histories, radiotherapy, salivary gland function and risk occupations were evaluated, but the data were presented as an abstract only.

Milosevic et al. (1997) undertook a cohort study on a population of 14–15-year-olds in the UK. Risk factors were identified in the cases using age, sex and place of education as matching criteria for the control group. Using a logistic regression model on the paired data they were able to demonstrate only borderline significance ($P = 0.055$) for carbonated beverages as a potential risk factor. Other acidic components of the diet were significant, excluding the use of ketchup or sauces and fruit juice as drinks. Despite evidence to the contrary (Bartlett and Smith 1995), regurgitation was not identified as a potential risk factor in this group of young people.

Wear at the cervical area was the subject of another case-control study by Bader et al. (1996). The authors acknowledged that the aetiology for these lesions is likely to be multi-factorial – a combination of erosion, abrasion and tooth flexure, so-called abfraction – a view supported by other workers (Yap and Neo 1995).

Prevalence studies – special populations

The earliest study to publish details of a prevalence survey was that of Sognnaes et al. (1972). These workers examined 10,000 extracted teeth from Southern California and showed that about 1700 teeth (18%) had erosive lesions, with incisor teeth most commonly affected. A similar survey (Robb et al. 1991), but this time on skulls dating back to Roman and Anglo-Saxon Britain, was carried out to look for evidence of this form of tooth wear. A total of 151 adult skulls were assessed for wear using the index of Smith and Knight (1984). A control group was made up of 947 subjects who formed part of a separate study to assess pathological tooth wear in a dentist-attending population in the south-east of England. Of the 151 skulls, 30 (19.9%) showed levels of wear greater than those in the popula-

tion as a whole. The site of the tooth surface loss led the authors to conclude that the causal factor was gastric regurgitation.

Most cases in this group had evidence of severe wear on the lingual surfaces of both upper and lower teeth. The wear patterns occurred in all age ranges, although they were more severe in the older groups, and affected both men (13 individuals) and women (9 individuals). In all three age groups, occlusal wear was greater in the skeletal populations than in the modern group and became more marked with age. This was to be expected, given the coarser diet of the historic group. Generally, the levels of lingual and buccal wear were the same in both populations, suggesting that the occlusal surfaces rather than the sides of the teeth bore the brunt of the coarser diet in the historic group. The cervical areas of the teeth were subject to less wear in the ancient population group.

A more recent study involving distinct ethnic groups in Northern Borneo (Milosevic and Lo 1996) found, as in the study by Robb et al. (1991), that explanatory factors again were different to those accepted as more prevalent in Western population groups. Although the sample in Borneo was a referred hospital population, the wear experienced reflected the aetiology. Thus, tobacco chewing and the crushing and eating of bones gave a distinctive pattern of wear, with more occlusal and buccal surfaces affected. The consumption of carbonated beverages and fresh fruit was low and not positively related to the tooth wear observed.

Another discrete cultural group, Saudi male military recruits, also presented with 'pronounced' dental erosion (Johansson et al. 1996). This was assessed not only clinically, but also from study casts and colour transparencies, using an index modified from Eccles (1979) to take into account the different types of wear (erosion, attrition and abrasion), as well as the surfaces affected. A questionnaire covered the topics of food and beverages consumed, medication taken, parafunctional and oral hygiene habits, stomach problems, reported bruxism and symptoms of a dry mouth. Unlike the findings of the study by Milosevic and Lo (1996), there was a strong relationship between the severity of tooth erosion in this group of young men and consumption of soft drinks, an average of 247 litres per person annually.

In the USA, a survey of incoming patients to the dental hospitals in Los Angeles and Boston (Xhonga-Oja and Valdmanis 1986) purported to look specifically at the prevalence of erosion in 527 patients (age range 14–80 years) of both sexes. However, the illustrations contained in the paper indicated that many of these lesions resembled abrasion rather than erosion. The prevalence of erosion as described by the authors was found to vary by city and by tooth type. Patients in Boston had a lower prevalence of erosion than the Los Angeles population, but minor erosion was a more frequent finding in Los Angeles. In the Boston population there was a lower prevalence of moderate erosion on anterior teeth, with the maximum frequency of severe erosion predominantly on the maxillary and mandibular molars. Interestingly, a slightly higher proportion of the Boston population had received fluoridated water (11% versus 0%), but a higher proportion of the Boston groups were frequent consumers of citrus fruits (16.9% versus 0.3%). Two of these three studies (Sognnaes et al. 1972, Xhonga-Oja and Valdmanis 1983) have not only been retrospective, but also the way in which the criteria on tooth wear were applied in them has cast doubt on the results, as presented for dental erosion exclusively.

A much larger study of adult patients (n = 1007) was undertaken in the south-east of England (Smith and Robb 1996) using the index of Smith and Knight (1984). This tooth wear index incorporates threshold levels to take into account wear that is acceptable at a given age and wear that is not, so-called *pathological* wear. The results of this study indicated that young people under 26 years of age have accelerated wear, as well as a significant proportion of the older age groups. This is of concern because, with greater retention of teeth into old age, a high prevalence of wear may impose a significant burden of treatment need in the subjects' advanced years.

A number of workers have investigated a link between exposure to acids in the workplace and the prevalence of dental erosion. The study by Tuominen and Tuominen (1991) looked at workers in four Finnish factories who were exposed to inorganic acid fumes. A sample of 186 workers was drawn from the factories. Of the 157 dentate workers, 76 worked in an environment containing acid fumes and 81 workers not

exposed to such conditions were used as the controls. The mouth prevalence of erosion was found to be 18.4% amongst the exposed workers and 8.6% in the controls. The affected workers had more eroded teeth than the controls, with upper anterior teeth especially involved. Petersen and Gormsen (1991) surveyed workers exposed to sulphuric acid fumes in a German battery factory. The prevalence of erosion was assessed after the method of ten Bruggen Cate (1968) amongst 61 dentate males in the age range 20–58 years. Evidence of erosion was found in 31% of the subjects, with 56% of the workers complaining about sharp and thin teeth and 29% complaining about short teeth. Painful teeth were reported by 17% of the subjects.

Anorexia and bulimia nervosa, potentially fatal disorders, are becoming more prevalent and are not confined to female populations, as is commonly assumed. Because of the frequency of vomiting seen in these patients, as well as the high consumption of acidic foods seen in some, it is likely that dental erosion would be a feature of the dentitions of such subjects. Eliciting a history can be difficult, not only in these patients, but also in patients who are alcoholics; all have a psychiatric component.

In a study of 17 anorexic patients (14 females, three males) by Hurst et al. (1977), a prevalence of 47% erosion was recorded. Loss of tooth tissue was greatest amongst the vomiters compared with the regurgitators, although there was no information given on the frequency of vomiting. Most of the subjects also ate large quantities of fruit regularly. A later paper from the USA (Roberts and Li 1987) looked at both bulimics and anorexics, with a mean age of 23 years and 28 years respectively, but without a control group (all were females). The prevalence of palatal erosion of maxillary anterior teeth was 35% for the anorexia patients and 33% for the bulimics. Similar results were recorded by Hellström (1977). Robb et al. (1995) and Milosevic and Slade (1989) divided up their study populations according to their eating disorder as well as including a control group. Both studies used the Smith and Knight index of tooth wear (1984) for assessment. In the former study all the experimental groups had significantly more wear than the control group. In the subgroups who vomited, there was significantly more wear of upper teeth. There was no reported difference between patients who routinely brushed their teeth after vomiting and those who did not. The authors commented that some of the clinical findings in this study were difficult to explain, but may have arisen as a consequence of the difficulty of obtaining an accurate history from some of these patients.

In the other study from the UK, Milosevic and Slade (1989) reported a prevalence of erosion of 6% for the control group of psychiatric patients without eating disorders and a range of 28% (bulimics with self-induced vomiting) to 42% (bulimics without self-induced vomiting) for those with eating disorders. Although the authors were unable to show a linear relationship between vomiting frequency, duration or total number of vomiting episodes and tooth wear, they did comment that the frequency of pathological tooth wear was significantly high in those bulimics who vomited, especially if the total number of vomiting episodes in a month was >1100. As with the study by Robb et al. (1995), more of those who vomited frequently had pathological tooth wear. In South Africa, a small study (Jones and Cleaton-Jones 1989) of bulimic women gave a similar prevalence rate for the 22 controls of 7% but a much higher prevalence of 69% for the 11 bulimics, albeit using a different index of erosion compared with the other studies.

Unlike the previous disorders, alcoholism tends to affect males more than females. In a study of 37 alcoholic patients with age- and sex-matched controls (Robb and Smith 1990) the amount of erosion was found to be worst in those who consumed alcohol continuously rather than in episodic binges, with 40% of the study group showing evidence of erosion on palatal surfaces of maxillary teeth.

Cross-sectional studies

A random sample of Swiss adults was selected in order to examine the prevalence of dental erosion (Lussi et al. 1991). Examinations of 391 people were carried out in their own homes using a scoring system modified from that of Linkosalo and Markkanen (1985). Of the total sample, 197 were aged 26–30 and 194 were between 46 and 50 years of age. With regard to

facial lesions, 7.7% of the younger group and 13.2% of the older group had one or more erosive lesions with involvement of dentine. For occlusal surfaces, 29.9% of the younger group and 42.6% of the older group had erosion involving dentine, with 3.2 and 3.9 teeth affected, respectively. Only 2% of subjects had lingual erosion and in these there was a correlation with chronic vomiting. For the remainder of the subjects, there was a statistically significant relationship between observed erosion and dietary habits such as intake of fruit juices, citrus or other fruits.

Population prevalence studies in children have only been reported in the UK. In 1992 a study examined 1035 14-year-old children for the presence of dental erosion (Milosevic et al. 1994). 51% of the sample were males and 49% were female. In all, 30% of the children had exposed dentine, mainly incisally and more commonly in females. In addition, 80 children (8%) also had exposed dentine on occlusal and/or lingual surfaces. A slight inverse relationship was found between the severity of tooth wear and levels of deprivation in the city studied, in that as the levels of deprivation worsened, so the prevalence of tooth wear increased. Conversely, in a study of 178 4- and 5-year-old children carried out in the West Midlands (Millward et al. 1994b), there was a positive correlation between socio-economic group and the prevalence of erosion, the children from the low socio-economic groups having less erosion. For example, 19% of children in the high socio-economic group had severe erosion (surface scoring 3 or 4 on the tooth wear index) compared with only 4% of children from a low socio-economic background. Overall, nearly half the children showed some erosion, with the most commonly affected site being the palatal surfaces of maxillary incisors.

The National Survey of Child Dental Health carried out in the UK in 1993 (O'Brien 1994) included for the first time an assessment of dental erosion of maxillary incisor teeth of a representative random sample of 5–15-year-old children. The index used was a modification of the Smith and Knight (1984) index, but it assessed the amount of tooth loss from the palatal surfaces of maxillary incisor teeth in both the primary and permanent dentitions. Results from the calibration exercise conducted during the dentists' training for the survey (standard deviation per unit ranging from 0.54 to 2.83) indicated that dentists found it difficult to agree in determining the presence of early wear of the enamel, so comparisons between countries on this basis may be suspect. As dentists from different countries did not examine the same children it is not possible to verify this from the calibrations, and variation may be random. However, it is suggested that the low levels of agreement between dentists in the case of enamel erosion are borne in mind when considering the results described in this chapter. Erosion into dentine and the dental pulp are easier to identify, and the importance of this in terms of treatment implications is considered to be greater. The results showed that over half the 5- and 6-year-old children had evidence of erosion, and in nearly a quarter, dentine was involved. Loss of tooth tissue was greatest on palatal surfaces of the incisors, with 52% of 5-year-olds affected, compared with only 18% presenting with buccal erosion. In the permanent dentition, for those over 11 years of age, nearly a quarter had evidence of erosion, with 2% of teenagers having wear into dentine.

A year later, a similarly conducted mainland UK survey on 1.5–4.5-year-old children was published, using the same criteria on erosion as the National Child Dental Health Survey (Hinds and Gregory 1995). However, the training of dentists for the school and pre-school children's dental health surveys differed; dentists working on the former survey attended a 2-day residential course while those working on the less complicated pre-school children's survey attended only a 1-day briefing and had less detailed written instructions. Overall, 10% of children had erosion of the buccal surfaces of their primary incisor teeth and 19% had erosion affecting the palatal surface. Erosion into dentine or pulp on the palatal surface affected 8% of children. Accompanying the oral health survey of these pre-school children was a large diet and nutrition enquiry (Gregory et al. 1995). Data from this survey indicated that there was a trend towards a relationship between the frequent consumption of sweetened drinks and carbonated beverages and dental erosion: 32% of 3.5–4.5-year-old children who consumed carbonated drinks (including low calorie carbonated drinks) had evidence of palatal surface erosion compared with 28% of the same age group who

consumed such drinks less frequently. The data on buccal surface erosion were 19% and 12% respectively. Also, a trend was observed between bedtime consumption of drinks and the prevalence of this form of tooth wear, with 41% of 3.5–4.5-year-old children who consumed drinks containing non-milk extrinsic sugars (NMES) – which includes fruit juices, squashes and carbonated drinks – showing evidence of palatal surface erosion compared with 30% of children who did not have drinks containing NMES.

Although these two UK-based surveys studied a continuum of ages – 1.5–4.5-year-old and 5–15-year-old children – the training of dentists for the collection of clinical data for each survey was different. Whilst the calibration data indicated some variability between examiners, the data on the more advanced wear appeared to endorse the clinical impression that tooth wear, measured in this age group as erosion, was clinically significant.

A study utilizing the same criteria as those from the national dental health surveys of young people (O'Brien 1994, Hinds and Gregory 1995), was undertaken in 3-year-old children in the north-west of England (Jones and Nunn 1995). A total sample of 135 children was examined by one calibrated examiner: 29% of children had erosion into dentine, primarily of the palatal surfaces of the maxillary incisors.

A later study on UK adolescents confirmed the widespread nature of erosion in young people's teeth (Bartlett et al. 1998) and raised important issues about the complex relationship between the possible aetiological factors. However, the authors did comment about the shortcoming of cross-sectional studies of this type when trying to demonstrate a relationship between the observed clinical effects and explanatory factors. In this school-based study of 11–14-year-old young people, 57% of the subjects had tooth wear, as measured by the Smith and Knight (1984) index, on more than 10 teeth, but involvement of dentine was rare. This latter finding contrasts with the studies by Millward et al. (1994a,b) and Milosevic et al. (1994) where dentine involvement was commoner in their study groups. However, there was closer agreement between the findings in this study and those of the National Child Dental Health Survey (O'Brien 1994) on the prevalence of erosion in this age group.

As part of the National Diet and Nutrition Survey programme in the UK, the results of the oral health survey second cohort, the over-65s, has been published recently (Steele *et al.* 1998). The survey was carried out on 753 free-living and 410 institutionalized elderly people. As well as an oral examination the survey included a 4-day weighed dietary record. Using criteria modified from Smith and Knight (1984), the survey reported prevalence data for wear, both coronal and cervical. Fifty-two per cent of the free-living sample had some evidence of coronal wear to a moderate degree, i.e. extensive exposure of dentine, but not necessarily indicating a need for treatment. This degree of wear was limited to surfaces with tooth-to-tooth contact, usually the incisal and occlusal edges. More severe and extensive wear was concentrated in a small proportion of the population, overall 15% were affected in the age range 65–85+ years. Moderate and severe wear was more prevalent in men than women, 60 and 42% respectively. Moderate to severe wear of coronal surfaces was more prevalent in the north of the country as compared with the south, a prevalence of 35% in the south-east of England compared with 65% for Scotland and the north of England. The pattern of coronal wear for the institutionalized population was similar to the free-living sample. Cervical wear affected 32% of the population. The regional differences for coronal wear were still present, as were the age differences, with more wear with increasing age a feature for these populations.

The 1998 National Adult Dental Health Survey of adults in the UK has incorporated a similar index of tooth wear into the oral health examination and results from this survey should be available in late 1999.

Measurement of wear

With the increasing trend for longevity, not only of the population but also of teeth, interest in the assessment of the impact of age and external forces on the teeth has grown. Whilst the assessment of tooth wear is not new, the very multitude of indices available is testament to the difficulties encountered in making such an assessment in a valid and reproducible way. A number of different indices or classifications of tooth wear exist today. One of the earliest was that of Broca (1879) and others are listed in Table 9.1.

Each successive author has modified or replaced criteria having found, presumably, deficiencies with existing indices (Donnachie and Walls 1995). Almost all the indices are applied with the intention of quantifying tooth tissue loss, often from a variety of causes, by a qualitative evaluation of wear as it presents clinically. On occasions this evaluation is combined with an estimate of the area of the tooth surface involved.

Whilst there may be different issues involved in the presentation of wear in children and

Table 9.1 Indices for the classification of tooth wear.

Authors	Sample	Type of evaluation
Broca (1879)	(Not available)	Qualitative
Lysell (1958)	Prehistoric skulls	Qualitative
Parma (1960)	(Not available)	Qualitative
Ten Bruggen Cate (1968)	Chemical factory	Qualitative: erosion
Hansson and Nilner (1975)	Shipyard workers	Qualitative: length reduction
Eccles (1979)	Dental hospital patients	Qualitative: area- and surface-specific
WHO (1979)	Screening surveys	Qualitative/length reduction
Egermark-Eriksson (1982)	Adolescents	Qualitative/length reduction
Sandin (1983)	Chemical industry	Qualitative erosion/abrasion
Smith and Knight (1984)	Dental hospital patients	Qualitative: area of wear facet
Linkosalo and Markkanen (1985)	Lactovegetarians	Qualitative: surface- and extent-specific
Carlsson *et al.* (1985)	Rats	Qualitative: area of wear facet
Oilo *et al.* (1987)	Brain-damaged people	Qualitative: based on need for treatment
Gourdon *et al.* (1987)	Stone diagnostic casts	Quantitative measurements
Johannson *et al.* (1996)	Young Saudi men	Qualitative and quantitative

adolescents as opposed to adults, new indices to take this into account have been slow to emerge. In the UK, a simple, qualitative index was devised to be used on index teeth, for speed of examination in the oral health survey component of the National Diet and Nutrition Survey of pre-school children, as well as the decennial children's dental health survey (O'Brien 1994). Whilst calibration of a large number of examiners has been a challenge, the experience gained from this has been used to devise a more appropriate screening index of erosion for use nationally in monitoring cross-sectional surveys of child and adolescent dental health in the UK. This is currently being piloted but has yet to be reported.

References

Aine L, Baer M, Maki M (1993) Dental erosion caused by gastroesophageal reflux disease in children. *J Dent Child* **60**: 210–14.

Asher C, Read MJF (1987) Early enamel erosion in children associated with the excessive consumption of citric acid. *Br Dent J* **162**: 384–7.

Bader JD, McClure F, Scurria MS et al (1996) Case control study of non-carious cervical lesions. *Community Dent Oral Epidemiol* **24**: 286–91.

Bartlett D, Smith BG (1995) Survey of children's dental health. *Br Dent J* **179**: 160.

Bartlett DW, Evans DF, Anggiansah A et al (1994) The relationship between gastroesophageal reflux and palatal dental erosion. *Gut* **35** (abstract no. 57).

Bartlett DW, Coward PY, Nikkah C, Wilson RF (1998) The prevalence of tooth wear in a cluster sample of adolescent school-children and its relationship with potential explanatory factors. *Br Dent J* **184**: 125–9.

Bishop K, Kelleher M, Briggs P, Joshi R (1997) Wear now? An update on the aetiology of tooth wear. *Quint Int* **28**: 305–13.

Broca P (1879) Instructions relatives a l'étude anthropologique du système dentaire. *Bull Soc Anthropol Paris* 128–63.

Carlsson GE, Johansson A, Lundqvist S (1985) Occlusal wear. A follow-up study of 18 subjects with extensively worn dentitions. *Acta Odont Scand* **43**: 83–90.

Donnachie MA, Walls AWG (1995) The tooth wear index: a flawed epidemiological tool in an ageing population group. *Community Dent Oral Epidemiol* **24**: 152–8.

Eccles JD (1979) Dental erosion of non-industrial origin. A clinical survey and classification. *J Prosth Dent* **42**: 649–53.

Eccles JD, Jenkins WG (1974) Dental erosion and diet. *J Dent* **2**: 153–9.

Ecclesiastes 9, Old Testament.

Egermark-Eriksson I (1982) Malocclusion and some functional recordings of the masticatory system in Swedish schoolchildren. *Swed Dent J* **6**: 9–20.

Gilmour AG, Beckett HA (1993) The voluntary reflux phenomenon. *Br Dent J* **175**: 368–72.

Gourdon AM, Buyle-Bodin Y, Woda A, Faraj M (1987) Development of an abrasion index. *J Prosthet Dent* **57**: 358–61.

Gregory J, Collins DL, Davies PSW et al (1995) *National Diet and Nutrition Survey: Children aged 1½ to 4½ years.* Volume 1: Report of the diet and nutrition survey. HMSO: London.

Hanson T, Nilner M (1975) A study of the occurrence of symptoms of diseases of the temporomandibular joint masticatory musculature and related structures. *J Oral Rehabil* **1**: 213–24.

Hellström I (1977) Oral complications in anorexia nervosa. *Scand J Dent Res* **85**: 71–86.

Hinds K, Gregory JR (1995) *National Diet and Nutrition Survey: Children aged 1½ to 4½ years.* Volume 2: Report of the dental survey. Office of Population Censuses and Surveys. HMSO: London.

Hurst PS, Lacey JH, Crisp AH (1977) Teeth, vomiting and diet: a study of the dental characteristics of seventeen anorexia nervosa patients. *Post Med J* **53**: 298–305.

Järvinen V, Meurman JH, Hyvarinen H et al (1988) Dental erosion and upper gastrointestinal disorders. *Oral Surg* **65**: 298–303.

Järvinen VK, Rytömaa II, Heinonen OP (1991) Risk factors in dental erosion. *J Dent Res* **70**: 942–7.

Johansson A-K, Johansson A, Birkhed D et al (1996) Dental erosion, soft drink intake and oral health in young Saudi men and development of a system for assessing erosive anterior tooth wear. *Acta Odont Scand* **54**: 369–77.

Jones RRH, Cleaton-Jones P (1989) Depth and area of dental erosions, and dental caries, in bulimic women. *J Dent Res* **68**: 1275–8.

Jones SG, Nunn JH (1995) The dental health of 3-year-old children in east Cumbria 1993. *Community Dent Health* **12**: 161–6.

Levine RS (1973) Fruit juice erosion – an increasing danger? *J Dent* **2**: 85–8.

10
Methodologies and instrumentation to measure tooth wear: future perspectives

Nicola X West and Klaus D Jandt

Introduction

There appears to be a general consensus that tooth wear has increased in prevalence and severity over recent decades. This conclusion could of course be artefactual and result from increased research and diagnosis in the area (Shaw and Smith 1994). Case report data on erosion due to acidic food stuffs are plentiful; however, it is only recently that well constructed surveys have been conducted that highlight the problem of dental erosion (Milosevic et al. 1993, Office of Population Censuses and Surveys 1993, Millward et al. 1994).

There are a number of possible explanations for the apparent increased incidence of excessive tooth wear. In many countries, a considerably greater number of teeth are retained into old age than was previously the case (Järvinen et al. 1991). Further, the aetiological factors themselves may have increased in prevalence (Imfeld 1996), notably dietary acid intake (National Food and Drink Survey Committee 1956–72), with a 56% increase in consumption of soft drinks in the UK over the past 10 years (Zenith International 1997). This equates to about 0.5 litre per person per day. However, amongst the young generations this is believed to be near 1 litre per day. Furthermore, gastro-oesophageal reflux disease (GORD) is known to affect 7% of the British population on a daily basis (Colin Jones 1996).

Measurement in vitro

The majority of the research on tooth wear has been based on in-vitro models, which are extremely useful for demonstrating the erosive propensity of a substance, but cannot replicate the oral environment with all its biological variations. Similar methods are difficult to apply in vivo, primarily because of controlling for numerous variables and difficulties in making accurate measurements of tooth substance loss. The in-vitro environment does have advantages in that it is possible to control variables such as exposure time, nature of the agent to be studied individually or in combination, tissue type, temperature and acidic concentration. Further, large numbers of teeth can be examined over relatively short periods of time, and a high level of standardization can be achieved. However, extrapolation to the oral environment is impossible to calculate and only trends and indications as to the true extent of tooth wear can be obtained.

Macroscopic changes

One method of measuring tooth wear and tooth wear potential is achieved by direct examination and assessment of a tooth or sample of dental hard tissue, with a scale required for the purpose of quantification.

A grading system for rats' teeth was devised by Restarski and co-workers (1945a, 1945b), and this was subsequently modified by other groups including McClure and Ruzicka (1946), Zipkin and McClure (1949), Holloway and co-workers (1958) and Hartles and Wagg (1962). Although widely used at the time, the system had limited sensitivity. A simplified grading system developed by McDonald and Stookey (1973) was more rapid, but again of only moderate sensitivity. Other indices for measuring wear are also found in the literature including one by Hooper (1995), giving a comprehensive grading system.

Whilst of value, macroscopic evaluations of tooth wear provide only an estimate of tooth tissue loss, as accurate tooth wear is impossible to determine visually.

Polarized light microscopy

Polarized light microscopy has been used extensively in the dental field, particularly looking at carious lesions. It has also been employed to assess erosion lesions, primarily to estimate the extent of subsurface loss with colour changes due to material porosity. Smith and Shaw (1987) investigated the effect of exposure of extracted primary teeth to fruit juices. Exposed windows of tooth tissue were examined macroscopically before sectioning for observation under polarized light. Although this is a useful methodology, meaningful qualitative data are difficult to obtain and only trends of tooth wear can be determined.

Surface profilometry

In a study of erosion brought about by sports drinks, Meurman et al. (1990) examined areas of bovine tooth specimens (1 × 3 mm) by different techniques. Loss of tooth material was measured by profilometry, driving a spherical diamond tip across the surface of the specimen using a load of 5 mg. This method has the advantage of allowing measurement of the actual depth of the erosion and also the dissolution rate of the enamel. Other researchers,

including Davis and Winter (1977, 1980), have used this technique to measure loss of dentine and enamel after potential erosive exposure. West et al. (1998a) investigated the effects of brushing desensitizing toothpastes, their solid and liquid phases and detergents on dentine and acrylic by this methodology, using a surfometer with 0.01 μm resolution of accuracy. Profilometry gives an accurate and reproducible measurement of surface loss, but only in a two-dimensional field.

Microhardness

Surface microhardness is another technique for assessing tooth wear. Instruments measure the difference between the depth of penetration of an indentor into a specimen under load. With the Wallace Micro Indentation Tester (H.W. Wallace, St James Road, Croydon, Surrey, UK) the ratio of the movement between the digital gauge and the table is 10:1 and a 0.002 mm dial gauge is used to measure indentation in units of 0.0002 mm, sensitivity being > 0.1 μm. The use of instrument coordinates on the specimen platform should ensure that indentations do not overlap. This technique was used by a number of researchers (Lussi et al. 1993, van Meerbeck et al. 1993, Attin et al. 1997, Dodds et al. 1997) to distinguish between tissue hardness characteristics before and after exposure to erosive factors.

West et al. (1998b) investigated the erosive potential of orange juice compared to water in a single blind, cross-over, randomized, single centre trial conducted according to good clinical practice (GCP). Microhardness of the human enamel specimens was determined and significant differences ($P <0.05$) were found between the exposed and unexposed sites for specimens exposed to orange juice but not for water. Further, variation in the results obtained from the microhardness of the enamel exposed to orange juice would suggest subsurface demineralization. Hence the possibilty of studying remineralization by this method could also be considered.

Grenby (1996) comments that hardness data are qualitative and may not measure the full extent of hard tissue loss by erosive attack.

Scanning electron microscopy

Scanning electron microscopy allows observation of the surface with high resolution and depth of field. However, the possibility of tissue shrinkage due to loss of fluid when the specimen is prepared for viewing and subsequent alteration of morphology must be borne in mind (Lambrechts *et al.* 1981). Following a similar technique to Davis and Winter (1977), Absi *et al.* (1992) found that dietary fluids (particularly red and white wine, citrus fruit juices, apple juice and yoghurt) readily produced etching effects on dentine in scanning electron microscopy studies. In another investigation of the effects of acids and dietary substances on root-planed and burred dentine in vivo (Addy *et al.* 1987), extracted teeth were cleaned in hypochlorite and 70% ethanol before being exposed for 5 min. Etching was assessed by sputter-coating the dried specimens with gold before examining them under the scanning electron microscope. Grading the severity of etching was on a scale from 0 (no tubules visible) to +++ (many tubules seen). Meurman and co-workers (1990) used a similar method, with microphotographs taken at magnifications of ×400 and ×2000.

More recently, Millward and co-workers (1995) described a replica impression technique of 'windows' on extracted teeth, examining castings by scanning electron microscopy after gold sputtering. The model is said to mimic conditions at the tooth surface in vivo and to be highly reproducible.

Another useful technique is environmental scanning electron microscopy, involving no sample preparation and allowing viewing on multiple occasions pre- and post-treatment (Farley and Shah 1991, Zammitti *et al.* 1997). The surface of specimens may also be analysed with an electron probe for further information.

The scanning electron microscope has the disadvantages of being expensive and requiring skill on the part of the operator. However, the technique is reproducible, the tooth surface reproduction is good and results may be both qualitative and quantitative (Grenby 1996). However, this technique will not yield as much information or be as detailed as many of the other methodologies available to assess tooth wear.

Microradiography

Longitudinal microradiographic methods for the measurement of mineral loss due to acid dissolution have been described by Bashir and Lagerlof (1996) and Klimek and co-workers (1996). In the latter study, the correlation between longitudinal microradiography and the results obtained by profilometry was very good. However, the total mineral loss expressed in micrometres measured by longitudinal microradiography was significantly higher ($P < 0.05$) than the depth of erosions measured by profilometry, indicating that there might be a subsurface demineralization in the eroded area.

The use of transverse microradiography for the detection and quantification of mineral loss due to acid erosion has been described by Hall *et al.* (1997) and Amaechi *et al.* (1998). In the former study, measurements made by profilometry were used as a 'gold standard' against which results were compared. Correlation coefficients for comparisons between microradiographic and profilometric data for both enamel and dentine specimens were very good. Sample *t* tests demonstrated that the microradiographic technique could detect early erosion, i.e. discriminate between erosion times of < 1 h. The authors concluded that transverse microradiography was a useful and acceptable method for the measurement of early mineral loss from thin sections of tooth tissue. Previously, this has been possible only by the use of longitudinal or wavelength-dependent microradiographic methods. These methods have traditionally used thick specimens and failed to detect mineral loss at the levels detected by transverse microradiography (Arends and ten Bosch 1992).

Digital image analysis

Between 1940 and 1990, various digital analysis techniques which had applications in vivo and in vitro were developed and published. With the increasing sensitivity and versatility of computer-aided evaluation and recording equipment, digital image analysis has improved in accuracy and reliability, as well as reducing time and labour requirements (Mistry and Grenby 1993). The sample is placed in a fixed position and imaged by a video camera. A feature, such as a ridge or other limit of eroded tissue, is chosen as a 'threshold' between different zones of attack which can be discerned, and its position is traced and stored. The area and depth of the damage to the enamel can then be calculated and statistical comparisons between different treatments performed. This technique is very precise and sensitive, and can be used both qualitatively and quantitatively (Grenby 1996). However, the equipment and programmes required are expensive and problems can arise from accurate location of the fixed reference points compared to the accuracy of measurement required.

Mayhall and Kageyama (1997) have described a new technique combining moire contourography and digital image analysis which allows the three-dimensional description of molar wear. Using this combination, it is possible to describe the amount of tooth substance lost in a given time, as well as the differing amounts of wear on individual cusps. The authors suggest that the moire technique can be used to describe small amounts of wear which hitherto were difficult to quantify. However, it is not recommended where the wear includes the greatest convexity of the crown or affects the central fossa. Further information on this technique is limited.

Iodide permeability

The iodide permeability test can be used to detect the very early stages of enamel demineralization (Bakos and Brudevold 1982). Lussi and co-workers (1993) evaluated this test as a method of measuring erosion, comparing it with the surface microhardness technique. However, the authors gave no clear verdict as to which of these two techniques was superior, leaving the impression that they may be complementary.

Synthetic hydroxyapatite powders/discs

The erosive potential of soft drink formulations can be determined using an enamel-like disc composed of ceramic (sintered) hydroxyapatite, measuring weight loss gravimetrically before and after exposure (Andon et al. 1992). However, comparison with human tooth response is impossible and this material is now rarely used for estimating erosion.

Calcium and phosphorus dissolution

Chemical methods of measuring erosion and erosive potential are extremely sensitive and have the advantage that it is easy to study variables such as exposure time and type of acid. However, they produce only quantitative data and do not exactly mirror conditions in vivo (Grenby 1996). Much of the research on the acidity and erosive potential of soft drinks has been based solely on measurements of oral or dental plaque pH (Birkhed 1984, Meurman et al. 1987), without using dental hard tissues, which is obviously disadvantageous with regard to estimating actual loss in the oral environment.

However, Grenby et al. (1989, 1990) developed a sensitive measurement of calcium and/or phosphorus dissolution from tooth tissue under the influence of potentially erosive agents under laboratory conditions. The initial calcium and phosphorus levels are subtracted from the final figures, giving the amount dissolved from the tooth mineral. It has been found that the well-known technique of atomic absorption spectroscopy (Grenby et al. 1990, Meurman et al. 1990) provides a reliable and sensitive means to estimate calcium in solution with little interference from other solutes.

Other methods

A number of technological advances have enabled other methodologies of tooth wear assessment to be considered. These include 3-D tomography, nuclear magnetic resonance, confocal laser scanning microscopy (Sönju Clasen et al. 1997) and atomic force microscopy (Parker et al. 1998). However, these techniques are unproved as yet and data are limited with regard to accurate assessment of tooth wear.

A non-destructive measurement of enamel thickness would provide the opportunity for both early diagnosis and longitudinal measurement of progressive enamel loss. Recognizing this, Huysmans and Thijssen (1998) investigated the potential of ultrasonic pulse echo measurements as a tool for monitoring enamel thickness. The results of their study supported the feasibility of the technique. However, further research is necessary to evaluate factors involved in reproducibility and determine clinical applicability. In a study originating from the same centre, Verdonschot and co-workers (1998) showed that decrease in thickness of sealed enamel could be monitored by measuring the fluorescence from a bonding agent mixed with a fluorescent dye.

Measurement in vivo

Accurate measurement of tooth wear in vivo over short periods of time is problematic for a number of reasons. Firstly, it is difficult to obtain fixed points from which to take measurements. Secondly, optical instruments able to measure minute changes in tooth morphology in vivo are unavailable as yet.

Macroscopic changes

Similar to in-vitro macroscopic examination, clinical grades of tooth wear severity are frequently used in clinical research. One of the early scales was devised by Eccles (1979). These early indices required diagnosis of aetiology, hence Smith and Knight proposed a new index in 1984 to assess each tooth surface susceptible to wear visually. Since then modifications of this index have been used to estimate tooth wear.

Whilst extremely useful for clinical diagnosis and treatment, these indices give only estimates of tooth wear and are difficult to standardize. Actual tooth loss is impossible to determine from macroscopic assessment.

Replica techniques

Replica techniques have been devised and these materials are now routinely used in scanning

electron microscopy to great effect in the study of tooth tissue (Absi et al. 1989). The choice of a positive replication material has varied over the years. The popular materials used at present to give an accurate negative replica are silicone-based dental impression materials and epoxy resin or Araldite to construct the positive specimens.

Replica techniques are limited by the accuracy of the impression material and often give information on morphological changes rather than measurements of hard tissue loss (Absi et al. 1989). Recently Bartlett and co-workers (1997) developed a method for measuring erosion in vivo by cementing metal disks to the palatal surfaces of upper incisor teeth covering not more than 5–10% of palatal tooth surface and free of occlusal contacts. Impressions were taken at 6-month intervals and tooth wear was estimated by scanning the impressions with a contacting laser profilometer to measure a change in depth around the disk using fixed reference points on the metal disks. Computer analysis produced a magnified image of the disk and adjacent tooth for measurement. This should reduce the number of errors, due to scanning an impression instead of the positive replica. However, the process of scanning is relatively lengthy, taking 1 h to scan each impression.

Chadwick and Mitchell (1998) suggested that electroconductive replicas fabricated from silicone impressions obtained at various times might be mapped using a computer-controlled probe, and compared using a surface matching and difference detection algorithm (SMADDA). However, dimensional changes inherent in such impression materials are still likely to be greater than the magnitude of tooth surface loss occurring in tooth wear.

Measurement in situ

A technique which has been cited as potentially useful in erosion research is the intra-oral cariogenicity test (ICT) described by Koulourides and Chien (1992). In this technique, slabs of enamel are mounted in the human mouth with intra-oral appliances and subjected to cariogenic or erosive conditions, after which demineralization can be recorded by microradiography and changes in microhardness. However, the limitations of the latter techniques have already been documented. Rugg-Gunn and co-workers (1998) utilized an upper removable appliance holding two bovine enamel slabs in the distal palatal region adjacent to the molar teeth, to measure erosion and compare the erosive potential of four drinks. The enamel slabs were removed from the appliance and inserted into the test drinks for 15 min four times per day for 6 days. Loss of enamel was quantified by profiling casts of the enamel slabs obtained before and after the test period. Samples were also measured with electron micrographs. Zero et al. (1998) also evaluated a new intra-oral dental erosion model, comparing it with an in-vitro erosion model. These authors constructed a palatal appliance to hold eight bovine enamel blocks which were evaluated by the surface microhardness test.

Whilst these techniques are far more realistic than in-vitro methods, it is hard to equate the response of bovine tissue to potential erosive agents to that of human tooth.

West and Addy (1996) described an in-situ model to measure tooth wear. An upper, acrylic, intra-oral appliance was constructed on a dental impression with clasps on the first molars for retention. This appliance permitted fixation of between one and four enamel samples (unerupted human third molars) palatally during a treatment period, whilst still allowing withdrawal and replacement in order to procure frequent measurements. Surface profiles of human enamel samples were made using the surfometer to measure across the area of tooth tissue exposed to the oral environment. A controlled method was thus devised to study erosion in situ caused by a single agent (orange juice) over a relatively short period of time, and to compare this with erosion produced by the same method applied in vitro (West et al. 1998b). A single centre, randomized, single blind cross-over clinical study was devised. Ten subjects wearing the intra-oral appliance retaining human enamel consumed 1 litre of orange juice per day for 15 days and a similar volume of water for the other leg of the trial.

A regimen was followed of wearing an intra-oral appliance fitted with an enamel sample from 9 am to 5 pm on each working day. Either 250 ml of orange juice (industrial standard orange juice supplied by SmithKline Beecham, Coleford, Gloucestershire, UK) or 250 ml of water was sipped over a period of 10 min at 9 am, 11 am, 1 pm and 3 pm. The drinks were consumed at room temperature and under supervision. The appliance and enamel sample were dipped in chlorhexidine gluconate 0.2% mouthrinse for 1 min at the beginning and end of the day to prevent plaque accumulation. The appliance was removed for 1 h over lunch (12–1 pm) and stored in saline. The appliance and sample were stored in isotonic saline at room temperature overnight. Only tea, coffee and water could be consumed while the appliance was place and no toothbrushing was allowed throughout the day. Volunteers were allocated a toothbrush and a conventional fluoride toothpaste to use morning and night throughout the trial. At the end of each study day the samples were taken from the appliances and the tape was removed. Surface profiles were again taken of each specimen and loss of tissue was determined by comparison with baseline readings. A safety margin of 20 µm loss of enamel was set, and if this was achieved subjects were removed from the study.

Results showed significantly more erosion on the enamel specimens when the subjects drank orange juice than when the same subjects consumed 1 litre of water per day over the same time period. The same investigation was performed in vitro. Again, orange juice was significantly more erosive; indeed it was in the order of 10 times that produced in situ.

One limitation of this type of surface profiling is that only measurements from flat surfaces can be obtained, requiring the aprismatic layer to be removed during specimen preparation. It is likely that the prismatic enamel exposed to the acid is more vulnerable than the aprismatic layer. However, it is nearly always the case that individuals exhibiting tooth wear have lost the aprismatic layer already. Also, ideally, specimen placement would have been on the labial or lingual aspects of the upper incisor teeth, as this is clinically the most frequent site of erosion from excessive acidic soft drink consumption. Whilst preliminary studies showed that this was technically possible, volunteer cooperation was compromised due to problems with regards to comfort, aesthetics and function. The palatal site was therefore chosen for volunteer acceptability and with the expectation that specimens would be contacted by the test fluids. However, providing that the above factors are fulfilled the siting of specimens is secondary to the aims and design of the study. Thus, the blind, controlled, randomized cross-over clinical trial design was chosen to compare the effects of two agents in an environment where most if not all other variables were standardized during both periods. Accepting the limitations of specimen siting, the study is one of the first of its kind to model erosion in situ by a single potential aetiological agent under highly controlled conditions.

Changes produced by water either in situ or in vitro were always well within the baseline measurement parameters ($\pm$ 0.3 µm) set down for the method and hence validated the clinical model in terms of reproducibility and accuracy in measurement. It is concluded that this method has confirmed the erosive potential of orange juice in situ, which previously had not been definitely proven as a major aetiological agent responsible for tooth erosion.

This model was used again in two subsequent clinical trials of similar design conforming to GCP (Hughes *et al*. 1999a,b, West *et al*. 1999), confirming the reproducibility of the technique and providing more data on the erosivity of fruit drinks on human enamel specimens. This research led to the formulation of a low erosive beverage now on sale in the UK.

Summary

To date, the measurement of tooth wear has been based largely on either case report data or cross-sectional epidemiological research. Such data only provide information on the total outcome measure of tooth wear, but cannot directly separate out specific aetiological agents. Certainly, case report data may provide information indicating the role of one particular factor in a single individual, e.g. erosion associated with behavioural eating disorders (Bargen and Austin 1937). Epidemiological data can only provide associations between possible variables and a particular condition. These studies measure tooth wear using clinical indices similar to those used in many disciplines of dentistry and as such are relatively crude and unable to detect minor changes in tooth morphology. This has meant that, to date, the clinical evaluation of potential aetiological agents in tooth wear has been difficult if not impossible to perform. In-vitro studies are plentiful. However, they cannot hope to replicate the oral environment, hence information obtained is limited.

In-situ models with human enamel appear to be the way forward in assessing tooth wear. Variables can be controlled to a large extent, which is extremely useful given the multifactorial aetiology and complexity of tooth wear. New technology appears to facilitate improved accuracy of measurement, but as yet the ultimate goal of tooth wear measurement and monitoring in true in vivo conditions has not been achieved.

New developments

In 1986 Gerd Binnig and Heinrich Rohrer were awarded the Nobel Prize in physics for their invention of the scanning tunnelling microscope (STM). One and a half decades after the introduction of the first STM (Binnig and Rohrer 1982, Binnig *et al*. 1982a,b,c) scanning probe microscopes (SPM or sometimes called SXM, where X refers to the physical or chemical property measured) are found in many modern laboratories working in the field of surface characterization of materials. The popularity of SPM methods is based on their high resolution in real space, the ability to probe the properties of a variety of materials, the relatively low costs compared with electron microscopes and the easy implementation of most SPM methods. In addition, SPM can be used for surface engineering, i.e. the purposeful creation and manipulation of structures on a microscopic scale.

In the early stages of its history STM was used to analyse surface structures of conductive materials, such as metals and semiconductors in ultra high vacuum (Binnig *et al*. 1983) with atomic resolution. Later, however, STM has also been shown to work well under a variety of other environmental conditions in situ such as in ambient air (Park and Quate 1986), water or other molecular liquids (Sonnenfeld and Hansma 1986, Akari *et al*. 1988, Manne *et al*. 1991).

The atomic force microscope (AFM) (Binnig *et al*. 1986) and other scanning probe microscopes (SPMs) can also be used under diverse environmental working conditions. This makes the AFM ideal for investigations of mineralized tissues such as enamel and dentine. Processes such as chemical reactions or erosion can be observed in real time on a microscopic scale with AFM. The flexibility of AFM is also reflected by the variety of measurable interactions such as van der Waals forces, or chemical forces between the probe of the AFM and the sample surface.

Today's scientists face the challenge to investigate structures and properties on ever smaller scales. This need arises from the decreasing structure sizes of functional units, e.g. in biomaterials systems such as drug delivery systems, or the understanding of wear processes of mineralized tissues on a microscopic scale. Scientists are especially interested in the microstructure, surface roughness, surface chemistry and mechanical properties of enamel and dentine. Furthermore, the exact amount of tooth wear must be measured and the aetiology of wear processes need to be explored. Finally, the effects of pellicle coatings on enamel or causes of dentine hypersensitivity are of special interest to researchers.

Although these processes manifest themselves on a macroscopic scale, their causes can be found on a microscopic scale. Some of these effects can be studied by traditional microscopic methods, such as optical microscopy (OM) or scanning electron microscopy (SEM). However, these methods often require sophisticated sample preparation methods, such as etching techniques or metal evaporation to the samples, which can lead to artefacts and the loss or change of detectable information in the sample structure and properties. SPM measurements can often be done without additional sample preparation, hence leaving the material and its properties in their original state.

The following section discusses the principles of SPM and its application in the investigation of tooth wear.

Scanning probe microscopes – principles, opportunities and limitations

In contrast to the optical or electron microscopes, SPMs do not use glass or magnetic lenses for producing an image, but extremely sharp tips (probes). Such a tip is brought very close (d = 0.1–10 nm) to the surface of the material to be investigated. The small distance between the tip and the material surface allows specific physical interactions to take place between them. The resolution of the SPM depends strongly on the shape of the tip. The smaller, i.e. sharper, the tip is, the smaller is the surface area sampled by this tip.

The second specific component of the SPM is a piezoelectric scanner. This scanner transfers electric signals supplied from the SPM control electronics into mechanical motion. During the scanning process the tip detects local variations in the physical property of interest, leading to an image of the measured physical property of the sample. In some systems the probe is attached to the piezo scanner whereas in other systems the sample is attached to the piezo unit, enabling a relative motion of probe and sample in both cases. The piezos are constructed in a way that enables a two-dimensional scanning motion in an x–y plane as well as a motion in z-direction to vary the distance between the probe and the sample.

Figure 10.1 shows the principle of an AFM. The AFM probe consists of a microfabricated pyramidal Si_3N_4 tip (radius ≈ 20 nm) which is attached to a flexible cantilever. If the tip is scanned over

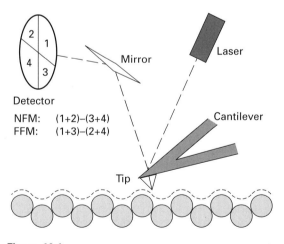

Figure 10.1

Schematic representation of an atomic force microscope (AFM). The four segment photo-detector is able to detect normal (NFM) and lateral or frictional forces (FFM) affecting the tip.

a sample surface the cantilever is deflected in z-direction due to the surface topography. A laser beam focused on and reflected from the rear of the cantilever to two adjacent photodiodes (wired in opposition) detects the deflection of the cantilever. The electrical differential signal of the photodiodes obtained from each point of the surface is processed by a computer and transferred into a topographic image of the surface. The main forces contributing to the cantilever deflection are repulsive van der Waals forces between the atoms within the tip and the atoms of the sample surface. In practice, however, other forces such as capillary or electrostatic forces may also contribute to the image data obtained.

The AFM can operate in different modes. In the constant force mode, the force (which is proportional to the cantilever deflection in z-direction) between the tip and the sample surface is kept constant via an electronic feedback loop. In this case an image is created from the tip height required to maintain a constant force over the surface. In constant force mode measurements additional to the surface topography can also be performed. As the tip is in permanent contact with the surface, the scanning motion of the system leads to some torsion of the cantilever in the lateral x–y plane as well. This torsion reflects the different frictional (mechanical) properties of a surface and can be monitored by the photodiodes. Measurements of this kind are called lateral force microscopy (LFM) (Mate et al. 1987) or frictional force microscopy (FFM). If the tip is modified with functional groups, such as -CH_3 (hydrophobic) or -COOH (hydrophilic) and the microscope is operated in the LFM mode, hydrophobic or hydrophilic areas on the sample surface can be detected with extreme resolution. This kind of experiment, which requires some experience in tip preparation, is therefore called chemical force microscopy (CFM) (Frisbie et al. 1994).

Frictional effects are not always welcome when performing AFM experiments, especially when very soft surfaces such as pellicle layers are to be imaged. Tapping mode (Digital Instruments 1995) utilizes an oscillating tip (frequencies 50–500 kHz) at a tip amplitude of about several tens of nm when the tip is not in contact with the surface. If the oscillating tip, which is driven by an oscillation piezo, is moved towards the surface it begins to touch or 'tap' the

surface. As a result of this surface contact, the tip amplitude is significantly reduced due to energy loss. The reduction of the oscillation amplitude is used to identify and measure surface topographic features. The average cantilever deflections are used as an input signal into the feedback loop similar to conventional contact mode AFM to maintain a constant average applied force.

Recently, nanoindentation and hardness testing with AFM have become available commercially (Digital Instruments 1997). The indentation process and the imaging are done with the same tip in subsequent steps. Probes used for this procedure have diamond tips. Special software makes it possible to indent distinct patterns in sample surfaces. Subsequently, the indentation mode is left, which automatically reactivates the tapping mode imaging and allows immediate observation of the results.

It should be emphasized that none of the methods mentioned here require any surface coating of the samples, i.e. AFM techniques are direct imaging techniques with extreme resolution. AFM is subject to artefacts caused by damage to fragile structures on the surface. In practice this means that extremely soft materials, such as pellicle or smear layers on top of a dental material or tissues, are difficult to image. Soft structures must be immobilized in order not to be swept away by the scanned tip and should be imaged in a fluid environment by using a so-called fluid cell, which contains the tip and the sample. Consequently capillary forces are reduced and soft samples can be imaged. The fluid cell also allows testing of the reaction of the sample exposed to different liquid chemical agents, such as acids.

Other common artefacts are caused by dull or multiple tips. Blurred or ghost (double) images are the result of imaging with low quality tips. If an artefact is suspected, the scan direction should be rotated and the magnification and the tip should be changed. If the observed structure is unaffected under consideration of the applied changes it is most likely not an artefact. More strategies to avoid artefacts can be found elsewhere (Jandt 1998).

Modern AFMs allow all sample sizes to be used. However, the typical scanning area is limited by the scanner to 1 nm^2 – 250 μm^2.

The *z*-range of SPM scanners is limited to about 6 µm, so that rougher samples or extremely curved samples cannot be imaged. Samples should therefore be flat, clean to avoid tip contamination, and not extremely soft. Like most microscopy methods SPM requires some experience.

Examples of SPM on mineralized tissue and other systems

This section gives brief examples of SPM investigations relevant to mineralized tissue and tooth wear. Naturally, these examples cannot cover all aspects of SPM in this field. Rather than explaining all details of the experiments, the basic concept of the measurements is explained. A linear grey scale where dark areas correspond to low surface regions and bright areas correspond to higher surface regions indicates the height in the AFM micrographs.

A detailed understanding of the enamel microscopic structure is of great importance for the understanding of tooth wear. The common approach for investigating the microscopic structure of enamel is a scanning electron microscopy (SEM) investigation in which the sample is exposed to a high vacuum. This results in dehydration of the enamel sample. Before the SEM investigation the enamel sample must be covered with a thin conducting gold layer to avoid electrical charging in the SEM. It is likely that such sample preparation leads to changes in the fine structure of the enamel surface, e.g. that details of the sample surface are altered or covered by the metal layer. AFM is carried out under ambient conditions without the need to apply a metal layer to the sample surface. Figure 10.2 shows an AFM micrograph of a natural enamel surface (Hooper S and Jandt KD, 1998, unpublished data). Prismatic and aprismatic enamel can be distinguished clearly and fine details within the prisms can be observed. The application of the AFM's fluid cell even allows imaging of enamel in liquids, e.g. to study the erosive effects of acidic liquids.

A second mineralized tissue of interest on a microscopic scale is dentine. In order to ensure good bonding between dentine and a dental bonding system, acid treatment of dentine is

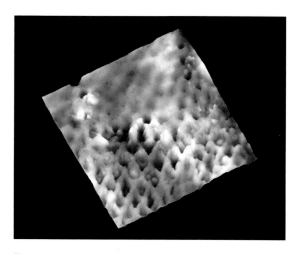

Figure 10.2

Natural enamel surface imaged with the AFM. The sample was taken from a premolar (buccal). The image size is 75 µm × 75 µm (z-range 2 µm). Clearly aprismatic (back) and prismatic (front) enamel can be distinguished.

commonly required as a first preparative step. Such treatment results in an erosive modification of the dentine surface structure on a microscopic scale. Depending on the duration of the acid treatment, modification or removal of the smear layer occurs, resulting in the exposure of the underlying tubules at the surface. Thus, a better understanding of the microstructure of treated dentine surfaces is of great importance for research focused on innovative methods of bonding between dentine and restorative materials. SEM investigations of treated dentine surfaces will dehydrate the dentine, which may lead to a significant change in the structure and properties of the sample; this can be avoided with AFM. Figure 10.3 shows an AFM micrograph of a dentine sample surface which was etched with Scotchbond 1 etching agent (3M Dental Products) for 40 s and subsequently rinsed with water for 30 s. The sample was obtained by cutting a section out of a molar. The micrograph shows the dentine tubules opened. Furthermore, the dentine surface shows a distinct surface roughness caused by the etching process. AFM allows the performance of a detailed analysis of the sample surface roughness. A detailed study of the

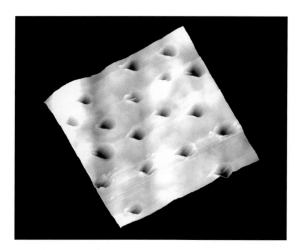

Figure 10.3

Dentine surface treated with Scotchbond 1 etching agent for 40 s. The surface shows open tubules and a distinct surface roughness due to the etching process. The image size is 30 × 30 μm (z-range 5 μm).

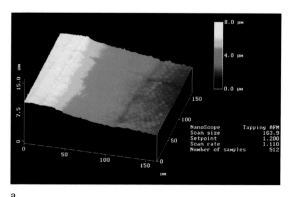

a

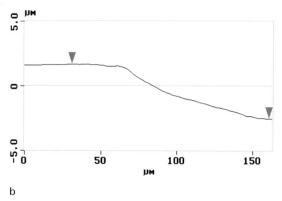

b

Figure 10.4

a AFM micrograph (image size 170 × 170 μm) of a flat ground enamel sample exposed in vitro to orange juice for a total time of 120 min. The left area of the sample was protected against erosion, the right sample area was exposed to fruit juice and, hence, eroded. A material loss of 4 μm caused by the erosive effects of the acids in the orange juice was measured. The erosion process has caused a material loss in the periphery of enamel prisms (right sample area).

b Surface profile of the sample shown in (a). Note that this profile was obtained through integration of all image data from (a) and not through a single profile scan line.

effects of conditioning agents on dentine can be found elsewhere (Silikas et al. 1999).

AFM is a very powerful metrological tool with unique precision, as illustrated in Figure 10.4a and b (Parker et al. 1998). A flat ground enamel sample was exposed to orange juice in vitro for four 10-min periods on 3 subsequent days. An area of the enamel sample was covered with a protective tape to obtain a reference area for surface profile measurements. The acids in the orange juice cause erosion (in this case a material loss of 4 μm) on the enamel surface which can be measured by AFM. In this example the material loss is relatively large. However, AFM is able to measure height differences in the order of the size of one atom (10^{-10} m). A second advantage of the method can be seen in Figure 10.4a. Surfometry gives a sample surface profile along one section line only, whereas AFM measurements produce high resolution images of the sample surface as well. Details such as characteristic etching patterns (reduced periphery of enamel prisms) and an increased surface free area caused by the erosive process can be assessed in addition to profiles and may allow better understanding of the morphological dimension of the erosive process.

The same method can potentially be used in clinical situations where the enamel samples are used with intra-oral appliances. In this case the enamel erosion caused in situ can be measured with the AFM. Figure 10.5a and b shows two examples of AFM measurements obtained in this way. As AFM is able to measure very small material losses it is potentially useful for the

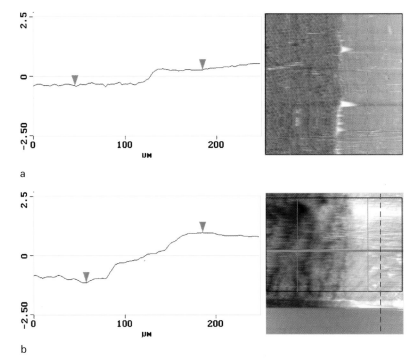

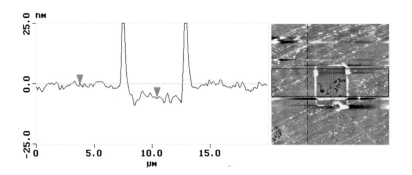

Figure 10.5

a and *b* Surface profiles (left) and corresponding AFM micrographs (image sizes 250 × 250 µm) of flat ground enamel samples exposed in situ to an orange drink for four 10-min periods daily. The right areas of the samples were protected against erosion, the left sample areas were exposed to the oral environment and, hence, eroded.

a After 2 days this sample shows an erosive material loss of 0.67 µm.

b After 5 days this sample shows an erosive material loss of 2.12 µm.

Figure 10.6

AFM surface profile section analysis (left) and the corresponding AFM micrograph (right, image size 20 × 20 µm) of an abraded fissure sealant surface. The abraded area is visible as a 'window' in the micrograph. Note the holes within the abraded area (Jandt KD, Parker DM, Hughes J et al, 1998, unpublished data).

detection of enamel erosion at a very early stage. This may lead to shorter clinical trials and hence a reduction of costs in this area.

An example of how information about mechanical properties of systems can be obtained and how AFM can be used to manipulate surfaces is shown in Figure 10.6 (Vowles RW and Jandt KD, 1998, unpublished data). In this example the system investigated is a dental material, but similar experiments can be carried out with mineralized tissues. A flat sample of a

fissure sealant (Delton, Dentsply Ltd, DeTrey GmbH, Konstanz, Germany) was first imaged in tapping mode to ensure that the sample was flat within 0.5 nm. Subsequently, a force of about 10^{-6} N, which is 1000 times larger than the forces applied in tapping mode, was applied with the tip to a small area of the sample. A mechanically stable tip with a diamond-like coating was used for this experiment. As a result of these larger forces the sample area is exposed to high frictional forces, which results in local abrasion.

The sample is scanned several times with the high forces and subsequently imaged in tapping mode again. The abraded surface area is shown in Figure 10.6. AFM also allows measurement of the material loss caused by abrasion very precisely. In this case the material loss measured was 5 nm.

These examples show that SPM has great potential in tooth wear research. Because of its flexibility SPM is able to explore areas that are not readily accessible with other microscopy methods. This method requires well-trained operators in order to rule out artefacts and in order to make use of its full potential. It is expected that SPM will play a major role in probing tooth wear in the future.

References

Absi EG, Addy M, Adams D (1989) Dentine hypersensitivity: the development and evaluation of a replica technique to study sensitive and nonsensitive cervical dentine. *J Clin Periodontal* **16**:190–5.

Absi EG, Addy M, Adams D (1992) Dentine hypersensitivity. The effects of toothbrushing and dietary compounds on dentine in vitro: a SEM study. *J Oral Rehabil* **19**:101–10.

Addy M, Absi EG, Adams D (1987) Dental hypersensitivity: the effects in vitro of acids and dietary substances on root planed and burred dentine. *J Clin Periodontol* **14**:274–9.

Akari S, Stachel M, Birk H et al (1988) Anomalous voltage dependence of tunnelling microscopy in WSe$_2$. *J Microsc* **152**:521.

Amaechi BT, Higham SM, Edgar WM (1998) The use of transverse microradiography to quantify mineral loss by erosion in bovine enamel. *Caries Res* **32**:351–6.

Andon MB, Kanerva RL, Rotruck JT et al (1992) Method of preventing tooth enamel erosion utilizing an acidic beverage containing calcium. US Patent. no 5,108,761.

Arends J, ten Bosch JJ (1992) Demineralization and remineralization evaluation techniques. *J Dent Res* **71**:924–8.

Attin T, Koidl U, Buchall W et al (1997) Correlation of microhardness and wear in differently eroded bovine dental enamel. *Arch Oral Biol* **42**:243–50.

Bakos Y, Brudevold F (1982) Effect of initial demineralisation on the permeability of human tooth enamel to iodine. *Arch Oral Biol* **27**:193–6.

Bargen JA, Austin LT (1937) Decalcification of teeth as a result of obstipation with long continued vomiting. Report of a case. *J Am Dent Assoc* **24**:1271–3.

Bartlett DW, Blunt L, Smith BG (1997) Measurement of tooth wear in patients with palatal erosion. *Br Dent J* **182**:179–84.

Bashir E, Lagerlof F (1996) The quantitative changes in mineral content of enamel exposed to citric acid in vitro. *Caries Res* **30**:279 (abstract).

Binnig G, Rohrer H (1982) Scanning tunnelling microscopy. *Hel Phys Acta* **55**:726.

Binnig G, Rohrer H, Gerber C, Weibel E (1982a) Surface studies by scanning tunnelling microscopy. *Phys Rev Lett* **49**:57.

Binnig G, Rohrer H, Gerber C, Weibel E (1982b) Tunnelling through a controllable vacuum gap. *Appl Phys Lett* **40**:178.

Binnig G, Rohrer H, Gerber C, Weibel E (1982c) Vacuum tunnelling, *Physica* **109** and **110B**:2075.

Binnig G, Rohrer H, Gerber C, Weibel E (1983) 7 × 7 Reconstruction on Si(111) resolved in real space. *Phys Rev Lett* **50**:120.

Binnig G, Quate CF, Gerber C (1986) Atomic force microscope. *Phys Rev Lett* **56**:930.

Birkhed D (1984) Sugar content, acidity and effect on plaque pH of fruit juices, fruit drinks, carbonated beverages and sport drinks. *Caries Res* **18**:120–7.

Chadwick RG, Mitchell HL (1998) Conduct of an algorithm in quantifying simulated palatal erosion. *J Dent Res* **77**:633 (abstract).

Colin Jones DG (1996) Gastro-oesophageal reflux disease. *Prescribers' J* **36**:66–72.

Davis WB, Winter PJ (1977) Dietary erosion of adult dentine and enamel protection with a fluoride toothpaste. *Br Dent J* **143**:116–19.

Davis WB, Winter PJ (1980) The effect of abrasion on enamel and dentine after exposure to dietary acid. *Br Dent J* **148**:253–6.

Digital Instruments (1995) Tapping mode imaging – applications and technology. Santa Barbara, CA 93103, USA.

Digital Instruments (1997) Nanoindentation and hardness testing with nanoscope SPMs. Santa Barbara, CA 93103, USA.

Dodds MWJ, Gragg PP, Rodriquez D (1997) The effect of some Mexican citric acid snacks on in vitro tooth enamel erosion. *Pediatr Dent* **19**:339–40.

Eccles JD (1979) Dental erosion of non-industrial origin. A clinical survey and classification. *J Prosthet Dent* **42**:649–53.

Farley AN, Shah JS (1991) High pressure scanning electron microscopy of insulating materials: a new approach. *J Microsc* **164**:107–26

Frisbie CD, Rozsnyai LF, Noy A et al (1994) Functional group imaging by chemical force microscopy. *Science* **265**:2071.

Grenby TH (1996) Methods of assessing erosion and erosive potential. *Eur J Oral Sci* **104**:207–14.

Grenby TH, Phillips A, Desai T et al (1989) Laboratory studies of the dental properties of soft drinks. *Br J Nutr* **62**:451–64.

Grenby TH, Mistry M, Desai T (1990) Potential dental effects of infants' fruit drinks studied in vitro. *Br J Nutr* **64**:273–83.

Hall AF, Sadler JP, Strang R et al (1997) Application of transverse microradiography for measurement of mineral loss by acid erosion. *Adv Dent Res* **11**:420–5.

Hartles RL, Wagg BJ (1962) Erosive effect of drinking fluids on the molar teeth of the rat. *Arch Oral Biol* **7**:307–15.

Holloway PJ, Mellanby M, Stewart RJC (1958) Fruit drinks and tooth erosion. *Br Dent J* **104**:305–9.

Hooper S (1995) Development of a new toothwear index. MSc, Bristol.

Hughes JA, West NX, Parker DM et al (1999a) Development and evaluation of a low erosive blackcurrant drink in vitro and in situ. 1. Comparison with orange juice. *J Dent* **27**: 285–9.

Hughes JA, West NX, Parker DM et al (1999b) Development and evaluation of a low erosive blackcurrant drink. 3. Final drink and concentrate, formulae comparisons in situ and overview of the concept. *J Dent* **27**: 345–50.

Huysmans MCD, Thijssen JM (1998) Ultrasonic measurement of enamel thickness: a tool for monitoring erosion. *Caries Res* **32**:292 (abstract).

Imfeld T (1996) Dental erosion. Definition, classification and links. *Eur J Oral Sci* **104**:151–5.

Jandt KD (1998) Developments and perspectives of scanning probe microscopy (SPM) on organic materials systems. *Mat Sci Eng R* **2**:221–95.

Järvinen VK, Rytömaa II, Meinonen OP (1991) Risk factors in dental erosion. *J Dent Res* **70**:942–7.

Klimek J, Ganss C, Jung M (1996) Quantification of the erosive effect of dietary acids by longitudinal microradiography and profilometry. *Caries Res* **30**:279 (abstract).

Koulourides T, Chien MC (1992) The ICT *in situ* experimental model in dental research. *J Dent Res* **71**(Sp. iss.):822–7.

Lambrechts P, Vanherle G, Davidson C (1981) A universal and accurate replica technique for scanning electron microscope study in clinical dentistry. *Micros Acta* **85**:45–58.

Lussi A, Jaeggi T, Scharer S (1993) The influence of different factors on in vitro enamel erosion. *Caries Res* **27**:387–93.

McClure FJ, Ruzicka SJ (1946) The destructive effect of citrate vs lactate ions on rats molar tooth surfaces *in vivo*. *J Dent Res* **25**:1–12.

McDonald JL, Stookey GK (1973) Laboratory studies covering the effect of acid containing beverages on enamel dissolution and experimental dental caries. *J Dent Res* **52**:211–16.

Manne S, Massie J, Elings VB et al (1991) Electrochemistry on a gold surface observed with the atomic force microscope. *J Vac Sci Tech* **B9**:950.

Mate CM, McClelland GM, Erlandson R, Chiang S (1987) Atomic-scale friction of a tungsten tip on a graphite surface. *Phys Rev Lett* **59**:1942.

Mayhall JT, Kageyama I (1997) A new, three-dimensional method for determining tooth wear. *Am J Phys Anthrop* **103**:463–9.

Meurman JH, Rytömaa I, Kari K et al (1987) Salivary pH and glucose after consuming various beverages, including sugar containing drinks. *Caries Res* **21**:353–9.

Meurman JH, Harkonen M, Naveri H et al (1990) Experimental sports drinks with minimal dental erosion effect. *Scand J Dent Res* **98**:120–8.

Millward A, Shaw L, Smith AJ (1994) Continuous intra-oral pH monitoring after consumption of acidic beverages. *J Dent Res* **73**:abstract no. 399.

Millward A, Shaw L, Smith AJ (1995) In vitro techniques for erosive lesion formation and examination in dental enamel. *J Oral Rehabil* **22**:37–42.

Milosevic A, Young P, Lennon MA (1993) The prevalence of tooth wear in 14 year old school children in Liverpool. *Community Dent Health* **11**:83–6.

Mistry M, Grenby TH (1993) Erosion by soft drinks of rat molar teeth assessed by digital image analysis. *Caries Res* **27**:21–5.

National Food and Drink Survey Committee (1956–72) *Household Food Consumption and Expenditure.* HMSO: London.

Office of Population Censuses and Surveys (OPCS) (1994) *Dental Caries Among Children in the United Kingdom in 1993.* Publication no. SS94/1.

Park SI, Quate CF (1986) Tunnelling microscopy of graphite in air. *Appl Phys Lett* **48**:112.

Parker DM, Finke M, Addy M et al (1998) Preliminary

investigation of measuring enamel erosion with atomic force microscopy. *J Dent Res* **77B**: 845.

Restarski JS, Gortner RA, McCay CM (1945a) A method of measuring the effects of acid beverages on the teeth of small laboratory animals. *Science* **102**:404.

Restarski JS, Gortner RA, McCay CM (1945b) Effect of acid beverages containing fluorides upon the teeth of rats and puppies. *J Am Dent Assoc* **32**:668–75.

Rugg-Gunn AJ, Maguire A, Gordon PH et al (1998) Comparison of erosion of dental enamel by four drinks using an intra-oral appliance. *Caries Res* **32**:337–43.

Shaw L, Smith A (1994) Erosion in children: an increasing clinical problem. *Dent Update* **4**:103–6.

Silikas N, Watts DC, England KER, Jandt KD (1999) Surface fine structure of treated dentin investigated with tapping mode atomic force microscopy (TMAFM). *J Dent* **27**:137–44.

Smith AJ, Shaw L (1987) Baby fruit juice and tooth erosion. *Br Dent J* **162**:65–7.

Smith BNF, Knight JK (1984) An index for measuring the wear of teeth. *Br Dent J* **156**:435–8.

Sönju Clasen AB, Øgaard B, Duschner H et al (1997) Caries development in fluoridated and non-fluoridated deciduous and permanent enamel in situ examined by microradiography and confocal laser scanning microscopy. *Adv Dent Res* **11**:442–7.

Sonnenfeld R, Hansma P (1986) Atomic-resolution microscopy in water. *Science* **232**:211.

Van Meerbeck B, Willems G, Celis JP et al (1993) Assessment by mono-indentation of the hardness and elasticity of the resin-dentin bonding area. *J Dent Res* **72**:1434–42.

Verdonschot EH, Huysmans MC, van Elswijk JF et al (1998) Measuring the decrease in thickness due to caries, erosion or abrasion of sealed enamel using a fluorescent bonding. *Caries Res* **32**:293 (abstract).

West NX, Addy M (1996) Method to investigate dietary erosion *in vivo*. *J Dent Res* **75**:1438.

West NX, Hughes J, Addy M (1998a) The effects of brushing desensitising toothpastes, their solid and liquid phases and detergents on dentine and acrylic. Studies in vitro. *J Oral Rehabil* **25**:885–95.

West NX, Maxwell A, Addy M et al (1998b) A method to measure clinical erosion: the effect of orange juice consumption on erosion of enamel. *J Dent* **26**:4 329–35.

West NX, Hughes JA, Parker DM et al (1999) Development and evaluation of a low erosive blackcurrant drink. 2. Comparison with a conventional blackcurrant juice drink and orange juice. *J Dent* **27**: 341–4.

Zammitti S, Habib C, Kugel G (1997) Use of environmental scanning electron microscopy to evaluate dental stain removal. *J Clin Dent* **8**:20–5.

Zenith International Market Research (1997) Tate and Lyle Industries Ltd, Philip Lyle Building, Whiteknights, Reading RG6 6BX, UK.

Zero DT, Barillas I, Hayes AL et al (1998) Evaluation of an intraoral model for the study of dental erosion. *Caries Res* **32**:312(abstract 132).

Zipkin I, McClure FJ (1949) Salivary citrate and dental erosion. *J Dent Res* **28**:613–26.

11

Etiology of enamel erosion: intrinsic and extrinsic factors

Domenick T Zero and Adrian Lussi

Introduction

Dental erosion is the physical result of a pathologic, chronic, localized loss of dental hard tissue that is chemically etched away from the tooth surface by acid and/or chelation without bacterial involvement (ten Cate and Imfeld 1996). Acids of intrinsic and extrinsic origin are thought to be the main etiologic factors. The specific contribution of dental erosion to tooth wear is complicated by the multifactorial nature of this disorder and the biological and behavioral modifying factors and cofactors. This chapter will review current knowledge on the etiology of dental erosion building on the published proceedings of the ILSI Europe Workshop on the 'Etiology, Mechanisms and Implications of Dental Erosion' published in the *European Journal of Oral Sciences* (Vol 104, No. 2, Part II, 1996). In reviewing this topic an attempt was made to critique the scientific evidence supporting the role of the various etiologic factors.

Intrinsic erosion

Intrinsic erosion can be considered less complicated than extrinsic erosion in that only endogenous acids of gastric origin are involved. Repeated direct contact of gastric contents with the teeth will result in demineralization of dental hard tissues. The dramatic nature of the disorder, which in some cases causes complete destruction of the dentition, supports the importance of early diagnosis and appropriate intervention, including preventive measures to preserve the remaining dentition. The dentist may be the first health care professional to become aware of an underlying medical or psychological disorder, requiring the need for referral to the appropriate medical specialist.

There is a wide array of medical and psychological disorders that may result in the introduction of gastric contents into the oral cavity. Due to the socially unacceptable nature of this activity, most individuals tend to be secretive and do not readily divulge information to health care professionals. This has most likely led to an under-reporting of the problem and also presents major hurdles to studying the pathogenesis of this disorder.

Any disorder or condition that results in gastric acid being introduced into the oral cavity can potentially cause dental erosion. Scheutzel (1996) has reviewed the intrinsic etiological factors associated with dental erosion, namely, vomiting, regurgitation and rumination. Each of these factors will be discussed under separate headings; however, it must be kept in mind that in many cases two or all three factors may be operational in the same individual.

Recurrent vomiting

Vomiting is the forceful expulsion of the gastric contents up to and out of the mouth as a result of strong, sustained contraction of the abdominal muscles and diaphragm (Lee and Feldman 1998). Järvinen *et al.* (1991) estimated that the risk of dental erosion was 31 times greater in individuals who vomited once per week or more than in individuals that vomited less frequently than once per week. Many disorders such as postoperative vomiting and motion sickness involve only transient vomiting, and thus cannot be directly linked to dental erosion. While it is generally believed that transient vomiting is not a significant cause of erosion, the cumulative effects of acid exposure on the dentition may be expressed later in life. Scheutzel (1996) compiled a comprehensive list of the many causes of vomiting. For the purposes of this review the causes of vomiting will be discussed under the headings: medical conditions, cyclic vomiting syndrome, side-effects of drugs, psychogenic vomiting syndrome, eating disorders, chronic alcoholism and binge drinking, and pregnancy-induced vomiting.

Medical conditions

Medical conditions that may cause vomiting include gastrointestinal disorders (peptic ulcer, hiatus hernia, gastric motility problems, intestinal obstruction, gastro-enteritis, food allergies), metabolic and endocrine disorders (diabetes mellitus, renal failure, hyperthyroidism, adrenal insufficiency), and neurological and central nervous system disorders (migraine headaches, Ménière's disease, intracranial neoplasms). Dental erosion has been associated with diabetes insipidus, hyperthyroidism, and chronic renal failure based on case reports (see Scheutzel 1996).

Cyclic vomiting syndrome (CVS) is characterized by recurrent attacks of severe vomiting that may last for periods of several hours to up to 10 days (Lee and Feldman 1998). This disorder of unknown etiology generally starts before age 5 and ceases by adolescence, although not in all cases. Milosevic (1998) reported a 'typical' pattern of palatal erosion in a 23-year-old female with an 18-year history of cyclic vomiting. The prevalence of CVS has been reported to be 1.9% in school children from Aberdeen, Scotland (Abu-Arafeh and Russell 1995).

Side-effects of drugs

The side-effects of drugs represent one of the most common causes of vomiting. A wide range of drugs has been associated with central emetic side-effects and secondary effects due to gastric irritation (Scheutzel 1996). The main classes of drugs with central emetic effects include dopamine agonists, opiate analgesics, digitalis preparations and cancer chemotherapeutic agents (Lee and Feldman 1998). Drugs that have secondary effects due to gastric irritation include aspirin, diuretics, and alcohol, which may also have a central emetic effect. Some of these drugs, such as opiate analgesics and cancer chemotherapeutic agents, may also have a hyposalivary side-effect that further increases the risk of erosion (see below). Furthermore, many individuals, especially the elderly, may be taking other drugs with hyposalivary side-effects (Handelman et al. 1986).

Psychogenic vomiting syndrome

Psychogenic vomiting syndrome involves recurrent vomiting, mainly in young women, that may be caused by an underlying emotional disturbance (Lee and Feldman 1998). It can be diagnosed by several clinical features associated with the vomiting: chronic or intermittent occurrence over a period of years; family history; occurs soon after commencement of a meal or just after completion; not accompanied by nausea and may be self-induced; may be of little concern to the patient; appetite usually normal; may subside after hospitalization.

Eating disorders

Eating disorders with a bulimic component are considered to be the major cause of dental erosion due to chronic vomiting (Scheutzel 1996). Anorexia nervosa and bulimia nervosa are widely recognized personality disorders that are most commonly found in young women between the ages of 20 and 30 years who are persistently overly concerned about their body shape and weight. The prevalence in this age group has been reported to be as high as 5%. Many anorexics and bulimics may be taking medications with hyposalivatory side-effects that may exacerbate the damage to their teeth caused by intrinsic and extrinsic acids.

The eating disorders take on different forms that influence the nature of the oral manifestations. The pattern of dental erosion tends to be highly variable, ranging from no detectable erosion to erosion affecting the entire dentition. Figure 11.1 shows an example of severe palatal erosion in a vomiting bulimic patient. Figure 11.2 shows an example of severe occlusal erosion in a vomiting anorexic patient.

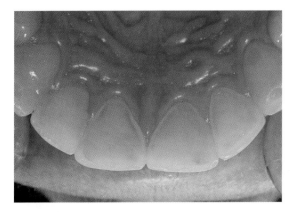

Figure 11.1

Severe palatal erosion in a 22-year-old bulimic female patient who vomited 3–4 times per week over a 5-year period.

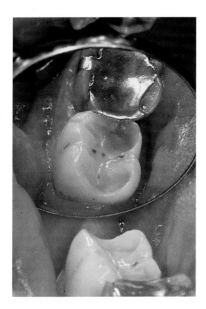

Figure 11.2

Severe occlusal erosion in a 26-year-old female anorexic patient with a history of chronic vomiting.

'Restrictive' or 'abstaining' anorexia nervosa is characterized by profound weight loss due to extreme dietary restriction and generally does not involve self-induced vomiting. This disorder has been associated more with dental erosion of the facial surfaces of the teeth due to a predisposition for excessive consumption of citrus fruits and juices (Hurst *et al.* 1977, Scheutzel 1996). 'Bulimic' or 'vomiting' anorexia nervosa is characterized by profound weight loss due to purging (self-induced vomiting and/or laxative abuse) in addition to dietary restriction. Bulimia nervosa involves repeated episodes of binge-eating and purging as well as dietary restriction, but without weight loss. Bulimics may purge by self-induced vomiting and/or laxative abuse. Certain forms of bulimia also include other abusive behavior, such as alcohol abuse, that may contribute to dental erosion.

The literature supporting a relationship between eating disorders and dental erosion is based on case reports (Stege *et al.* 1982, Roberts and Li 1987) and observational epidemiological studies (Hellström 1977, Hurst *et al.* 1977, Jones and Cleaton-Jones 1989, Milosevic and Slade 1989, Robb *et al.* 1995, Milosevic and Dawson 1996, Milosevic *et al.* 1997a, Rytömaa *et al.* 1998). Milosevic and Slade (1989) could not establish a linear association between frequency, duration or total number of vomiting episodes in a case-control (age-matched) study of bulimic and anorexic patients. However, they did conclude that pathological tooth wear was more frequent when the total number of vomiting episodes was greater than 1100. Jones and Cleaton-Jones (1989) observed erosion in 69% of a group of bulimic women and only 7% of a matched control group. More recent case-control studies have also reported a higher prevalence of tooth wear in vomiting bulimics than in controls (Robb *et al.* 1995, Rytömaa *et al.* 1998). In the latter study, erosion was nearly six times more frequent among bulimics than controls.

Another form of self-induced vomiting that does not involve an eating disorder has been described in the literature. Bishop and Deans (1996) described a horse jockey who repeatedly vomited to control body weight for occupational reasons. This may also be a problem in other occupations that require low body weight such as dancers and models.

Chronic alcoholism and binge drinking

Chronic alcoholism and binge drinking are problems that pervade many countries around the world. The secretive nature of these afflictions and self-denial of the problem may hamper clinical diagnosis. The lifetime prevalence of alcohol dependence in a representative sample of US adults was estimated to be 13.3% (Grant 1997). Men were found to be significantly more likely than women to abuse alcohol. Alcohol can have both a central emetic effect and secondary effects due to gastric irritation (Lee and Feldman 1998). Excessive alcohol intake may also lead to chronic problems with gastro-esophageal reflux (Smith and Robb 1989, Scheutzel 1996).

Several case reports have linked chronic alcoholism with dental erosion (Simmons and Thompson 1987, Smith and Robb 1989, O'Sullivan and Curzon 1998). Two case-control studies have also found a relationship between alcohol consumption and dental erosion (Robb and Smith 1990, Hede 1996). The extent of dental erosion appears to be related to frequency and duration of alcohol abuse. Robb and Smith (1990) reported more pathological tooth wear in individuals who drank continuously than in binge drinkers.

Dental erosion due to alcohol abuse may be caused by both intrinsic factors (vomiting and regurgitation) and extrinsic factors, depending on the type of alcoholic drinks that are ingested. Wines have a low pH (2.8–3.8), while spirits tend to have a more neutral pH (6.5–6.9) (Sorvari and Rytömaa 1991). However, drinks that combine spirits with acidic citrus mixers will also have a low pH. A recent report has raised concerns about the use of low pH alcoholic soft drinks (alcopops) by teenagers and young adults in the UK (O'Sullivan and Curzon 1998).

Pregnancy-induced vomiting

Pregnancy-induced vomiting is a common experience affecting 50–90% of all pregnant women, usually during the first trimester (Broussard and Richter 1998); because of the transient nature of this problem it is generally not considered to be a major risk factor (Scheutzel 1996). However, in cases where the vomiting is prolonged and occurs during multiple pregnancies, the cumulative effects may result in clinically detectable erosion (Stafne and Lovestedt 1947). Hyperemesis gravidarum is a condition characterized by intractable vomiting so severe as to cause dehydration, electrolyte and metabolic disturbances, nutritional deficiency and even weight loss, necessitating hospitalization. Hyposalivation secondary to dehydration may increase the risk of dental erosion. The evidence linking dental erosion with pregnancy-induced vomiting is mostly anecdotal. Evans and Briggs (1994) reported on a clinical case of a 29-year-old patient with palatal erosion who had severe, prolonged vomiting during two pregnancies.

Regurgitation

Recently, considerable attention has been given to the possibility that gastro-esophageal reflux disease (GERD) may be an important risk factor for dental erosion (Bartlett et al. 1996b). GERD is a term used to describe individuals with any symptomatic clinical condition or histopathologic alteration that results from gastro-esophageal reflux (Kahrilas 1998). The most common symptoms of GERD include heartburn, acid regurgitation, and dysphagia. GERD can only be considered as a contributing factor in dental erosion when the gastro-esophageal reflux (GER) is accompanied by regurgitation. Regurgitation occurs when the acid reflux passes through the upper esophageal sphincter into the pharynx. The refluxate needs to come in direct contact with teeth to have an erosive effect. Figure 11.3 shows an example of a patient with severe palatal erosion who chronically regurgitated due to a malfunction of the esophageal sphincter.

Regurgitation can be differentiated from vomiting because it occurs without nausea, retching or abdominal contractions. Studies have shown that the refluxate is a heterogeneous mixture of gastric acid, small amounts of undigested food particles and pepsin, as well as bile acids, and trypsin when there is accompanying duodenogastric reflux (Kahrilas 1998). Pepsin is considered to be a coparticipant in acid-induced damage to the esophageal mucosa and thus important in the pathogenesis of GERD. Interestingly, the role of pepsin and the other

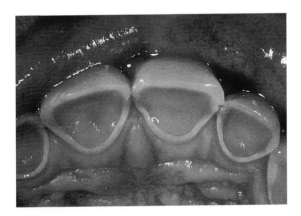

Figure 11.3

Severe palatal erosion in a 31-year-old female patient who chronically regurgitated because of a malfunction of the esophageal sphincter.

digestive enzymes in the etiology of dental erosion has not been investigated (see below).

There is an interesting parallelism between GERD and dental erosion in regard to salivary secretion. Saliva is important in esophageal clearance and neutralization of acidic refluxate, and diminished salivary function is considered a contributing factor in GERD (Kahrilas 1998). Gastro-esophageal reflux occurring during sleep when salivary flow is diminished has been associated with markedly prolonged acid clearance from the esophagus. Chronically diminished salivary function caused by cigarette smoking has been linked with prolonged esophageal clearance and GERD (Kahrilas 1998). Individuals with salivary dysfunction may be in double jeopardy because of an increased risk of GERD and greater susceptiblity to erosion due to prolonged acid clearance from the mouth.

Gastro-esophageal reflux has been associated with dental erosion based on case reports (White et al. 1978, Eccles 1982, Taylor et al. 1992, Bartlett and Smith 1996, Dodds and King 1997, Gregory-Head and Curtis 1997) and observational epidemiological studies (Järvinen et al. 1988, Meurman et al. 1994, Gudmundsson et al. 1995, Schroeder et al. 1995, Bartlett et al. 1996a, Böhmer et al. 1997, Bartlett et al. 1998). All the observational studies supported a relationship between dental erosion and gastro-esophageal reflux with the exception of the study by Gudmundsson and co-workers.

In a group of patients diagnosed with reflux esophagitis or duodenal ulcer, 20% were found to have dental erosion (Järvinen et al. 1988). Schroeder et al. (1995) found a significantly higher prevalence of dental erosion in patients with gastro-esophageal reflux (55%) than in patients without reflux (10%). Meurman et al. (1994) reported that 24% of patients diagnosed with gastro-esophageal reflux disease had dental erosion. Bartlett and co-workers (1996a) observed that 64% of patients with palatal dental erosion were found to have pathological gastro-esophageal reflux. In a group of institutionalized intellectually disabled individuals identified with dental erosion, 65.5% were diagnosed with gastro-esophageal reflux disease (Böhmer et al. 1997).

The studies by Gudmundsson et al. (1995) and Bartlett et al. (1996a) also included intra-oral pH monitoring along with esophageal pH monitoring – attempting to connect gastro-esophageal reflux directly with a drop in the pH in the oral cavity. Gudmundsson et al. (1995) could not associate periods of low intra-oral pH with episodes of gastro-esophageal reflux in a population of 14 adolescent patients. They did report that the patients with erosion had significantly lower salivary buffering capacity than controls and suggested that this predisposed them to dental erosion of dietary origin. In contrast, Bartlett et al. (1996a) were able to find a moderate correlation ($r = 0.47$) between the percentage of time that the distal esophageal pH was < 4 and the pH of the mouth was < 5.5 in a population of 36 patients (age range 15–74 years) with dental erosion.

Differences in the experimental design in these studies may explain the contradictory results. Bartlett and co-workers did not attempt to connect episodes of esophageal reflux directly with changes in intra-oral pH. Gudmundsson et al. (1995) measured intra-oral pH in the sublingual area adjacent to the lower first molar, while Bartlett et al. (1996a) measured intra-oral pH with a pH-sensitive radio-telemetric device placed in the palatal area. The location of the pH sampling used in the latter study is more congruous with the pattern of dental erosion associated with gastro-esophageal reflux.

Rumination

Rumination is a syndrome consisting of repetitive, effortless regurgitation of undigested food from the stomach within minutes after a meal, which is then rechewed, reswallowed or sometimes expectorated (Malcolm et al. 1997). This disorder can be found in infants with a typical onset between 3 and 6 months of age. There is a relatively high prevalence (6–10%) in mentally challenged institutionalized patients. Up to 20% of bulimics have been reported to ruminate, possibly as a means of weight control. More recently this disorder has been increasingly described in adults with normal intelligence and may go undiagnosed for several years while patients are under medical care. Only 11 cases of rumination with dental consequences have been reported in the dental literature (Scheutzel 1996). Dental erosion may present in different locations of the dentition depending on the ruminating behavior, which may involve retention of regurgitated material in the palate or buccal vestibule and different chewing patterns.

Summary of evidence linking intrinsic factors with dental erosion

The evidence linking dental erosion and endogenous acid as presented above is primarily by association of the clinical presentation of the disorder and the individuals' medical condition as documented in case reports and more recently several observational epidemiological studies. Very little is known about the pathogenesis of erosion caused by intrinsic factors (discussed below). The best evidence comes from case-control studies that have associated frequent vomiting with increased risk of dental erosion. Järvinen et al. (1991) reported that the risk of dental erosion was 31 times greater in patients who vomited once a week or more. Case-control studies also support the connection between dental erosion and chronic alcoholism (Robb and Smith 1990, Hede 1996) and eating disorders (Jones and Cleaton-Jones 1989, Milosevic and Slade 1989, Robb et al. 1995, Rytomaa et al. 1998).

The relationship between regurgitation and dental erosion is not as strong as that for vomiting. In a case-control study of Finnish adults, Järvinen and co-workers (1991) found that the

risk of erosion was 10 times greater in patients who exhibited gastric symptoms (acid taste in the mouth, belching, heartburn, stomach-ache, gastric pain on awakening) once a week or more. The specific link with gastro-esophageal reflux disease (GERD) is even more tenuous, because not all cases of GERD result in the refluxate reaching the oral cavity. Furthermore, GERD is frequently associated with other conditions that also involve vomiting, such as bulimia nervosa, chronic alcoholism, and pregnancy.

Many of the studies connecting GERD with dental erosion are limited by problems with experimental design, such as small sample size and sample selection bias. The heterogeneous expression of the GERD is also problematic. The studies mentioned above used different means to establish a diagnosis of gastro-esophageal reflux: patient-reported symptoms (Bartlett et al. 1998); endoscopic examination (Järvinen et al. 1988); ambulatory esophageal pH monitoring (Gudmundsson et al. 1995, Schroeder et al. 1995, Bartlett et al. 1996a, Böhmer et al. 1997), and esophageal histopathologic examination in addition to all of the above methods (Meurman et al. 1994). The two studies that attempted to link GER directly with regurgitation of acidic material into the oral cavity (Gudmundsson et al. 1995, Bartlett et al. 1996a) have reported conflicting results.

The only evidence connecting rumination with dental erosion is from several case reports. However, there is a dated study that attempted to measure the intra-oral pH in a ruminating patient with severe palatal erosion who held regurgitated gastric material against his palate (Lange 1940). The pH of the tongue was found to fall to pH 3.7 during rumination, while the pH of the buccal vestibule remained at pH 6.5.

Understandably, there has been very little in-vitro investigation of the pathogenesis of erosion caused by intrinsic factors. While earlier studies have shown that hydrochloric acid can demineralize teeth (Elsbury 1952), the effects of vomit and regurgitated material on teeth have not been systematically studied. The gastric acid as measured in the stomach can be below pH 1, and thus has the potential to cause dental erosion. There is only limited evidence of the actual pH of vomit and regurgitated material as it comes into the mouth.

Milosevic et al. (1997a) were able to obtain samples of vomit collected and frozen by vomiting bulimics ($n = 6$). The pH of the vomit ranged from 2.9 to 5.0 with a mean of 3.8. The time interval between last food intake and vomiting ranged generally from 10–20 min with one subject vomiting 4 h after eating. These subjects were part of a follow-up study involving 20 eating disorder subjects of whom 60% were reported to have worsening tooth erosion. Unfortunately, the subjects who were willing to provide samples of vomit did not include any of the subjects who exhibited dental erosion, suggesting that additional investigation is warranted in this area.

Since there is little scientific information in this area, this does permit some room for speculation as to factors that influence the erosive potential of vomit. The type and volume of the food consumed and the time between last food intake before vomiting are possible factors affecting the pH and composition of vomit, and thus its erosive potential. Also, the use of antacids and drugs which block acid secretion (H_2 receptor antagonists and proton pump inhibitors) will raise the pH of gastric contents, as will the hypersalivation that precedes and accompanies vomiting. Vomit and refluxate also contain pepsin and other digestive enzymes that may be involved in the pathogenesis of dental erosion by disrupting the integrity of the acquired pellicle and breaking down salivary mucins, thus reducing their tooth-protecting properties. As discussed above, pepsin is considered to be a coparticipant in acid-induced esophageal damage in GERD by disrupting the integrity of the mucosal barrier.

Extrinsic factors

The extrinsic factors related to dental erosion include acids of environmental, dietary or medicinal origins. This topic has been reviewed by Zero (1996), and thus this treatment will be limited to an overview of the subject.

Environmental (occupational) factors

Any industrial processing procedure that exposes workers to acidic fumes or aerosols has the potential to cause dental erosion. The incisal edges of anterior teeth are primarily affected. Mouth breathing is considered to be a contributing factor. An increased rate of tooth wear of posterior teeth has also been reported. Sulfuric, nitric, and hydrochloric acids have all been implicated on the basis of evidence from in-vitro studies (Elsbury 1952), cross-sectional studies (Petersen and Gormsen 1991, Chikte et al. 1998), and case-control studies (ten Bruggen Cate 1968, Tuominen and Tuominen 1991, 1992). Occupations involved with galvanizing, electroplating, metal and glass etching, printing and mouth pipetting laboratory acids – as well as munitions, battery, fertilizer, and chemical manufacturing – are all at risk of dental erosion unless appropriate safeguards are taken. Artisans and hobbyists working with inorganic acids are also potentially at risk of dental erosion, especially since these activities are unregulated.

Professional wine tasting has recently been identified as an occupational risk factor for dental erosion. The pH of wine was reported to range from 2.8 to 3.8 (Sorvari and Rytömaa 1991). Ferguson et al. (1996) reported that New Zealand wines ranged in pH from 3.3 to 3.8, with tartaric and malic acids accounting for 95% of the total acids present. Lactic acid may also be present, depending on the degree of malto-lactic fermentation.

Chaudhry et al. (1997) published a case report of a 52-year-old British wine merchant with extensive palatal erosion, who had been a professional wine taster over a 23-year period during which time he tasted an average of 30 wines a day. A study of 19 Swedish wine tasters who usually tested 20–50 different wines 5 days per week found that 74% had dental erosion (Wiktorsson et al. 1997). These authors reported an association between the severity of the damage to the teeth and the number of years as a wine taster.

Several case reports have associated competitive swimmers using improperly pH-regulated swimming pools with dental erosion (Savad 1982, Centerwall et al. 1986). Gas chlorinated swimming pools require daily pH monitoring and adjustment to maintain pool water in the recommended pH range of 7.2–8.0. This can also be a problem for recreational swimmers who swim on a regular basis. Figure 11.4 shows the clinical appearance of the anterior teeth of a 48-year-old

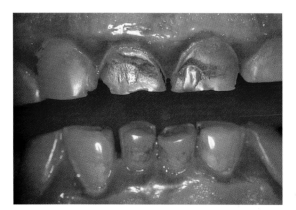

Figure 11.4

Unusual tooth wear pattern in a 48-year-old male patient who swam daily in a gas-chlorinated swimming pool. He had a habit of taking the pool water into his mouth and spraying it out between his teeth. He was later informed that the pool was not properly pH regulated for a period of several months.

physician who swam in a chlorinated pool where the pH had not been properly regulated. He had the habit of squirting pool water through his teeth while he swam, which resulted in an unusual wear pattern of his maxillary anterior teeth.

Diet

The diet has been the most extensively studied etiologic factor in dental erosion. This can partly be explained because it is amenable to the full spectrum of applied research methodologies, i.e. clinical, animal, and in-vitro investigation. More importantly, dietary factors represent the greatest risk to the broadest segment of the population due to the general consumption of acidic foods and beverages, and thus must be considered the most important of the extrinsic factors. Evidence obtained from each of the experimental approaches will be presented in summary form. The different dietary factors that have been implicated in dental erosion are listed in Box 11.1, based on the strength of evidence supporting their role in dental erosion.

Clinical studies implicating dietary factors have involved clinical trials (Thomas 1957, Stabholz *et*

> **Box 11.1** Evidence supporting erosive potential of dietary factors
>
> - Citrus fruit juices and other acidic fruit juices (1–6)
> - Acidic carbonated beverages (1–6)
> - Acidic uncarbonated beverages (1–6)
> - Acidic sports drinks (2,3,5,6)
> - Citrus fruits and other acidic fruits and berries (2,3,5,6)
> - Salad dressing (2,6)
> - Vinegar conserves (2)
> - Wines (3,6)
> - Acidic fruit-flavored candies (3,6)
> - Cider (4)
> - Acidic herbal teas (6)
>
> (1) Clinical trials, (2) epidemiological studies, (3) case reports, (4) experimental clinical studies, (5) animal studies, (6) in-vitro studies.

al. 1983), observational epidemiological studies (Linkosalo and Markkanen 1985, Järvinen *et al.* 1991, Lussi *et al.* 1991, Millward *et al.* 1994, Johansson *et al.* 1997, Milosevic *et al.* 1997b,c) experimental clinical studies (Imfeld 1983, Meurman *et al.* 1987, Gedalia *et al.* 1991, Lussi *et al.* 1997) and numerous case reports (Stafne and Lovestedt 1947, Eccles and Jenkins 1974, High 1977, Asher and Read 1987, Smith and Shaw 1987, Milosevic 1997). (See Zero (1996) for more complete listing of references.)

The clinical trials, although limited in number and scope, provide the most direct evidence that frequent exposure to acidic juices and beverages can result in dental erosion. Based on the epidemiological studies, acidic fruits and juices, carbonated and uncarbonated beverages, sports drinks, and vinegar conserves have been associated with causing erosion. Experimental clinical studies involving intra-oral pH measurements after drinking or rinsing with acidic beverages (ciders, citric fruit juices, fruit juice drinks, flavored drinks, diet drinks) indicated that most acidic beverages cause only transient lowering of the pH of oral fluids. Grapefruit juice, which had the highest level of titratable acid, was the only beverage that resulted in a prolonged pH depression. Rinsing was found to cause a lower and more prolonged pH depression than drinking. Unusual or excessive consumption of specific dietary substances such as lemon juice, orange juice, carbonated cola beverage, orange cordial and fruit-flavored drinks have been implicated on the basis of case reports.

Animal models have been used widely to evaluate the erosive potential of different food and beverages (McClure 1943, Miller 1952, Holloway *et al*. 1958, Stephan 1966, Sorvari 1989, Mistry and Grenby 1993). In-vitro studies (Miller 1907, Rytömaa *et al*. 1988, Grenby *et al*. 1989, Meurman *et al*. 1990, Lussi *et al*. 1993, 1995, Sorvari *et al*. 1996, Grando *et al*. 1996, Maupomé *et al*. 1998) have gained considerable favor because of the relative ease of use, permitting comparison of large numbers of foods and beverages under well controlled conditions. However, the interpretation of animal and in-vitro studies is confounded by differences in experimental design and methodology among the studies and concerns over their clinical relevance (Zero 1996). Despite these limitations some general conclusions can be drawn from these studies:

1. All the acidic foods and beverages that have been identified in clinical studies as etiologic factors in erosion have been confirmed in animal and in-vitro studies (see Box 11.1).
2. Citric, phosphoric, malic, and tartaric acids are the main dietary acids associated with erosion. The relative erosive potential of these organic acids has not been established because of inconsistencies in the findings among the studies (Meurman and ten Cate 1996).
3. The pH of a dietary substance alone is not predictive of its potential to cause erosion. Other parameters modify the erosive potential of foods and beverages (see Box 11.2). The titratable acid content is considered more important than pH level, and calcium chelating properties may greatly enhance the erosive potential of food and beverages. Calcium, phosphate, and fluoride content have a protective effect. Yogurt is a good example of a food with a low pH (3.8), yet it has no erosive potential due to its high calcium and phosphate content (Lussi *et al*. 1993). Other physical properties and chemical properties can affect adherence to the enamel surface and stimulation of salivary flow (see below).
4. Some beverages appear to be less erosive than others within the same class. It may be possible to reduce the erosive potential of beverages by modifying the amount and type of acid used in beverage formulations, e.g. using malic acid instead of citric acid, and supplementing with calcium and phosphate (Grenby 1996).

Several models have been proposed to predict the erosive potential of beverages based on just their chemical properties. Larsen (1973) suggested that erosion potential could be calculated on the basis of the degree of saturation with respect to both hydroxyapatite and fluorapatite, by determining the pH, calcium, phosphate, and fluoride content of a beverage. Lussi and co-workers (1993) incorporated baseline pH, titratable acidity, fluoride, and phosphate content into their model to predict the erosion potential of beverages. A later study (Lussi *et al*. 1995) determined that this approach was predictive of the in-vitro erosion capacity of different beverages with accuracy in the range of 7%.

Medicaments

The frequent use of acidic medications that come in direct contact with teeth has been identified as an etiologic factor in dental erosion. Acetylsalicylic acid (aspirin) (Sullivan and Kramer 1983), liquid hydrochloric acid (Smith 1989), ascorbic acid (vitamin C) (Giunta 1983), iron tonics (James and Parfitt 1953), cocaine (Kapila and Kashani 1997), acidic oral hygiene products (Bhatti *et al*. 1994) or products with calcium chelators (Rytömaa *et al*. 1989), acidic saliva substitutes (Smith 1989) and salivary flow stimulants (Rytömaa *et al*. 1989), and hospital

---

Box 11.2 Parameters influencing the erosive potential of foods and beverages

- pH
- Total acid level (titratable acid)
- Type of acid (pKa)
- Calcium chelating properties
- Calcium, phosphate and fluoride concentration
- Physical and chemical properties affecting adherence to the enamel surface and stimulation of salivary flow

Box 11.3 Evidence supporting role of acidic medications

- Aspirin (2)
- Liquid hydrochloric acid (3)
- Ascorbic acid (vitamin C) (3,6)
- Cocaine (3)
- Iron tonics (6)
- Acidic oral hygiene products or products with calcium chelators (6)
- Acidic saliva substitutes and salivary flow stimulants (6)
- Hospital mouth-cleaning aids (6)

(1) Clinical trials, (2) epidemiological studies, (3) case reports, (4) experimental clinical studies, (5) animal studies, (6) in-vitro studies.

Box 11.4 Evidence supporting role of lifestyle (behavioral) factors

- Healthier life style – diets high in acidic fruits and vegetables (2,3)
- Excessive consumption of acid foods and drinks (2,3)
- Night-time baby bottle feeding with acidic beverages (3)
- Strenuous sporting activities (3)
- Dieting (3)
- Oral hygiene practices (2,3,5,6)

(1) Clinical trials, (2) epidemiological studies, (3) case reports, (4) experimental clinical studies, (5) animal studies, (6) in-vitro studies.

mouth-cleaning aids (Meurman *et al.* 1996) have been implicated in dental erosion based on case reports and/or laboratory studies (see Box 11.3).

Lifestyle (behavioral factors)

The clinical expression of dental erosion is highly variable, with some individuals experiencing total destruction of their teeth and others maintaining most of their tooth structure throughout a lifetime. Biological factors are likely to account for some of the variability (discussed below); however, differences in lifestyle and behavior must also be considered important in the etiology of dental erosion (Zero 1996).

Box 11.4 lists the different lifestyle factors associated with erosion that have been reported in the literature (Zero 1996). Abusive or unusual behaviors have been linked to erosion based primarily on case reports. Frequent and excessive consumption of specific dietary substances such as citrus fruits, lemon juice, orange juice, fruit squashes, cola-flavored soft drinks, and citrus-flavored drinks have all been implicated. Unusual eating, drinking, and swallowing habits (e.g. holding an acid beverage in the mouth before swallowing) increase the contact time of an acidic substance with the teeth and thus increase the risk of erosion. Figure 11.5 shows severe erosion of the facial surface of the upper anterior teeth due to the subject placing a lemon slice under the upper lip while long distance running. Figure 11.6 shows an example of facial

erosion in a patient who consumed 10–15 sugar-free acidic candies per day. The patient was also found to have a low salivary buffering capacity and low unstimulated flow rate.

Bedtime consumption of acid beverages is also considered to be a risk factor, especially for children. Several reports have suggested that the recent dramatic increase in consumption of acidic fruit juices, fruit drinks and carbonated beverages may be leading to a higher prevalence of erosion, especially in young children and adolescents. The use of illegal designer drugs by teenagers at 'raves' has been associated with increased risk of erosion due to excessive

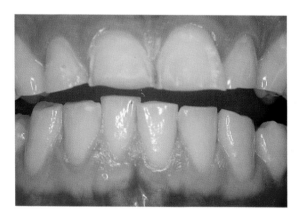

Figure 11.5

Severe erosion of the facial surface of the upper anterior teeth in a 27-year-old male patient who placed lemon slices under his upper lip while long distance running.

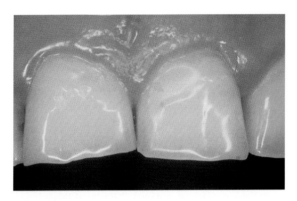

Figure 11.6

Mild facial erosion in a 25-year-old female patient who consumed 10–15 sugar-free candies per day. The patient was found to have a low unstimulated salivary flow rate and buffering capacity.

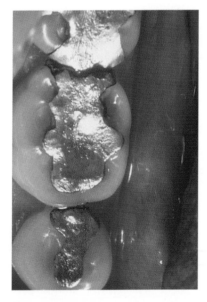

Figure 11.7

Occlusal erosion in a 35-year-old female patient, which was associated with excessive consumption of fruits, apple juice and orange juice.

consumption of acidic beverages in combination with the hyposalivatory side-effects of the drugs.

A healthier lifestyle that includes a diet high in acidic fruits and vegetables may subject teeth to an increased risk of erosion. Frequent dieting

with high consumption of citrus fruits and fruit juices as part of a weight-reducing plan may also be a risk factor. Figure 11.7 shows an example of occlusal erosion due to excessive consumption of acidic fruits, apple juice and orange juice. Strenuous sporting activities and exercise may lead to higher risk of erosion if frequent intake of acidic sport drinks, fruit juices and other acidic beverages is used for fluid and energy replacement. This problem may be compounded by decreased salivary flow secondary to increased fluid loss associated with strenuous exercise.

Health-conscious individuals also tend to have better than average oral hygiene. While good oral hygiene is of proven value in the prevention of periodontal disease and dental caries, frequent tooth brushing with abrasive oral hygiene products may render teeth more susceptible to dental erosion. Erosion is not generally found under areas covered by plaque, which is most likely due to the ability of plaque to buffer acids. The pellicle is also considered to have a protective role against acid dissolution. There is some evidence that the frequent removal of the pellicle by toothbrushing with dentifrice may render the enamel surface more susceptible to acid erosion. However, this potentially detrimental effect of the abrasive component of dentifrice products may be offset by the protective and reparative effect of fluoride. Concerns have also been raised regarding frequent professional cleaning with abrasive prophylaxis paste and professional and home tooth-whitening procedures. While these concerns are not supported by clinical studies, the counter argument can be made that there is a lack of information available to the dental profession on the long-term safety of these procedures.

Dynamics of dental erosion

Very little is known about the natural history of the erosion process. Most laboratory investigations of erosion have focused solely on the consequences of the immediate effects of exposing teeth to an acid challenge. However, the clinical expression of erosion suggests that the erosion process is much more complex. Figure 11.8 represents a conceptual model of the dynamic nature of the erosion process. Based on

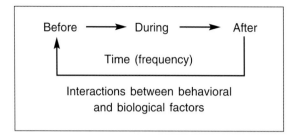

Figure 11.8

Diagram of the dynamic nature of the erosion process.

this model the erosion process is influenced by what goes on **before**, **during** and **after** the erosive challenge. The variable clinical expression of erosion can be explained by the complex interplay between behavioral and biological factors occurring over **time**. The behavioral factors have been discussed above. The biological factors have been reviewed previously (Meurman and ten Cate 1996, Zero 1996) (see Box 11.5).

Box 11.5 Biological modifying factors

- Saliva – flow rate, composition, buffering capacity, pH
- Acquired pellicle – diffusion-limiting properties and thickness
- Tooth composition and structure
- Dental anatomy and occlusion
- Anatomy of oral soft tissues in relationship to the teeth
- Physiological soft tissue movements

What goes on before an erosive challenge will determine the acid susceptibility of the tooth surface at the time of the acid challenge. The factors that influence the acid solubility of enamel at a particular tooth site will be discussed below and include: post-eruptive age of the tooth; previous loss of surface enamel due to tooth wear (erosion, abrasion, attrition, demastication); status of the acquired pellicle; previous exposure to topical fluoride; and an adaptive response to prior acid challenges.

1. Enamel undergoes a maturation process where teeth become more acid-resistant as they age (Brudevold 1948). Newly erupted teeth may be more susceptible to erosion than mature teeth. While no direct comparison of the erosion susceptibility of deciduous teeth and permanent teeth has been made, there is suggestive evidence that this may be the case (Meurman and ten Cate, 1996). This may explain in part why frequent exposure of young children to acidic beverages may result in rapid progress of erosion.

2. Previous loss of surface enamel due to tooth wear (erosion, abrasion, attrition, demastication) may actually increase susceptibility to subsequent erosive challenges. Based on research on the dissolution behavior of enamel, it has been established that intact surface enamel has a higher fluoride content and is more acid-resistant than subsurface enamel. Laboratory studies have shown that abraded enamel is more acid-soluble than unabraded enamel (Brudevold 1948). Thus, it may be hypothesized that the rate of loss of tooth material is not constant over time. Once the surface layer is lost, teeth may become more susceptible to subsequent erosive challenges, and erosion may progress more rapidly once the surface layer has been lost.

3. The presence of the acquired pellicle is known to protect enamel from erosion. The pellicle, which rapidly forms again after removal, must undergo a maturation process that may require 7 days to attain optimal protective properties (Zahradnik *et al.* 1976, Nieuw Amerongen *et al.* 1987). Any procedure that removes or reduces the thickness of the pellicle may compromise its protective properties and accelerate the erosion process. Procedures such as toothbrushing with abrasive dentifrice products, professional cleaning with prophylaxis paste, and tooth-whitening procedures will remove the pellicle and may render teeth more susceptible to erosion (Zero 1996). As discussed above, digestive enzymes in vomit and refluxate also may be involved in disrupting the integrity of the acquired pellicle. There remains the need for a better understanding of how quantitative and qualitative differences in the nature of the acquired pellicle can modify the erosion process.

4. While it is well established that topical fluoride treatment can increase acid resistance of enamel, the clinical effectiveness of fluoride against erosion has not been adequately investigated. There is an intuitive basis for assuming that professionally applied and home-use fluoride will diminish the effects of an erosive challenge (Meurman and ten Cate 1996). For the purposes of this discussion, fluoride treatment before an erosion challenge may decrease enamel susceptibility to a subsequent erosive challenge.

5. Enamel is known to undergo an adaptive process to acid challenge that renders it more resistant to future acid attack (Koulourides 1986). This process involves the loss of the more acid-soluble mineral phase, and the formation of larger more acid-resistant crystals, which is enhanced by the presence of fluoride. The adsorption of organic material into enamel defects (subsurface pellicle) is also thought to be part of the adaptation process (Bibby 1971).

Immediately before an erosive challenge to the teeth, increased salivary flow due to psychogenic stimulation in anticipation of a food or drink may serve a protective role. There is also a hyper-salivatory response that often precedes vomiting that is under the control of the 'vomiting center' of the brain (Lee and Feldman 1998). Increased secretion of mucins may serve to coat the teeth and offer protection against dietary and gastric acids (Mannerberg 1963).

During an erosive challenge the main factors are the nature of the erosive agent and the duration of contact with enamel at a particular site. The different intrinsic and extrinsic erosive factors have been reviewed above. The parameters influencing the erosive potential of dietary agents are well established (Box 11.2). However, the parameters that influence the erosive potential of intrinsic factors have received little attention. The type and volume of the food consumed, the time since the last food intake, and the use of antacids and drugs that block gastric acid secretion are possible factors affecting the pH and composition of vomit and refluxate, and thus their erosive potential.

During an erosive challenge the critical factor is the length of time that the erosive agent maintains conditions that are undersaturated with respect to enamel at a particular site. Obviously, the duration of a particular episode of exposure to an erosive agent, such as vomit or an acidic beverage, is of paramount importance. The physical and chemical properties of an erosive agent, particularly the total level of acid or titratable acidity, affects how long the erosive agent will maintain undersaturated conditions at the tooth surface. As discussed earlier, grapefruit juice – which has a very high level of titratable acid compared with other beverages – results in a prolonged pH depression at the tooth surface. There also appear to be differences in the ability of beverages to adhere to enamel (Ireland et al. 1995). The more adherent an acidic substance is to the tooth surface, the greater the contact time and risk of erosion.

There are also interactions between the physical and chemical properties of the erosive agent and the biological and behavioral factors that can modify the extent of erosion. The biological factors that come into play during an erosive challenge involve mainly the salivary protective mechanisms – dilution and clearance of an erosive agent from the mouth, neutralization and buffering of acids, and slowing down the rate of enamel dissolution through common ion effect by salivary calcium and phosphate. The salivary gland function of an individual and the chemical properties of an erosive agent will determine the extent of the salivary stimulation. For example, citric acid, which is found in many fruit juices and beverages, is a strong gustatory stimulant. Other biological factors include the anatomy of the teeth and soft tissues that may influence the retention/clearance pattern of erosive agents. The proximity of tooth surfaces to the salivary duct orifices is of over-riding importance. Also, soft tissue movements of the tongue and buccal mucosa, and swallowing patterns, can influence clearance rate.

Numerous studies have examined the relationship between various salivary parameters and the risk of dental erosion (Mannerberg 1963, Hellström 1977, Woltgens et al. 1985, Järvinen et al. 1991, Meurman et al. 1994, Gudmundson et al. 1995, Milosevic and Dawson 1996, Bartlett et al. 1998, Rytömaa et al. 1998). Overall, these studies support the protective value of saliva, with the strongest association found between dental erosion and low salivary flow rate and low buffering capacity.

Several studies have confirmed the importance of saliva in clearing and neutralizing acids on the surfaces of teeth. Bashir and Lagerlöf (1996) reported a correlation between the rate of clearance of citric acid and the minimum degree of salivary saturation with respect to hydroxyapatite during the first 5 minutes after rinsing with 2% citric acid. This research group had earlier found differences in the clearance pattern of citric acid from different tooth sites in the mouth and suggested that this may explain the clinical distribution of erosion caused by dietary extrinsic factors (Bashir et al. 1995). Millward and co-workers (1997) monitored the pH at the surface of teeth of healthy volunteers after drinking 1% citric acid. They observed that the pH recovered to above pH 5.5 within 2 min at a site adjacent to the palatal surface of the upper central incisor and within 4–5 min at the upper first molar.

During an erosive challenge, behavioral factors also can modify the erosion process. The manner in which dietary acids are introduced into the mouth (gulping, sipping, use of a straw) will affect which teeth are contacted by the erosive challenge and possibly the clearance pattern (Millward et al. 1997). The consumption of other foods and drinks in conjunction with an erosive agent can neutralize and help to clear acid substances from the mouth. Night-time exposure to erosive agents may be particularly destructive because of the absence of salivary flow. Two examples of this are bedtime baby bottle feeding with acidic beverages and gastro-esophageal reflux with regurgitation during sleep.

After an erosive challenge, biological and behavioral factors again modify the extent of permanent damage to the teeth. An erosive attack can result in the irreversible loss of the outer surface layer of enamel. However, there is also destruction of subsurface enamel mineral, which may be still at a reversible stage. Biological and behavioral factors can influence whether the softened tooth structure is subsequently permanently lost or if it is repaired (remineralized).

There is evidence that acid-eroded enamel is more susceptible to abrasion and attrition than intact enamel. Therefore, for some undefined period of time until repair takes place, functional and parafunctional hard and soft tissue contact with softened enamel may accelerate loss of enamel. The importance of the tongue in this regard has long been the subject of speculation. Holst and Lange (1939) considered mechanical abrasion caused by the tongue to be a contributing factor in erosion caused by vomiting. In support of this contention, Järvinen et al. (1992) observed that in a population of referred patients with dental erosion the most severe erosion was found on the palatal surfaces of teeth touched by the tongue. Observations from animal studies also provide support in that beverages produced erosion mainly on the lingual surfaces of rat molar teeth in areas where the tongue contacts the teeth (Stephan 1966). The size of the tongue in relationship to the size of the dental arches and physiologic tongue movements may account for some of the biologic variability observed among different individuals. Malocclusion and parafunctional habits (bruxism) of erosion-softened enamel can also greatly accelerate the tooth wear process.

There continues to be controversy over whether or not oral hygiene practices after an erosive challenge are helpful or harmful. Several studies have shown that after an erosive challenge the loss of tooth substance is accelerated by toothbrushing (Davis and Winter 1980, Kelly and Smith 1988). However, the presence of fluoride in a dentifrice may serve a protective role. Bartlett and co-workers (1994) have reported that fluoride-containing dentifrice reduces the amount of tooth wear compared with non-fluoride dentifrice. The timing of oral hygiene practices is particularly important for patients who vomit frequently. There are conflicting reports in the literature on the harmful effects of toothbrushing shortly after vomiting in patients with anorexia and bulimia nervosa (Scheutzel 1996). The positive effects of toothbrushing, such as promoting the clearance of gastric acids and introducing fluoride into the oral cavity, may offset the potentially harmful effects. Furthermore, many patients may not brush the palatal surfaces of teeth while performing oral hygiene anyway. Other behaviors that either stimulate salivary flow (such as chewing gum) or that directly help to neutralize acids (such as rinsing with sodium bicarbonate) may counter the destructive effects of vomiting and may also be beneficial against dietary acids.

After an erosive challenge, saliva also plays a reparative role by providing mineral substrate and organic material to fill in microscopic defects created by the erosion process. Once the erosive agent is neutralized and/or cleared from the tooth surface, the deposition of salivary calcium and phosphate can lead to remineralization of some of the lost tooth structure. There is some evidence that acid-softened enamel can reharden after short-term in-situ exposure to saliva (Gedalia *et al.* 1991, Zero *et al* 1994) and that dairy products (Gedalia *et al.* 1991) and fluoride (Zero *et al.* 1994) can enhance the rehardening process.

A discussion of the dynamic nature of erosion is not complete without including the time component. Similar to dental caries, a model can be proposed for the erosion process where there is a dynamic equilibrium between enamel surface demineralization and repair and adaptation. It can be hypothesized that there is a threshold that, if exceeded, may allow the rapid progress of dental erosion. As illustrated in Figure 11.8 the length of time between erosive challenges determines if there is sufficient time for repair and adaptation of the affected enamel. Based on this threshold hypothesis, if the frequency and strength of the acid challenge are greater than the process of repair and adaptation, dental erosion will manifest clinically. This threshold is subject to individual variability and is influenced by the biological and behavioral factors discussed earlier.

The above discussion of the dynamics of dental erosion is intended to provide some insight into the complexity of dental erosion. The nature of the erosive agent and the duration and frequency of the challenge are of greatest importance. However, behavioral practices occurring before, during and after an erosive challenge can greatly modify the extent of permanent damage to the enamel surface. Likewise, biological factors, especially saliva, can have a major impact on the outcome of an erosive challenge to the teeth. The relative importance of stimulated saliva immediately before and during the challenge, and of unstimulated saliva after the challenge is not well understood.

Conclusions

Tooth wear is a cumulative lifetime process, which to a large extent is irreversible. There are many intrinsic and extrinsic factors that may contribute to erosion. It is unlikely that any one etiologic factor operates in total isolation from the other factors. Primarily the strength and frequency of the erosive challenge to the teeth affect the clinical expression of dental erosion. However, biological and behavioral factors can greatly modify the destructive potential of an erosive agent. The etiology of enamel erosion must be considered in terms of a dynamic process that occurs over time. What occurs before, during and after an erosive challenge will determine if permanent and progressive loss of tooth structure will take place. The other causes of tooth wear, i.e. abrasion and attrition, are accelerated by erosion and vice versa.

The loss of some tooth structure over time due to the normal wear and tear of using our teeth can be considered as physiologic. The question that still remains unanswered is: what rate of tooth wear is considered to be pathologic? What we consider an acceptable rate of tooth wear should be driven to some extent by our expectations of how long we live and whether we will keep our teeth for our entire lifetime. There are no epidemiological data available as to the extent that dental erosion is contributing to the need for restorative treatment or tooth loss. However, based primarily on case reports and limited epidemiological data, it is apparent that severe cases of erosion can totally compromise the dentition. With caries and periodontal disease now regarded as preventable, the dental profession has the opportunity to focus some of its attention on other disorders, such as erosion, that can compromise the function, esthetics and comfort of our teeth. A first step may require that dental professionals be better trained in how to properly diagnose dental erosion at an early stage and how to monitor the progress of dental erosion.

A philosophical question that must be posed is this – should the dental profession be more proactive in the prevention of erosion through public education and chair-side education of patients, or should we continue with the practice of waiting until the patient presents in the dental chair with obvious irreversible damage to their dentition? It can be argued that the dental profession should become more proactive in informing and educating patients with regard to the consequences and causes of erosion (tooth wear) and how to prevent or minimize the problem.

In addition to general public and patient education, there is a need to target certain groups of patients on the basis of their medical history. For example, patients with medical disorders that are associated with vomiting, such as patients undergoing cancer chemotherapy, should be advised on how to minimize damage to their teeth. We need to work more closely with our medical colleagues to alert them to the dental consequences of frequent vomiting, regurgitation and rumination. Patients with salivary dysfunction must be considered as a high risk population for dental erosion and need to be counselled on the dangers of gastric and dietary acid.

References

Abu-Arafeh I, Russell G (1995) Cyclical vomiting syndrome in children: a population-based study. *J Pediatr Gastroenterol Nutr* **21**: 454–58.

Asher C, Read MJF (1987) Early enamel erosion in children associated with excessive consumption of citric acid. *Br Dent J* **162**: 384–7.

Bartlett D, Smith B (1996) Clinical investigations of gastro-oesophageal reflux: Part 1. *Dent Update* **23**: 205–8.

Bartlett DW, Smith BGN, Wilson RF (1994) Comparison of the effect of fluoride and non-fluoride toothpaste on tooth wear *in vitro* and the influence of enamel fluoride concentration and hardness of enamel. *Br Dent J* **176**: 346–8.

Bartlett DW, Evans DF, Anggiansah A *et al* (1996a) A study of the association between gastro-oesophageal reflux and palatal dental erosion. *Br Dent J* **181**: 125–31.

Bartlett DW, Evans DF, Smith BG (1996b) The relationship between gastro-oesophageal reflux disease and dental erosion. *J Oral Rehabil* **23**: 289–97.

Bartlett DW, Coward PY, Nikkah C *et al* (1998) The prevalence of tooth wear in a cluster sample of adolescent schoolchildren and its relationship with potential explanatory factors. *Br Dent J* **184**: 125–9.

Bashir E, Lagerlöf F (1996) Effect of citric acid clearance on the saturation with respect to hydroxyapatite in saliva. *Caries Res* **30**: 213–17.

Bashir E, Gustavsson A, Lagerlöf F (1995) Site specificity of citric acid retention after an oral rinse. *Caries Res* **29**: 467–9.

Bhatti SA, Walsh TF, Douglas WI (1994) Ethanol and pH levels of proprietary mouthrinses. *Community Dent Health* **11**: 71–4.

Bibby BG (1971) Organic enamel material and caries. *Caries Res* **5**: 305–22.

Bishop K, Deans RF (1996) Dental erosion as a consequence of voluntary regurgitation in a jockey: a case report. *Br Dent J* **181**: 343–5.

Böhmer CJ, Klinkenberg-Knol EC, Niezen-de Boer MC et al (1997) Dental erosions and gastro-oesophageal reflux disease in institutionalized intellectually disabled individuals. *Oral Dis* **3**: 272–5.

Broussard CN, Richter JE (1998) Nausea and vomiting of pregnancy. *Gastroenterol Clin North Am* **27**: 123–51.

Brudevold F (1948) A study of the phosphate solubility of the human enamel surface. *J Dent Res* **27**: 320–9.

Centerwall BS, Armstrong CW, Funkhouser GS et al (1986) Erosion of dental enamel among competitive swimmers at a gas-chlorinated swimming pool. *Am J Epidemiol* **123**: 641–7.

Chaudhry SI, Harris JL, Challacombe SJ (1997) Dental erosion in a wine merchant: an occupational hazard? *Br Dent J* **182**: 226–8.

Chikte UM, Josie-Perez AM, Cohen TL (1998) A rapid epidemiological assessment of dental erosion to assist in settling an industrial dispute. *J Dent Assoc S Afr* **53**: 7–12.

Davis WB, Winter PJ (1980) The effect of abrasion on enamel and dentine after exposure to dietary acids. *Br Dent J* **148**: 253–6.

Dodds AP, King D (1997) Gastroesophageal reflux and dental erosion: case report. *Pediatr Dent* **19**: 409–12.

Eccles JD (1982) Erosion affecting the palatal surfaces of upper anterior teeth in young people. *Br Dent J* **152**: 375–87.

Eccles JD, Jenkins WG (1974) Dental erosion and diet. *J Dent* **2**: 153–9.

Elsbury WB (1952) Hydrogen-ion concentration and acid erosion of the teeth. *Br Dent J* **93**: 177–9.

Evans R, Briggs P (1994) Tooth-surface loss related to pregnancy-induced vomiting. *Primary Dent Care* **1**: 24–6.

Ferguson MM, Dunbar RJ, Smith JA et al (1996) Enamel erosion related to winemaking. *Occup Med* **46**: 159–62.

Gedalia I, Dakuar A, Shapira L et al (1991) Enamel softening with Coca-Cola and rehardening with milk or saliva. *Am J Dent* **4**: 120–2.

Giunta JL (1983) Dental erosion resulting from chewable vitamin C tablets. *J Am Dent Assoc* **107**: 253–6.

Grando LJ, Tames DR, Cardoso AC et al (1996) In vitro study of enamel erosion caused by soft drinks and lemon juice in deciduous teeth analyses by stereomicroscopy and scanning electron microscopy. *Caries Res* **30**: 373–8.

Grant BF (1997) Prevalence and correlates of alcohol use and DSM-IV alcohol dependence in the United States: results of the National Longitudinal Alcohol Epidemiologic Survey. *J Stud Alcohol* **58**: 464–73.

Gregory-Head B, Curtis DA (1997) Erosion caused by gastroesophageal reflux: diagnostic considerations. *J Prosthod* **6**: 278–85.

Grenby TH (1996) Lessening dental erosive potential by product modification. *Eur J Oral Sci* **104**: 221–8.

Grenby TH, Phillips A, Desai T et al (1989) Laboratory studies of the dental properties of soft drinks. *Br J Nutr* **62**: 451–64.

Gudmundsson K, Kristleifsson G, Theodors A et al (1995) Tooth erosion, gastroesophageal reflux, and salivary buffer capacity. *Oral Surg Oral Med Oral Pathol* **79**: 185–9.

Handelman SL, Baric JM, Espeland MA et al (1986) Prevalence of drugs causing hyposalivation in an institutionalized geriatric population. *Oral Surg Oral Med Oral Pathol* **62**: 26–31.

Hede B (1996) Determinants of oral health in a group of Danish alcoholics. *Eur J Oral Sci* **104**: 403–8.

Hellström I (1977) Oral complications in anorexia nervosa. *Scand J Dent Res* **85**: 71–86.

High AS (1977) An unusual pattern of dental erosion. *Br Dent J* **143**: 403–4.

Holloway PJ, Mellanby M, Stewart RJC (1958) Fruit drinks and tooth erosion. *Br Dent J* **104**: 305–9.

Holst JJ, Lange F (1939) Perimylolysis. A contribution towards the genesis of tooth wasting from non-mechanical causes. *Acta Odontol Scand* **1**: 36–48.

Hurst PS, Lacey LH, Crisp AH (1977) Teeth, vomiting and diet: a study of the dental characteristics of seventeen anorexia nervosa patients. *Postgrad Med J* **53**: 298–305.

Imfeld T (1983) Acidogenic and erosive potential of soft drinks and mineral waters, In: *Monographs in Oral Science, Vol II, Identification of Low Caries Risk Dietary Components*, 165–74. Karger: Basel, Switzerland.

Ireland AJ, McGuinness N, Sherrif M (1995) An investigation into the ability of soft drinks to adhere to enamel. *Caries Res* **29**: 470–6.

James PMC, Parfitt GJ (1953) Local effects of certain medicaments on the teeth. *BMJ* **2**: 1252–3.

Järvinen V, Meurman JH, Odont D et al (1988) Dental erosion and upper gastrointestinal disorders. *Oral Surg Oral Med Oral Pathol* **65**: 298–303.

Järvinen V, Rytömaa I, Heinonen OP (1991) Risk factors in dental erosion. *J Dent Res* **70**: 942–7.

Järvinen V, Rytömaa I, Meurman JH (1992) Location of dental erosion in a referred population. *Clin Sci* **26**: 391–6.

Johansson AK, Johansson A, Birkhed D et al (1997) Dental erosion associated with soft-drink consumption in young Saudi men. *Acta Odontol Scand* **55**: 390–7.

Jones RRH, Cleaton-Jones P (1989) Depth and area of dental erosions, and dental caries, in bulimic women. *J Dent Res* **68**: 1275–8.

Kahrilas P (1998) Gastroesophageal reflux disease and its complications. In: Feldman M, Scharschmidt B, Sleisenger M, eds, *Sleisenger and Fordtran's Gastrointestinal and Liver Disease: Pathophysiology, Diagnosis, Management*, 6th edn, 498–517. Saunders: Philadelphia.

Kapila YL, Kashani H (1997) Cocaine-associated rapid gingival recession and dental erosion. A case report. *J Periodontol* **68**: 485–8.

Kelly MP, Smith BGN (1988) The effect of remineralizing solutions on tooth wear in vitro. *J Dent* **16**: 147–9.

Koulourides T (1986) Implications of remineralization in the treatment of dental caries. *Higashi Nippon Dent J* **5**: 1–20.

Lange F (1940) Rumination as a cause of perimylolysis. *Acta Odontol Scand* **2**: 202–8.

Larsen MJ (1973) Dissolution of enamel. *Scand J Dent Res* **81**: 518–22.

Lee M, Feldman M (1998) Nausea and vomiting. In: Feldman M, Scharschmidt B, Sleisenger M, eds, *Sleisenger and Fordtran's Gastrointestinal and Liver Disease: Pathophysiology, Diagnosis, Management*, 6th edn, 117–27. Saunders: Philadelphia.

Linkosalo E, Markkanen H (1985) Dental erosion in relation to lactovegetarian diet. *Scand J Dent Res* **93**: 436–41.

Lussi A, Schaffner M, Hotz P et al (1991) Dental erosion in a population of Swiss adults. *Community Dent Oral Epidemiol* **19**: 286–90.

Lussi A, Jäeggi T, Schärer S (1993) The influence of different factors on *in vitro* enamel erosion. *Caries Res* **27**: 387–93.

Lussi A, Jäeggi T, Jäeggi-Schärer S (1995) Prediction of the erosive potential of some beverages. *Caries Res* **29**: 349–54.

Lussi A, Portmann P, Burhop B (1997) Erosion on abraded dental hard tissues by acid lozenges: an in situ study. *Clin Oral Invest* **1**: 191–4.

Malcolm A, Thumshirn MB, Camilleri M et al (1997) Rumination syndrome. *Mayo Clin Proc* **72**: 646–52.

Mannerberg F (1963) Saliva factors in cases of erosion. *Odontol Revy* **14**: 156–66.

Maupomé G, Diez-de-Bonilla J, Torres-Villasenor G et al (1998) *In vitro* quantitative assessment of enamel microhardness after exposure to eroding immersion in cola drink. *Caries Res* **32**: 148–53.

McClure FJ (1943) The destructive action, in vivo, of dilute acids and acid drinks and beverages on the rat's molar teeth. *J Nutr* **26**: 251–9.

Meurman JH, ten Cate JM (1996) Pathogenesis and modifying factors of dental erosion. *Eur J Oral Sci* **104**: 199–206.

Meurman JH, Rytömaa I, Kari K et al (1987) Salivary pH and glucose after consuming various beverages, including sugar containing drinks. *Caries Res* **21**: 353–9.

Meurman JH, Harkonen M, Naveri H et al (1990) Experimental sports drinks with minimal dental erosion effect. *Scand J Dent Res* **98**: 120–8.

Meurman JH, Toskala J, Nuutinen P et al (1994) Oral and dental manifestations in gastroesophageal reflux disease. *Oral Surg Oral Med Oral Pathol* **78**: 583–9.

Meurman JH, Sorvari R, Pelttari A et al (1996) Hospital mouth-cleaning aids may cause dental erosion. *Spec Care Dentist* **16**: 247–50.

Miller CD (1952) Enamel erosive properties of fruits and various beverages. *J Am Diet Assoc* **28**: 319–24.

Miller WD (1907) Experiments and observations on the wasting of tooth tissue erroneously designated as erosion, abrasion, denudation, etc. *Dent Cosmos* **49**: 109–24.

Millward A, Shaw L, Smith AJ et al (1994) The distribution and severity of tooth wear and the relationship between erosion and dietary constituents in a group of children. *Inter J Paediat Dent* **4**: 152–7.

Millward A, Shaw L, Harrington E et al (1997) Continuous monitoring of salivary flow rate and pH at the surface of the dentition following consumption of acidic beverages. *Caries Res* **31**: 44–9.

Milosevic A (1997) Sports drinks hazard to teeth. *Br J Sports Med* **31**: 28–30.

Milosevic A (1998) Toothwear: aetiology and presentation. *Dent Update* **25**: 6–11.

Milosevic A, Dawson LJ (1996) Salivary factors in vomiting bulimics with and without pathological tooth wear. *Caries Res* **30**: 361–6.

Milosevic A, Slade PD (1989) The orodental status of anorexics and bulimics. *Br Dent J* **167**: 66–70.

Milosevic A, Brodie DA, Slade PD (1997a) Dental erosion, oral hygiene, and nutrition in eating disorders. *Int J Eating Disorders* **21**: 195–9.

Milosevic A, Lennon MA, Fear SC (1997b) Risk factors associated with tooth wear in teenagers: a case control study. *Community Dent Health* **14**: 143–7.

Milosevic A, Kelly MJ, McLean AN (1997c) Sports supplement drinks and dental health in competitive swimmers and cyclists. *Br Dent J* **182**: 303–8.

Mistry M, Grenby TH (1993) Erosion by soft drinks of rat molar teeth assessed by digital image analysis. *Caries Res* **27**: 21–5.

Nieuw Amerongen AV, Oderkerk CH, Driessen AA (1987) Role of mucins from human whole saliva in the protection of tooth enamel against demineralization in vitro. *Caries Res* **21**: 297–309.

O'Sullivan EA, Curzon MEJ (1998) Dental erosion associated with the use of 'alcopop' – a case report. *Br Dent J* **184**: 594–6.

Petersen PE, Gormsen C (1991) Oral conditions among German battery factory workers. *Community Dent Oral Epidemiol* **19**: 104–6.

Robb ND, Smith BGN (1990) Prevalence of pathological toothwear in patients with chronic alcoholism. *Br Dent J* **169**: 367–9.

Robb ND, Smith BG, Geidrys-Leeper E (1995) The distribution of erosion in the dentitions of patients with eating disorders. *Br Dent J* **178**: 171–5.

Roberts MW, Li SH (1987) Oral findings in anorexia nervosa and bulimia nervosa: a study of 47 cases *J Am Dent Assoc* **115**: 407–10.

Rytömaa I, Meurman JH, Koskinen J (1988) *In vitro* erosion of bovine enamel caused by acidic drinks and other foodstuffs. *Scand J Dent Res* **96**: 324–33.

Rytömaa I, Meurman JH, Franssila S, Torkko H (1989) Oral hygiene products may cause dental erosion. *Proc Finn Dent Soc* **85**: 161–6.

Rytömaa I, Järvinen V, Kanerva R, Heinonen OP (1998) Bulimia and tooth erosion. *Acta Odontol Scand* **56**: 36–40.

Savad EN (1982) Enamel erosion ... multiple cases with a common cause? *J NJ Dent Assoc* **53**: 32, 35–7, 60.

Scheutzel P (1996) Etiology of dental erosion–intrinsic factors. *Eur J Oral Sci* **104**: 178–90.

Schroeder PL, Filler SJ, Ramirez B et al (1995) Dental erosion and acid reflux disease. *Ann Intern Med* **122**: 809–15.

Simmons MS, Thompson DC (1987) Dental erosion secondary to ethanol-induced emesis. *Oral Surg Oral Med Oral Pathol* **64**: 731–3.

Smith AJ, Shaw L (1987) Baby fruit juice and tooth erosion. *Br Dent J* **162**: 65–7.

Smith BGN (1989) Toothwear: aetiology and diagnosis. *Dent Update* **16**: 204–12.

Smith BGN, Robb ND (1989) Dental erosion in patients with chronic alcoholism. *J Dent* **17**: 219–21.

Sorvari R (1989) Effects of various sport drink modifications on dental caries and erosion in rats with controlled eating and drinking pattern. *Proc Finn Dent Soc* **85**: 13–20.

Sorvari R, Rytömaa I (1991) Drinks and dental health. *Proc Finn Dent Soc* **87**: 621–31.

Sorvari R, Pelttari A, Meurman JH (1996) Surface ultrastructure of rat molar teeth after experimentally induced erosion and attrition. *Caries Res* **30**: 163–8.

Stabholz A, Raisten J, Markitziu A et al (1983) Tooth enamel dissolution from erosion or etching and subsequent caries development. *J Pedodont* **7**: 100–8.

Stafne EC, Lovestedt SA (1947) Dissolution of tooth substance by lemon juice, acid beverages and acids from other sources. *J Am Dent Assoc* **34**: 586–92.

Stege P, Visco-Dangler L, Rye L (1982) Anorexia nervosa: review including oral and dental manifestations. *J Am Dent Assoc* **104**: 648–52.

Stephan RM (1966) Effects of different types of human foods on dental health in experimental animals. *J Dent Res* **45**: 1551–61.

Sullivan RE, Kramer WS (1983) Iatrogenic erosion of teeth. *J Dent Child* **50**: 192–6.

Taylor G, Taylor S, Abrams R et al (1992) Dental erosion associated with asymptomatic gastroesophageal reflux. *J Dent Child* **182**: 182–5.

Ten Bruggen Cate HJ (1968) Dental erosion in industry. *Br J Ind Med* **25**: 249–66.

Ten Cate JM, Imfeld T (1996) Dental erosion, summary. *Eur J Oral Sci* **104**: 241–4.

Thomas AE (1957) Further observations on the influence of citrus fruit juices on human teeth. *NYS Dent J* **23**: 424–30.

Tuominen M, Tuominen R (1991) Dental erosion and associated factors among factory workers exposed to inorganic acid fumes. *Proc Finn Dent Soc* **87**: 359–64.

Tuominen M, Tuominen R (1992) Tooth surface loss and associated factors among factory workers in Finland and Tanzania. *Community Dent Health* **9**: 143–50.

White DK, Kayes RC, Benjamin RN (1978) Loss of tooth structure associated with chronic regurgitation and vomiting. *J Am Dent Assoc* **97**: 833–5.

Wiktorsson AM, Zimmerman M, Angmar-Mansson B (1997) Erosive tooth wear prevalence and severity in Swedish winetasters. *Eur J Oral Sci* **105**: 544–50.

Wöltgens JMH, Vingerling P, DeBlieck-Hogervorst JMA (1985) Enamel erosion and saliva. *Clin Prev Dent* **7**: 8–10.

Zahradnik RT, Moreno EC, Burke EJ (1976) Effect of salivary pellicle on enamel subsurface demineralization in vitro. *J Dent Res* **55**: 664–70.

Zero DT (1996) Etiology of dental erosion – extrinsic factors. *Eur J Oral Sci* **104**: 162–77.

Zero DT, Fu J, Scott-Anne K et al (1994) Evaluation of fluoride dentifrices using a short-term intraoral remineralization model. *J Dent Res* **73** (Special issue) 272 (abstract).

12

Development of an in-situ model to study dental erosion

Bennett T Amaechi, Susan M Higham and W Michael Edgar

Introduction

Dental erosion, described as the loss of hard tissue from the tooth surface by a chemical process in the absence of dental plaque (Eccles 1979), is a problem which is increasing in prevalence (Nunn 1996). It is now the focus of increasing interest and has assumed new importance in the field of dental research. It is speculated that dental erosion is an area of research and clinical practice that will undoubtedly expand in the next decade (ten Cate and Imfeld 1996).

Demineralization of tooth tissue by erosion is caused by frequent contact between the tooth surface and acids – the source of the acid may be extrinsic or intrinsic. Extrinsic causes of erosion involve acidic foods/beverages and exposure to acidic environments such as acid fumes in industries and poorly maintained swimming pools (Zero 1996). Erosion by intrinsic factors is caused by gastric acid reaching the teeth as a result of vomiting, regurgitation, gastro-oesophageal reflux or rumination, and this is usually seen in such problems as bulimia nervosa or anorexia nervosa (Scheutzel 1996).

Studies on dental erosion in humans have been limited for ethical reasons and as a result many of the studies have been carried out either in vitro or with experimental animals. However, experimental models using animals are not the most appropriate for the study of human dental erosion, because they are far removed from the biological conditions and variations found in the human oral environment. A more suitable model for the study of erosion would be an in-situ model in human subjects. In-situ models provide solutions to many of the problems encountered by other methods, as testing is performed on slabs of human enamel which are worn in a human subject's mouth. In this way important factors found in the oral environment – saliva, pellicle, food intake, toothbrushing and the movement of the soft tissues in relation to the teeth – are all taken into account. In-situ models are widely accepted as being closely related to the natural oral environment and have the advantage that clinically relevant results may be obtained relatively quickly and at much reduced cost compared with full clinical trials.

Existing in-situ erosion models

The in-situ model systems currently in use in some centres to assess erosion involve the attachment of a tooth slab on removable appliances worn by volunteer subjects (Sadler et al. 1997, Addy et al. 1998, Rugg-Gunn et al. 1998, Zero et al. 1998). These models are subject to a number of problems. The volunteer subjects may discontinue the wearing of the appliance when not under supervision because of the discomfort and inconvenience associated with these appliances. The compliance of the subjects is an important variable in in-situ studies. The appliance places the tooth slabs in the way of the surrounding structures, thereby subjecting the slabs to shear forces/abrasion from these tissues. This would rather exacerbate the eroded lesion (Smith 1975) giving false results in these studies. Most of these appliances are removed from the mouth during eating, oral hygiene procedures and/or the erosion protocol, and this obviously excludes the enamel slabs from the normal everyday activities inside the mouth. It is also well established that the presence of such a removable appliance changes the ecology of the oral cavity (Brill *et al*. 1977).

Current lesion quantification methods

An important aspect of an in-situ model is the method of quantification of the lesions produced. This can only be achieved with a validated method which is quantitative and sensitive enough to measure a small change in mineral content of a tooth sample. Different methods, such as grading (Eccles 1979), scoring (Reussner *et al*. 1975), tooth wear index (Smith and Knight 1984), surfometry (Addy *et al*. 1998), atomic force microscopy (Parker *et al*. 1998), surface profilometry (Davis and Winter 1980), digital image analysis (Mistry and Grenby 1993) and impression-taking (Millward *et al*. 1995), are presently in use to measure erosion. Grenby (1996) made a detailed review of the various techniques which have been developed and published since the 1940s for the assessment of dental erosion. However, these methods have one common limitation in that they cannot quantify the mineral loss and actual depth of mineral loss (lesion depth) in an eroded lesion. Erosion does not only lead to ad integrum loss of enamel, but also to a slight undersurface mineral loss (Meurman and ten Cate 1996), and the surface of an eroded lesion is hypomineralized (Imfeld 1996). Hence, the lesion depth in an eroded lesion is the depth of the erosion-formed crater plus the depth of the surface softening and undersurface mineral loss. The systems of grading, scoring and tooth wear index (TWI) are subjective and do not give quantitative data, while profilometry, impression-taking, surfometry, atomic force microscopy and digital image analysis measure the area and the depth of the erosion defect.

The aim of this study therefore was to develop a simple in-situ model which provides minimal discomfort to the subjects, and use this to investigate the possible remineralization of early eroded enamel lesion by saliva, and to examine the influence of saliva in the site-specificity of dental erosion. Most individuals exposed to the established erosion-causing factors (Scheutzel 1996, Zero 1996) achieve a balance status, free of erosion, alongside the demineralization and remineralization continuum. This may imply that some intrinsic factors which vary among individuals may be involved in the pathogenesis of dental erosion. Saliva is known to have many properties that can serve a protective function against dental erosion (Mandel 1987), but the influence of saliva on the development and progression of erosion has not been investigated fully. It is envisaged that since it has been established both in vitro and in vivo (Mühlemann *et al*. 1964, Gängler and Hoyer 1984, Collys *et al*. 1993) that etched and softened enamel can be remineralized on exposure to saliva, early enamel erosion may be remineralizable by saliva. It has also been established that the thickness and the velocity of the salivary film varies in different locations in the oral cavity (Dawes 1993), hence it has been speculated that this may influence the remineralizing power of saliva at different sites in the mouth.

Materials and methods

An in-situ caries model has been developed and used by the Cariology Research Group in Liverpool (Manning and Edgar 1992) over many years. This model was modified to produce an erosion model, by combining the expertise we have gained in the use of in-situ models together with the techniques we have developed for the in-vitro production and quantification of eroded lesions, in order to overcome the problems associated with the existing erosion models (such as discomfort from the model which may lead to poor compliance, as discussed above). The development of the in-situ erosion model for the remineralization of eroded enamel lesions described in this chapter was undertaken in a series of stages.

Lesion production technique

The first stage involved the in-vitro production of the eroded lesions. In most studies eroded lesions are produced in vitro by simply immersing a tooth into an acidic solution or drink for a prolonged period of time. This exaggerates the erosive effects of these items due to the absence of the modifying influence of the salivary factors that would be present in vivo. Moreover, the method clearly favours titratable acidity and hence is not reliable for differentiating the erosive potentials of different agents. An in-vitro technique using a cycling method to simulate the conditions that exist in the immediate environment of the tooth in vivo was developed (Amaechi et al. 1999a). A significant reduction in the degree of erosion was observed in specimens treated with artificial saliva when compared with those treated with water or by single continuous immersion in orange juice. Thus the artificial saliva reduced the degree of erosion by protecting and/or remineralizing the lesion being formed.

Lesion quantification method

In order to quantitatively assess the mineral loss and the depth of mineral loss (lesion depth) of the eroded lesions, a two-step image analysis technique was developed (Amaechi et al. 1998a) by modification of the transverse microradiography (TMR) technique used in the field of cariology for the quantification of subsurface carious lesions in demineralization and remineralization studies. The two-step image analysis technique has been demonstrated to be a sensitive and accurate method for detection and quantification of mineral loss due to acid erosion in several studies as follows.

Validation of the lesion production and quantification methods

The sensitivity and reproducibility of the techniques for production and quantification of eroded lesions were comfirmed by their application in a number of studies, as described below.

Xylitol and fluoride study

Pure orange juice was supplemented with either 25% xylitol, 0.5 ppm fluoride or combined xylitol/fluoride (in the same concentrations) and the influence of these agents on the development of dental erosion caused by pure orange juice was investigated in vitro. In this study, xylitol and fluoride produced an additive effect in the reduction of dental erosion caused by pure orange juice (Amaechi et al. 1998b). Xylitol and fluoride used separately did not show a significant reduction in mineral loss by erosion, but this was considered to be due to the concentrations used.

Enamel type, temperature and exposure time study

Other factors affecting the development and progression of early enamel erosion such as enamel type, temperature and exposure time were also investigated in vitro (Amaechi et al. 1999b). In this particular study, the erosive potential of pure orange juice was less pronounced at a lower temperature and increased with an increased exposure time. Erosion progressed twice as fast in bovine permanent enamel as in human permanent enamel, and 1.5 times more rapidly in human deciduous than in human permanent enamel.

Effect of pellicle thickness on erosion

The two-step image analysis technique was also applied in a novel study (Amaechi et al. 1998c) in which the thickness of acquired salivary pellicle formed in vivo on enamel samples at different sites within the dental arches was measured. Early enamel erosion was then produced in vitro on these pellicle-bearing enamel samples and on control samples without pellicle. A significantly lower degree of erosion was observed in slabs with pellicle when compared with those without pellicle. Pellicle thickness varied significantly at different sites within the dental arches and among individuals. An inverse relationship was observed between the degree of erosion and pellicle thickness. This study thus suggests that the variation in pellicle thickness within the arches may be a determinant factor for the site-specificity of dental erosion, and also confirmed that pellicle does protect the teeth from erosion.

In-vitro erosion remineralization study

A further step was taken to examine the possible remineralization of early enamel erosion by natural saliva and saliva substitutes in vitro (Amaechi *et al*. 1998d). Using the same quantitative technique (Amaechi *et al*. 1998a), mineral loss and lesion depth were observed to be significantly lower in remineralized groups when compared with the control (unremineralized) group. This showed that early enamel erosion is remineralizable and that this can be achieved not only by natural saliva but by any solution at a neutral pH containing an adequate level of calcium, phosphate and fluoride. The greatest remineralization ability was exhibited by the natural saliva. Although the defect formed by erosion persisted, the surface softening and undersurface demineralization was completely remineralized in a significant percentage of the samples.

A pilot in-situ study

Having established that the mineral loss and the lesion depth produced by acid erosion can be reliably and accurately quantified by a two-step image analysis technique using TMR, and that early enamel erosion can be remineralized, a pilot in-situ study was conducted to determine the possible in-vivo remineralization of early eroded enamel lesions by stimulated saliva in human subjects (Higham *et al*. 1998). In this study, enamel slabs were bonded with Right-On® orthodontic composite (TP Orthodontics, LaPorte) on to the palatal surface of the upper right central incisor of five healthy volunteers who chewed a sugar-free gum four times daily ad libitum. Following intra-oral exposure for 4 weeks, no significant difference was observed in mineral loss and lesion depth between the control and the remineralized samples, although a lower numerical value for both parameters was observed in remineralized samples. The enamel slabs were coated with a double layer of acid-resistant nail varnish, except for the lesions and the bottom of the slab with which it was cemented to the tooth surface. Following intra-oral exposure, it was observed that the nail varnish coating on the buccal surface of the slab facing the oral tissues

was totally worn off, indicating an abrasive action by shear forces, possibly from the food during mastication and frequent rubbing of the tongue over the slab. As the surfaces of eroded lesions are hypomineralized (Imfeld 1996), and it has been shown that erosion decreases the wear resistance of dental hard tissues (Davis and Winter 1980), thus rendering them more susceptible to the effects of mechanical abrasion (Smith 1975), it was speculated that the net gain in mineral following remineralization was the difference between the mineral gained from the saliva remineralizing effect and that lost by abrasion of the lesion. Thus the non-significant difference in mineral loss and lesion depth between the control and the remineralized samples observed in this study may be attributed to the above observation. This demonstrated the need for a more advanced in-situ model for the study of enamel erosion which would provide protection against further abrasion of the eroded lesion.

Construction of the new in-situ erosion model

With regard to the above observation in the pilot study, an in-situ model – with a device to protect the eroded lesion under study from further abrasion and of appropriate size to provide minimal interference with normal oral functions – was constructed. This model was then used to re-investigate the possible remineralization of early eroded enamel lesion by saliva, and to examine the influence of saliva in the site-specificity of dental erosion.

Lesions and slabs production

Human premolars freshly extracted for orthodontic reasons were collected, cleaned of all debris and soft tissue and examined for caries, cracks or enamel malformations. Five suitable teeth were selected and polished with wet pumice to remove organic contaminants (such as acquired salivary pellicle) from the buccal surface. Each tooth was then coated with two layers of an acid-resistant nail varnish (Max Factor®), except for a window of exposed enamel measuring approximately 6 × 1 mm in a mesio-distal orientation on

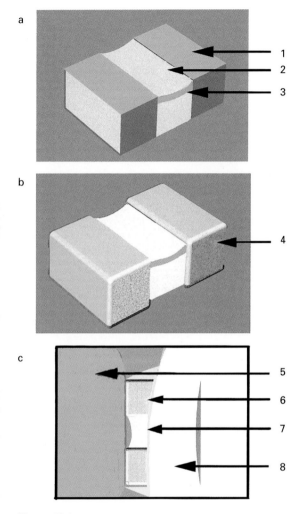

Figure 12.1

Diagram of the in-situ erosion model.

a Lesion-bearing enamel slab: 1 = sound enamel surface; 2 = eroded enamel lesion; 3 = undersurface demineralization.

b The model (the slab with the built-in protective device) 4 = composite resin protective device.

c Illustration of the contact of the model with oral structure (tongue) and the lesion protection: 5 = oral structure; 6 = in-situ model cemented on tooth surface; 7 = the cementing composite; 8 = natural tooth.

with a water-cooled diamond saw (Well, Walter Ebner, Germany). Each section/slab bore the eroded lesion bounded on both ends by sound enamel (Figure 12.1a) to be used as a reference during image analysis (Amaechi *et al.* 1998a). The slabs were then sterilized by gamma irradiation (Amaechi *et al.* 1999c).

Protective device

Following sterilization, the sound enamel surfaces adjacent to the lesion and their adjoining sides of the slab were covered with a thin layer of composite resin (Dyract, De Trey Dentsply, Konstanz, Germany), approximately 0.5 mm thick, forming loops of composite over the two ends of the slab (Figure 12.1b). The composite was freshly mixed in accordance with the manufacturer's instructions, and the setting was photo-initiated with 3M Curing Light XL3000 (3M Dental Products, St Paul, Germany) applied for 40 s. The loop formation provided retention for the composite, as the enamel surfaces were not etched. Etching would cause demineralization of the enamel surfaces and can produce an erosion-like lesion, while an intact enamel surface is needed for the use of TMR in quantification of the eroded lesion. Further retention for the composite was provided by the bonding of the loop to the composite used for cementation of the model to the natural tooth surface (Figure 12.1c).

Remineralization procedure

Five healthy adult subjects (three males, two females) aged between 22 and 35 years were selected. Each subject was examined clinically by the same clinician to ensure that (1) sufficient surface was present behind (palatal) the point of occlusion of the incisal edge of the lower incisors with the palatal surface of the upper incisors to avoid interference with occlusion and movements, and (2) there was no evidence of active erosion of the natural teeth. The consent of the subjects and the approval of the local ethics committee were obtained. The two eroded enamel slabs (now in-situ models) from one tooth allocated to one subject were randomly

the buccal surface. Early enamel erosion was produced on each tooth (Amaechi *et al.* 1999a). Following this, four sections used as controls and two enamel slabs (3 mm length × 2 mm width × 1 mm height) were cut from each tooth assigned to the palatal surface of the upper right lateral incisor and the lingual surface of the lower right lateral incisor of each of the five subjects taking part in the study.

Intra-oral procedure

The models were cemented to the surface of their respective tooth using Right-On® orthodontic composite following acid-etching of both the natural tooth surfaces and the bottom of the models. The excess composite material that spilled out from the sides of the model was used to cover the sides, bevelling it to permit a comfortable streamline (non-catching) movement when the model came in contact with soft tissue surfaces (e.g. tongue) (Figure 12.1c). The bonding of the cementing composite to the loop composite provided a further retention for the protective device (composite loop) (Figure 12.1c).

Experimental regime

Following cementation of the models, the subjects were provided with sugar-free chewing gum (Wrigley, Plymouth, Devon, UK) which they chewed four times daily, for 20 min on each occasion. They were asked to continue their normal dietary intake and usual oral hygiene measures with a fluoridated toothpaste twice daily. The models were removed after intraoral exposure for 28 days by debonding with an orthodontic bracket remover.

Sample processing

Four sections bearing the eroded lesion bounded at both ends by sound enamel surfaces were cut from each model with a water-cooled diamond saw (Well). The composite resin of the protective device was carefully and gently detached from the enamel surface of the sections, but most of the composite came off easily during sectioning. The sections (both control and remineralized), approximately 250 µm in thickness, were mounted on brass anvils with nail varnish allowed to harden overnight, and polished to

give planoparallel specimens of 80 µm thickness using a diamond disc. The specimens were mounted on a microradiographic plate-holder bearing an aluminium stepwedge (25 µm steps). The microradiographs were taken with a 20-min exposure on Kodak high-resolution plates (Type 1A) using a Cu(Kα) X-ray source (Philips BV, Eindhoven, The Netherlands) operating at 25 kV and 10 mA at a focus–specimen distance of 30 cm. The plates were developed using standard techniques.

Lesion quantification

The microradiographs of the specimens were examined with a Leica DMRB optical light microscope (Leica, Wetzlar, Germany). The image was captured at a magnification of 20×/0.40 via a CCD video camera (Sony, Tokyo, Japan) connected to a computer (Viglen PC, London, UK). The lesion parameters (integrated mineral loss and lesion depth) were quantified by the two-step image analysis technique (Amaechi *et al.* 1998a) using a software package (TMRW v.1.22, Inspektor Research Systems BV, Amsterdam, The Netherlands) based on the work described by de Josselin de Jong *et al.* (1987).

Statistical analysis

Statistical analysis of the data was performed with the Biosoft Stat-100 package, with a level of significance prechosen at 0.05. The values of the lesion parameters for the control samples of each tooth were the average values of the four sections cut from the tooth before model construction, while the values of the lesion parameters for each model slab were the average values of the four sections cut from it following oral exposure. Using paired Student's *t* tests, the mean ($n = 5$) value ($\pm$ SD) of the mineral loss (ΔZ) and lesion depth (Id) for the lesions placed in each position (upper palatal and lower lingual surfaces) after intra-oral exposure was compared with that of the control. ΔZ and Id for lesions positioned palatally were also compared with those of the lesions positioned lingually by *t* tests.

Davis WB, Winter PJ (1980) The effect of abrasion on enamel and dentine after exposure to dietary acid. *Br Dent J* **148**:253–6.

Dawes C (1993) The ebb and flow of the salivary tide. In: Bowen WH, Tabak L, eds, *Cariology for the Nineties*, 133–41. University of Rochester Press: Rochester.

De Josselin de Jong E, ten Bosch JJ, Noordman J (1987) Optimised microcomputer guided quantitative microradiography on dental mineralised tissue slices. *Phys Med Biol* **32**:887–99.

Eccles JD (1979) Dental erosion of non-industrial origin: a clinical survey and classification. *J Prosthet Dent* **42**:649–53.

Edgar WM (1998) Sugar substitutes, chewing gum and dental caries – a review. *Br Dent J* **184**:29–32.

Gängler P, Hoyer I (1984) *In vivo* remineralization of etched human and rat enamel. *Caries Res* **18**:336–43.

Grenby TH (1996) Methods of assessing erosion and erosive potential. *Eur J Oral Sci* **104**:207–14.

Hector MP, Sullivan A (1992) Migration of erythrosin-labelled saliva during unilateral chewing in man. *Arch Oral Biol* **37**:757–8.

Hicks MJ, Silverstone LM (1984a) Acid-etching of caries-like lesions of enamel: a polarized light microscopic study. *Caries Res* **18**:315–26.

Hicks MJ, Silverstone LM (1984b) Acid-etching of caries-like lesions of enamel: a scanning electron microscopic study. *Caries Res* **18**:327–35.

Higham SM, Amaechi BT, Milosevic A, Edgar WM (1998) *In situ* remineralisation of eroded enamel lesions by stimulated saliva. *J Dent Res* **77**(Sp. issue B):716 (abstract 678).

Imfeld T (1996) Dental erosion. Definition, classification and links. *Eur J Oral Sci* **104**:151–5.

Ingram GS, Edgar WM (1994) Interactions of fluoride and non-fluoride agents with the caries process. *Adv Dent Res* **8**:158–65.

Mandel ID (1987) The functions of saliva. *J Dent Res* **66**(Special issue):623–7.

Manning RH, Edgar WM (1992) Intraoral models for studying de- and remineralisation in man: methodology and measurement. *J Dent Res* **71**(Sp. issue):895–900.

Mellberg JR (1992) Hard tissue substrates for evaluation of cariogenic and anti-cariogenic activity *in situ*. *J Dent Res* **71**(Sp. issue):913–19.

Meurman JH, Frank RM (1991) Scanning electron microscope study of the effect of salivary pellicle on enamel erosion. *Caries Res* **25**:1–6.

Meurman JH, ten Cate JM (1996) Pathogenesis and modifying factors of dental erosion. *Eur J Oral Sci* **104**:199–206.

Millward A, Shaw L, Smith AJ et al (1994) The distribution and severity of tooth wear and the relationship between erosion and dietary constituents in a group of children. *Int J Paediatr Dent* **4**:151–7.

Millward A, Shaw L, Smith AJ (1995) In vitro techniques for erosive lesion formation and examination in dental enamel. *J Oral Rehabil* **22**:37–42.

Mistry M, Grenby TH (1993) Erosion by soft drinks of rat molar teeth assessed by digital image analysis. *Caries Res* **27**:21–5.

Mühlemann HR, Lenz H, Rossinsky K (1964) Electron microscopic appearance of rehardened enamel. *Helv Odontol Acta* **8**:108–11.

Nunn JH (1996) Prevalence of dental erosion and the implications for oral health. *Eur J Oral Sci* **104**:156–61.

Parker DM, Finke M, Addy M et al (1998) Preliminary investigation of measuring enamel erosion with atomic force microscopy. *J Dent Res* **77**(Sp. issue B):845 (abstract 1708).

Reussner GH, Coccodrilli G, Thiessen R (1975) Effects of phosphates in acid-containing beverages on human tooth erosion. *J Dent Res* **54**:365–70.

Robb ND, Smith BGN, Geidrys-Leeper E (1995) The distribution of erosion in the dentitions of patients with eating disorders. *Br Dent J* **178**:171–5.

Rugg-Gunn AJ, Maguire A, Gordon, PH et al (1998) Comparison of erosion of dental enamel by four drinks using an intra-oral appliance. *Caries Res* **32**:337–43.

Sadler JP, Hall AF, Creanor SL et al (1997) An *in situ* model to study erosion in enamel and dentine. *Caries Res* **31**:318 (abstract 113).

Scheutzel P (1996) Etiology of dental erosion – intrinsic factors. *Eur J Oral Sci* **104**:178–90.

Smith BGN (1975) Dental erosion, attrition and abrasion. *Practitioner* **214**:347–55.

Smith BGN, Knight JK (1984) An index for measuring the wear of teeth. *Br Dent J* **156**:435–8.

Ten Cate JM (1984) The effect of fluoride on enamel de- and remineralization *in vitro* and *in vivo*. In: Guggenheim B, ed, *Cariology Today*, 231–6. International Congress, Zurich, 1983: Karger. Basel.

Ten Cate JM, Imfeld T (1996) Preface. *Eur J Oral Sci* **104**:149.

Verbeeck RMH, De Maeyer EAP, Marks LAM et al (1998) Fluoride release process of (resin-modified) glass-ionomer cements versus (polyacid-modified) composite resins. *Biomaterials* **19**:509–19.

Watanabe S (1992) Salivary clearance from different regions of the mouth in children. *Caries Res* **26**:423–7.

Zero DT (1996) Etiology of dental erosion – extrinsic factors. *Eur J Oral Sci* **104**:162–77.

Zero DT, Barillas I, Hayes A et al (1998) Evaluation of an intraoral model for the study of dental erosion. *Caries Res* **32**:312 (abstract 132).

13
Chemistry of demineralization and remineralization of enamel and dentine

Jacob M ten Cate

Introduction

In recent decades researchers have shown a marked interest in studying the processes of demineralization and remineralization of the dental hard tissues. While originally the focus was on the pathogenesis of the acid dissolution of the mineral phase of enamel leading to demineralization, subsequently mineral deposition (remineralization) during periods of physiological pH also became the subject of many investigations (Koulourides et al. 1961, ten Cate and Arends 1977). Increased knowledge about the reactions at the enamel–oral fluid interface has led to the understanding that dental caries is the result of the combination of demineralization of the tooth mineral – during periods of reduced pH after carbohydrate fermentation - and remineralization from saliva and plaque after the pH is restored. When the two processes are in balance no net mineral loss occurs at the tooth surface, but when the magnitude of one exceeds the other, this will lead to net demineralization or, alternatively, to remineralization of previously formed white spot lesions. The notion that loss of tooth mineral can be compensated by mineral deposition has considerable consequences in operative and preventive dentistry. It implies that non-restorative clinical strategies have become a realistic option, which, given the iatrogenic nature of restorative treatment, is currently widely supported. Also the dentine tissue, as the locus of (de)mineralization, has received considerable attention for two reasons. Firstly, during the caries process the

decay will at some stage pass the enamel–dentine junction. Secondly, the tooth root is covered by a thin layer of cementum on top of the dentine and caries in this part of the tooth thus affects the dentine almost immediately (Nyvad and Fejerskov 1982).

About 2000 citations on de/remineralization can be found in the dental literature using Medline search profiles. Most of these articles cover phenomenological aspects and only a few deal with more basic, mechanistic topics. This chapter deals with some aspects of the demineralization and remineralization of enamel and dentine.

Chemical rationale for demineralization and remineralization

The inorganic phase of enamel consists of the calcium phosphate mineral hydroxyapatite (HAP). This mineral is the least soluble in a range of calcium phosphates which are found in nature. Hydroxyapatite crystals in the body contain a large number of foreign ions, such as sodium, potassium, zinc, strontium, fluoride or (bi)carbonate ions. The solubility of the apatite mineral depends on both the presence of these impurities and the pH of the environment. At low pH the saturation concentration of calcium and phosphate ions with respect to apatite is higher than at high pH. pH is therefore the driving force for dissolution and precipitation of hydroxyapatite. Apart from these thermodynamic considerations other factors play a role – such as the 'nucleators' for precipitation: supersaturated solutions do not precipitate unless this precipitate can form onto a surface. In enamel or dentine in contact with saliva or plaque fluid, mineral deposition onto the hydroxyapatite crystallites may occur.

The mineral composition of saliva and plaque fluid is given in Table 13.1. The calcium and phosphate content, and in particular the pH of these liquids, determine whether enamel and dentine will dissolve or alternatively whether mineral may precipitate.

Figure 13.1 shows the relationship between the saliva and plaque fluid calcium and phosphate levels and the saturation lines for enamel and dentine. This figure may be used to explain caries and remineralization. At neutral pH saliva and plaque fluid are supersaturated with respect to HAP. Consequently mineral will precipitate if a suitable precipitation nucleus is available. After the consumption of fermentable sugars, acids are formed in the plaque. With this decrease in

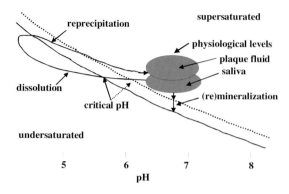

Figure 13.1

Solubility isotherm for enamel (solid line) and dentine (broken line), with some of the processes occurring during demineralization and remineralization.

pH the calcium and/or phosphate concentration needed for saturation increases and in the pH range below 5.6 the tissues will dissolve to maintain saturation. As a result of the dissolution

Table 13.1 Calcium, phosphate and fluoride levels in human stimulated whole saliva and plaque fluid.

Source	Parameters		
Saliva	*Approximate concentration ranges (mmol/l)*		
Calcium	0.75–1.75		
Phosphate	2.0–5.0		
Fluoride	0.0005–0.005		
Calculated ion product (expressed as –log(PI))			
HAP	50.5 to 53.4	pK (solubility product) = 54.6	
FAP	48.4 to 52.3	59.6	
Plaque fluid*	*Mean (mmol/l)*		
Calcium ion	0.85		
Phosphate	11.5		
Fluoride	0.0049		
Calculated ion product (expressed as –log(PI))			
HAP	51.2		
FAP	49.1		
Plaque fluid†	*'Caries free'*	*'Caries susceptible'*	
Calcium ion	5.1	5.1	
Phosphate	15.8	14.9	
pH	5.95	5.63	
Calculated ion product (expressed as –log(PI))			
HAP	47.9	50.9	

Solutions commonly used are as follows. Remineralization: calcium, phosphate, 1.5, 0.9 mmol/l, pH 7.0; ionic product HAP, 50.8. Demineralization: calcium, phosphate, 1.5, 0.9 mmol/l, pH 5.0; ionic product HAP, 62.9.
*Carey *et al.* 1986.
†Margolis *et al.* 1988.

of mineral the phosphate and hydroxyl ions released will neutralize the acids, thus slowing down the decrease in pH. Moreover with decreasing pH the fermentation (rate of acid formation) by oral bacteria is slowed down. During the recovery phase the plaque gradually becomes supersaturated with HAP and mineral will reprecipitate. Ideally, this occurs at the sites 'damaged' during the demineralization. The composition of the apatite then formed depends on the composition of the solution from which it is precipitated, in this case the plaque fluid. For instance, if fluoride is present this will 'co-precipitate' to form a fluoridated hydroxyapatite. In summary, this periodic cycling of pH results in a step-by-step modification of the chemical composition of the outer layers of enamel, which become somewhat less soluble with time. This process is known as the post-eruptive maturation of the enamel.

Enamel

Although enamel is a hard and dense material it possesses local differences in porosity and acid solubility. In restorative dentistry this property is used to create a rough surface for the retention of restorative materials. In caries pathogenesis it implies that acids selectively dissolve enamel and create pathways for diffusion. Thus, acids can penetrate deep into enamel and dissolve tooth mineral locally, rather than dissolving the enamel layer by layer. The latter type of mineral dissolution is known as erosion and is caused by acids at low pH (in the range 1–3).

Acid diffusion through enamel and the resultant formation of subsurface white spot lesions (Figure 13.2) offers the possibility of mineral redeposition from saliva and plaque fluid into the porosity of the lesion. This process of remineralization of a lesion depends on the degree of supersaturation of saliva and plaque fluid, the presence of enamel crystallites for the mineral to be precipitated onto, and the presence of either stimulators or inhibitors of crystal growth.

Clinical remineralization data are limited to a few citations on the reversal of white spot lesions observed during clinical trials (Backer Dirks 1966). Most data available come from

Figure 13.2

Microradiograph of artificial incipient lesion in enamel.

laboratory studies in which lesions are immersed in 'artificial' saliva, usually with a composition stoichiometric to hydroxyapatite (Silverstone and Poole 1968, ten Cate and Arends 1977). In reality in vivo (i.e. in saliva or plaque fluid), the solution composition is considerably more complex: the solution is not stoichiometric to apatite, calcium ions are partly bound to organic molecules or complexed with anionic species. Given these factors it is difficult to determine the 'real' remineralization potential of the oral fluid, and thus to conclude whether the in-vitro studies over- or under-score the possible rates of remineralization of lesions (see Table 13.1).

In addition, the role of inhibitors should be considered. From enamel or plaque fluid a protective layer of proteins is formed onto the enamel, the acquired enamel pellicle, which has been reported to inhibit demineralization (Zahradnik et al. 1977). By a similar mode of action, inhibitors will slow down the remineralization (Zahradnik 1979). It has been observed previously that enamel remineralization can be completely inhibited by a short treatment with a crystallization inhibitor of the bisphosphonate type (Ten Cate et al. 1981).

Promotors of crystallization, on the other hand, will stimulate mineral deposition, particularly when, as for fluoride, the ions are incorporated into the crystallite lattice and result in a lower solubility. In that case the newly formed crystals, or at least the outer layer of a crystal 'behaving' as a new crystal, will follow the thermodynamics of a crystal of lower solubility, i.e. showing a higher difference in solution supersaturation (expressed as 'ion product') and solubility (expressed as solubility product). Consequently mineral deposition onto this crystal will be even more accelerated (Ten Cate 1990).

In the case of enamel remineralization the rate is not determined by the conditions in the outside solutions, but at the crystallite surface. With the small pores in an enamel lesion, diffusion of mineral ions from the outside solution (saliva or plaque fluid) to the site of precipitation may be a limiting factor (Ten Cate and Arends 1978, Featherstone et al. 1987). In recent years there has been discussion as to whether calcium is a rate limiting factor in remineralization (Ten Cate 1994, Dawes 1996), a question that remains in spite of the concomitant development of extra calcium-containing dentifrices. Sullivan et al. (1997) investigated whether the use of brushite-containing dentifrices increases the levels of free calcium ions in plaque fluid. They showed that brushing with this dentifrice does introduce additional, exogenous calcium into the oral environment, which could improve remineralization of teeth in combination with fluoride.

With regard to the process of enamel remineralization, the current consensus view is that mineral deposition occurs either at the outer surface, as part of the continuous demineralization and remineralization process, or as a regrowth of apatite crystallites in previously formed white spot enamel lesions. Mineral deposition takes place as crystal growth, rather than as de novo precipitation of mineral or mineralization of the organic matrix (Arends and ten Cate 1981).

Remineralization is enhanced by various forms of fluoride treatment, such as fluoridation of drinking water, the use of fluoride dentifrices, fluoride slow-release devices or fluoride-releasing restorations. The chemical rationale for each of these actions is similar, the presence of an elevated level of ionic fluoride. Clinical, in situ as well as laboratory studies have shown a dose response between the fluoride concentrations in, for example, a dentifrice and the observed caries preventive effect. In part this is attributed to the effect of fluoride on remineralization (Stookey et al. 1993, Zero 1995).

Dentine

In many demineralization and remineralization studies, dentine is treated in a similar way to enamel, with the focus on the mineral component of the tissue and with very little attention given to the possible role of the organic matrix. This is surprising, as 50 vol% of dentine consists of collagen and other organic components.

The role of the organic matrix on the demineralization and remineralization process has been investigated in a number of studies. These aimed to investigate how the organic matrix is affected during demineralization, both in vitro and in situ, and if its presence affects the remineralization of the dentine. During in-vitro demineralization of dentine it was observed that the non-collagenous components are readily liberated from the tissue. During the acid phase the molecules remain 'trapped' by the lesion material, but they are released when the pH is neutralized (Klont and ten Cate 1990). This would imply that many of these molecules, which have been shown to have an effect on mineralization, are not present inside the lesion to interfere with a subsequent remineralization step.

In studies with alternating demineralization and enzyme-induced collagenolysis, the dissolution of mineral components and solubilization of the organic matrix takes place in parallel. The quantity of exposed enzyme-degradable collagen in dentine was proportional to the calcium released during demineralization. The degradability of collagen was found to be substantially less in subsurface lesions than in erosive lesions. This was consistent with the observation that collagen is covered with apatite and can only be broken down enzymatically when the apatite is first removed by demineralization (Klont and ten Cate 1991a).

Kleter et al. (1994) investigated the effect of matrix degradation on the rate of demineralization of dentine lesions. Bovine root dentine specimens were alternately demineralized and incubated with a bacterial collagenase. The demineralization was carried out in media creating caries and erosive lesions. Under all conditions, the demineralization was found to be accelerated when the matrix was degraded by collagenase. This observation supports the hypothesis that the presence of an organic matrix inhibits the demineralization of the underlying mineralized dentine.

A similar study pertaining to remineralization had been reported previously by Klont and ten Cate (1991b). In their study, subsurface and erosive dentinal lesions were created with an in-vitro system. Both types of lesion were then subjected to remineralization and/or treated with collagenase buffer solution. The results indicated that remineralization of erosive lesions is surface-controlled and that of subsurface lesions is diffusion-controlled, similar to the results previously shown for enamel lesions (Ten Cate and Arends 1978). Also it was found that the removal of collagen before remineralization did not affect the rate of mineral deposition in the root lesions. Nevertheless, remineralization in those lesions where accessible collagen had not been removed resulted in a significant reduction in the amount of (post remineralization) degradable collagen. These observations suggest that remineralization did not occur by nucleation of mineral on the organic matrix, but rather by growth of residual crystals in the partially demineralized root tissue.

Kawasaki and Featherstone (1997) also studied the effects of collagenase treatment on demineralization and remineralization of dentine in a pH-cycling model. Collagenase was added to either the demineralizing solution or the remineralizing solution. Results were obtained by histological assessment of the dentine specimens and by chemical analysis of the solutions. Surface erosion was observed only in the groups with collagenase in the remineralizing solution combined with severe demineralization challenge. However, the collagenase treatment did not lead to differences among the groups in calcium and phosphate uptake and loss in the pH-cycling solutions. The conclusion that collagenase primarily works during the remineralization phase is not surprising given the pH optimum for the enzyme.

While the number of in-vitro studies on the role of the organic matrix in dentine caries is limited, virtually no studies deal with the intra-oral fate of the organic matrix when exposed to plaque and saliva under in-vivo conditions. Van Strijp *et al.* (1992) placed completely demineralized dentine specimens covered by a retentive gauze in partial dentures of volunteers. After 7 weeks in vivo, the specimens were analysed for the amounts of denatured and native collagen. With this mass balance approach it was calculated that between 1 and 47 wt% of the collagen was denatured and solubilized. Only about 0.5 wt% of the available collagen was present as denatured matrix. These findings indicate that collagen – once denatured – is rapidly solubilized and released into the oral cavity.

Mineral aspects

Although the mineral component of dentine and enamel is – in simple terms – described as hydroxyapatite, a better description is a carbonated apatite. During the mineralization of the dental hard tissue, carbonate is abundantly available and this explains the high content of carbonate in the apatites of enamel and dentine. The carbonate level of dentine is higher than that of enamel, presumably because of the small size of the dentine crystallites. As a result the solubility behaviour of dentine, and to a lesser extent enamel, is different from that of hydroxyapatite. In both cases an experiment with powdered tissue in carbonate-free media would result in the dissolution of carbonate apatite and the concomitant reprecipitation of stoichiometric apatite. Moreno and Aoba (1991) concluded that demineralization experiments involving dentine and enamel should be performed in carbonate-containing media to get realistic values for the dissolution parameter of the two tissues.

The rate of dissolution during demineralization of the tissue is not only controlled by such thermodynamic considerations, the size of the crystallites is also a regulating factor. As with any crystalline material, the rate of dissolution is determined by the solution-exposed crystallite surface. On that basis alone the dissolution of dentine crystallites could be a factor of 100 greater than enamel. The remineralization and fluoride acquisition of dentine is affected similarly by this phenomenon.

Various data were accumulated to calculate that the rate of mineral loss of dentine at pH = 5.0 is three times the corresponding value for enamel (Ten Cate 1994). A similar finding was obtained from a pH-cycling study with alternate exposure to remineralization (in total 21 h/day) and demineralization (in total 3 h/day) (Ten Cate *et al.* 1995). Some data from the literature on the

Table 13.2 Data on rate of demineralization of dentine.

Reference	Condition	Rate of demineralization (g Ca/mm²/s)
Featherstone *et al.* 1987	In-vitro demineralization, pH 5.0, lactate/MHDP	3.1×10^{-11}
Nyvad *et al.* 1989	In situ	1.1×10^{-11}
Hoppenbrouwers *et al.* 1987	In-vitro demineralization	2.4×10^{-11}
Ten Cate *et al.* 1995	pH-cycling (demineralization data only)	1.7×10^{-10}

rate of demineralization of dentine are presented in Table 13.2.

The acid susceptibility of dentine is also affected by the history of the dentinal tissue. A number of studies reported that apatite crystallites in carious dentine were considerably larger than in dentine that had not been exposed to the oral cavity or been subject to demineralization and remineralization processes. An earlier study reported that the rate of in-vitro dentine demineralization was reduced by 25–40%, for bovine and human dentine respectively, after a 7-week intraoral exposure period with no additional fluorides being administered. With fluoride dentifrice usage this value was increased to 70% (Ten Cate *et al.* 1987).

Nyvad *et al.* (1997) placed dentinal specimens in partial dentures and followed lesion formation for a period of 3 months, after which a preventive regime of brushing and fluoride treatment was initiated. A microradiographic analysis of the specimens revealed that a mineralized band was formed inside the lesions, presumably at the site of the original lesion's front. This phenomenon was studied in greater detail under better controlled laboratory conditions by Damen *et al.* (1998), who confirmed this hypothesis.

Remineralization of lesions extending through enamel into the underlying dentine

Remineralization studies have been conducted with enamel and dentine, but always as separate tissues. In the development of caries lesions will at some stage pass the dentine–enamel junction, extending through the enamel into the dentine. Often this is a clinical indication for restorative treatment. However, there is also the possibility

that lesions into the dentine can still be remineralized. This question was addressed recently in a laboratory experiment (Ten Cate *et al.* 1998). The aim of the project was to study whether lesions into the dentine can still be remineralized, and to determine the relative remineralization efficacy of enamel and the underlying dentine. The study was performed with 'single sections', thin sections taken perpendicular to the outer surface and covered on all sides with a protective varnish. One surface was exposed by cutting the varnished specimens parallel to the dentine–enamel junction. Lesions were formed in undersaturated calcium phosphate-containing solutions and periodically microradiographed to monitor the demineralization. Demineralization was stopped when the lesions were well into the dentine. Next the lesions were put in a remineralization medium and followed for up to 200 days. Again microradiographs were taken at regular intervals. The results showed that both enamel and dentine were remineralized (Figure 13.3). Quantitative analysis of the percentage remineralization showed no significant differences between enamel and dentine at various locations.

Conclusion

This chapter has addressed a number of topics regarding the chemistry of demineralization and remineralization of enamel. This topic is in fact too large to allow a complete and comprehensive review within the scope of this book. Therefore some *capita selecta* were chosen. Moreover, many reviews have been published dealing with demineralization and remineralization, particularly the effect of fluoride on these processes. As stated in the introduction, most articles are more phenomenological than

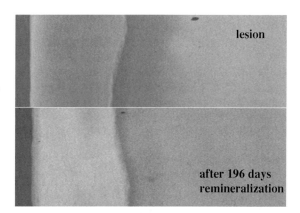

Figure 13.3

Microradiographs of lesions extending into the dentine and their remineralization during 196 days in a remineralizing solution, indicating that remineralization of dentine is also possible underneath enamel.

fundamental, even though many models have been developed which deal with specific parts of the overall problem. Also in many studies hydroxyapatite is used as a model for enamel to overcome the biological variation of the tissue. The mouth is difficult to simulate in a laboratory experiment; thus many investigators now perform intra-oral or so-called in-situ experiments (for a review see White 1992). Although the latter are more representative of the conditions in vivo, with presumably the advantage that results better describe the events in vivo, the description usually does not allow reactions to be followed in well-defined physical or chemical terms.

It should be an interesting task to bridge this gap in knowledge in the coming years.

References

Arends J, ten Cate JM (1981) Tooth enamel remineralization. *J Crystal Growth* **53**: 135–47.

Backer Dirks O (1966) Posteruptive changes in dental enamel. *J Dent Res* **45**: 503–11.

Carey C, Gregory T, Rupp W et al. (1986) The driving forces in human dental plaque fluid for demineralisation and remineralisation of enamel mineral. In: Leach SA, ed, *Factors Relating to Demineralisation and Remineralisation of the Teeth*, 163–73. IRL Press: Oxford.

Damen JJM, Buijs MJ, ten Cate JM (1998) Fluoride-dependent formation of mineralized layers in bovine dentin during demineralization in vitro. *Caries Res* **32**: 435–40.

Dawes C (1996) Salivary calcium as a limiting factor for enamel remineralization. *Caries Res* **30**: 268–9 (abstract).

Featherstone JDB, McIntyre JM, Fu J (1987) Physicochemical aspects of root caries progression. In: Thylstrup A, Leach SA, Qvist V, eds, *Dentine and Dentine Reactions in the Oral Cavity*, 127–37. IRL Press: Oxford.

Hoppenbrouwers PMM, Driessens FCM, Borggreven JMPM (1987) The mineral solubility of human tooth roots. *Arch Oral Biol* **32**: 319–22.

Kawasaki K, Featherstone JDB (1997) Effects of collagenase on root demineralization. *J Dent Res* **76**: 588–95.

Kleter GA, Damen JJM, Everts V et al. (1994) The influence of the organic matrix on demineralization of bovine root dentin in vitro. *J Dent Res* **73**:1523–9.

Klont B, ten Cate JM (1990) Release of organic matrix components from bovine incisor roots during in vitro lesion formation. *J Dent Res* **69**: 896–900.

Klont B, ten Cate JM (1991a) Susceptibility of the collagenous matrix from bovine incisor roots to protolysis after in vitro lesion formation. *Caries Res* **25**: 46–50.

Klont B, ten Cate JM (1991b) Remineralization of bovine incisor root lesions in vitro: the role of the collagenous matrix. *Caries Res* **25**: 39–45.

Koulourides T, Cueto H, Pigman W (1961) Rehardening of softened enamel surfaces on human teeth by solutions of calcium phosphates. *Nature* **189**: 226–7.

Margolis HC, Duckworth JH, Moreno EC (1988) Composition of pooled resting plaque fluid from caries-free and caries-susceptible individuals. *J Dent Res* **67**: 1468–75.

Moreno EC, Aoba T (1991) Comparative solubility study of human dental enamel, dentin, and hydroxyapatite. *Calcif Tissue Int* **49**: 6–13.

Nyvad B, Fejerskov O (1982) Root surface caries: clinical, histopathological and microbiological features and clinical implications. *Int Dent J* **32**: 311–26.

Nyvad B, ten Cate JM, Fejerskov O (1997) Arrest of root surface caries in situ. *J Dent Res* **76**: 1845–53.

Silverstone LM, Poole DFG (1968) The effect of saliva and calcifying solutions upon the histological appearance of enamel caries. *Caries Res* **2**: 87–96.

Stookey GK, DePaola PF, Featherstone JDB et al (1993) A critical review of the relative anticaries efficacy of sodium fluoride and sodium monofluorophosphate dentifrices. *Caries Res* **27**: 337–60.

Sullivan RJ, Charig A, Blake-Haskins J et al (1997) In vivo detection of calcium from dicalcium phosphate dihydrate dentifrices in demineralized human enamel and plaque. *Adv Dent Res* **11**: 380–7.

Ten Cate JM (1990) In vitro studies on the effects of fluoride on de- and remineralization. *J Dent Res* **69**: 614–19.

Ten Cate JM (1994) In situ models, physico-chemical aspects. *Adv Dent Res* **8**: 125–33.

Ten Cate JM, Arends J (1977) Remineralization of artificial enamel lesions in vitro. *Caries Res* **11**: 277–86.

Ten Cate JM, Arends J (1978) Remineralization of artificial enamel lesions in vitro. II. Determination of activation energy and reaction order. *Caries Res* **12**: 213–22.

Ten Cate JM, Jongebloed WL, Arends J (1981) Remineralization of artificial enamel lesions in vitro. IV. The influence of fluorides and disphosphonates on short and long term remineralization. *Caries Res* **15**: 60–70.

Ten Cate JM, Jongebloed WL, Simons YM et al. (1987) Adaptation of dentin to the oral environment. In:

Thylstrup A, Leach SA, Qvist V, eds, *Dentine and Dentine Reactions in the Oral Cavity*, 67–76. IRL Press: Oxford.

Ten Cate JM, Buijs MJ, Damen JJM (1995) pH-cycling of enamel and dentin lesions in the presence of low concentrations of fluoride. *Eur J Oral Sci* **103**: 362–7.

Ten Cate JM, Exterkate RAM, Flissebaalje TD (1998) Remineralization of lesions extending into the dentine. *Caries Res* **32**: 282.

Van Strijp AJP, Klont B, ten Cate JM (1992) Solubilization of dentin matrix collagen in situ. *J Dent Res* **71**: 1498–502.

White DJ (1992) The comparative sensitivity of intra-oral, in vitro, and animal models in the 'Profile' evaluation of topical fluorides. *J Dent Res* **71**: 884–94.

Zahradnik RT (1979) Modification by salivary pellicles of in vitro enamel remineralization. *J Dent Res* **58**: 2066–73.

Zahradnik RT, Propas D, Moreno EC (1977) In vitro enamel demineralization by *Streptococcus mutans* in the presence of salivary pellicles. *J Dent Res* **56**: 1107–10.

Zero DT (1995) In situ caries models. *Adv Dent Res* **9**: 214–30.

14

Mechanical tooth wear: the role of individual toothbrushing variables and toothpaste abrasivity

Margaret L Hunter and Nicola X West

Introduction

Brushing with toothpaste is arguably the most common form of oral hygiene practised by individuals in developed countries (Frandsen 1986). However, incorrect or over-vigorous brushing with an abrasive is considered to be a prime aetiological agent in the development of lesions at the neck of the tooth. This association is supported by studies reporting an increase in cervical abrasive lesions in individuals who brush their teeth more often, for longer, and use a scrubbing technique rather than a less damaging method (Levitch et al. 1994).

It is generally accepted that, in vitro, toothbrushing with abrasives can cause loss of dental hard tissue (Sangnes 1976), while little damage occurs with toothbrushing alone (Manly 1944, Mannerberg 1960, Manly et al. 1965, Bjorn and Lindhe 1966a, Absi et al. 1992).

It is encouraging to note that in Europe, over the last decade, there has been a general trend toward reduced toothpaste abrasivity without loss of cleaning efficacy. This may be mostly due to the increased use of high-performance abrasives such as hydrated silica (Wulknitz 1997).

Toothbrushing and abrasion

Abrasion, derived from the Latin verb *abradere* (to scrape off), describes the wearing away of a substance or structure through mechanical processes such as grinding, rubbing or scraping.

In the dental context, Imfeld (1996) has defined abrasion as the pathological wearing away of dental hard tissue through abnormal mechanical processes involving foreign objects or substances repeatedly introduced in the mouth and contacting the teeth. In contrast, the term attrition is used to describe the physiological wearing away of dental hard tissues as a result of tooth-to-tooth contact without the intervention of foreign substances (Imfeld 1996).

Little is known of the epidemiology of abrasion, most knowledge coming from examination of skeletal remains. As yet, no investigation has established prevalence rates in any sample which could be considered representative of a population group (Hand et al. 1986).

Xhonga and co-workers (1972) considered that between 18 and 29% of the population were affected, whereas Bergstrom and Lavestedt (1979) stated that 31% of individuals had cervical abrasion defects. The latter authors noted that the prevalence of both superficial and deep lesions becomes more frequent with age. In their 1986 study, Hand and co-workers found that 56% of the dentate elderly population had some cervical abrasion lesions. Abrasion was found on 16% of teeth, 5% of lesions being deeper than 1 mm. Consistent with brushing with toothpaste being the primary aetiological agent, people with fewer mobile, carious and calculus-covered teeth demonstrated increased cervical abrasion. In an early report, Ervin and Bucher (1944) stated that the actual number of abrasion lesions per mouth ranged from 2.0 in young people to 4.0 in older individuals.

Abrasion lesions can occur on any tooth, but commonly present on the buccal cervical region of incisors, canines and premolars in both jaws (Orchardson and Collins 1987). Addy *et al.* (1987) have observed that the position of teeth within the dental arch is relevant to the distribution of abrasion lesions, teeth in buccal misalignment being more susceptible to wear and trauma than those displaced lingually.

Although several authors have expressed concern that habitual mechanical cleaning may damage oral hard and soft tissues (McConnell and Conroy 1967, Bergenholtz 1972) few studies have demonstrated the origin and extent of such damage. This probably reflects the practical difficulties associated with establishing reliable experimental conditions in man (Niemi *et al.* 1984). In the 1940s, two reports from the USA indicated that oral hygiene procedures could lead to a high prevalence of toothbrushing abrasion (Kitchin 1941, Ervin and Bucher 1944). However, more recent studies have usually concentrated on gingival abrasions (Phaneuf *et al.* 1962, Ash 1964).

Opinion tends to favour the view that soft tissue damage is caused by the toothbrush, whereas hard tissue loss is largely a function of toothpaste abrasives (Sangnes 1976). Other agents operating in vivo, notably dietary acid, may greatly enhance the action of toothpaste abrasives on enamel and dentine (Rees and Davis 1975, Davis and Winter 1980).

Several individual toothbrushing variables potentially influence the abrasion of dental hard tissues during toothbrushing (Kitchin 1941, Sangnes 1976, Saxton and Cowell 1981). These include:

- Brushing technique
- Bristle stiffness
- Brushing force
- Time spent brushing
- Frequency of brushing.

Brushing technique

Vertical and horizontal toothbrushing techniques are associated with fundamental differences in the contact relationship of brush and tooth surface. Manly (1944) found that, in vitro, cross-brushing produced 2–3 times as much dentine wear as longitudinal brushing, an observation supported by Bergström and Lavestedt (1979). This phenomenon is explained by the work of Bjorn and Lindhe (1966b) who found that horizontal brushing produced a prolonged contact duration between bristles and tooth surface. As a result of their observations, Bergström and Lavestedt (1979) recommended the use of a rolling technique or vertical strokes. However, Padbury and Ash (1974) found that a simulated roll action in vitro produced greater loss of tissue than a scrub motion, although they did comment that the scrub motion was thought to produce unsightly grooving in vivo.

Limited data are available on abrasion due to power brushing. In their 1993 study, Schemehorn and co-workers found that rotary brushing with the Interplak brush (Bausch and Lomb, 106 London Road, Kingston upon Thames, Surrey, UK) produced 3.5 times more dentine abrasion than a manual brush when a 'raw' abrasive system was used. Conversely, this electrical brushing technique was not excessively abrasive when used with the Interplak or a conventional toothpaste.

The review and consensus report of the World Workshop in Periodontics (Hancock 1996) concluded that, although there was growing evidence that some of the new designs of power brush were more effective than manual toothbrushes in terms of their ability to remove plaque, no analogous data were available with regard to hard and soft tissue abrasion.

Bristle stiffness

Toothbrush bristles show enormous variation with regard to material, stiffness, orientation, dimensions and their placement on the brushhead. Until now, the British Standards Institution (1987) has graded filament stiffness as soft, medium and hard. This categorization is based on parallel aligned, multi-tufted, flat trim toothbrushes containing filaments of the same material and diameter. However, in more recently developed brushes, filaments vary in diameter and tip shape, tufts may not be parallel, and different materials may be combined. Further, neck and head angulation, as well as the nature of the handle, are by no means uniform.

The interaction between the filaments and toothpaste may also be important. A hard brush might logically be expected to be more abrasive than a soft one when tested with a standard paste in vitro. However, unpublished preliminary studies by Addy and Dyer would indicate that this is not so due to the ability of hard filaments to retain more paste than soft ones.

Brushing force

Although not the most significant cause of abrasion, brushing force is thought to be of great relevance (Padbury and Ash 1974). Early work by Phaneuf and co-workers (1962) and Frostell and Lindström (1964) suggested that dentine wear is proportional to the force applied to the brush, although this varies with the individual area of the arch being cleaned (Alexander et al. 1977). More recently, Saxton and Cowell (1981) stated that brushing force could be an extremely important factor in the dynamics of abrasion. This view has yet to be confirmed with supporting data.

In vivo, it is difficult to measure and standardize the force applied to a brush, while measurements of force in vitro do not compare as well as might be expected. In an in-vivo experiment to measure force applied during horizontal brushing, Mannerberg (1960) estimated that males created a force of 539 g while females created one of 478 g. In contrast, Phaneuf and co-workers (1962) found that, on average, the brushing force for hand-brushing was 318 g.

In attempts to reduce wear and trauma to teeth and gingival tissues, Spieler (1996) recently described the first toothbrush to allow users to monitor and standardize their brushing pressure, while Savill and co-workers (1998) have described a toothbrush specifically designed to combine optimal plaque control with oral hard and soft tissue care (Mentadent Adaptor toothbrush, Unilever, Port Sunlight, Bebington, Wirral L63 3JW, UK). This latter has a brush-head which consists of a polypropylene core, which is surrounded at the sides by a flexible thermoplastic elastomer. Embedded into the elastomer are a number of what are described as 'flex caps'

into which the outer bristle tufts are inserted. Bristle tufts are also inserted into the central polymer core of the head and the bristles are arranged into a cup shape to mimic the profile of the teeth. In use, the elastomer flexes, allowing the bristles to adapt to the contours of the teeth.

In many of the newer power brushes introduced during the 1990s, bristle movement is prevented when a brushing force in the region of 100–200 g is reached. This represents a significant reduction in brushing force compared with that exerted with manual brushes. However, the effect of such forces on abrasion of hard and soft tissues has yet to be elucidated clinically.

Time spent toothbrushing

Time spent brushing the teeth also appears to play an important role in the multifactorial aetiology of abrasion. Evidence indicates that the average brushing time is 60 s (Emling et al. 1981), although this is extremely variable. Some studies report average brushing times of < 56 s (Rugg-Gunn and MacGregor 1978, MacGregor et al. 1986), while others quote brushing times of between 56 and 70 s (MacGregor and Rugg-Gunn 1979, Emling et al. 1981, Saxer et al. 1983). MacGregor and Rugg-Gunn (1985) showed that in the 13-year-old age group approximately 33 seconds were spent on brushing. In addition, not all teeth or tooth surfaces receive equal attention; it is known that some teeth are brushed for longer periods than others (MacGregor and Rugg-Gunn 1979), particularly those at the start of the brushing cycle, such as premolars and canines.

Frequency of toothbrushing

Sangnes (1976) and Bergström and Lavestedt (1979) have stated that the frequency of toothbrushing and the contact time between tooth and brush may influence the degree of wear observed. It has been suggested that little benefit to periodontal health is achieved if the teeth are brushed more than twice per day and that frequency in excess of this may encourage dental abrasion (Sheiham 1977).

Toothpaste abrasivity

Toothpastes are complex formulations, and a fine balance has to be achieved in order to provide cosmetic and oral health benefits whilst limiting chemical and/or physical damage to teeth. Toothpaste abrasives used both currently and over the last decade include: diatomaceous earth, calcium carbonate, dicalcium phosphate, hydrated or anhydrous insoluble sodium metaphosphate, silica, aluminium oxide, calcium pyrophosphate, alumina and pumice. These are known to vary in cleaning/abrasion characteristics (Barbakow et al. 1987), although no overall ranking has been published. It should be emphasized that chemically identical abrasives such as hydrated silica or calcium carbonate can produce different cleaning/abrasion characteristics. Similarly, a mixture of chemically different abrasives may result in effects differing markedly from those of the individual components (Wulknitz 1997).

Miller first documented the abrasive properties of toothpastes in 1907. Since that time, many investigators have studied the concept of abrasion of dental hard tissue by these products (Manly 1944, Mannerberg 1960, Frostell and Lindström 1964) and concern has been expressed regarding their potential for tooth-wear. For example, Hirschfeld (1939) considered that, in order to obtain good cleaning properties and stain removal, toothpastes may abrade tooth structure to an unacceptable degree. Later, Bull and co-workers (1968) emphasized that it was important to consider this problem when selecting an abrasive or mixture of abrasives, bearing in mind that actual cleansing requirements vary from person to person. In contrast, Davis and Winter (1980) considered that abrasives had a minimal effect on enamel, their effect being more pronounced on dentine. This is in agreement with the opinion of the British Standards Institution (1981).

Bjorn and co-workers (1966) noted that when undiluted, all toothpastes were capable of abrading human dentine in vivo, their relative abrasivity being unchanged on dilution with saliva. In-vitro studies have demonstrated that there is wide variation in the depth of abrasion depending on which toothpaste is used. Those containing diatomaceous earth and so-called 'smokers toothpastes' are particularly abrasive (Addy et al.

1991). In contrast, the tartar control toothpastes are not excessively abrasive, because they work by adsorption of pyrophosphate to the surface rather than by removal of the surface calcium phosphate (Manson et al. 1991).

The investigation of toothpaste abrasivity in vitro and in vivo

Abrasion is likely to increase with increased toothpaste abrasivity (Bergstrom and Lavestedt 1979), wear resistance rapidly increasing as the tissue hardness approaches that of the abrasive (Wright and Stevenson 1967). Measurement of mean particle size is thought to be a highly reliable method of predicting abrasion (Bull et al. 1968, Sangnes 1976), while the role of particle concentration is more controversial. Manly (1944) stated that the rate of abrasion was fairly independent of particle concentration, a change in the latter merely altering the thickness of the abrasive layer. In comparison, Bjorn and Lindhe (1966a) found that the relative concentration of particles per square unit brushing surface was the determining factor with regard to the rate of abrasion.

Techniques employed for the measurement of abrasivity of toothpastes in vitro have included:

- Gravimetric changes in dental tissues and substitutes (Sexson and Phillips 1951)
- Recording radioactive calcium released from irradiated teeth (Wright and Stevenson 1967, Stookey and Muhler 1968)
- Scanning electron microscopy (Wictorin 1972)
- Surface profilometry (Manly 1944, Bouchal 1966)
- Replication techniques (Mannerberg 1960)
- Digital imaging analysis (Mistry and Grenby 1993).

It is tempting to criticize any of the available techniques as being poor imitations of the oral environment. However, as methods can be standardized, it is possible to investigate products extensively, at reasonable cost and without too many technical difficulties (Addy et al. 1991).

In 1991, Addy and co-workers described a simple and reproducible method for comparing the abrasivity of toothpastes in vitro. In this technique, blocks of acrylic, 43 mm^2 cut from 3-mm thick sheets of the optically clear polymethylmethacrylate product Perspex (ICI, Macclesfield, UK) were prepared to fit into a template secured in the well of an electric motor-driven reciprocal action toothbrushing machine. The brushes, heads removed from compact medium texture toothbrushes (Oral B 35, Oral B, Aylesbury, UK), were replaced for each product tested. These were loaded with 100 g and positioned to pass approximately through the middle of the specimens. Brushing with water or a slurry of toothpaste consisting of 5 g of product in 20 ml of water was carried out for 12,500 cycles (25,000 strokes, equivalent to brushing for 4 h) or 25,000 cycles (50,000 strokes, equivalent to brushing for 8 h). For each experiment 40 ml of slurry was placed into the shallow reservoir. This was agitated to resuspend the ingredients every 20 min and replaced every hour. When brushing was complete, specimens were washed thoroughly under running tap water and allowed to bench dry. Surface profiles were then made with a profilometer (Surfometer SF200; Planer Industries, Middlesex, UK), attached to a micro-computer. Recordings were made across three zones at right angles to the direction of brushing, including both unbrushed peripheries. The measurements were expressed as mean loss in micrometres.

The use of acrylic as a substitute for dental hard tissues may be criticized, as it is chemically inert to ingredients such as detergents, which may affect the mechanical action of abrasives. Indeed, recent work by West et al. (1998) has shown that the liquid phase containing the detergent (often sodium lauryl sulphate) is capable of removing the dentine smear layer, thereby exposing the dentinal tubules. However, tests in vitro using dental tissues alone are not devoid of problems. Specimens can never be accurately standardized, particularly as they are obtained from different individuals and different tooth types, and are altered by numerous factors during their period in the mouth. Hardness values of different specimens may be similar, but their susceptibility to abrasion may vary greatly (Davis 1978). Gravimetric results are considerably influenced by hydration of the specimens (Davis 1978) and radiolabelling significantly alters the susceptibility of both enamel and

dentine to abrasion (Davis 1975, Davis and Hefferen 1975). It would therefore seem pertinent to employ several different materials for tests in vitro.

Clinical studies are problematic for a number of reasons. In vivo, tooth wear is multifactorial in origin and there is currently no evidence to show which factors are dominant. Studies are also hampered by problems related to volunteer compliance and sensitivity of measurement (Saxton and Cowell 1981). Practical problems arise because wear is a slow process which requires precision equipment for measurement. The progression of lesions on hard tissues and restorations has been estimated at as much as 7 μm per week in some individuals (Xhonga et al. 1972), although a more frequently quoted figure is about 1 μm per week (Cowell and Allen 1979).

Methods used clinically have been based on either comparison of tooth profiles over time or comparison of surface marks such as scratches (Cowell and Allen 1979). Mannerberg (1960) observed scratches appearing and disappearing on the tooth surface, thereby demonstrating a plastic flow of tissue with remineralization. However, the quantitative relationship between scratching and increased abrasion cannot be held true for all abrasive systems: alumina, for example, abrades without scratching (Cowell and Allen 1979). Similar tissue flow was observed by Absi (1989) using a replica technique. In a 6-year study, Mannerberg (1960) demonstrated scratches on enamel and concluded that habitual toothbrushing was the causative factor.

Standards for toothpaste abrasivity

In 1974, a British Standard for toothpaste was drawn up in an attempt to prevent the manufacture of toothpastes which could conceivably produce harmful effects not easily recognized by the user. This was subsequently revised in 1981 (British Standards Institution 1981) primarily to incorporate surface profilometry as an alternative method of abrasivity measurement. The primary test method for abrasivity, which was developed from basic research undertaken at the National Engineering Laboratory, involves a radio-tracer technique of wear resistance. In this technique, extracted human permanent teeth are irradiated, subjected to simulated brushing, and the abrasivity value is calculated on the basis of the measurement of radioactivity transferred to the toothpaste. The surface profile method employs an identical brushing programme, but relies for its measurement of abrasivity on a highly accurate measurement of the depth of the abraded groove. In order to minimize the effects of the variability of tooth substance between one tooth and another, both methods produce results expressed as a ratio of the abrasivity of the test paste to that of a standard reference paste. Alternative substrates to human enamel and dentine have been examined, but have been found unsuitable. The standard sets upper limits for abrasivity: for dentine, the abrasivity of the test paste should not exceed twice that of the standard reference paste, while for enamel, the abrasivity: value for the test paste should not exceed four times that of the BSI paste. In cases of dispute, or if the results achieved by the surface profile method fall between the reduced limits for that method (1.5 $\times$ abrasivity of the reference paste for dentine and 3 $\times$ abrasivity of the reference paste for enamel) and the normal limits, the abrasivity of the toothpaste is determined by the radio-tracer method. A similar system is in operation in the USA, where most toothpastes have a radioactive dentine abrasivity (RDA) between 50 and 150 (Pader 1988). These regulations safeguard dental hard tissue from abrasion to a certain extent, yet even today there is no standard accepted by the profession above which there is damage and below which there is safety. A calculation by Saxton and Cowell (1981) suggests that a lower limit of 55 RDA allows cleaning to occur with minimal abrasion.

Cleaning power and abrasivity of European toothpastes

The major anti-stain effects of toothpastes on the European market are still due to abrasivity. Bleaching by peroxides is restricted for consumer products in the EU due to the regulations of the European Cosmetics Directive. Wulknitz (1997) recently evaluated 41 toothpastes available to European consumers in 1995 for cleaning efficacy in comparison with dentine

abrasivity (RDA value). In order to assess cleaning efficacy, a modified pellicle cleaning ratio (PCR) measurement method was developed. Slabs cut from bovine incisors were subjected to a 5-day tea-staining procedure prior to standardized brushing and brightness measurement by a chromametric technique. No product exceeded an RDA value of 200, the majority (80%) having an RDA value below 100. Only three products exceeded the pyrophosphate standard in cleaning power, with just one of these having an RDA lower than 100. Most products (73%) had a PCR value between 20 and 80.

The correlation between cleaning power and dentine abrasion was low ($r = 0.66$). Factors such as abrasive type, particle surface and size, as well as the chemical influence of other toothpaste ingredients, may explain this. Some major trends could be shown on the basis of abrasive types. Most of the hydrated silica-based toothpastes had good or very good cleaning values combined with low to moderate dentine abrasivity. A lower PCR:RDA ratio was found in some products containing calcium carbonate or aluminium trihydrate as the only abrasive. The addition of other abrasives, such as aluminium oxide (polishing alumina), showed improved cleaning power. Sequestrants such as sodium tripolyphosphate or phosphonates such as AHBP also improved the PCR:RDA ratio without being abrasive. The data for some special anti-stain products did not differ significantly from standard products.

While it is encouraging to note that in Europe, over the last decade, there has been a general trend toward reduced abrasivity, it should be borne in mind that dentine abrasivity should not be regarded as the sole safety criterion for the abrasivity of toothpastes. Comparison of data shows that enamel abrasivity values can differ substantially without major changes in abrasion on dentine (Wulknitz 1997).

Summary

Assessing the role of various parameters in the origin of abrasion lesions, Bergström and Lavestedt (1979) found that toothpaste abrasivity correlated with abrasion lesions less well than did brushing technique and brushing frequency.

A variety of opinions exists as to the contribution of toothbrush and/or toothpaste action in the production of abrasion lesions. It is generally accepted that abrasion can be produced by toothbrushing in vitro if abrasives are used (Sangnes 1976), while little damage occurs with toothbrushing alone (Manly 1944, Mannerberg 1960, Manly et al. 1965, Bjorn and Lindhe 1966a, Absi et al. 1992). In contrast, Saxton and Cowell (1981) suggested that brushing made a substantial contribution to the amount of dentine removed and that the addition of a toothpaste abrasive was not a major factor in the progression of cervical lesions. This statement is lacking in support and contradicts evidence from in-vitro studies (Miller 1907, Tainter and Epstein 1942, Manly 1944, Manly et al. 1965, Bjorn and Lindhe 1966a).

References

Absi EG (1989) Studies on the aetiology, appearance, and treatment of hypersensitive dentine. PhD Thesis, University of Wales.

Absi EG, Addy M, Adams D (1992) The effects of toothbrushing and dietary compounds on dentine *in vitro*: a SEM study. *J Oral Rehabil* **19**: 101–10.

Addy M, Mostafa P, Newcombe RG (1987) Dentine hypersensitivity: the distribution of recession, sensitivity and plaque. *J Dent* **15**: 242–8.

Addy M, Goodfield S, Harrison A (1991) The use of acrylic to compare the abrasivity and stain removal properties of toothpastes. *Clinical Materials* **7**: 219–25.

Alexander JF, Safir AI, Gold W (1977) The measurement of the effect of toothbrushing on soft tissue abrasion. *J Dent Res* **56**: 722–7.

Ash MM Jr (1964) A review of the problems and results of studies on manual and power toothbrushes. *J Periodontol* **35**: 202–13.

Barbakow F, Lutz F, Imfeld T (1987) Abrasives in dentifrices and prophylaxis pastes. *Quint Int* **18**: 17–22.

Bergenholtz A (1972) Mechanical cleaning in oral hygiene. In: Frandsen A, ed, *Oral Hygiene*, 27–60. Munksgaard: Copenhagen.

Bergström J, Lavestedt S (1979) An epidemiologic approach to toothbrushing and dental abrasion. *Community Dent Oral Epidemiol* **7**: 57–64.

Bjorn H, Lindhe J (1966a) Abrasion of dentine by toothbrush and dentifrice. *Odont Revy* **17**: 17–27.

Bjorn H, Lindhe J (1966b) On the mechanics of toothbrushing. *Odont Revy* **17**: 10–16.

Bjorn H, Lindhe, J. Grondahl HG (1966) The abrasion of dentine by commercial dentifrices. *Odont Revy* **17**: 109–20.

Bouchal AW (1966) The abrasiveness of dentifrices. *Proceedings of the Scientific Section of the Toilet Goods Association* **45**: 2–5.

British Standards Institution (1981) Specification for toothpastes (BS 5136). 2 Park Street, London W1A 2BS.

British Standards Institution (1987) Determination of stiffness of the tufted area of toothbrushes (BS 5757) 1987. 2, Park Street, London W1A 2BS.

Bull WH, Callender RM, Pugh BR, Wood GD (1968) The abrasion and cleaning properties of dentifrices. *Br Dent J* **125**: 331–7.

Cowell CR, Allen RW (1979) A comparison of dentine wear on prepared tooth sections in vivo using two toothpastes. *Br Dent J* **140**: 339–42.

Davis WB (1975) Reduction in dentine wear resistance by irradiation and effects of storage in aqueous media. *J Dent Res* **54**: 1078–81.

Davis WB (1978) The cleansing, polishing and abrasion of teeth and dental products. *Cosmetic Science* **1**: 39–81.

Davis WB, Hefferen JJ (1975) The effects of irradiation on wear resistance, microhardness and acid solubility of dentine. *J Dent Res* **54**: L150 (abstract).

Davis WB, Winter PJ (1980) The effect of abrasion on enamel and dentine after exposure to dietary acid. *Br Dent J* **148**: 253–6.

Emling RC, Flickinger KC, Cohen DW, Yankell SI (1981) A comparison of estimated versus actual brushing time. *Pharmacol Ther Dent* **6**: 93–8.

Ervin JC, Bucher EM (1944) Prevalence of tooth root exposure and abrasion among dental patients. *Dental Items of Interest* **66**: 760–9.

Frandsen A (1986) Mechanical oral hygiene practices. In: Löe H, Kleinman DV, eds, *Dental Plaque Control Measures and Oral Hygiene Practices*, 93–116. Oxford University Press: Northants.

Frostell G, Lindström G (1964) Undersokning av nagra av den svenska marknadens tandkramer Del 1. *Odont Foren T* **28**: 211–48.

Hancock EB, ed. (1996) Prevention. World Workshop in Periodontics. *Ann Periodontol* **1**: 223–55

Hand JS, Hunt RJ, Reinhardt JW (1986) The prevalence and treatment implications of cervical abrasion in the elderly. *Gerodontics* **2**: 167–70.

Hirschfeld I (1939) The toothbrush. Its use and abuse. In: *Dental Items of Interest*, 1–27, 262–7, 358–465, 484–95. Kimpton: Edinburgh.

Imfeld T (1996) Dental erosion. Definition, classification and links. *Eur J Oral Sci* **104**: 151–5.

Kitchin P (1941) The prevalence of tooth root exposure and the relation of the extent of such exposure to the degree of abrasion in different age classes. *J Dent Res* **20**: 565–81.

Levitch LC, Bader JD, Shugars DA, Heymann HO (1994) Non-carious cervical lesions. *J Dent* **22**:195–207.

McConnell D, Conroy CW (1967) Comparisons of abrasion produced by stimulated versus a mechanical toothbrush. *J Dent Res* **46**: 1022–7.

MacGregor IDM, Rugg-Gunn AJ (1979) A survey of toothbrushing sequence in children and young adults. *J Periodont Res* **14**: 225–30.

MacGregor IDM, Rugg-Gunn AJ (1985) Toothbrushing duration in 60 uninstructed young adults. *Community Dent Oral Epidemiol* **13**: 121–2.

MacGregor IDM, Rugg-Gunn AJ, Gordon PH (1986) Plaque levels in relation to the number of toothbrushing strokes in uninstructed English schoolchildren. *J Periodont Res* **21**: 557–82.

Manly RS (1944) Factors influencing tests on the abrasion of dentin by brushing with dentifrice. *J Dent Res* **23**: 59–72.

Manly RS, Wiren J, Manley PJ, Keene RC (1965) A method for measurement of abrasion of dentin by toothbrush and dentifrice. *J Dent Res* **44**: 533–40.

Mannerberg F (1960) Appearance of tooth surfaces as observed in shadowed replicas, in various age groups, in long term studies, after toothbrushing, in cases of erosion and after exposure to citrus fruit juice. *Odont Revy* **11** (Suppl 6): 1–116.

Manson S, Levan A, Crawford R et al (1991) Evaluation of tartar control dentifrices in *in vitro* models of dentine sensitivity. *Clin Prev Dent* **12**: 6–9.

Miller WD (1907) Experiments and observation on the wasting of tooth tissue erroneously designated as erosion, abrasion, denudation, etc. *Dental Cosmos* **49**: 109–24.

Mistry M, Grenby TH (1993) Erosion by soft drinks of rat molar teeth assessed by digital image analysis. *Caries Res* **27**: 21–5.

Niemi ML, Sandholm L, Ainamo J (1984) Frequency of gingival lesions after standardized brushing as related to stiffness of toothbrush and abrasiveness of dentifrice. *J Clin Periodontol* **11**: 254–61.

Orchardson R, Collins WJN (1987) Clinical features of hypersensitive teeth. *Br Dent J* **162**: 253–6.

Padbury AD, Ash MM Jr (1974) Abrasion caused by three methods of toothbrushing. *J Periodontol* **45**: 434–8.

Pader M (1988) *Oral Hygiene Products and Practice*, 200. Marcel Dekker: New York.

Phaneuf EA, Harrington JH, Ashland AB et al (1962) Automatic toothbrush: a new reciprocating action. *J Am Dent Assoc* **65**: 12–25.

Rees DA, Davis WB (1975) An in vitro method for assessing dentine and enamel loss. *J Dent Res* **54** (Sp. issue): (abstract no. 341).

Rugg-Gunn AJ, MacGregor IDM (1978) A survey of toothbrushing behaviour in children and young adults. *J Periodont Res* **13**: 382–9.

Sangnes G (1976) Traumatization of teeth and gingivae related to habitual tooth cleaning. Review article. *J Clin Periodontol* **3**: 94–103.

Savill G, Grigor J, Huntingdon E (1998) Toothbrush design: adapting for the future. *Int Dent J* **48** (Suppl 1): 519–25.

Saxer UP, Emling R, Yankell SL (1983) Actual versus estimated toothbrushing time and toothpaste used. *Caries Res* **17**:179–80.

Saxton CA, Cowell CR (1981) Clinical investigation of the effects of dentifrices on dentine wear at the cementoenamel junction. *J Am Dent Assoc* **102**: 38–43.

Schemehorn B, Ball T, Bloom B (1993) A model to determine the relative abrasiveness of rotary toothbrushes. *J Dent Res* **72** (abstract no. 2478).

Sexson JC, Phillips RW (1951) Studies on the effects of abrasives on acrylic resins. *J Prosthet Dent* **1**: 454–71.

Sheiham A (1977) Preventive control of periodontal disease. In: Klavan B et al, eds, *International Conference on Research into the Biology of Periodontal Disease*, 308–9. University of Illinois.

Spieler EL (1996) Preventing toothbrush abrasion and the efficacy of the Alert toothbrush: a review and patient study. *Compendium of Continuing Education in Dentistry* **17**: 478–80, 482, 484–5.

Stookey GK, Muhler JC (1968) Laboratory studies concerning the enamel and dentine abrasion properties of common dentifrices and polishing agents. *J Dent Res* **47**: 524–32.

Tainter ML, Epstein S (1942) A standard procedure for determining abrasion by dentifrices. *J Am Coll Dent* **9**: 353.

West N, Addy M, Hughes J (1998) Dentine hypersensitivity: the effects of brushing desensitizing toothpastes, their solid and liquid phases and detergents on dentine and acrylic: studies in vitro. *J Oral Rehabil* **25**:885–95.

Wictorin L (1972) Effect of toothbrushing on acrylic resin veneering material. II. Abrasive effect of selected dentifrices and toothbrushes. *Acta Odont Scand* **30**: 338–95.

Wright KHR, Stevenson JI (1967) The measurement and interpretation of dentifrice abrasiveness. *J Soc Cosmetic Chemists* **18**: 387–411.

Wulknitz P (1997) Cleaning power and abrasivity of European toothpastes. *Adv Dent Res* **11**: 576–9.

Xhonga FA, Wolcott RB, Sognnaes RF (1972) Dental erosion II: Clinical measurement of dental erosion progress. *J Am Dent Assoc* **84**: 557–82.

15

Interplay of erosion, attrition and abrasion in tooth wear and possible approaches to prevention

Jukka H Meurman and Rita Sorvari

Introduction

Tooth wear is produced by non-carious destructive processes and is likely to be a multifactorial phenomenon (Smith 1975, Eccles 1982, Meurman and ten Cate 1996). In most cases, mechanical tooth wear (abrasion and attrition) and chemical dissolution (erosion) act simultaneously (Smith and Knight 1984a, Nunn et al. 1996). In the clinical situation it is often difficult to determine the part played by a specific causative factor in a single patient with tooth wear (Pindborg 1970, Lewis and Smith 1973). Chemically softened tooth surface becomes liable to mechanical wear which emphasizes the need to focus on the interaction of these pathological mechanisms (Davis and Winter 1980). As long ago as 1907, Miller had pointed out the importance of different aetiological factors in the 'wasting of tooth tissue'.

In the past and in primitive cultures even extensive tooth wear could be considered a normal phenomenon due to the roughness of food; in ancient skulls drastic wear can also be seen in persons who died young (Varrela and Varrela 1991). Normally, tooth wear increases with age, which is a physiological process, but the increasing incidence of natural tooth retention into older age today has resulted in a wider prevalence of severely worn dentition than previously seen in modern man (Johansson and Omar 1994).

Over the last two decades, interest in tooth wear has increased, and the various aetiological aspects of dental erosion in particular have been investigated (Eccles and Jenkins 1974, Linkosalo and Markkanen 1985, Wöltgens et al. 1985, Asher and Read 1987, Järvinen et al. 1988, Rytömaa et al. 1988, Sorvari 1989b, Westergaard et al. 1993, Meurman et al. 1994). Nevertheless, the complex interplay of erosion, attrition and abrasion is not clear. This chapter will briefly review relevant literature on the topic and discuss which aspects, in particular, require further attention and more research. Finally, guidelines and recommendations for controlling and preventing tooth wear are presented.

Clinical and epidemiological studies

Attrition

Many studies have been published on attrition in anthropological materials but investigations describing the contemporary epidemiological status are seldom found (for reviews see: Johansson 1992, Varrela 1996). On the other hand, attrition has been described as a prerequisite for balanced occlusion. This form of tooth wear can be considered physiological (Begg 1954).

Lambrechts et al. (1989) investigated the normal progression and rate of occlusal contact area wear over a period of 4 years in young adults and observed a steady wear of 29 μm per year in molars, 15 μm per year in premolars. High bite force and bruxism have been suggested to influence attrition (Waltimo *et al.* 1994). In a longitudinal study extending over 13 years in 39 patients aged 5–18 years, the maximal anterior bite force was found to be the strongest background factor for horizontal tooth wear (Nyström *et al.* 1990). Johansson *et al.* (1991, 1993a) investigated the significance of some factors associated with tooth wear in selected Saudi Arabian and Swedish samples and found no correlation between subjects from different geographic and/or climatic areas and the severity of tooth wear. Nevertheless, low salivary buffer capacity and low secretion rate were significantly correlated with high wear (Johansson *et al.* 1993c). Attrition is greatly increased if other causes of tooth wear act simultaneously (Lewis and Smith 1973). For example, workers from Tanzania who were exposed to industrial and environmental stone dust have been shown to have significantly more wear than controls (Tuominen and Tuominen 1991). Similarly, exposure to acid fumes in the work environment is known to be associated with increased tooth wear in which the erosive component adds to the attrition (ten Bruggen Cate 1968, Tuominen *et al.* 1991). It is known that deciduous teeth are less wear-resistant than permanent teeth, probably because of differences in their chemical and physical structure. However, the concept of 'normality' in tooth attrition requires further study.

Abrasion

Toothbrushing is the principal cause of tooth abrasion, which is enhanced by use of abrasive dentifrice (Kuroiwa *et al.* 1994). Interestingly, abrasive toothpastes have been used for over 2000 years, as stain removal requires a degree of abrasivity (Forward 1991). Cervical abrasion of teeth has been particularly linked to the use of abrasive dentifrice (Volpe *et al.* 1975, Teaford and Tylenda 1991). Nordbo and Skogedal (1982) investigated the rate of abrasion in a 26-month study using micrometer measurements and observed an average rate of tooth substance loss of 0.2 μm per day in 20 subjects who brushed their teeth either with a conventional toothpaste or with a non-abrasive dentifrice. The hardness of toothbrushes and abrasivity of toothpastes have been areas of great concern among manufacturers of oral hygiene products. The reader is advised to turn to the specific regulations in this respect (British Standards Institution 1981) (see also Chapter 14).

The prevalence of abrasion lesions has been extensively studied in selected patients but a general picture with regard to the population level is still lacking (Radentz *et al.* 1976, Sangnes and Gjermo 1976, Hand *et al.* 1986, Bergström and Eliasson 1988, Smith and Robb 1996, Smith *et al.* 1997). In the USA, cervical abrasion has also been termed 'cervical erosion' which, on the other hand, reflects the complex aetiology and interplay of the different pathological mechanisms acting simultaneously. Acids have also been shown to enhance dental abrasion in vitro and, like attrition, it is modified by erosion (Eccles 1982, Attin *et al.* 1998). In individual patients strange biting habits such as biting nails, pens and other foreign objects are occasionally identified as causes of tooth abrasion (see Chapter 7).

Erosion

Sognnaes *et al.* (1972) reported dental erosion in 18% of a random sample of 10,000 extracted teeth. The same group also assessed that erosion would progress at an average rate of approximately 1 μm per day (Xhonga *et al.* 1972). Xhonga and Valdmanis (1983) then investigated erosion in 527 dental hospital patients (age range 14–80 years) and reported prevalence figures up to 25%. More recently, the prevalence figure was 16% in an epidemiological study by Lussi *et al.* (1991) investigating two randomly selected groups of 391 Swiss adults. However, differential diagnosis between erosion and attrition is difficult (Eccles and Jenkins 1974, Eccles 1979).

In general, the prevalence figures in erosion studies show large differences, ranging from a very low percentage to almost 100%, depending on the population examined (Nunn 1996). For example, lactovegetarians have been reported to be at high risk of erosion. According to a study by Linkosalo and Markkanen (1985), the main factors in these individuals were low salivary flow rate and high consumption of vinegar products, citrus fruits and acidic berries. Another group of patients often cited in this context is patients suffering from anorexia and/or bulimia.

These are well-defined psychiatric disorders known to cause dental erosion due to frequent vomiting (Hellström 1977, Scheutzel and Meermann 1994, Robb *et al.* 1995, Rytömaa *et al.* 1998). Severe cases of these eating disorders can result in total destruction of the dentition. Gastrointestinal disorders that cause regurgitation of gastric contents into the mouth, or which are associated with an increased output of gastric acid in general, have also been shown to render the patient liable to dental erosion (Järvinen *et al.* 1988, 1992, Meurman *et al.* 1994, Schroeder *et al.* 1995, Scheutzel 1996, Lazarchik and Filler 1997). This may also happen in children (O'Sullivan *et al.* 1998). Recently, Johansson *et al.* (1997) showed erosion to be

associated particularly with the consumption of soft drinks in a study of young Saudi men.

Acidic erosion enhances both abrasion and attrition of the dentition, but it is difficult to distinguish the exact pathogenic role of each of these factors in a single case of tooth wear (Figures 15.1–15.3). However, erosion seems to play an increasing role due to altered lifestyle, such as the increased consumption of acidic beverages, use of special diets and increasingly prevalent episodes of acid regurgitation (Anon 1980, Dwyer 1988, Zero 1996). Multicentric population studies should therefore be established in order to survey the significance of the problem in general. The various aetiological factors of tooth wear – together with dental, medical, socio-economical,

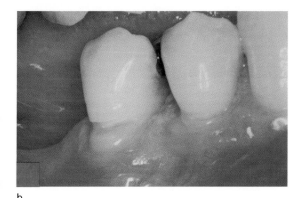

a

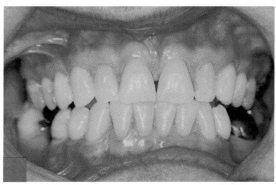

b

Figure 15.1

Dentition of a 45-year-old woman with a history of eating acidic berries frequently. *a* Good oral hygiene is obvious. *b* Cervical abrasion has been induced.

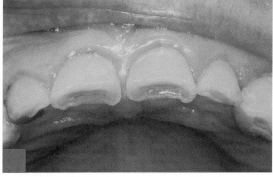

Figure 15.2

Shortened maxillary incisors with eroded occlusal surfaces in a 57-year-old woman following a lactovegetarian diet.

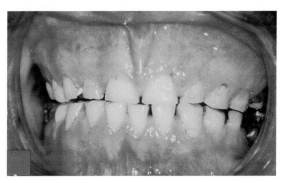

Figure 15.3

Worn dentition of a 30-year-old man. The patient's case history revealed frequent use of an acidic sport drink and high bite force.

dietary and lifestyle aspects – should be taken into account (see Chapter 11).

Animal studies

Teaford and Oyen (1989) examined the rate of molar tooth wear in monkeys given diets of different composition for up to 4 years. These authors found significant differences between animals on soft versus hard food. Sorvari *et al.* (1989b) have investigated dental erosion in a rat model. The earlier studies focused on assessing the effects of acidic drink on rat teeth and means of modifying their detrimental impact (Sorvari and Kiviranta 1988, Sorvari *et al.* 1988, Sorvari 1989a). More recently, the interplay between erosion and attrition was shown by feeding rats different diets for 6 weeks: the effects of soft and rough food, as

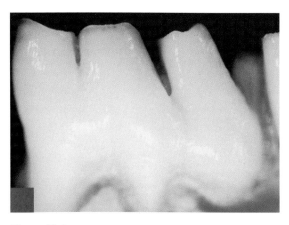

Figure 15.4

Intact lingual surface of the right first mandibular molar of a rat given soft food and distilled water. Soft tissues are removed.

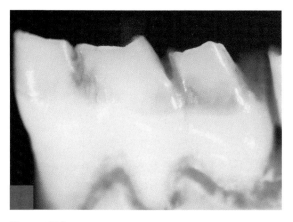

Figure 15.6

Lingual surface with effects of attrition; the rat was given rough food and distilled water.

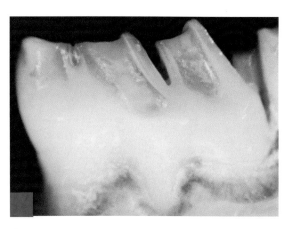

Figure 15.5

Eroded enamel with exposed dentine in the cuspal parts of the mandibular molar of a rat given sport drink (pH 3.2) and soft food. Samples were stained with Schiff's reagent before investigation under a stereomicroscope.

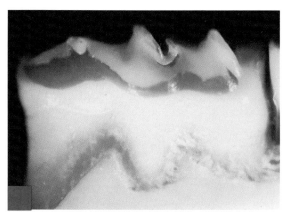

Figure 15.7

Tooth surface with extensive tissue loss due to simultaneous erosion and abrasion. The rat was given rough food and sport drink for 6 weeks.

well as an acidic sport drink, were studied (Sorvari *et al.* 1996). It was shown that tooth wear was greatest in the animals that received both rough food and an acidic drink, in comparison with cases where either attrition or erosion was generated (Figures 15.4–15.7). It was further shown that tooth wear could be diminished if fluoride was added to the drink. Interestingly, erosion alone appeared to leave dentinal tubules exposed, while erosion with attrition seemed to cause mostly occluded tubules. This finding may explain why patients with erosion often complain about increased sensitivity of the teeth (see Chapter 27).

It seems that animal models could be developed further to assess more precisely the different aetiological factors causing tooth wear. Animal studies may also help in testing various preventive measures against tooth wear. Compared with in-vitro experiments, animal studies are more biological and the results are more reliable because they take the complex environment of the mouth into account. Nevertheless, man is not a rat and caution should be used when applying results derived from animal experiments to human clinical practice.

Experimental in-vitro studies

Several in-vitro models have been presented to study pathological mechanisms of tooth wear (for reviews see: Niemi 1987, Joint Working Group FDI/ISO/TC 1991, Grenby 1996). However, the methods introduced mainly focus on only one aspect of the phenomenon at a time, and the complex interplay between erosion, attrition and abrasion has not been mimicked. Similarly, the complexity of the oral environment is difficult to simulate in vitro and protective factors that modify tooth wear are mostly neglected in the study models. Thus, in-vitro studies can be performed when the testing of a certain factor or a new product under simplified conditions is called for. Such studies can provide the first-line assessment of a new method, for example. If experimental models are used to investigate the various aetiological aspects and pathogenic mechanisms of tooth wear, their limitations must be borne in mind. In the future artificial mouths may provide better means of simulating the pathological processes acting in tooth wear.

Protective factors and prevention

Boxes 15.1 and 15.2 summarize the aspects that need consideration in the diagnosis and prevention of tooth wear. Without the lubricating effect of saliva, tooth wear apparently proceeds more rapidly than if saliva is present in the mouth. This

---

Box 15.1 Factors contributing to tooth wear.

Abrasion
- Biting habits
- Use of mechanical oral hygiene aids (e.g. hard-bristle toothbrush)
- Abrasive dental restorations and prostheses

Attrition
- Bruxism
- Malocclusion
- Diet (hard and coarse food items)
- Environmental hazards (e.g. stone dust)

Erosion
- Acids in diet (food items, drinks; frequency of intake)
- Acidic medicines (e.g. ascorbic acid)
- Gastro-oesophageal regurgitation, dyspepsia and peptic ulcer disease
- Anorexia and bulimia
- Other medical disorders leading to frequent vomiting (e.g. malignant disease, renal disease, liver disease)
- Acids in environment (e.g. industrial, work-related)

Box 15.2 Aspects considered in the prevention of tooth wear of different aetiology.

Abrasion
- Counselling about harmful biting habits
- Instruction as to the proper selection and use of oral hygiene aids
- Selection of non-abrasive dental materials

Attrition
- Adjustment of occlusion, preparation of splints and mouth guards
- Dietary counselling
- Work hygiene and counselling on environmental factors

Erosion
- Dietary counselling
- Selecting medicines with minimal side-effects on teeth
- Treatment of medical disorders and diseases
- Administration of salivary replacement therapy and antacids in selected cases
- Work hygiene and counselling on environmental factors

also applies to the experimental model systems used to study tooth wear (Wöltgens *et al.* 1985, Järvinen *et al.* 1991, Meurman and Frank 1991, Imfeld 1996, Meurman and ten Cate 1996). Another aspect is the chemical composition and physical structure of dental tissue under strain, together with craniofacial morphology and bite force (Kiliriadis *et al.* 1995). However, the fluoride content of enamel is a factor most often investigated in this respect. Davis and Winter (1977) showed that the application of fluoride toothpaste slurry for as little as 1 min protected teeth from erosion and abrasion in vitro. Recently, Attin and co-workers (1998) concluded that the application of sodium fluoride solutions immediately before toothbrushing significantly reduced abrasion of eroded dentine in vitro. Sorvari *et al.* (1994) found no difference between fluoride varnish and fluoride solution in this respect. The authors emphasized the key role of fluoride in modifying the process of erosion in general (Figure 15.8).

As regards prevention of attrition, early diagnosis and treatment of bruxism and malocclusion have been mentioned, and abrasion can be prevented by avoiding vigorous toothbrushing with a hard brush (Pindborg 1970, Schweitzer-Hirt *et al.* 1978, Eccles 1982, Johnson and Sivers 1987). The use of occlusal splints has also been shown to retard attrition (Carlsson *et al.* 1985). The simultaneous effects of erosion, attrition and abrasion accelerate the process of tooth wear in a single patient and care should be taken to avoid such situations. Brushing devices should be selected on an individual basis, so as to avoid hard-bristle brushes in patients with dry mouth or other known risk factors for tooth wear (Murtomaa and Meurman 1992). Mouth cleaning aids should not contain harmful components that are detrimental to tooth tissue (Rytömaa *et al.* 1989, Meurman *et al.* 1996).

If the cause of tooth wear is evident – as, for example, in patients with anorexia or other medical conditions – then the proper treatment of the underlying disease is the only remedy and means of prevention with regard to the progress of tooth wear. Patients with dry mouth should be instructed to drink enough in order to avoid dehydration and ensure salivary secretion. The patient's medication may also need consideration and modification. However, the diagnosis and treatment of these conditions are beyond the scope of this chapter and the reader is therefore

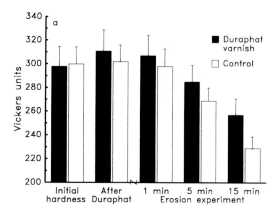

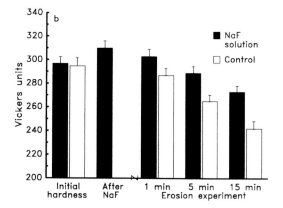

Figure 15.8

Enamel microhardness values of human tooth specimens measured initially after fluoride treatment, and after exposure to cola beverage. Test areas were (*a*) covered with Duraphat varnish for 24 h or (*b*) immersed in NaF solution for 48 h. Controls were not treated with fluoride (Sorvari *et al.* 1994: *Caries Res* **28**: 227–32).

advised to turn to other sources in this regard (Sreebny 1996).

Patients with frequent acid regurgitation and vomiting should be advised to avoid brushing their teeth immediately after the episode in order to prevent the extra burden of abrasion on teeth. Such patients may also benefit from rinsing their mouth with fluoride solution, the use of fluoride tablets and lozenges, and topical use of antacids (Meurman *et al.* 1988). As stated, the diagnosis and treatment of bruxism and malocclusion constitute the cornerstone for preventing pathological attrition. In order to prevent further progression of existing trauma in these patients, occlusal splints may be recommended, together with topically applied fluoride gels. With regard to abrasion, its cause must be eliminated to avoid further progress. Proper instruction in selecting and using various oral hygiene products and counselling on detrimental biting habits (e.g. on foreign objects) are the only means of preventing abrasion. Severe cases need restorative therapy, irrespective of the reason for tooth wear. The selection of dental restorative and prosthodontic materials must be based on knowledge of their physicochemical properties, so that materials best suited for the particular needs of individual patients with tooth wear can be used.

Finally, the interplay of erosion, attrition and abrasion is not well understood, in spite of a vast amount of literature on the topic. However, most studies have focused on only one aspect of tooth wear at a time, totally neglecting the complex pathology encountered in the clinical situation. Therefore, experimental models should be developed in order to assess the role of each of these factors in the process. Clinical indexes to measure tooth wear and simple dental office guidelines for differential diagnosis should also be developed (Smith and Knight 1984b, Johansson et al. 1993b, Nunn et al. 1996). Comprehensive multicentric studies are also required, to gain information on the prevalence and incidence of tooth wear at the population level, so that strategies for prevention and treatment can be developed further (Box 15.3).

Box 15.3 Summary of suggestions for further studies and guidelines on tooth wear

- Epidemiological, multicentric population studies on the prevalence and incidence of tooth wear
- Continuing surveys on selected groups (e.g. subjects on special diets or medications, bruxism and malocclusion patients, patients suffering from upper gastrointestinal disorders and other medical illnesses linked to tooth wear; anorexia and bulimia patients)
- Development of comprehensive in-vitro methods to study the interplay of different factors and defensive systems of tooth wear
- Development of animal models for the study of tooth wear
- Development of standardized protocols for testing various products, foodstuffs and drinks with regard to their effect on dental tissues
- Construction of guidelines and preparation of materials for counselling on tooth wear, at both the individual and population levels

---

References

Anon (1980) Erosion of teeth by acid. *Lancet* **2**: 353.

Asher C, Read MJF (1987) Early enamel erosion in children associated with the extensive consumption of citric acid. *Br Dent J* **16**: 384–7.

Attin T, Zirkel C, Hellwig E (1998) Brushing abrasion of eroded dentin after application of sodium fluoride solutions. *Caries Res* **32**: 344–50.

Begg PR (1954) Stone Age man's dentition. *Am J Orthod* **40**: 298–12.

Bergström J, Eliasson S (1988) Cervical abrasion in relation to toothbrushing and periodontal health. *Scand J Dent Res* **96**: 405–11.

British Standards Institution Specification for Toothpastes (1981) BS5 139.

Carlsson GE, Johansson A, Lundqvist S (1985) Occlusal wear. A follow-up study of 18 subjects with extensively worn dentitions. *Acta Odontol Scand* **43**: 83–90.

Davis WB, Winter PJ (1977) Dietary erosion of adult dentine and enamel, Protection with fluoride toothpaste. *Br Dent J* **143**: 116–19.

Davis WB, Winter PJ (1980) The effect of abrasion on enamel and dentine after exposure to dietary acid. *Br Dent J* **148**: 253–6.

Dwyer JT (1988) Health aspects of vegetarian diets. *Am J Clin Nutr* **48**: 712–38.

Eccles JD (1979) Dental erosion of non-industrial origin. A clinical survey and classification. *J Prosthet Dent* **42**: 649–53.

Eccles JD (1982) Tooth surface loss from abrasion, attrition and erosion. *Dental Update* **9**: 373–81.

Eccles JD, Jenkins GN (1974) Dental erosion and diet. *J Dent* **2**: 153–9.

Forward GC (1991) Role of toothpastes in the cleaning of teeth. *Int Dent J* **41**: 164–70.

Grenby TH (1996) Methods of assessing erosion and erosive potential. *Eur J Oral Sci* **104**: 207–14.

Hand JS, Hunt RJ, Renhardt JW (1986) The prevalence and treatment implications of cervical abrasion in the elderly. *Gerodontics* **2**: 167–70.

Hellström I (1977) Oral complications in anorexia nervosa. *Scand J Dent Res* **85**: 71–86.

Imfeld T (1996) Prevention of progression of dental erosion by professional and individual prophylactic measures. *Eur J Oral Sci* **104**: 215–20.

Järvinen V, Meurman JH, Hyvärinen H, Rytömaa I (1988) Dental erosion and upper gastrointestinal disorders. *Oral Surg Oral Med Oral Pathol* **65**: 298–303.

Järvinen VK, Rytömaa II, Heinonen OP (1991) Risk factors in dental erosion. *J Dent Res* **70**: 942–7.

Järvinen V, Rytömaa I, Meurman JH (1992) Location of dental erosion in a referred population. *Caries Res* **26**: 391–6.

Johansson A (1992) A cross-cultural study of occlusal tooth wear. *Swed Dent J* **16** (Suppl): 86.

Johansson A, Omar R (1994) Identification and management of tooth wear. *Int J Prosthodont* **7**: 506–16.

Johansson A, Fareed K, Omar R (1991) Analysis of possible factors influencing the occurrence of occlusal tooth wear in a young Saudi population. *Acta Odontol Scand* **49**: 139–45.

Johansson A, Haraldson T, Omar R et al (1993a) An investigation of some factors associated with occlusal tooth wear in a selected high-wear sample. *Scand J Dent Res* **101**: 407–15.

Johansson A, Haraldson T, Omar R et al (1993b) A system for assessing the severity and progression of occlusal tooth wear. *J Oral Rehabil* **20**: 125–31.

Johansson A, Kiliriadis S, Haraldson T et al (1993c) Covariation of some factors associated with occlusal tooth wear in a selected high-wear sample. *Scand J Dent Res* **101**: 398–406.

Johansson AK, Johansson A, Birkhed D et al (1997) Dental erosion associated with soft drink consumption in young Saudi men. *Acta Odontol Scand* **55**: 390–7.

Johnson GK, Sivers JE (1987) Attrition, abrasion and erosion: diagnosis and therapy. *Clin Prev Dent* **9**: 12–16.

Joint Working Group FDI/ISO/TC 106 I: Toothpaste (1991) *Toothpastes, Requirements, Test Methods.* Federation Dentaire International: London.

Kiliriadis A, Johansson A, Haraldson T et al (1995) Craniofacial morphology, occlusal trains, and bite force in persons with advanced occlusal tooth wear. *Am J Orthod Dentofacial Orthop* **107**: 286–92.

Kuroiwa M, Kodaka T, Kuroiwa M, Abe M (1994) Brushing-induced effects with and without a non-fluoride abrasive dentifrice on remineralization of enamel surfaces etched with phosphoric acid. *Caries Res* **28**: 309–14.

Lambrechts P, Braem M, Vuylsteke-Wauters M, Vanherle G (1989) Quantitative in vivo wear of human enamel. *J Dent Res* **68**: 1752–4.

Lazarchik DA, Filler SJ (1997) Effects of gastrointestinal reflux on the oral cavity. *Am J Med* **103**: 107S–13S.

Lewis KJ, Smith BGN (1973) The relationship of erosion and attrition in extensive tooth tissue loss. Case reports. *Br Dent J* **135**: 400–3.

Linkosalo E, Markkanen H (1985) Dental erosions in relation to lactovegetarian diet. *Scand J Dent Res* **93**: 436–41.

Lussi A, Schaffner M, Hotz P, Suter P (1991) Dental erosion in a population of Swiss adults. *Community Dent Oral Epidemiol* **19**: 286–90.

Meurman JH, Frank RM (1991) Scanning electron microscopic study on the effect of salivary pellicle on enamel erosion. *Caries Res* **25**: 1–6.

Meurman JH, ten Cate JM (1996) Pathogenesis and modifying factors of dental erosion. *Eur J Oral Sci* **104**: 199–206.

Meurman JH, Kuittinen T, Kangas M, Tuisku T (1988) Buffering effect of antacids in the mouth – a new treatment of dental erosion? *Scand J Dent Res* **96**: 412–17.

Meurman JH, Toskala J, Nuutinen P, Klemetti E (1994) Oral and dental manifestations in gastroesophageal reflux disease. *Oral Surg Oral Med Oral Pathol* **78**: 583–9.

Meurman JH, Sorvari R, Pelttari A et al (1996) Hospital mouth-cleaning aids may cause dental erosion. *J Spec Care Dent* **16**: 247–50.

Miller WD (1907) Experiments and observations on the wasting of tooth tissue variously designated as erosion, abrasion, chemical abrasion, denudation, etc. *Dental Cosmos* **69**: 225–47.

Murtomaa H, Meurman JH (1992) Mechanical aids in the prevention of dental diseases in the elderly. *Int Dent J* **42**: 365–72.

Niemi ML (1987) Risk factors of gingival injuries in plaque removal by toothbrushing. *Proc Finn Dent Soc* **84** (Suppl): 19–24.

Nordbo H, Skogedal O (1982) The rate of cervical abrasion in dental students. *Acta Odontol Scand* **40**: 45–7.

Nunn JH (1996) Prevalence of dental erosion and the implications for oral health. *Eur J Oral Sci* **104**: 156–61.

Nunn J, Shaw L, Smith A (1996) Tooth wear – dental erosion. *Br Dent J* **180**: 449–52.

Nyström M, Könönen M, Alaluusua S et al (1990) Development of horizontal tooth wear in maxillary anterior teeth from five to 18 years. *J Dent Res* **69**: 1765–70.

O'Sullivan EA, Curzon MEJ, Roberts GJ et al (1998) Gastroesophageal reflux in children and its relationship to erosion in primary and permanent teeth. *Eur J Oral Sci* **106**: 765–9.

Pindborg JJ (1970) *Pathology of Dental Hard Tissues.* Munskgaard: Copenhagen.

Radentz WH, Barnes GP, Cutright DE (1976) A survey of factors possibly associated with cervical abrasion of tooth surfaces. *J Periodontol* **47**: 148–54.

Robb ND, Smith BGN, Geidrys-Leeper E (1995) The distribution of erosion in the dentitions of patients with eating disorders. *Br Dent J* **178**: 171–5.

Rytömaa I, Meurman JH, Koskinen J et al (1988) In vitro erosion of bovine enamel caused by acidic drinks and other foodstuffs. *Scand J Dent Res* **96**: 324–33.

Rytömaa I, Meurman JH, Franssila S, Torkko H (1989) Oral hygiene products may cause dental erosion. *Proc Finn Dent Soc* **85**: 161–6.

Rytömaa I, Järvinen V, Kanerva R, Heinonen OP (1998) Bulimia and tooth erosion. *Acta Odontol Scand* **56**: 36–40.

Sangnes G, Gjermo P (1976) Prevalence of oral soft and hard tissue lesions related to mechanical toothcleansing procedures. *Community Dent Oral Epidemiol* **4**: 77–83.

Scheutzel P (1996) Etiology of dental erosion – intrinsic factors. *Eur J Oral Sci* **104**: 178–90.

Scheutzel P, Meermann R (1994) *Anorexie und Bulimie aus Zahnärztlicher Sicht.* Urban and Schwarzenber: Munchen.

Schroeder PL, Filler SJ, Ramirez B et al (1995) Dental erosion and acid reflux disease. *Ann Intern Med* **122**: 809–15.

Schweitzer-Hirt CM, Schait A, Schmid R et al (1978) Erosion und Abrasion des Schmelzes. Eine experimentelle Studie. *Schweiz Monatsschr Zahnheilkd* **88**: 497–529.

Smith BGN (1975) Dental erosion, attrition and abrasion. *Practitioner* **214**: 347–55.

Smith BGN, Knight JK (1984a) A comparison of patterns of tooth wear with aetiological factors. *Br Dent J* **157**: 16–19.

Smith BGN, Knight JK (1984b) An index for measuring the wear of teeth. *Br Dent J* **156**: 435–8.

Smith BG, Robb ND (1996) The prevalence of toothwear in 1007 dental patients. *J Oral Rehabil* **23**: 232–9.

Smith BG, Bartlett DW, Robb ND (1997) The prevalence, etiology and management of tooth wear in the United Kingdom. *J Prosthet Dent* **78**: 367–72.

Sognnaes RF, Wolcott RB, Xhonga FA (1972) Dental erosion. I. Erosion-like patterns occurring in association with other dental conditions. *J Am Dent Assoc* **84**: 517–76.

Sorvari R (1989a) Effects of various sport drink modifications on dental caries and erosion in rats with controlled eating and drinking pattern. *Proc Finn Dent Soc* **85**: 13–20.

Sorvari R (1989b) *Sport Drink Studies with an Animal Model. Special Reference to Dental Caries and Erosion.* University Printing Office, Original Reports 10/1989: University of Kuopio.

Sorvari R, Kiviranta I (1988) A semiquantitative method of recording experimental tooth erosion and estimating occlusal wear in the rat. *Arch Oral Biol* **33**: 217–20.

Sorvari R, Kiviranta I, Luoma H (1988) Erosive effect of a sport drink mixture with and without addition of fluoride and magnesium on the molar teeth. *Scand J Dent Res* **96**: 226–31.

Sorvari R, Meurman JH, Alakuijala P, Frank RM (1994) Effect of fluoride varnish and solution on enamel erosion in vitro. *Caries Res* **28**: 227–32.

Sorvari R, Pelttari A, Meurman JH (1996) Surface ultrastructure of rat molar teeth after experimentally induced erosion and attrition. *Caries Res* **30**: 163–8.

Sreebny LM (1996) Xerostomia: diagnosis, management and clinical complications. In: Edgar WM, O'Mullane DM, eds, *Saliva and Oral Health,* 43–66. British Dental Association: London.

Teaford MF, Oyen OJ (1989) Differences in the rate of molar wear between monkeys raised on different diets. *J Dent Res* **68**: 1513–18.

Teaford MF, Tylenda CA (1991) A new approach to the study of tooth wear. *J Dent Res* **70**: 204–7.

Ten Bruggen Cate HJ (1968) Dental erosion and industry. *Br J Ind Med* **25**: 249–66.

Tuominen M, Tuominen R (1991) Tooth surface loss among people exposed to cement and stone dust in the work environment in Tanzania. *Community Dent Health* **8**: 233–8.

Tuominen ML, Tuominen RJ, Fubusa F, Mgalula N (1991) Tooth surface loss and exposure to organic and inorganic acid fumes in workplace. *Community Dent Oral Epidemiol* **19**: 217–20.

Varrela TM (1996) Plaque related diseases in different dietary environments. An anthropological study of five ethnically different human skeletal samples from bronze age to new era. *Annales Universitatis Turkuensis* **Series D**: 252.

Varrela J, Varrela TM (1991) Dental studies of a Finnish skeletal material: a paleopathologic approach. *Tandlaegebladet* **95**: 283–90.

Volpe AR, Mooney R, Zumbrunnen C et al (1975) A long term clinical study evaluating the effect of two dentifrices on oral tissue. *J Periodontol* **46**: 113–18.

Waltimo A, Nyström M, Könönen M (1994) Bite force and dentofacial morphology in men with severe dental attrition. *Scand J Dent Res* **102**: 92–6.

Westergaard J, Moe D, Pallesen U, Holmen L (1993) Exaggerated abrasion/erosion of human dental enamel surfaces: a case report. *Scand J Dent Res* **101**: 265–9.

Wöltgens JMH, Vingerling P, de Blieck-Hogervorst JMA, Bervoets DJ (1985) Enamel erosion and saliva. *Clin Prev Dent* **7**: 8–10.

Xhonga FA, Valdmanis S (1983) Geographic comparisons of the incidence of dental erosion: a two centre study. *J Oral Rehabil* **10**: 269–77.

Xhonga FA, Wolcott RB, Sognnaes RF (1972) Dental erosion II. Clinical measurements of dental erosion progress. *J Am Dent Assoc* **84**: 577–82.

Zero DT (1996) Etiology of dental erosion – extrinsic factors. *Eur J Oral Sci* **104**: 162–77.

16
Wear in the mouth: the tribological dimension

Lawrence H Mair

Introduction

It is common to classify dental wear as abrasion, attrition and erosion. These are not wear processes in their own right, but describe the clinical outcomes of a number of underlying events. In addition, it is well known that the majority of clinical cases do not fit neatly into one of the three classified conditions (Smith and Knight 1984). An alternative approach to the study and diagnosis of wear is to consider the fundamental mechanisms that give rise to the clinical conditions (Mair *et al.* 1996).

The parent discipline for the study of wear is **tribology**, which investigates the relationship between lubrication, friction and wear. Tribologists recognize that wear occurs because of the need to dissipate the kinetic energy between moving surfaces (Stolarski 1990). In the stomatognathic system it is necessary to dissipate the energy developed by the muscles of mastication both during and between masticatory events. A proportion of the energy can be absorbed by shearing the inter-molecular bonds within the lubricating system (saliva, plaque and pellicle) (Davies and Baker 1972). The remaining energy will be transformed into heat (through friction), or transferred to the periodontal complex and teeth. Therefore, some of the energy results in viscoelastic compression of the periodontal membrane, whilst the remainder is transferred to the molecules of the occlusal surface. This causes damage at a microscopic level and eventually manifests as wear or fracture.

The lubricating system within the mouth is very important as it absorbs some of the kinetic energy, thereby reducing the potential for damage to the periodontium and teeth. The condition of the periodontium determines whether the additional energy gives rise to wear or trauma from occlusion.

Wear

Wear is the overall effect of a number of inter-related processes. Tribologists describe these with the following five terms (Zum Gahr 1987). **Abrasion** describes the process whereby the surfaces are rubbed away either by direct contact (*two body* abrasion), or by an intervening slurry of abrasive particles (*three body* abrasion). If one of the surfaces is a liquid or gas then the process is termed **erosion**. Surfaces with a high attraction between them may experience adhesive wear. Molecular disruption beneath the surface causes subsurface damage as a result of **fatigue**. All the previous mechanisms may be potentiated by chemical effects which weaken the forces of attraction between surface molecules. Formerly known as corrosion, this process is now known as **tribochemical wear**. The most important feature is that as soon as the weakened molecules have been rubbed away the next layer of the surface is exposed to the chemical attack. For historical reasons two of these terms (*abrasion* and *erosion*) are used in dentistry, but with completely different meanings (Mair 1992).

Two body abrasion

This occurs because at a microscopic level no surfaces are smooth and therefore they contact

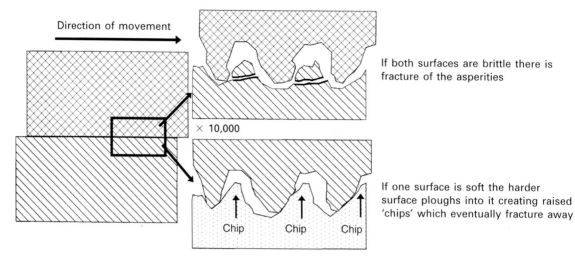

Figure 16.1

Two body abrasion in direct surface-to-surface wear.

by the meeting of their asperities (Figure 16.1). During movement the asperities must either fracture or deform. Alternatively, if one surface is relatively soft, then the hard surface will plough into it, raising up 'chips' which eventually fracture away (Abebe and Appl 1988). In time all the asperities fracture and the cumulative effect of microscopic loss manifests as wear. Two body abrasion can be recognized because it results in mating surfaces, that is, surfaces that remain in intimate contact throughout the movement which gives rise to wear. In the mouth these conditions occur predominantly during non-masticatory tooth movement and are particularly prevalent in bruxism (Figure 16.2). If foreign bodies are habitually held between the teeth then these can abrade both surfaces resulting in characteristic defects (Figure 16.3).

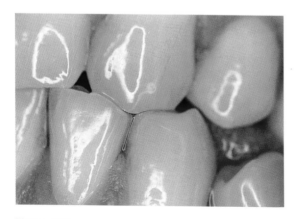

Figure 16.2

The mating of the incisal edges in lateral excursion.

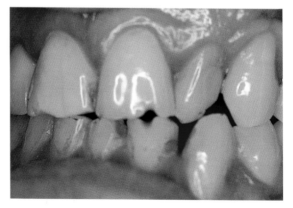

Figure 16.3

Notches on the upper and lower incisors caused by two body wear of the teeth against carpentry nails held by the patient.

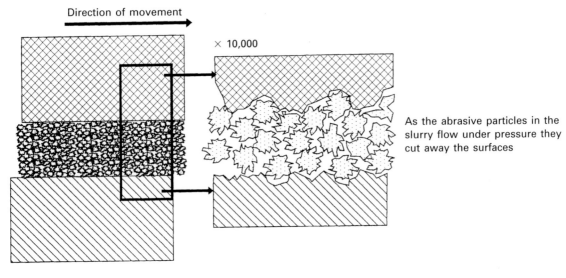

Direction of movement

× 10,000

As the abrasive particles in the slurry flow under pressure they cut away the surfaces

Figure 16.4

Three body abrasion by an abrasive slurry – early stage.

Three body abrasion

Three body abrasion occurs as a result of an intervening slurry of abrasive particles (Figure 16.4). The pressure between the surfaces is transferred to the particles which then cut away the asperities. In the mouth this type of wear occurs during mastication and is prevalent in

patients who eat an abrasive diet such as granary bread or fresh salads (the latter often contain fine silica particles from the soil). It can be divided into two stages – early and late (Mair *et al*. 1996).

During the early stage, when the occlusal surfaces are separated by the food bolus, the abrasive particles act as a slurry and abrade the whole surface. However, they preferentially abrade the surface in the food shedding pathways. This process is very common in restorations with buccal or palatal extensions because these take the main force of the masticatory slurry (Figure 16.5). In composite filling materials the slurry preferentially abrades the softer polymer matrix, exposing the filler particles (Figure 16.6). An important feature of early three body abrasion is that the surfaces do not mate as there is no direct contact between them. The process tends to hollow out the softer regions on a surface. In the mouth this can cause a step between enamel and dentine on the incisal edge or occlusal surface (Figure 16.7).

As the teeth begin to approximate during the later stages of mastication, the remaining slurry particles became lodged in pits and grooves within the surfaces (Figure 16.8). These particles are then scratched across the opposing surface.

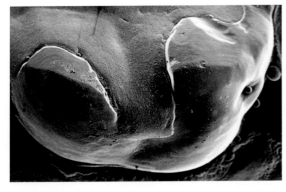

Figure 16.5

Scanning electron micrograph (SEM) of three body abrasion of a posterior composite restoration caused by the masticatory slurry which is forced out through the palatal extension.

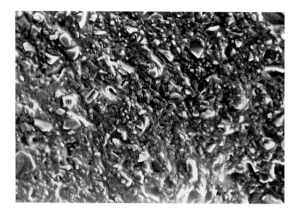

Figure 16.6

SEM of an epoxy model of the occlusal surface of a composite restoration showing filler particles exposed by preferential wear of the polymer matrix by the masticatory slurry. Space bar = 100 μm.

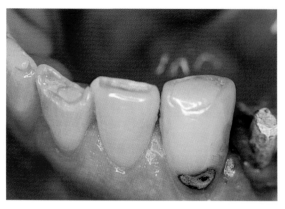

Figure 16.7

Three body abrasion causing hollowing out of the dentine on the lower incisors. There is a dentine groove on the lateral incisor and the slurry has also affected the restorations in the central and canine.

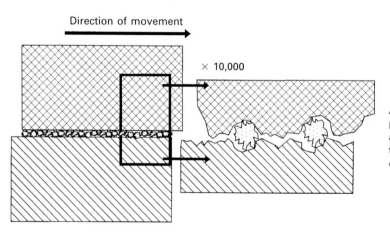

Figure 16.8

Three body wear – late stage. This occurs as the teeth begin to approximate during mastication.

If both surfaces are of similar morphology then the abrasive particles may transfer between scratches and cause more or less equal loss of both surfaces. Figure 16.9 shows the scratch marks on the enamel of an occlusal surface. This process is similar to the process of lapping whereby abrasive particles are made into an abrasive layer by suspension in the grooves of a lap wheel (Pugh 1973). Surfaces that are subject to this type of wear will mate because the abrasive particles have effectively become part of the surface.

Fatigue wear

Some of the movement of the surface molecules is transferred to the subsurface causing rupture of inter-molecular bonds and a zone of subsurface

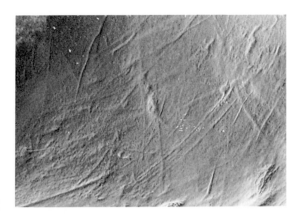

Figure 16.9

SEM showing scratches on the occlusal enamel.

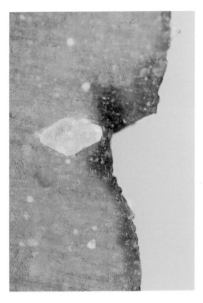

Figure 16.11

Incident light micrograph showing a zone of subsurface damage, stained with silver nitrate, on the palatal surface of an anterior composite restoration. The outline of the lower incisor can be seen.

damage (Figure 16.10). Eventually micro-cracks form within the subsurface and, if these coalesce to the surface, then there can be loss of a fragment of material. A method has been developed to stain subsurface damage in composites that have been removed from the mouth for replacement (Wu and Cobb 1982, Mair 1991). Figure 16.11 shows the damaged zone on the palatal surface of a large proximal composite restoration. This type of wear is prevalent in areas where there is heavy compression of the surface. It is likely to be a feature of non-masticatory tooth wear. Very recently similar zones of subsurface damage have been stained in enamel under wear facets (Figure 16.12).

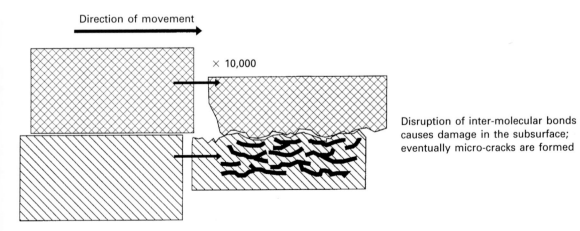

Figure 16.10

Fatigue in the subsurface. If the micro-cracks coalesce to the surface a fragment of surface is displaced.

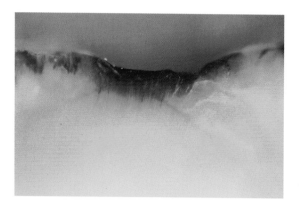

Figure 16.12

A zone of subsurface damage, stained with silver nitrate, in the enamel and dentine under an occlusal wear facet on a lower molar.

most important thing to understand is that acids weaken only the surface molecules. These are then rubbed away by the movement of the surfaces and immediately the underlying (previously unaffected) surface is attacked by the acid (Figure 16.13). Although acid corrosion is acknowledged to be an important aetiological factor in many cases of tooth wear, it must be remembered that wear is, by definition, surface loss occurring as a result of movement between surfaces. Therefore it should be possible to identify the moving surfaces. Sometimes the effect of the acid may allow a relatively non-abrasive food bolus to act as an effective third body. In other cases the weakened surface molecules may allow enamel and dentine to be rubbed away by soft tissues such as the tongue (Figure 16.14).

Tribochemical wear (dental erosion)

To some extent this is not a wear process in its own right; it is caused when chemicals weaken the inter-molecular bonds of the surface and therefore potentiate the other wear processes. In the mouth this effect is normally caused by acids, which may be extrinsic (such as dietary acids) or intrinsic resulting from gastric reflux (Järvinen *et al.* 1991, Bartlett *et al.* 1996). The

Adhesive wear

This occurs when there is a high attraction between surfaces such that cold welds occur between the asperities. As the movement continues these micro-welds fracture, but not along their original line of fusion. The overall effect is that plates of one surface build up on the other surface (Teer and Arnell 1975). Although this type of wear is normally associated with metals it has

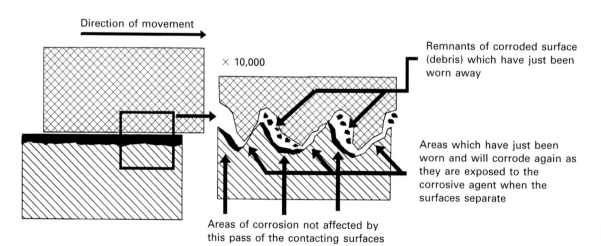

Direction of movement

× 10,000

Remnants of corroded surface (debris) which have just been worn away

Areas which have just been worn and will corrode again as they are exposed to the corrosive agent when the surfaces separate

Areas of corrosion not affected by this pass of the contacting surfaces

Figure 16.13

Tribochemical wear.

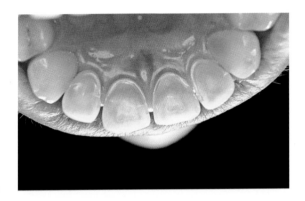

Figure 16.14

Tribochemical wear of the palatal surface of a patient with voluntary gastric reflux (bulimia).

been shown to occur between two surfaces of polymethylmethacrylate (Vaziri *et al.* 1998).

Lubrication

The oral lubricants consist of saliva, plaque and pellicle. Together they form a boundary lubrication system, because the thickness of the lubricant layer is insufficient to prevent asperity contact through the film. In general the effectiveness of boundary lubricants is more influenced by their chemical properties than their viscosity (Teer and Arnell 1975). This is especially important in the case of tribochemical wear which takes place because the chemical properties of the lubricant influence the reaction of fresh surface (exposed by the last pass of the abrading surface) to the corrosive agents. The presence of even a minute film of lubricant can protect this freshly exposed surface from the acid, thereby preventing its removal during the next pass of the abrading surface. The buffering capacity of saliva and plaque is important in minimizing the corrosive effects of acids whilst the pellicle may act as a protective layer (Milosevic and Dawson 1996). In addition to these effects the presence of the lubricant influences how much of the kinetic energy is absorbed by shearing of the inter-molecular bonds in the lubricant and how much is transferred to the teeth.

Wear of dental materials

Most dental materials can be considered to have two or more phases. Composites, ionomers and their various hybrids consist of filler particles embedded in a polymer or hydrogel matrix. Amalgam consists of the unreacted amalgam alloy particles surrounded by the reaction alloys. Sintered porcelain consists of the frit particles surrounded by the fusion matrix. The important factor which determines the wear potential of these materials appears to be the relative difference in hardness between various phases. This is because three body wear, by the masticatory slurry, tends to remove the softer phases. In the case of composites and ionomers this causes the filler particles to be denuded of, and ultimately displaced from, their supporting matrix (Figure 16.6). This process is much less likely to happen with porcelains because the fusion matrix is almost as hard as the original particles in the frit. Amalgams have a relatively good wear resistance because of their ductility. Movement of the surface molecules causes flattening of the wear facets which reduces the coefficient of friction and maximizes the effect of the oral lubricants (Figure 16.15).

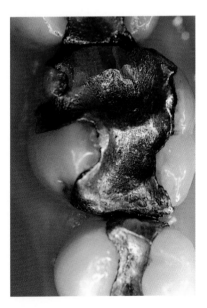

Figure 16.15

Wear facets on an amalgam restoration. The areas of wear are much smoother than the surrounding enamel (which is corroded).

Differential diagnosis

A key to the diagnosis of wear in the mouth is to check to see if there are mating surfaces. If this is the case then it must be the result of direct surface-to-surface wear. However, it is important to realize that this could have been potentiated by chemical effects (tribochemical wear) or by trapped abrasive particles during the late stages of mastication. There are often wear facets on the tooth surface which correspond to the shape of the opposing surface. This type of wear is often indicative of non-masticatory wear such as occurs during thegosis or bruxism (Mair *et al*. 1996). If the surfaces do not mate then either three body abrasion or chemical corrosion must be responsible. If there is any sign of this type of wear on composite fillings it is indicative of wear by abrasive particles, because these materials are resistant to acid corrosion.

Tribologists recognize that the individual mechanisms of wear seldom occur in isolation, most cases being a combination of two or more processes. However, every case of wear has a cause and it is hoped that this brief description of the tribological dimension will help researchers and clinicians to identify the mechanisms which are active in individual cases.

References

Abebe M, Appl FC (1988) Theoretical analysis of the basic mechanics of the abrasive processes. Part 1: General model. *Wear* **126**, 251–66.

Bartlett DW, Evans DF, Anggiansah A, Smith BG (1996) A study of the association between gastro-oesophageal reflux and palatal dental erosion. *Br Dent J* **181**: 125–31.

Davies RT, Baker AJS (1972) Theory and basic principles of lubrication. In: Evans GG et al, eds, *Lubrication in Practice*, 7–13. Macmillan Press: Basingstoke.

Järvinen VK, Rykömaa II, Heinonen OP (1991) Risk factors in dental erosion. *J Dent Res* **70**: 942–7.

Mair LH (1991) Staining of *in vivo* subsurface degradation in composite resins with silver nitrate. *J Dent Res* **70**: 215–20.

Mair LH (1992) Wear in dentistry – a review of current terminology. *J Dent* **20**: 140–4.

Mair LH, Stolarski TA, Vowles RW, Lloyd CH (1996) Wear: mechanisms, manifestations and measurement. Report of a workshop. *J Dent* **24**: 141–8.

Milosevic A, Dawson LJ (1996) Salivary factors in vomiting bulimics with and without pathological toothwear. *Caries Res* **30**: 361–6.

Pugh B (1973) *Friction and Wear*, 141–72. Newnes-Butterworths: London.

Smith BGN, Knight JK (1984) A comparison of patterns of tooth wear with aetiological factors. *Br Dent J* **157**: 16–19.

Stolarski TA (1990) *Tribology in Machine Design*, 19–23. Heinemann: Oxford.

Teer DG, Arnell RD (1975) Wear. In: Halling J, ed, *Principles of Tribology*, 94–126. Macmillan: London.

Vaziri M et al (1988) An investigation into the wear of polymeric materials. *Wear* **122**: 329–42.

Wu W, Cobb EN (1981) A silver staining technique for investigating wear of restorative dental composites. *J Biomed Mater Res* **15**: 343–8.

Zum Gahr K-H (1987) *Microstructure and Wear of Materials*, 80–131. Elsevier: Amsterdam.

17
Variations in pellicle thickness: a factor in tooth wear?

Anne Beate Sønju Clasen, Matthias Hannig and Torleif Sønju

Introduction

Tooth erosion is a chemical dissolution of tooth minerals caused by acids other than those produced by oral bacteria (Dahl and Øilo 1996). Loss of tooth mineral due to a combined action of acid and the rubbing force of the tongue against tooth surfaces has been described by Holst and Lange (1939) as perimylolysis. Clinically it is difficult to assign affected enamel surfaces to erosion, perimylolysis, abrasion or attrition; because of the uncertain aetiology use of the term tooth wear has been suggested (Smith *et al*. 1997).

Recent studies indicate that tooth wear may be an increasing problem in adolescent populations in Western countries (Lussi *et al*. 1991, Milosevic *et al*. 1994). Increased intake of acidic beverages has been suggested as an important factor (O'Brien 1994). A recent in-situ study by West *et al*. (1998) showed that prolonged drinking of orange juice resulted in mineral loss, but this was only a tenth of the loss achieved in vitro. It was shown earlier that acid may dissolve parts of the enamel pellicle (Mayhall 1970). Prolonged drinking of acidic beverages may therefore remove parts of the enamel pellicle. It is not known how 'normal drinking' may affect the ultrastructure and the thickness of the enamel pellicle. Orange juice may reduce the enamel pellicle, whereas milk may increase the enamel pellicle. Milk proteins form micelle structures (Rollema 1992) which may have similar chemical properties to the globular structures observed in the buccal pellicle (Lie 1977, Hannig 1997) and in parotid saliva (Rykke *et al*. 1997).

The acquired enamel pellicle reduces the effect of acid attacks (Moreno and Zahradnik 1979) and therefore enamel erosion (Meurman and Frank 1991, Hannig 1998) (see also Chapter 3). Earlier studies (Sønju and Rølla 1973, Rykke *et al*. 1990) led to the belief that the pellicle is of a uniform thickness on all tooth surfaces in the oral cavity. A recent study by Hannig (1997) indicated differences in pellicle thickness on the buccal and palatal surfaces of the teeth. The pellicle formed on various palatal surfaces consisted only of a granular layer (Hannig 1997) with a similar appearance to the basal layer of the buccal pellicle as described by Lie (1977). The often observed wear of palatal surfaces has lead to the hypothesis that the palatal surfaces may be less protected because of a thinner enamel pellicle. Milosevic and Dawson (1996) suggested that a thinner palatal pellicle could be the result of tongue rubbing.

The aim of the first part of the study was to investigate if some beverages could change the thickness of the enamel pellicle by 'normal drinking'. The second aim of the study was to investigate if the thinner palatal enamel pellicle is a result of the rubbing action of the tongue.

Materials and methods

Variations in pellicle thickness caused by drinking some beverages

In the first part of the study one subject carried pumiced enamel pieces in an appliance on the palatal side of the upper first molar. The pieces had no prior contact with saliva and were not further exposed to the oral environment after the drinking experiments. Four specimens with 2-h palatal acquired enamel pellicle were exposed to orange juice by the subject drinking 100 ml in 20 s. Twelve pieces were subjected to milk (3.4% fat), milk and water, and milk and orange juice (pH = 3.7) by the subject drinking 100 ml of the respective beverages in 20 s. Four enamel pieces were exposed to the oral environment for 30 or 60 min, after the consumption of 100 ml of milk by the subject.

After removal from the appliance, the enamel pieces were rinsed in 0.1 mM phosphate buffer (pH = 7.2) and processed for transmission electron microscopy (TEM) or subjected to Auger electron spectroscopic analyses and depth profiling by argon ion sputtering.

Pellicle thickness on various tooth surfaces

In the second part of the study pellicle was allowed to form, subjected to or protected from the rubbing action of the tongue on pumiced enamel pieces. The pieces were carried on the buccal, lingual and palatal sides of the first upper and lower molars in appliances fitted for the study subjects' jaws. To eliminate contact with the tongue during pellicle formation, enamel pieces were covered with orthodontic bands (for Auger analyses) or pellicle was allowed to be formed in enamel slots 0.3-mm wide and 0.5-mm deep (for TEM examinations). Six study subjects carried the enamel pieces on the various oral sites as described, for 2 h. After removal from the appliances, the pieces were rinsed in phosphate buffer and examined by TEM or Auger analysis as described above.

Transmission electron microscopy

After rinsing, the enamel pieces were fixed in 3% glutaraldehyde solution for 2 h. Post fixation, dehydration, embedding, decalcification, sectioning and contrasting were performed as described by Sønju Clasen et al. (1997). The TEM examinations were performed in a Philips TEM 201 electron microscope (Philips, The Netherlands) at a magnification $\times$ 30,000. The adsorbed pellicles, both in the slots and on the unprotected surfaces, were analysed with respect to their ultrastructure and thickness.

Auger analysis

After rinsing, the enamel specimens were air-dried. The adsorbed protein films were subjected to Auger electron spectroscopy and depth profiling by argon ion sputtering as described by Skjørland et al. (1995). The sequential sputtering time was $\frac{1}{20}$ min (i.e. 3 s), using an argon ion beam of 3 kV energy and 100 μA/cm^2 ion current density. The detection of nitrogen and oxygen on the enamel surfaces was taken as an indication of the presence of organic material. A sudden change to low levels of nitrogen coincident with a sudden increase in calcium was taken as the beginning of the enamel surface.

Results

Variations in palatal pellicle thickness caused by some beverages

The TEM examination of 2-h palatal pellicle subjected to 100 ml orange juice in 20 s is shown in Figure 17.1. The Auger analysis with depth profiling showed a sputtering time of 0.2 min.

TEM examination of the pellicle formed by the subject drinking 100 ml milk in 20 s is shown in Figure 17.2a. The sputtering time of the 'milk' pellicle was 0.7 min. TEM illustrations of 'milk' pellicle (formed by drinking 100 ml milk in 20 s and thereafter carried in the mouth for 30 min and 1 h) are presented in Figure 17.2b and c.

TEM examination of pellicle formed by drinking milk followed by either 100 ml of water or 100 ml of orange juice both showed a similar palatal pellicle consisting only of an electron-dense basal layer. The sputtering time of the 'milk' pellicle subjected to water was 0.3 min and the sputtering time of the 'milk' pellicle subjected to orange juice was 0.4 min.

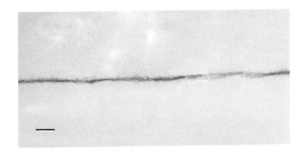

Figure 17.1

Two-hour palatal enamel pellicle subjected to drinking of orange juice. An electron-dense basal layer can be seen (bar represents 100 nm).

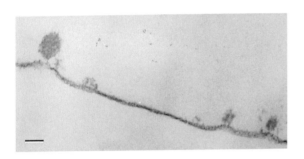

a

b

Figure 17.2

Pellicle formed on palatal pumiced enamel specimen by drinking milk (bar represents 100 nm).

a Immediately removed from mouth; a basal layer with some globular structures can be seen.

b Carried on the palatal side of the upper first molar for 30 min; only an electron-dense layer can be seen.

c Carried on the palatal side of the upper first molar for 1 h; only an electron-dense layer can be seen.

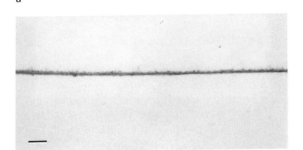

c

Pellicle thickness on various tooth surfaces

Figure 17.3a–d shows the results of the TEM examination of pellicle formed on enamel surfaces and in enamel slots on buccal and palatal sides of the upper first molars. TEM illustrations of the buccal pellicle (upper jaw) are representative of the ultrastructural picture of both the buccally and lingually formed pellicles of the lower jaw. The pellicles consisted of a granular electron-dense basal layer closest to the enamel surface with a second globular layer on top. In contrast, palatal pellicles were characterized by a basal layer without globules. The

ultrastructure of the various enamel pellicles was not significantly different when formed on the surface or in the enamel slots. Figure 17.4 shows the results of the Auger analyses of pellicle formed on enamel pieces with or without orthodontic band coverage on buccal and palatal sides of the upper first molars.

Discussion

It is suggested that the acquired enamel pellicle protects the enamel by reducing the effect of acid attacks in vivo. Therefore it is of interest to investigate whether nutritional components

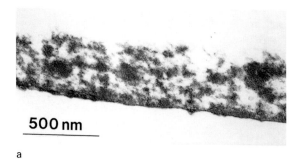

a

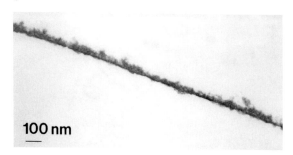

b

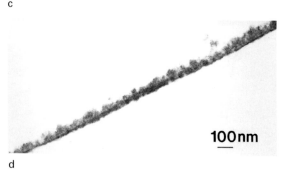

c

d

Figure 17.3

Acquired enamel pellicle of salivary origin formed at various sites.
a Buccal side of the upper first molar.
b Buccal side of the upper first molar in enamel slots.
c Palatal side of the upper first molar.
d Palatal side of the upper first molar in enamel slot.

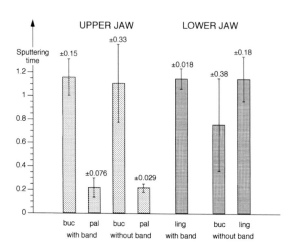

Figure 17.4

Relative pellicle thickness on various tooth surfaces. The columns represent the time needed to remove the pellicle by argon ion sputtering. buc, buccal; pal, palatal; ling, lingual.

influence the pellicle thickness in situ. Millward *et al.* (1997) showed that the pH on the palatal surface of the first permanent molar dropped to about 2.5 after drinking 100 ml of 1% citric acid solution. The mean time for drinking 100 ml was 18 s. Therefore a similar situation was chosen for the study described here to see if this would influence the palatal enamel pellicle in situ. TEM examination of the 2-h palatal pellicle subjected to orange juice drinking did not reveal significant changes in the pellicle thickness or its ultra-structure. When this was compared with untreated enamel pellicle (Figures 17.1 and 17.3c) loss of some granular structures could be observed. A continuous and dense pellicle layer covered the enamel surface. The Auger analyses confirmed a pellicle thickness representative of the basal pellicle layer as shown earlier by Skjørland *et al.* (1995).

The lipoproteins in milk have been shown to form micelles (Rollema 1992). In the oral cavity protein aggregates of a globular structure have been observed in the second layer of the buccal pellicle (Lie 1977, Hannig 1997). Globular struc-tures have been observed in parotid saliva and because of their similarity to milk micelles they have been called micelle-like structures (Rølla and Rykke 1994, Rykke *et al.* 1997). It was therefore of interest to see if the palatal pellicle thickness could be increased by 'normal drinking' of milk. Nyvad and Fejerskov (1984) were able to increase the buccal enamel pellicle by frequent rinses with milk or cream. TEM examination of the palatal 'milk pellicle' showed a dense basal pellicle layer with some globular structures on top. The sputtering time of the milk pellicle was increased compared with the sputtering time of the basal pellicle layer. This may be explained by the sputtering of a globular structure and then the basal layer.

Both TEM examinations and Auger analyses showed that 'normal drinking' of either tap water or orange juice after drinking milk removed the few globular structures from the basal layer. Therefore it is not likely that it is possible to increase the palatal pellicle thickness by drinking milk except for a very short time. Although no significant reduction of the pellicle thickness could be observed after 'normal drinking' of orange juice, it is possible that acids have an effect on both pellicle and enamel even in such a short time. The study by Millward et al. (1997) suggests such an effect, whereas the study by Hannig (1998) showed protection of the enamel covered by in-vitro pellicle. Further studies of the effect of prolonged and frequent intake of acidic beverages on palatal enamel pellicle in situ and the effect on the enamel are needed.

The palatal tooth surfaces seem to be more prone to tooth wear than other surfaces in the mouth (Milosevic et al. 1994). Salivary clearance times on palatal tooth surfaces after intake of acidic beverages are longer than on other surfaces, and this shows a strong relationship to the clinical observations of more pronounced tooth wear on palatal surfaces (Smith and Shaw 1993, Millward et al. 1997). Palatal tooth wear has been presented as a combination of the rubbing action of the tongue and acid against the tooth surfaces and this has been termed perimylolysis (Holst and Lange 1939). Tooth wear may also be a consequence of repeated episodes of vomiting and regurgitation (Milosevic and Dawson 1996), where the tongue may retain acids in less accessible crypts. In-vitro acquired enamel pellicle has been shown to reduce acid attacks and enamel erosion (Meurmann and Frank 1991), but a recent study could not confirm this protective effect in vivo (Milosevic and Dawson 1996).

In the study described in this chapter, TEM examination of 2-h pellicle on various tooth surfaces showed a dense granular pellicle close to the enamel surface. On all buccal surfaces and on the lingual surface in the lower jaw, the pellicle also had a second-layer consisting of what seemed to be globular structures. The pellicles formed on the palatal side of the upper first molars consisted only of a dense granular basal layer and had no second globular layer. The TEM examination showed a palatal pellicle thickness that was only 20–25% of the buccal pellicle thickness. The results of the Auger analyses confirmed the results of the TEM examinations. These results also corroborate an earlier study of pellicle formation (Skjørland et al. 1995). The results of both TEM examinations and Auger analyses showed that the pellicles formed on enamel surfaces protected from tongue rubbing were not significantly different from the pellicles formed when the surfaces were unprotected. Therefore these results do not support the hypothesis that tongue rubbing is an influential factor in pellicle thickness.

Distinct differences in ultrastructure and thickness of the acquired enamel pellicle were found between the palatal and the buccal and lingual surfaces. A second globular layer was not formed on the palatal enamel pellicle. It is not known if the second layer protects the enamel surface more than the dense basal layer alone. Further studies may elucidate this aspect. As the thickness of the palatal enamel pellicle is not influenced by tongue rubbing, it is also unlikely that perimylolysis initiates tooth wear. It is more likely that tooth wear is initiated by erosion. Several studies indicate that erosion, rather than attrition or abrasion, is the major cause of tooth wear (Smith and Knight 1984, Järvinen et al. 1988, Aine et al. 1993).

The thinner pellicle on palatal enamel surfaces may be a result of the locally available salivary proteins (Hannig 1997). Recent findings indicate that saliva from parotid glands and saliva from palatal glands is essentially different (Veerman et al. 1996). Based on the assumption made by Collins and Dawes (1987), that the teeth are covered by a salivary film, Dawes et al. (1989) calculated the film velocity in the upper posterior region to be 7 mm/min. They suggested that the velocity was greatly increased for a very short time during each swallow. It therefore cannot be ruled out that a thinner palatal pellicle may be a result of shearing forces from the salivary film acting on the pellicle during swallowing. The results from the drinking experiments in this study indicate that swallowing may have an effect on the palatal enamel pellicle. The globules that appeared after drinking milk were removed during an additional oral exposure time of 30–60 min. Busscher and van der Mei (1997) suggested that a detachment of adhering plaque on the enamel pellicle is likely to take place in the salivary conditioning film.

Further studies are required to quantify the eventual difference in protective effect between the thicker and the thinner enamel pellicle.

References

Aine L, Baer N, Maki M (1993) Dental erosions caused by gastrooesophageal reflux disease in children. *ASDC J Dent Child* **60**: 210–14.

Busscher HJ, van der Mei HC (1997) Physico-chemical interactions in initial microbial adhesion and relevance for biofilm formation. *Adv Dent Res* **11**: 24–32.

Collins LMC, Dawes C (1987) The surface area of the adult human mouth and thickness of the salivary film covering the teeth and oral mucosa. *J Dent Res* **66**: 1300–2.

Dahl BL, Øilo G (1996) Wear of teeth and restorative materials. In: Öwall B, Käyser AF, Carlsson GE, eds, *Principles and Management Strategies*, 187–200. Mosby-Wolfe: London.

Dawes C, Watanabe S, Piglow-Lecomte P, Dibdin GH (1989) Estimation of the velocity of the salivary film at some different locations in the mouth. *J Dent Res* **68**: 1479–82.

Hannig M (1997) Transmission electron microscopic study of in vivo pellicle formation on dental restorative materials. *Eur J Oral Sci* **105**: 422–33.

Hannig M (1998) Die Protektive Wirkung der Pellikel bei der Schmelzerosion durch verschiedene Säuren. *ZWR* **107**: 421–6.

Holst JJ, Lange F (1939) Perimylolysis. A contribution towards the genesis of tooth wasting from non-mechanical causes. *Acta Odontol Scand* **1**: 36–48.

Järvinen V, Meurman JH, Hyvärinen H et al (1988) Dental erosion and upper gastrointestinal disorders. *Oral Surg Oral Med Oral Pathol* **65**: 298–303.

Lie T (1977) Scanning and transmission electron microscope study of pellicle morphogenesis. *Scand J Dent Res* **85**: 217–31.

Lussi A, Schaffner M, Hotz P, Suter P (1991) Dental erosion in a population of Swiss adults. *Community Dent Oral Epidemiol* **19**: 286–90.

Mayhall CW (1970) Concerning the composition and source of the acquired enamel pellicle of human teeth. *Arch Oral Biol* **15**: 1327–41.

Meurmann JH, Frank RM (1991) Scanning electron microscopic study of the effect of salivary pellicle on enamel erosion. *Caries Res* **25**: 1–6.

Millward A, Shaw L, Harrington E, Smith AJ (1997) Continuous monitoring of salivary flow rate and pH at the surface of the dentition following consumption of acidic beverages. *Caries Res* **31**: 44–9.

Milosevic A, Dawson LJ (1996) Salivary factors in vomiting bulimics with and without pathological tooth wear. *Caries Res* **30**: 361–6.

Milosevic A, Young P, Lennon MA (1994) The prevalence of tooth wear in 14 year old school children in Liverpool. *Community Dent Health* **11**: 83–6.

Moreno EC, Zahradnik RT (1979) Demineralization and remineralization of dental enamel. *J Dent Res* **58**: 896–902.

Nyvad B, Fejerskov O (1984) Experimentally induced changes in ultrastructure of pellicle on enamel in vivo. In: ten Cate JM, Leach SA, Arends J, eds, *Bacterial Adhesion and Preventive Dentistry*, 143–51. IRL Press: Oxford.

O'Brien M (1994) *Dental health in the United Kingdom 1993*. Office of Population Censuses and Surveys. HMSO: London.

Rølla G, Rykke M (1994) Evidence for presence of micelle-like protein globules in human saliva. *Colloids Surfac [B] Biointerfaces* **3**: 177–82.

Rollema HS (1992) Proteins. In: Fox PF, ed, *Advanced Dairy Chemistry*, 111–40. Elsevier Applied Science: London.

Rykke M, Sønju T, Rølla G (1990) Interindividual and longitudinal studies of amino acid composition of pellicle collected in vivo. *Scand J Dent Res* **98**: 129–34.

Rykke M, Young A, Rølla G et al (1997) Transmission electron microscopy of human saliva. *Colloids Surfac [B] Biointerfaces* **9**: 257–67.

Skjørland K, Rykke M, Sønju T (1995) Rate of pellicle formation in vivo. *Acta Odontol Scand* **53**: 358–62.

Smith BGN, Knight JK (1984) A comparison of patterns of tooth wear with etiological factors. *Br Dent J* **157**: 16–19.

Smith AJ, Shaw L (1993) Comparison of rate of clearance of glucose from various oral sites following drinking with a glass, feeder cup and straw. *Med Sci Res* **21**: 617–19.

Smith BGN, Bartlett DW, Robb ND (1997) The prevalence, aetiology and management of tooth wear in the United Kingdom. *J Prosthet Dent* **78**: 367–72.

Sønju T, Rølla G (1973) Chemical analyses of the acquired enamel pellicle formed in two hours on cleaned human teeth in vivo. *Caries Res* **7**: 30–8.

Sønju Clasen AB, Hannig M, Skjørland K, Sønju T (1997) Analytical and ultrastructural studies of pellicle on primary teeth. *Acta Odontol Scand* **55**: 339–43.

Veerman ECI, van den Keybus PAM, Vissink A, Nieuw Amerongen AV (1996) Human glandular salivas: their separate collection and analysis. *Eur J Oral Sci* **104**: 346–52.

West NX, Maxwell A, Hughes JA et al (1998) A method to measure clinical erosion: the effect of orange juice consumption on erosion of enamel. *J Dent* **26**: 329–35.

18

Wettability of dental enamel by soft drinks as compared to saliva and enamel demineralization

Henk J Busscher, Wieke Goedhart, Jan Ruben, Rolf Bos and Henny C van der Mei

Introduction

Several studies have shown that excessive consumption of soft drinks can lead to erosion of enamel surfaces in the oral cavity (Järvinen et al. 1991, West et al. 1998). Most soft drinks have an acidic pH combined with a reasonable buffer capacity (Lussi et al. 1993) that leads to demineralization of the enamel surface. In vivo, however, salivary flow rates increase within 1 min after drinking acidic soft drinks from 0.15 ml/min at rest to around 1.5 ml/min. Usually, salivary flow rates return to the normal resting level within 6 min. Consequently, the pH drop at the enamel surface to below pH 5.5 (the critical pH for enamel dissolution) lasts less than 5 min (Millward et al. 1997).

The return of the enamel surface pH to normal levels depends on the ability of saliva to displace the soft drink from the enamel surface. Ireland et al. (1995) described how the thermodynamic work of adhesion of several drinks and enamel (W_A) varied significantly, as calculated from contact angle (θ) and surface tension (γ_{lv}) measurements according to the equation:

$$W_A = \gamma_{lv} (1 + \cos \theta)$$

Consumption of soft drinks with a lower ability to stick to the enamel surface than saliva ($W_A = 124$ mJ/m²) was suggested to be preferable, as these drinks were presumably more easily displaced by saliva. Such drinks would be, for instance, unsweetened orange juice ($W_A = 105$ mJ/m²), a carbonated diet cola ($W_A = 106$ mJ/m²), but not carbonated cola 1 ($W_A = 130$ mJ/m²) or blackcurrant juice ($W_A = 141$ mJ/m²).

The analysis by Ireland et al. (1995) employed equilibrium contact angles and neglected contact angle hysteresis (Neumann and Good 1972), i.e. the difference in contact angle between an advancing and a receding liquid front. Displacement of a soft drink film by an advancing saliva front would require use of an advancing saliva contact angle versus a receding soft drink contact angle (Figure 18.1).

This chapter reports advancing and receding contact angles of soft drinks, water and saliva on enamel and compares their adhesion to enamel. For a selected soft drink predictions on the displacement of a soft drink film by saliva and vice versa will be verified by microhardness measurements.

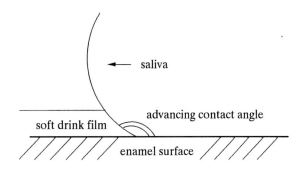

Figure 18.1

A saliva front advances over an enamel surface to displace a soft drink film.

Materials and methods

Enamel, saliva and soft drinks

The outer 50–100 μm of the surface of freshly extracted bovine incisors was removed by grinding and polishing to remove not only the pellicle but also the outer mineral layer, which in general shows the greatest variation in chemical constituents. Final enamel surface preparation for contact angle and microhardness measurements was done by polishing in a 0.05 μm Al_2O_3 slurry in water. Saliva was obtained (unstimulated, human whole saliva) from a healthy male volunteer. Soft drinks were commercially purchased and decarbonated prior to use by sonication, and are listed in Table 18.1.

Acidity and buffer capacity

The pH of soft drinks was measured with a PHM84 pH meter (Radiometer, Copenhagen, Denmark) with an accuracy of 0.1 pH unit. A combined glass electrode was used to determine the pH of 15 ml of the various soft drinks at room temperature. The electrode was stabilized in a pH of 7.00 and pH of 4.01 buffer solution. The pH was registered when the display was stable for 5 s.

The buffer capacity (β, mol/l) is defined as the number of moles of strong base or acid required to cause a one unit increase or decrease in the pH of 1 litre of liquid, and was measured by adding small amounts (0.1 ml) of either a 0.05 M KOH solution or a 0.05 M HCl solution to 15 ml of a soft drink under constant stirring at 250 rpm, until the pH had changed one unit.

Surface tensions

Surface tensions of decarbonated soft drinks, water and saliva were measured from the profile of axisymmetric liquid drops (60–100 μl) on FEP-Teflon surfaces. Droplets were viewed with a contour monitor and the profile coordinates were fitted to the Laplace equation of capillarity (Rothenberg et al. 1983) to obtain the liquid surface tension γ_{lv} (Noordmans and Busscher

1991). This method is preferable to tensiometry for surfactive components containing liquids, such as carbonated cola, saliva, etc.

Contact angles

Advancing and receding contact angles of the decarbonated soft drinks, water and saliva were also measured with a contour monitor. Droplets were positioned on the enamel surface with a microsyringe, and measurements were taken with the needle in the droplets, while slowly moving the sample. In this way, one side of a droplet reflects the contact angle of an advancing liquid front while the opposite side is a receding liquid front. All contact angles were measured on five different enamel samples.

Microhardness

The microhardness indentation values were measured with a Leitz miniload microhardness tester with a Knoop diamond at a load of 500 g, which was applied for 10 s. Hardness measurements were taken on polished bovine enamel and on bovine enamel exposed to saliva or a soft drink to create a film, and subsequent partial immersion in the selected soft drink or saliva, respectively. Instead of partial immersion, experiments were also done with 100 μl of soft drink or saliva droplets placed on the film. On each enamel sample, five indentations were made on the differently exposed sections of the surface and the average value was calculated.

Results and discussion

Table 18.1 summarizes the properties of the soft drinks measured as compared with water and saliva. The pH of the soft drinks all ranged between 2 and 3, while for most drinks the buffer capacity was comparable with that of saliva. Surface tensions of the decarbonated soft drinks were closer to water than to saliva and generally above 65 mJ/m². Equilibrium contact angles of the soft drinks, water and saliva were not signif-

Table 18.1 pH, buffer capacity (β), surface tension and advancing (A), equilibrium (E) and receding (R) contact angles on polished bovine enamel of various soft drinks, water or pooled human whole saliva.

Soft drink	pH	Buffer capacity (mol/l)		γ_{lv} (mJ/m^2)	Contact angle (degrees)		
		β_{HCl}	β_{KOH}		A	E	R
Carbonated cola 1	2.6	0.03	0.004	69.3	73 ± 3	46 ± 7	41 ± 7
Carbonated diet cola	2.9	0.02	0.008	71.9	68 ± 9	46 ± 6	38 ± 6
Carbonated cola 2	2.5	0.04	0.005	72.2	71 ± 13	46 ± 4	33 ± 6
Carbonate 1	3.0	0.02	0.01	65.3	74 ± 5	45 ± 5	40 ± 7
Carbonate 2	2.9	0.001	0.01	70.9	68 ± 9	46 ± 6	35 ± 7
Water	4.5	0.0001	0.00001	71.8	66 ± 13	45 ± 5	39 ± 15
Saliva	7.1	0.05	0.002	57.9	71 ± 12	51 ± 11	38 ± 10

*± indicates SD over five enamel samples.

Table 18.2 Work of adhesion of soft drinks, water and saliva on dental enamel (mJ/m^2) calculated based on advancing $W_{A,ADV}$ and receding $W_{A,REC}$ contact angles, together with the work of displacement of a soft drink by saliva, D_{drink}, or of saliva by soft drinks, D_{saliva}. A positive displacement energy D_{drink} or D_{saliva}, indicates that displacement of a soft drink or saliva film, respectively, is thermodynamically unfavourable.

Soft drink	$W_{A,ADV}$	$W_{A,REC}$	D^*_{drink}	$D^\dagger_{saliva}$
Carbonated cola 1	90	122	45	14
Carbonated diet cola	99	129	52	5
Carbonated cola 2	96	133	56	8
Carbonate 1	83	115	38	21
Carbonate 2	97	129	52	7
Water	101	128	51	3
Saliva	77	104	–	–

*$D_{drink} \equiv W_{A,REC,drink} - W_{A,ADV,saliva}$
†$D_{saliva} \equiv W_{A,REC,saliva} - W_{A,ADV,drink}$

icantly different, and the advancing and receding contact angles varied little amongst the drinks. Receding contact angles were on average 30° lower than the advancing angles.

Works of adhesion reflect differences in surface tension and contact angle and as a consequence they varied most between the drinks (Table 18.2). Works of adhesion based on advancing contact angles for the soft drinks were in excess of that for saliva, similar to the works of adhesion based on receding contact angles, which all reflected a higher value than calculated from the advancing angles.

As a soft drink film must recede under the influence of an advancing saliva front, and a salivary film must recede upon the approach of an advancing soft drink front, the works of displacement D_{drink} and D_{saliva} can be calculated. The values listed in Table 18.2 seem to indicate that thermodynamically it is more difficult to displace a soft drink film by saliva than it is to displace a salivary film by a soft drink.

In Table 18.3 it can be seen that the presence of a salivary film on the enamel surface for up to 3 h hardly affected the microhardness, while exposure to a cola film led to significant surface softening. Also, immersion of enamel with a

Table 18.3 Indentation lengths of polished bovine enamel (absolute, in μm) and after film formation and subsequent exposure to saliva or carbonated cola 1 (relative to the value for polished enamel, μm).

Polished enamel	After film exposure		After subsequent immersion		After subsequent droplet	
185 ± 8	1 min saliva*	−3	3 h in cola	+31	5–30 min, cola	−13
	3 h saliva	+5				
	1 min cola†	+9	3 h in saliva	−13	5–30 min, saliva	+5
	3 h cola	+32				

*Displacement of salivary film by cola requires 14 mJ/m^2 (see Table 18.2).
†Displacement of cola film by saliva requires 45 mJ/m^2 (see Table 18.2).

salivary film in cola led to significant surface softening, indicating that the salivary film was displaced by immersion in cola. In addition, the cola film was displaced by immersion in saliva, as hardening of the enamel surface, previously etched by cola, was observed. It can be concluded that the displacement phenomena of salivary or soft drink films by immersion in a soft drink or saliva, respectively, did not obey surface thermodynamical analyses based on works of adhesion. This was probably due to interference by hydrostatic pressures and a potential miscibility of the fluids.

Interference by hydrostatic pressures can be eliminated by placing microdroplets of one fluid on a film of the other fluid. In this experimental set-up (see also Table 18.3), hardening occurred under a cola droplet placed on a salivary film, indicating that cola displaced the salivary film, which only required 14 mJ/m², but at the same time the etching effect of the cola in contact with the enamel remained to be followed by the remineralization action of saliva still present. Alternatively, a saliva droplet on a cola film still left minor softening by the soft drink film, indicating that a saliva droplet cannot displace the soft drink film, as it requires 45 mJ/m².

Although the displacement experiments carried out with a displacing droplet were more in line with surface thermodynamical analyses than those involving immersion, it is concluded that displacement hypotheses using surface thermodynamics may be complicated by miscibility problems, while it is not clear whether immersion or droplet experiments represent the events occurring in the oral cavity in vivo.

References

Ireland AJ, McGuinnes N, Sheriff M (1995) An investigation into the ability of soft drinks to adhere to enamel. *Caries Res* **29**: 470–6.

Järvinen VK, Rytömaa II, Heinonen OP (1991) Risk factors in dental erosion. *J Dent Res* **70**: 942–7.

Lussi A, Jäggi K, Schärer N (1993) The influence of different factors on in vitro enamel erosion. *Caries Res* **27**: 387–93.

Millward A, Shaw L, Harrington E, Smith AJ (1997) Continuous monitoring of salivary flow rate and pH at the surface of the dentition following consumption of acidic beverages. *Caries Res* **31**: 44–9.

Neumann AW, Good RJ (1972) Thermodynamics of contact angles – heterogeneous solid surfaces. *J Colloid Interface Sci* **38**: 341–58.

Noordmans J, Busscher HJ (1991) The influence of droplet volume and contact angle on liquid surface tension measurements by axisymmetric drop shape analysis-profile (ADSA-P). *Colloids Surfaces* **58**: 239–49.

Rothenberg Y, Boruvka L, Neumann AW (1983) Determination of surface tension and contact angle from the shapes of axisymmetric fluid interfaces. *J Colloid Interface Sci* **93**: 169–83.

West NX, Maxwell A, Hughes J et al (1998) A method to measure clinical erosion: the effect of orange juice consumption on erosion of enamel. *J Dent* **26**: 329–35.

19
Restorative management of the worn dentition

Paul A King

Introduction

The effects of tooth wear can present in a variety of forms and severity (Figure 19.1) depending on the aetiological factors responsible. Although to some extent the severity of tooth wear is age dependent (Steele *et al.* 1996), a significant number of younger patients are experiencing tooth wear, usually erosive in nature (O'Brien 1993; Nunn *et al.* 1996) (Figure 19.2). It is generally agreed that prevention of further tooth wear should form the basis of any ongoing lifelong dental management. However, in some situations it may also become necessary to consider intervenient restorative treatment (Williams 1987, Smith *et al.* 1997). The clearest indications are where:

- The patient feels that the appearance of the teeth is unacceptable
- Normal function is disrupted due to the loss of tooth tissue and/or ongoing pulp sensitivity which does not respond to conservative measures
- There is progressive tooth wear which may result in pulp necrosis and/or teeth becoming difficult to restore.

A broad range of restorative treatment options are possible with today's materials and techniques and usually range between:

- Conventional fixed restorations
- Removable onlay/overlay prostheses
- Minimal preparation adhesive restorations.

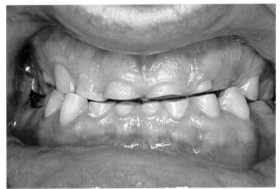

a

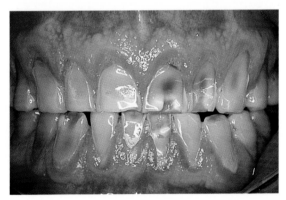

b

Figure 19.1

Patients (middle-aged) presenting with moderate/severe tooth wear.

(*a*) Tooth wear mainly attrition.
(*b*) Tooth wear mainly abrasion.

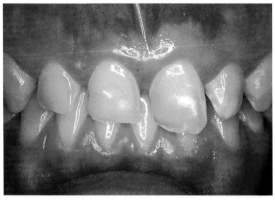

a

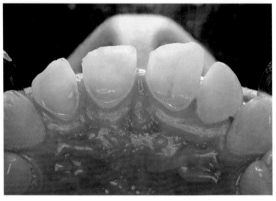

b

Figure 19.2

Young patient (aged 17 years) exhibiting severe localized tooth wear, mainly erosive in nature.

(*a*) Labial view.
(*b*) Palatal view.

This chapter will illustrate and discuss some of the conventional methods used to restore the worn dentition as well as the newer, less invasive and minimal preparation adhesive techniques now available to the dental surgeon.

Conventional fixed restorations

Conventional fixed restorations, usually in the form of porcelain-fused-to-metal (PFM) and all metal crowns, have been used for many years for restoring worn and broken down teeth. The clinical performance of conventional crown restorations has been reasonably well documented, and in general tolerable survival times have been demonstrated (Schwartz *et al.* 1970, Walton *et al.* 1986, Fyffe 1992). Unfortunately, studies have not assessed risk factors specifically associated with the various forms of tooth wear, although there is general agreement that restorations in patients exhibiting distinct parafunctional clenching and grinding habits have a higher risk of failure compared with other types of tooth wear.

Tooth preparation for conventional crown restorations is an invasive procedure, especially if porcelain is required to satisfy aesthetic demands, and as a consequence may further compromise an already damaged dentition. Pulp necrosis, tooth fracture, loss of cementation and marginal caries can all occur following the placement of crown restorations, which will often complicate any subsequent repair or replacement, resulting in possible premature tooth loss (Eckerbom *et al.* 1992, Jackson *et al.* 1992). This is particularly the case if crowns are prescribed for the younger patient.

Notwithstanding some of the risk factors described, these type of restorations are extensively used and offer an effective way of restoring worn and missing teeth, allowing a degree of versatility with regard to appearance and occlusal form. One of the potential advantages of this treatment approach is the ability to use provisional crowns for a period of time, thus providing the opportunity for clinician and patient to assess appearance and function and make any modifications as necessary.

Often complicating the restoration of worn teeth is the need to recreate inter-occlusal space lost as a result of compensatory eruption of opposing teeth during the process of tooth wear (Berry and Poole 1976). This is often the case with anterior teeth and if not addressed will result in a compromised finish (Figure 19.3). In these circumstances there are a number of well-established conventional restorative techniques available to overcome the difficulties of reduced crown height and lack of inter-occlusal space (Ricketts and Smith 1993). The main options either individually or in combination are:

*   Opposing tooth reduction
*   Elective endodontic treatment and post retention

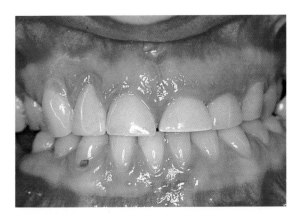

Figure 19.3

Anterior crowns constructed to conform to the existing worn teeth without recreation of lost inter-incisal space resulting in poor aesthetics and retention form.

- Occlusal adjustment (retruded arc of mandibular closure)
- Periodontal surgical crown lengthening
- Localized orthodontic tooth movement (Dahl appliance)
- Overall increase in occlusal vertical dimension.

For an adequate restoration of good appearance and durable function, the role of opposing tooth reduction, elective pulp extirpation and post retention, occlusal adjustment, and periodontal surgical crown lengthening alone may be of limited help and can compromise remaining tooth structure and periodontal support. Periodontal surgical crown lengthening is capable of dramatically improving available coronal tooth structure for adequate crown preparation (Figure 19.4) and is often required when restoring more severe forms of tooth wear. However, it is an invasive procedure with postoperative sensitivity and can create a number of subsequent restorative difficulties, such as interproximal spacing and placement of crown margins on root surfaces (Briggs and Bishop 1997).

One of the more satisfactory and conservative ways of recreating space, particularly in situations of localized anterior tooth wear, is by orthodontic tooth movement. A number of techniques can be used to achieve this which

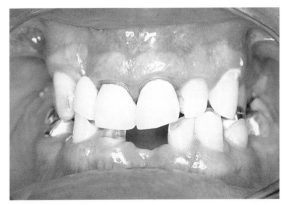

a

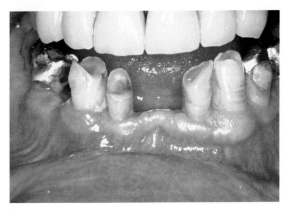

b

Figure 19.4

Periodontal surgical crown lengthening on worn lower anterior teeth prior to the construction of a fixed bridge prosthesis.

(a) Before surgery.
(b) After surgery.

have been reviewed by Ricketts and Smith (1994), with a fixed or removable cobalt–chromium-based anterior bite-plane being the more established method of today. The so called 'Dahl appliance', described after the author, achieves space recreation by a combination of anterior tooth intrusion and posterior tooth extrusion (Dahl et al. 1975, Dahl and Krogstad 1982). This localized orthodontic treatment provides the opportunity to maximize the appearance and function of the subsequent crowns and preserves tooth tissue (Figure 19.5).

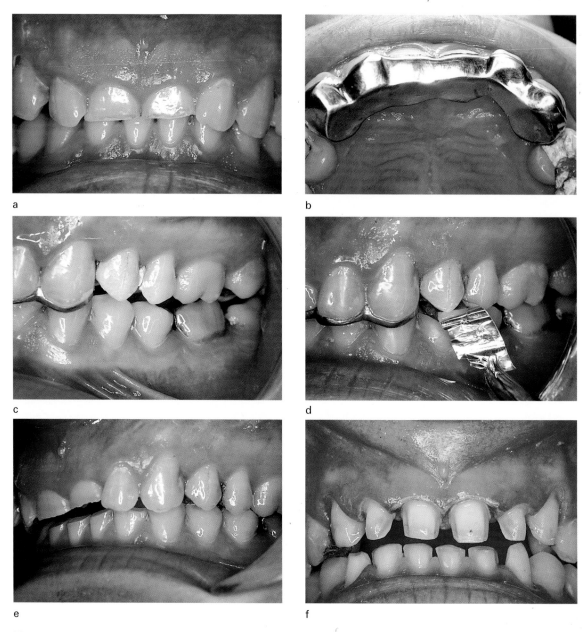

a

b

c

d

e

f

Figure 19.5

The use of an orthodontic Dahl appliance to recreate lost inter-incisal space prior to the restoration of worn anterior teeth with porcelain-fused-to-metal (PFM) crowns.

(a) Localized anterior tooth wear.
(b) Dahl appliance cemented in place.
(c) Initial space in posterior quadrants.
(d) Regained posterior tooth contacts after 6 months.
(e) Inter-incisal space recreated following the removal of the Dahl appliance.
(f) Following periodontal surgical crown lengthening teeth prepared for PFM crowns with optimum retention and resistance form.

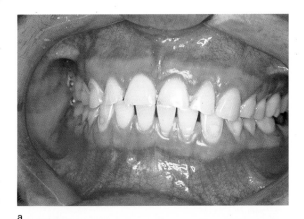

a

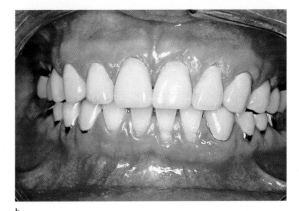

b

Figure 19.6

Generalized tooth wear restored with PFM crowns in the anterior and posterior segments at an overall increase in occlusal vertical dimension.

(*a*) Before restoration.
(*b*) After restoration.

In certain situations where there is generalized tooth wear and sufficient indications to consider crown restorations for the posterior teeth, a full mouth crown reconstruction at an overall increase in occlusal vertical dimension will usually provide adequate space for anterior restorations (Figure 19.6). This situation will avoid the need for an anterior orthodontic appliance, as well as preserving valuable incisal and occlusal tooth tissue. Although excellent and predictable results can be achieved by this method, the process is relatively complex and requires a number of carefully planned stages, appropriate operator skills and knowledge, time, and good technical laboratory support (Ibbetson and Setchell 1989a, 1989b). As a consequence this form of treatment may not be accessible for many patients.

It is possible to achieve an increase in occlusal vertical dimension with the use of a removable posterior onlay prosthesis in combination with anterior fixed crown restorations. This approach relies heavily on patient compliance and may result in an unpredictable outcome for the anterior restorations due to adverse occlusal loads if the removable prosthesis is not used periodically. If a removable prosthesis is being considered to provide posterior occlusal support in this situation, then it may be more sensible and predictable to restore the worn anterior teeth with the same removable prosthesis.

Removable onlay/overlay prostheses

The use of a removable onlay/overlay prosthesis can be a valuable means of rehabilitating patients with moderate/severe tooth wear, particularly when there are also missing strategic teeth to be replaced. This form of treatment has been advocated by a number of clinicians (Brown 1980, Licht and Leveton 1980, Graser 1990, Basker *et al*. 1993, Watson 1997) for patients with more severe forms of tooth wear. This approach provides a relatively simple, non-invasive and cost-effective way to achieve improvements in appearance and function of the dentition.

The construction of a provisional acrylic resin removable prosthesis is recommended initially, allowing the opportunity to carry out modifications to the shape, position and occlusal relationship of the prosthetic teeth and soft tissues, as well as assessing the patient's tolerance of a removable prosthesis (Figure 19.7). It is advisable to avoid any significant tooth preparation at this stage, but if this treatment approach is to be continued in the longer term then subsequent prostheses, often incorporating a cobalt–chromium framework, will usually require some tooth preparation in order to optimize appearance, fit and retention.

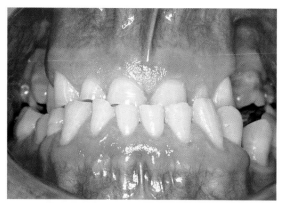

a

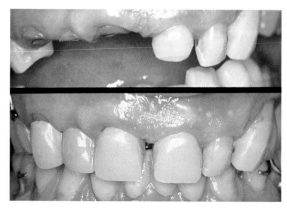

a

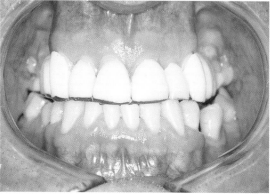

b

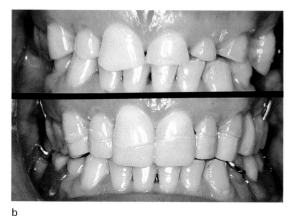

b

Figure 19.7

Moderate/severe tooth wear with an unfavourable occlusal relationship initially restored with a provisional onlay/overlay removable prosthesis to assess appearance and function.

(*a*) Before restoration.
(*b*) After restoration with removable prosthesis.

Figure 19.8

(*a*) Before and after gingival fitting anterior tooth facings on removable prostheses.
(*b*) Before and after butt-fitting anterior tooth facings on removable prostheses.

Space demands are usually greatest in the anterior region, both in the vertical and labio-lingual dimensions, and will be influenced by the amount of sound tooth structure remaining and changes to the occlusal vertical dimension. Unless modified by tooth reduction or extraction the available space will determine whether or not an anterior labial flange can be used, or alternatively gingival fitting and/or butt-fitting tooth facings (Figure 19.8). The final decision may to

some extent depend on the patient's aesthetic demands and desire to avoid or limit any necessary tooth reduction.

There are some well-established advantages in retaining teeth as overdenture abutments, such as maintenance of alveolar bone and support, improved sensory feedback and masticatory performance and reduced psychological trauma of tooth extraction (Basker *et al.* 1993). Some disadvantages also exist, particularly if patients

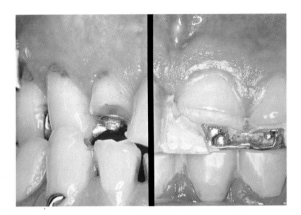

Figure 19.9

Fracture and wear of acrylic resin facings on removable prostheses often demonstrated in patients with parafunctional clenching/grinding habits.

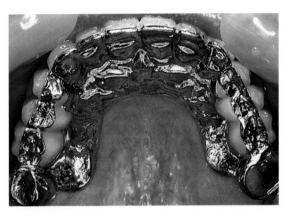

Figure 19.10

The use of a metal framework incorporating incisal and occlusal coverage used to strengthen removable onlay/overlay prostheses for patients demonstrating significant parafunctional clenching/grinding habits.

are unable to establish and maintain adequate oral and denture plaque control. In this situation the abutment teeth will be at an increased risk of primary dental disease, although the daily application of a non-acidulated fluoride gel may reduce the risk of root surface caries (Toolson and Taylor 1989, Ettinger and Jakobsen 1997).

Maintenance demands are relatively high for this form of prosthesis (Ettinger and Jakobsen 1997), with material wear and fracture being common, particularly in patients exhibiting parafunctional clenching/grinding habits (Figure 19.9). The use of extensive metal frameworks, including incisal and occlusal coverage (Figure 19.10), may reduce the regularity of repair, but increases the clinical and technical complexity when repair or replacement eventually becomes necessary. This complexity may be further exacerbated if copings and precision attachments have been utilized on abutment teeth to increase retention and stability of the prosthesis (Basker *et al.* 1993).

While for certain situations this form of treatment offers a satisfactory way of restoring the worn dentition, for many patients difficulties arise in adapting both functionally and psychologically to a removable prosthesis and this approach is often seen as a last resort.

Minimal preparation adhesive restorations

Since the introduction to the dental profession of the acid-etch technique using phosphoric acid by Buonocore in 1955, and an early form of Bis-GMA-based composite resin by Bowen in the early 1960s, there has been significant progress in the development of adhesive materials and techniques within dentistry. With the additional development of glass ionomer cements, dentine bonding agents, silane primers and composite resin luting cements it is now possible to produce acceptable adhesive bonds between enamel and dentine tooth tissue and a variety of materials such as composite resins, ceramics and metal alloys suitable for use in situations where restoration of the worn dentition is necessary (McClean and Wilson 1977, Calamia 1985, Toh *et al.* 1987, Saunders 1989, Banks 1990, Duke 1993, Willems *et al.* 1993).

This final section will highlight the range of adhesive materials available to the dental surgeon and discuss how they may be applied when restoring the dentitions of patients with moderate to severe tooth wear. The following areas will be discussed:

- Cervical tooth wear
- Anterior tooth wear
  - palatal tooth wear
  - incisal/palatal tooth wear
  - labial/incisal/palatal tooth wear
- Posterior (generalized) tooth wear.

Cervical tooth wear

Cervical tooth wear lesions are common and present in a variety of forms depending on the type and severity of the causative factors. Not all lesions require restoration, but if aesthetics, sensitivity, or prevention of further tooth wear dictates then some form of adhesive restoration will usually be most suitable.

A plethora of tooth-coloured restorative materials is now available. Materials can either be composite resin or glass ionomer-based, or a combination of both – either in a layered technique, with the individual materials or one of the newer resin-modified glass ionomer cements. The choice of materials can be bewildering, with new materials and techniques seemingly introduced to the market on a weekly basis (Willems *et al.* 1993).

There are a number of approaches to bonding restorations to cervical tooth tissue (Watson and Bartlett 1994). For lesions with margins that are still confined to enamel the use of a microfine or polishable densified composite resin, in conjunction with acid-etched enamel, will produce good aesthetic and durable results. Unfortunately, most cervical lesion margins are not confined to enamel and usually involve root cementum and dentine. In this situation dentine bonding is required, usually in the form of a dedicated dentine bonding agent in combination with a composite resin or alternatively a glass ionomer cement with inherent bonding properties to both dentine and enamel.

In situations where aesthetics are paramount then a polishable composite resin combined with a dentine bonding agent are often the materials of choice. However, despite ongoing improvements questions remain as to the longer term durability of dentine bonding agents, which may result in micro-leakage and characteristic marginal discolouration of the restoration.

Where lesions are not as visually prominent and involve more of the root surface, often partly below the gingival margin, then a glass ionomer material may prove to be more durable. The dynamic bond of glass ionomer cements to both dentine and enamel through an ionic exchange provides the opportunity for continual repair of the adhesive bond at the tooth and cement interface. There is also the possible additional benefit of fluoride ion release from the glass ionomer cement reducing the possibility of marginal caries in susceptible individuals.

Although much improved over recent years, the colour properties of conventional glass ionomer cements are not ideal. However, in deeper cervical lesions it is possible to consider a layered technique combining the adhesive properties of the glass ionomer cement with the superior colour properties of a polishable composite resin. This can be carried out in one visit or preferably following a minimum set time of 24 hours; the superficial portion of the glass ionomer cement restoration can be reduced and a layer of composite resin added.

The new generation of light-activated resin-modified glass ionomer materials attempt to combine some of the better properties of composite resin and conventional glass ionomer cements. Certainly the command set, improved colour and easier finishing of some of these newer materials allow the opportunity to provide very acceptable conservative restorations for cervical tooth wear lesions. Only longer term observation and assessment will determine how durable these newer materials will ultimately prove.

Anterior tooth wear

Although tooth wear can generally affect the whole dentition it is often localized to the anterior teeth, and the maxillary anterior teeth in particular.

Palatal tooth wear

This pattern of tooth wear is usually characteristic of acid erosion, possibly combined with a degree of attrition, and is the type more commonly seen in the younger age groups. Often, the labial and incisal surfaces are relatively intact and the main indications for restorative treatment are to offer some resistance to further palatal tooth wear which will reduce the risk of significant enamel fractures to the weakened incisal edges and pulp tissue inflammation.

The use of resin-bonded palatal metal alloy veneers is an acceptable method to manage this form of tooth wear (Darbar 1994, Hussey *et al.* 1994) and has been shown to be a relatively durable technique (Nohl *et al.* 1997). Either heat-treated gold alloys or nickel–chromium alloys, as used in resin-bonded bridge frameworks, are currently the cast metal alloys of choice. The decision as to which of the two materials to use is based on the improved bond strength of resin to nickel–chromium alloys versus the easier working properties and wear characteristics of the gold alloys.

Tooth preparation is minimal, usually restricted to smoothing the incisal and palatal peripheral enamel margins. Laboratory fabrication of the metal alloy veneers is either directly on a refractory working cast, or by a wax/resin 'lift off' technique.

When restoring worn anterior teeth, creation of inter-occlusal space is usually required in order to accommodate the thickness of the restoring material. As the tooth structure is already compromised, avoiding further tooth reduction to create space is obviously advantageous. Orthodontic tooth movement using an anterior Dahl appliance has been described as a method of achieving inter-occlusal space. Although this is a predictable method, there are some disadvantages, not least the increased treatment time and extra laboratory procedures. An alternative approach, based on similar principles to the Dahl appliance, is to deliberately design and construct the palatal veneers in such a manner that they are cemented initially high in occlusion. Expected tooth movement is enhanced if a positive cingulum contact can be achieved with the occluding lower incisor teeth in an attempt to direct orthodontic forces along the long axis of the contacting teeth. This method would appear to contradict traditional occlusal teaching, but to date has proved to work well in these particular circumstances.

Luting cements are usually resin-based and used in combination with the manufacturer's dentine bonding agent where appropriate. The use of an opaque resin-based cement will overcome any potential greying of the incisal third caused by the underlying palatal metal veneer. Rubber dam isolation is used when necessary and occasionally gingival retraction cord in situations where there has been excessive tooth wear in the cervical region. By including metal coverage of the palatal veneers onto the incisal edges, location during cementation is made somewhat easier and this design will also offer some increased resistance to shearing loads. An example of the use of resin-bonded metal alloy palatal veneers is illustrated in Figure 19.11.

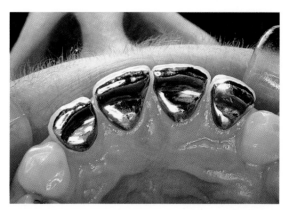

a

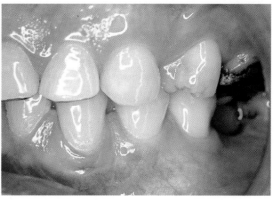

b

Figure 19.11

The use of nickel–chromium alloy resin-bonded palatal veneers to restore localized palatal tooth wear for maxillary incisor teeth.

(*a*) Palatal view of veneers.
(*b*) Labial view demonstrating re-establishment of posterior occlusal contacts.

Incisal/palatal tooth wear

Although the use of metal alloy palatal veneers is an excellent conservative method of managing localized anterior tooth wear, it is not possible to improve the appearance of lost incisal and labial tooth tissue. In these circumstances, it is feasible to build up the incisal portion of the tooth with a polishable composite resin and then construct a resin-bonded metal alloy palatal veneer to cover both the palatal tooth tissue and composite resin (Foreman 1988, Creugers and Kayser 1992). However, potential difficulties arise with this technique, in that it is difficult to know where to finish the composite resin build up palatally and the adhesive bond of the metal alloy palatal veneer will be somewhat compromised because of the reduction in available tooth enamel.

An alternative and very conservative approach is to restore both the incisal and palatal tooth surfaces with direct acid-etch retained composite resin at an increase in occlusal vertical dimension to accommodate the thickness of the restorative material (Darbar and Hemmings

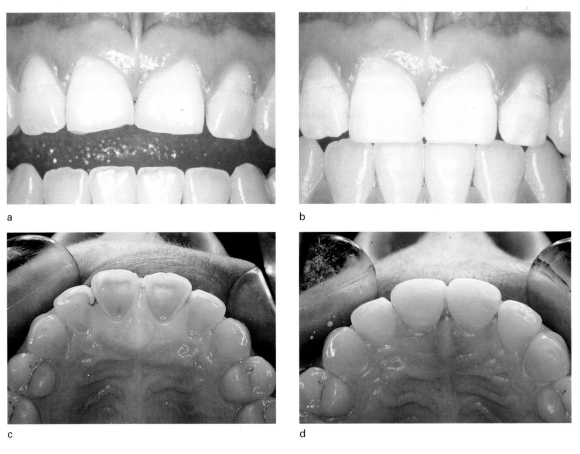

a

b

c

d

Figure 19.12

Restoration of incisal and palatal aspects of worn upper anterior teeth with direct composite resin restorations.

(*a*) Labial view before restoration.
(*b*) Labial view after restoration.
(*c*) Palatal view before restoration.
(*d*) Palatal view after restoration.

1997). This particular technique is relatively straightforward and avoids the need for laboratory support; although the longer term durability can be unpredictable, particularly when restoring lower anterior teeth. However, the technique provides the opportunity for repair or replacement, and allows the possibility of more involved and complex procedures in the form of conventional crowns to be considered at a later date once inter-occlusal space has been gained. An example of this particular technique is shown in Figure 19.12.

Alternatives to using direct composite resins are available in the form of indirect densified composite resins, with the potential advantages being the improved physical properties and better control over occlusal and interproximal contour (Briggs *et al*. 1994). Modified porcelain laminate veneer restorations of both the incisal and palatal worn tissue have also been described by a number of clinicians (Milosevic 1990, McLundie 1991). There are, however, potential difficulties with both these techniques in that it is often very difficult to disguise the junction between the incisal porcelain or indirect composite resin with the remaining tooth structure on the labial aspect of the tooth. When using porcelain, it is also necessary to create greater inter-occlusal space to provide sufficient bulk of material to reduce the risk of material fracture. Theoretically both these indirect techniques should be more durable than using direct composite resin, although to date there is no scientific clinical evidence to confirm this assumption. Figure 19.13 illustrates the use of modified porcelain laminate and gold alloy veneers to restore worn upper anterior teeth.

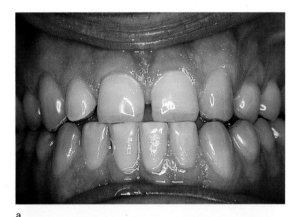

a

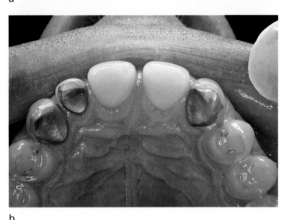

b

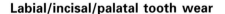

Figure 19.13

Resin-bonded porcelain laminate veneers used to restore the incisal and palatal aspects of maxillary central incisor teeth, with resin-bonded gold alloy palatal veneers used for the remaining worn anterior teeth.

(*a*) Labial view after treatment.
(*b*) Palatal view after treatment.

Labial/incisal/palatal tooth wear

A number of adhesive approaches have been recommended for the restoration of teeth with lost tooth structure on all three major surfaces. These have included the use of a labial porcelain laminate veneer in conjunction with a metal alloy veneer for the palatal surface (Cheung and Dimmer 1988, Bishop *et al*. 1996), a resin-bonded minimal ceramic crown (Holmes and Dan Sneed 1990), or an adhesive metal–ceramic crown restoration (Bishop *et al*. 1997). All these techniques are relatively complex and would

normally require some inter-occlusal space creation prior to completion of the restoration. In these circumstances consideration should be given to the provision of a more conventional full coverage crown.

In certain situations it is possible to restore all tooth surfaces with direct composite resin at an increased occlusal vertical dimension in an attempt to initially recreate lost inter-occlusal space (Figure 19.14). Once completed a decision can be taken either to continue with the

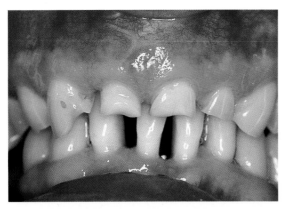

a

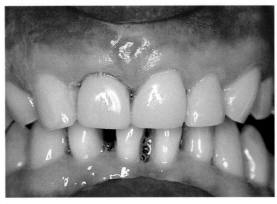

b

Figure 19.14

Direct acid-etch retained composite resin used to restore the labial, incisal and palatal aspects of worn maxillary incisor teeth at an initial increase in occlusal vertical dimension.

(a) Before treatment.
(b) After treatment.

composite resin restorations or alternatively to convert them into conventional crowns conforming to the newly established occlusion. This approach is often more acceptable to the patient compared with the use of a metal-based Dahl appliance, and has the additional advantage of not committing the patient to conventional crown restorations.

Posterior (generalized) tooth wear

Tooth wear affecting posterior teeth in isolation is rare, and is usually part of a generalized condition affecting the whole dentition. Occasionally the pattern of tooth wear is such that individual posterior teeth may require restoring, and it is possible in these situations to consider some of the adhesive materials and techniques described earlier. If aesthetics is not paramount then the use of a resin-bonded heat-treated gold alloy restoration can be advantageous (Crawford and Aboush 1993). Alternatively, if aesthetics dictate then a resin-bonded ceramic or indirect composite resin onlay can be considered. These techniques are helpful where retention and resistance form for conventional crowns are particularly compromised, and there is a desire to avoid adjunctive treatments such as periodontal surgical crown lengthening.

In situations of generalized tooth wear where there are indications to consider a full mouth reconstruction of the dentition, then the use of adhesive onlay restorations in the posterior quadrants can be of value in certain circumstances (Rawlinson and Winstanley 1988). Restoring posterior quadrants with adhesive onlays is a conservative method, although on occasions it is not always possible to create sufficient inter-occlusal space by opening the vertical dimension alone, particularly if opposing occluding surfaces in the molar regions need to be restored. In these circumstances some occlusal tooth reduction may also be necessary. Where space is at a premium the selection of a gold alloy as opposed to porcelain will be advantageous. Because of the normal arc of mandibular closure there will often be more space available in the premolar regions, allowing the opportunity to use more aesthetic tooth-coloured restorations. The space created by restoring the posterior quadrants, at an overall increase in occlusal vertical dimension, will provide the opportunity to successfully restore the worn anterior teeth either by conventional or adhesive methods (Figures 19.15 and 19.16).

In selected cases it is possible to consider a full mouth reconstruction of the worn dentition using resin-bonded ceramic restorations. However, the longer term durability, particularly of the posterior onlay restorations, still remains unpredictable and characteristically small fracture lines can appear in time which may eventually result in a catastrophic

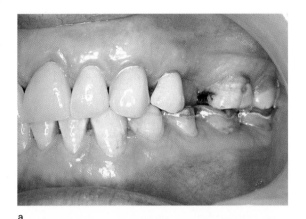

a

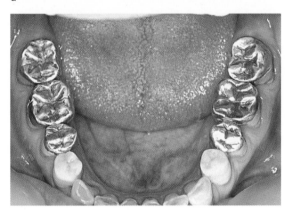

b

Figure 19.15

Resin-bonded gold alloy and indirect composite resin onlays used to restore the mandibular posterior teeth in conjunction with conventional PFM crowns for the maxillary anterior teeth at an increase in occlusal vertical dimension.

(*a*) Labial view of restorations in occlusion.
(*b*) Occlusal view of mandibular resin-bonded onlays.

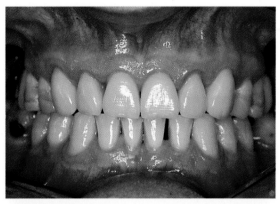

a

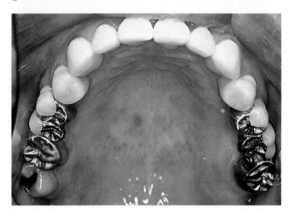

b

Figure 19.16

Reconstruction of a worn maxillary dentition using modified resin-bonded laminate porcelain veneers for the anterior teeth, and resin-bonded bridges and onlays for the posterior teeth at an overall increase in occlusal vertical dimension.

(*a*) Labial view of restorations.
(*b*) Occlusal view of restorations.

failure. This is more likely to be the outcome for patients who exhibit parafunctional clenching/grinding habits. The use of a full coverage occlusal splint to be worn chiefly at night may offer some protection to vunerable restorations.

An occasional alternative to laboratory-manufactured restorations for full mouth rehabilitation is to consider a technique (Roessler 1990)

using direct acid-etch retained composite resin materials at an increase in occlusal vertical dimension. This will of course involve greater clinic time and the need ideally to restore multiple teeth in one session in order to control the increase in occlusal vertical dimension. The longer term durability is likely to be inferior to indirect materials and techniques, but if appropriate, would have the advantage of being easier to repair and maintain on a piecemeal basis.

New techniques bring with them new difficulties and challenges, and the use of adhesive onlay restorations in managing the worn dentition is no exception to this fact. Temporization following tooth preparation can be problematic. Procedures involving complete resin bonding of the temporary restoration to the underlying tooth tissue may compromise the subsequent adhesive bond for the final restoration. There is also a risk of damage to the tooth preparation during the removal of the interim resin lute. Conversely, avoiding this approach by using a less adhesive material or technique may result in the early loss of any temporary restorations, with the possible consequences of unplanned tooth movement. Although not ideal, laboratory-manufactured acrylic or composite resin quadrant splinted temporary restorations, cemented with a composite resin lute to spot-etched enamel, have proved to be reasonably reliable in these circumstances.

Checking the occlusal relationship at the try-in stage can also be difficult due to the relative lack of retention of the restorations before cementation. It is therefore critical that accurate jaw records are secured and transferred to the working casts on at least a semi-adjustable articulator so that any occlusal form manufactured in the laboratory will be close to the clinical situation. Time and attention to detail at this stage will always be productive, and will usually reduce the need for any major adjustment to the restorations following cementation. Removal of all the residual composite resin lute following the final cemention of the restorations can also prove to be problematic and time-consuming, particularly in the proximal regions.

Despite some of these present limitations, as ceramic and resin technology improves – and stronger, less abrasive, castable materials become available – it may become more realistic to consider resin-bonded ceramic restorations as routine when managing patients with generalized tooth wear.

Conclusions

A wide range of treatment options exist when considering the restoration of the worn dentition, ranging from the more conventional fixed and removable prosthodontic approach to some of the newer, less invasive and minimal preparation adhesive techniques now available to the dental surgeon. While a number of the minimal preparation adhesive methods would appear to offer significant advantages over more traditional measures, only time and careful clinical evaluation will dictate whether these become the accepted treatment patterns of tomorrow.

References

Banks RG (1990) Conservative posterior ceramic restorations: A literature review. *J Prosthet Dent* **63**:619–26.

Basker RM *et al.* (1993) *Overdentures in General Dental Practice*. 3rd edn. British Dental Association: London.

Berry DC, Poole DFG (1976) Attrition: possible mechanisms of compensation. *J Oral Rehabil* **3**:201–6.

Bishop K, Bell M, Briggs P, Kelleher M (1996) Restoration of a worn dentition using a double-veneer technique. *Br Dent J* **180**:26–9.

Bishop K, Priestley D, Deans R, Joshi R (1997) The use of adhesive metal– ceramic restorations as an alternative to conventional crown and bridge materials. *Br Dent J* **182**:101–16.

Bowen RL (1963) Properties of a silica-reinforced polymer for dental restorations. *J Am Dent Assoc* **66**:57–64.

Briggs P, Bishop K (1997) Fixed restorations in the treatment of tooth wear. *Eur J Prosthodont Restor Dent* **5**:175–80.

Briggs P, Bishop K, Kelleher M (1994) The use of indirect composite for the management of extensive erosion. *Eur J Prosthodont Restor Dent* **3**:51–4.

Brown KE (1980) Reconstruction considerations for severe dental attrition. *J Prosthet Dent* **44**:384–8.

Buonocore MG (1955) A simple method of increasing the adhesion of acrylic filling materials to enamel surfaces. *J Dent Res* **34**:849–53.

Calamia JR (1985) Etched porcelain veneers: the current state of the art. *Quint Int* **16**:12–15.

Cheung SP, Dimmer, A (1988) Management of the worn dentition: a further use for the resin-bonded cast metal restoration. *Restor Dent* **4**:76–8.

Crawford PJM, Aboush YEY (1993) The use of adhesively retained gold onlays in the management of dental erosion in a child: a 4-year case report. *Br Dent J* **175**:414–16.

Creugers HC, Kayser AF (1992) The use of adhesive metal partial crowns to restore attrition defects: a case report. *Quint Int* **23**:245–8.

Dahl BL, Krogstad O (1982) The effect of a partial bite raising splint on the occlusal face height. An X-ray cephalometric study in human adults. *Acta Odontol Scand* **40**:17–24.

Dahl BL, Krogstad O, Karlsen K (1975) An alternative treatment in cases with advanced attrition. *J Oral Rehabil* **2**:209–14.

Darbar UR (1994) Treatment of palatal erosive wear by using oxidised gold veneers: a case report. *Quint Int* **25**:195–7.

Darbar UR, Hemmings KW (1997) Treatment of localised anterior tooth wear with composite restorations at an increased occlusal vertical dimension. *Dent Update* **24**:72–5.

Duke ES (1993) Adhesion and its application with restorative materials. *Dent Clin North Am* **37**:329–39.

Eckerbom M, Magnusson T, Martinsson T (1992) Reasons for and incidence of tooth mortality in a Swedish population. *Endodont Dent Traumatol* **8**:230–4.

Ettinger RL, Jakobsen J (1997) Denture treatment needs of an overdenture population. *Int J Prosthodont* **10**:355–65.

Foreman PC (1988) Resin-bonded acid-etched onlays in two cases of gross attrition. *Dent Update* **15**:150–3.

Fyffe HE (1992) Provision of crowns in Scotland – a ten year longitudinal study. *Comm Dent Health* **9**:159–64.

Graser GN (1990) Removable partial overdentures for special patients. *Dent Clin North Am* **34**:741–57.

Holmes R, Dan Sneed W (1990) Treatment of severe chemomechanical erosion using castable ceramic restorations and a new dentin/enamel bonding system: a case report. *Quint Int* **21**:863–7.

Hussey DL, Irwin CR, Kime DL (1994) Treatment of anterior tooth wear with gold palatal veneers. *Br Dent J* **176**:422–5.

Ibbetson RJ, Setchell DJ (1989a) Treatment of the worn dentition 1. *Dent Update* **16**:247–53.

Ibbetson RJ, Setchell DJ (1989b) Treatment of the worn dentition 2. *Dent Update* **16**:300–7.

Jackson CR, Skidmore AE, Rice RT (1992) Pulpal evaluation of teeth restored with fixed prostheses. *J Prosthet Dent* **67**:323–5.

Licht WS, Leveton EE (1980) Overdentures for treatment of severe attrition. *J Prosthet Dent* **43**:497–500.

McLean JW, Wilson AD (1977) The clinical development of the glass-ionomer cements. Formulations and properties. *Aust Dent J* **22**:31–6.

McLundie AC (1991) Localised palatal tooth surface loss and its treatment with porcelain laminates. *Restor Dent* **7**:43–4.

Milosevic A (1990) The use of porcelain veneers to restore palatal tooth loss. *Restor Dent* **6**:15–18.

Nohl FSA, King PA, Harley KE, Ibbetson RJ (1997) Retrospective survey of resin-retained cast metal palatal veneers for the treatment of anterior palatal tooth wear. *Quint Int* **28**:7–14.

Nunn J, Shaw L, Smith A (1996) Tooth wear – dental erosion. *Br Dent J* **180**:349–52.

O'Brien M (1993) *Children's Dental Health in the United Kingdom*. HMSO: London.

Rawlinson A, Winstanley RB (1988) The management of severe dental erosion using posterior occlusal porcelain veneers and an anterior overdenture. *Restor Dent* **4**:10–16.

Ricketts NJ, Smith BGN (1993) Minor axial tooth movement in preparation for fixed prostheses. *Eur J Prosthodont Restor Dent* **1**:145–9.

Ricketts NJ, Smith BGN (1994) Clinical techniques for producing and monitoring minor axial tooth movement. *Eur J Prosthodont Restor Dent* **2**:5–9.

Roessler DM (1990) Amalgam and composite resin as an alternative to crown and bridgework in the rehabilitation of an extensively debilitated dentition. Case report. *Aust Dent J* **36**:1–4.

Saunders WP (1989) Resin bonded bridgework: a review. *J Dent* **17**:255–65.

Schwartz NL, Whitsett LD, Berry TG, Stewart JL (1970) Unserviceable crowns and fixed partial dentures: lifespan and causes for loss of serviceability. *J Am Dent Assoc* **81**:139–401.

Smith BG, Bartlett DW, Robb ND (1997) The prevalence, etiology and management of tooth wear in the United Kingdom. *J Prosthet Dent* **78**:367–72.

Steele JG, Walls AW, Ayatollahi SM, Murray JJ (1996) Major clinical findings from a dental survey of elderly people in three different English communities. *Br Dent J* **180**:17–23.

Toh CG, Setcos JC, Weinstein AR (1987) Indirect dental laminate veneers – an overview. *J Dent* **15**:117–24.

Toolson LB, Taylor TD (1989) A 10-year report of a longitudinal recall of overdenture patients. *J Prosthet Dent* **62**:179–81.

Walton JN, Gardner FM, Agar JR (1986) A survey of crown and fixed partial denture failures. Length of service and reasons for replacement. *J Prosthet Dent* **56**:416–21.

Watson RM (1997) The role of removable prostheses and implants in the restoration of the worn dentition. *Eur J Prosthodont Restor Dent* **5**:181–6.

Watson TF, Bartlett DW (1994) Adhesive systems: composites, dentine bonding agents and glass ionomers. *Br Dent J* **176**:227–31.

Willems G, Lambrechts P, Braem M, Vanherle G (1993) Composite resins in the 21st century. *Quint Int* **24**:641–58.

Williams DR (1987) A rationale for the management of advanced tooth wear (ATW). *J Oral Rehabil* **14**:77–89.

20

Toothbrushes: benefits versus effects on hard and soft tissues

Fridus Van der Weijden and Monique M Danser

Introduction

Natural cleaning of the dentition is considered to be almost non-existent. The natural physiological forces that clean the oral cavity are insufficient to remove all dental plaque. Plaque, to be controlled, must be removed frequently by physical methods. Hence the dental community continues to encourage proper oral hygiene and more effective use of mechanical cleaning devices (Cancro and Fischman 1995). Maintenance of oral hygiene has been an objective of man since the dawn of civilization. The use of the chewing stick (Figure 20.1) to clean the dentition is an example of an ancient pre-Islamic custom that continues to be used today. Most historians trace the development of the first toothbrushes to 1498 AD in China. The Dutchman Cornelis van Solingen (1614–87) gave probably the oldest 'picture' of a toothbrush. In the 1698 edition of his book we find the picture of a toothbrush combined with a tongue-scraper (Figure 20.2). The bristle brush was reinvented in the late 18th century, and by the first part of the 20th century, in the USA a family toothbrush was

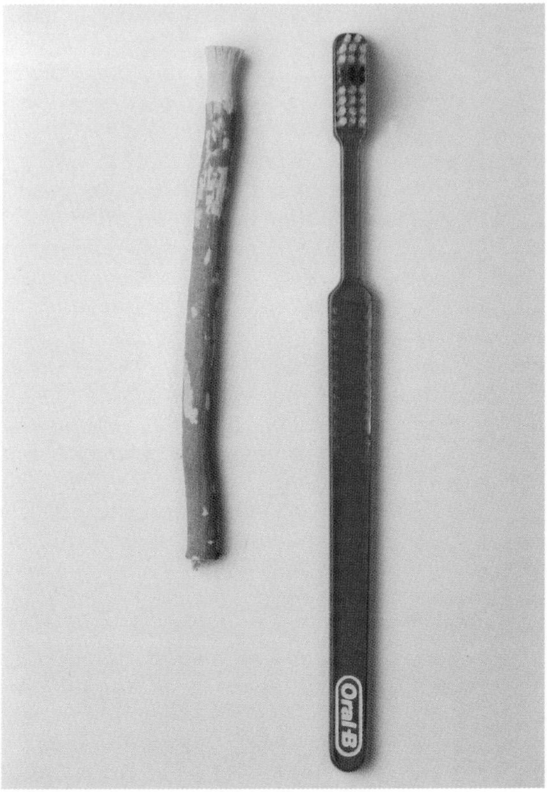

Figure 20.1

Primitive toothbrush (miswak or siwak).

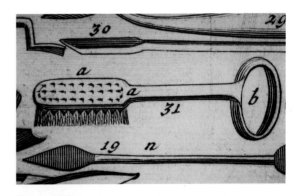

Figure 20.2

Toothbrush with tongue-scraper designed by Cornelis van Solingen (with thanks to Utrecht Universiteits Museum).

common even among the poor. In the late 1930s, nylon filaments began to replace natural bristles, and wood and plastic replaced bone handles. This made toothbrushes inexpensive enough for virtually everybody to own one. During the past 30 years oral hygiene has improved and in industrialized countries 80–90% of the population brush their teeth once or twice a day (Saxer and Yankell 1997) (see also Chapter 14).

Benefit of oral hygiene

Bacterial plaque on teeth is considered the direct cause of periodontal diseases and caries. In the absence of plaque, disease will not occur. One practical approach to control both diseases simultaneously is to eliminate bacterial plaque at daily intervals (Löe 1979).

Oral hygiene will act as a non-specific suppressor of plaque mass. Such a therapeutic approach is based on the rationale that any decrease in plaque mass will benefit the inflamed tissues adjacent to bacterial deposits. This non-specific control of the periodontal microbiota is effective in the majority of cases where access to the plaque deposits is possible (Listgarten 1988). Diminishing the plaque mass, as a result of good oral hygiene, will reduce the injurious load on the tissues. Some residual inflammation may persist, but is unlikely to be of sufficient magnitude to contribute to progressive tissue destruction.

The significance of oral hygiene in the prevention of oral diseases has long been stressed in the dental literature. However, the impact of this message upon the prevalence of these diseases has been small and it is apparent that these diseases still constitute a serious problem today (Pilot and Miyazaki 1991). Proper mechanical cleansing of the teeth by brushing, flossing and/or the use of toothpicks can remove plaque thoroughly from the teeth, but correct oral hygiene techniques require an extended period of training for patient motivation and dexterity. One possible way to overcome the limitations associated with manual brushing is to develop a mechanical brushing device, and as early as 1855 the Swedish clockmaker Frederick Wilhelm Tornberg patented a mechanical toothbrush (Scutt and Swann 1975).

Electric toothbrushes

The first electric toothbrushes came much later and were introduced in the 1960s. They provided a brush-head capable of a variety of motions driven by a power source. Over time such devices have become established as a valuable alternative to manual methods of toothbrushing. The first electric brushes mimicked the back-and-forth motion commonly used with a manual toothbrush. When first introduced there were many reports of the effectiveness of such devices. In 1986, an international workshop on oral hygiene concluded that up to that time neither powered nor manual toothbrushes removed more plaque, regardless of the brushing method (Löe and Kleinmann 1986). At that time, only what are now known as conventional electric toothbrushes were available. This first generation of electric toothbrushes had a brush-head designed as a manual toothbrush and a (combined) horizontal and vertical motion. Because of the lack of clear superiority and many problems of mechanical breakdown, powered toothbrushes fell out of favour, and during the late 1960s they gradually disappeared from the market. However, powered brushes continued to be recommended for the handicapped and for persons with reduced manual dexterity. Over the last decade a new generation of electric toothbrushes has become available and they can be conveniently categorized into two distinct types. Firstly, there has been a move towards more (oscillating) rotary action brushes, instead of the traditional side-to-side motion (Walmsley 1997). The rotary motion can be either the motion of the whole head, or of the individual tufts moving in a counter-clockwise direction. Secondly, there are brushes which operate with a brush-head motion at a higher frequency (Johnson and McInnes 1994). It has been shown that this new generation of brushes, featuring an oscillating or high frequency action, removes plaque significantly more effectively in the approximal area than do conventional manual toothbrushes (for review see van der Weijden et al. 1998a). This led (in the 1996 World Workshop in Periodontics) to the careful conclusion that limited evidence suggested that electric brushes provide additional benefit compared with manual brushes (Hancock 1996).

Effects on hard and soft tissues

At the start of this century, toothbrushing was not common and was correlated with a degree of fear because of its newness. Many published papers focused on the side-effects of toothbrushes and even questioned the safety of regular use. Thompson, in 1927, described injuries to gingival margins from toothbrushing. He believed that it was better to have a diet that encouraged chewing coarse food than to brush teeth to gain tooth cleanliness (Gillette and van House 1980). In contrast, there were also many reports in support of the need for oral hygiene. Toothbrushing is now the most common means of oral prophylaxis and in the light of its potential benefits to oral health the adverse effects or damage caused by toothbrushing can be regarded as insignificant.

However, it would be an exaggeration to conclude that toothbrushing is totally harmless. It has been known for a long time that toothbrushing has some unwanted effects on the gingiva and hard tooth tissues. The simple act of cleaning away dental deposits from teeth requires that the toothbrush–dentifrice combination possesses some level of abrasivity. The filaments must have a degree of stiffness to create sufficient abrasion to dislodge plaque deposits. This stiffness has to be balanced against potential detrimental effects to dental hard and soft tissues. In the oral cavity, four tissues are at risk from the abrasive effect of toothbrushing. These are the enamel, dentine, gingival tissues and alveolar mucosa.

Three types of damage seem to predominate:

- Epithelial abrasion (Figure 20.3)
- Gingival recession with root surface exposure (Figure 20.4)
- Cervical abrasion of cementum and dentine (Figure 20.5).

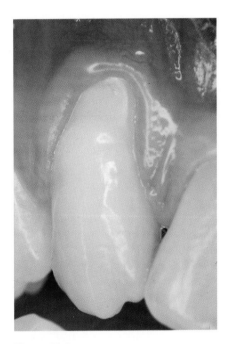

Figure 20.4

Gingival recession as a result of traumatic brushing.

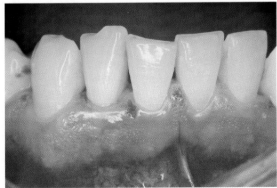

Figure 20.3

Gingival abrasion due to toothbrushing.

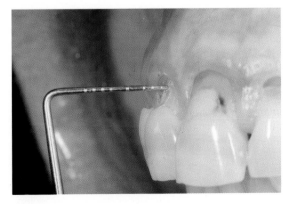

Figure 20.5

Cervical abrasion due to brushing.

To date, few scientific data have been available to help in understanding the risks associated with toothbrush abrasion. In particular, research into the abrasion of hard tissues is difficult. First of all the effect usually takes years to become visible. Secondly various factors have been regarded as responsible for the damage caused, namely: material-oriented factors such as dentifrice abrasivity and brush quality; and individual-oriented factors such as brushing habit, brushing frequency and the position of the teeth within the arch (Bergström and Lavstedt 1979).

Manly (1944) believed that the toothbrush causes little hard tissue abrasion compared with dentifrice. Radentz et al. 1976 reported cervical abrasion in exactly half their 80 subjects and they also thought that the type of dentifrice and brush had no effect on abrasion, nor did brushing technique or frequency. However, Reisstein et al. (1978) found that toothbrushing with dentifrice abraded cementum more than toothbrushing with a saline solution, but neither method abraded enamel.

Effect on enamel and dentine – in vitro

Enamel is not as susceptible to toothbrush wear in vitro as less calcified structures (Bull et al. 1968, Stookey and Muhler 1968). Slop (1986) used an in-vitro model to investigate to what extent the enamel will wear down as a result of brushing. Although some wear was observed, there appeared to be no potential danger for extensive abrasion of enamel. The abrasivity of a modern dentifrice on enamel is such that after about 50 000 brush strokes an average layer of about 0.5 µm enamel is removed. Assuming in practice that a tooth is brushed with 25 strokes twice daily, the toothbrush/dentifrice abrasivity will remove in a life time about 10–15 µm of the 2-mm thick enamel. This suggests that toothbrushing with a dentifrice per se constitutes little risk to the integrity of the enamel. Kuroiwa et al. (1993) found some abrasion of enamel with a dentifrice containing abrasive; however, toothbrushing without dentifrice seemed to protect the enamel surface via the formation of a mineral protective membrane. The hardness of enamel may have some influence on the wear caused. Thus the

presence of tooth erosion has been shown to increase the rate of enamel abrasion in an animal model (Attin et al. 1997). Dental erosion is usually attributed to such factors as the excessive drinking of fruit juices, the ingestion of medication with a low pH or working in an acid environment (Radentz et al. 1976). In such a case toothbrushing may increase the loss of enamel. In fact, tooth erosion can be observed even in young populations and should be considered a risk factor associated with tooth abrasion (Milosevic et al. 1997). A controversial theory of cervical loss enamel is that of Lee and Eakle (1984). They suggested that lateral forces can create tensile stresses that disrupt hydroxyapatite crystals in enamel, thereby allowing small molecules, such as those of water, to penetrate and render the crystals more susceptible to chemical attack and further mechanical deterioration.

As with enamel, little is known about the abrasion of dentine. This holds true for both manual and electric toothbrushes (Harrington and Terry 1964). One approach to evaluate dentine abrasion by toothbrushing has been to assess the relative dentine abrasion in vitro, using a model which has been developed at Indiana University (USA) and approved by the ADA. This method was developed primarily to assess the abrasiveness of dentifrices (Hefferren 1976, Schemehorn et al. 1993). To date no studies are available which specifically evaluated different manual toothbrushes with regard to dentine abrasivity; however, a number of studies have evaluated electric toothbrushes.

The results of several studies carried out in Indiana (Schemehorn et al. 1993, van der Velden et al. 1993, Schemehorn and Zwart 1996) indicate that oscillating/rotating electric toothbrushes are safe with respect to dentine abrasion. Recent studies carried out in Zurich (Imfeldt and Sener 1998a) apparently using the same model appear to contradict these findings. The origin of these differences could be the result of minor but trivial deviations from the original model and should be the object of future studies.

Cervical abrasion – in vivo

Although the etiology of cervical abrasion is not fully understood as yet, it has become clear that toothbrushing plays an important part. Only a few studies concerning cervical lesions due to toothbrushing have been reported in the dental literature. The lack of control of the frequency and force of brushing and also the exact criteria for the observations do not permit definite conclusions to be drawn. In a large epidemiological study Bergström and Lavstedt (1979) investigated the prevalence and severity of abrasive lesions in the light of individual toothbrushing technique and toothbrushing frequency and also of the stiffness of the toothbrush and abrasivity of the dentifrice. They differentiated between superficial and deep cervical lesions. Of the sample taken from a population in Sweden (aged 18–65 years) 31% of the subjects exhibited either superficial or deep lesions, of whom 12% had deep lesions. There appeared to be a slight predominance for the left side in both jaws. A strong correlation to abrasion was found for the variable brushing techniques (horizontal, vertical, roll, or combination) and brushing frequency (number of times per day), whereas the influence exerted by bristle stiffness (soft, medium, hard) and dentifrice abrasivity (low, medium and high) were rather weak. The age of the subject exhibited the strongest correlation to abrasion, where age may be interpreted as an expression for the toothbrushing consumption of the individual.

Toothbrush abrasion is usually located at the cervical area on the facial surfaces of teeth prominent in the arch. Premolars and canines are most commonly affected, second and third molars are least affected. The notch-shaped lesion usually begins at the cemento–enamel junction and extends a short distance apically. Extensive lesions can involve the pulp. Lesions are initiated by horizontal brushing with a brush with firm bristles. Although not all studies agree, contributory factors seem to be time, force of application, dentifrice and prominence of the tooth in the arch. Abrasion occurs only in the presence of gingival recession, also probably caused by the brushing technique where the cemento–enamel junction becomes exposed. Occasionally, multiple parallel grooves are present rather than just one groove. Cervical hypersensitivity may accompany the lesion (Gillette and van House 1980) (see Chapter 21).

Sangnes and Gjermo (1976) observed concomitant gingival and dental lesions in the same individual in more than half of the cases studied, indicating a common etiology. However, some cases with hard tissue lesions but no retraction of the gingiva were also observed. This suggests that individual factors in the oral environment may influence the development of the lesions.

Effect on soft tissue – in vitro

To date there have been few if any in-vitro models to assess the possible damaging effects of toothbrushes on soft tissues and certainly none that could be reliably extrapolated to clinical outcome. Human skin, mucosa or gingiva can be obtained, but tissue from animals is more readily available in in-vitro studies (Addy 1998). Alexander et al. (1977) studied the effect of toothbrushing on soft tissue abrasion by assessing the amount of protein removed during brushing of hamster cheek pouch tissue. They found that with increasing brushing pressure and number of strokes, there was a corresponding rise in the amount of tissue protein removed. They concluded that their method was sensitive in detecting the effects of brush load, number of strokes applied and the texture of the brush.

More recently a model was introduced by Imfeldt and Sener (1998b) in which a dead pig jaw is brushed for a specified amount of time with different brushing forces. Several concerns have to be expressed about such a model. Firstly, the reproducibility of the system has not been addressed as yet, and standardization problems can be envisaged. Secondly, it is difficult to translate this model back to the situation in vivo, as brushing at a specific spot for >30 s would implicate a brushing time of at least 14 min, which is not common daily practice (for review see van der Weijden et al. 1993). Thirdly, because the model employs non-vital tissue, it does not have natural defence systems nor the normal potential for repair. Therefore the relevance to the clinical situation in vivo must be questioned. The same criticisms also apply to the model introduced by Alexander et al. (1977). Therefore both models offer only the possibility of evaluating the relative gingival abrasive potential of brushes, which may be useful while developing new designs. True in vivo studies are needed to assess the effect in the clinical situation.

Effect on gingiva – in vivo

Findings indicate that brushing increases the degree of keratinization of the gingiva (which in the past was considered to be protective) and that natural bristles are slightly more effective in this respect than synthetic bristles (Stahl *et al.* 1953). In an animal experiment, Plagmann *et al.* (1978) subjected guinea pigs to cleaning with two different manual toothbrushes three times weekly for 4 weeks. Depending on the brush type they found different epithelial lesions which differed in depth of the lesion. Abbas *et al.* (1990) showed that mechanical oral hygiene basically is a traumatic procedure for the periodontium. They observed increased bleeding upon probing scores shortly after oral hygiene procedures. Trauma to soft tissues can result in gingival recession (Gorman 1967, Paloheimo *et al.* 1987, Vekalahti 1989, Källestål and Uhlin 1992, Löe *et al.* 1992, Khocht *et al.* 1993, Serino *et al.* 1994) and gingival abrasion (Alexander *et al.* 1977, Breitenmoser *et al.* 1979, Sandholm *et al.* 1982). Gingival abrasion takes two forms: inflammation of the gingival margin, and inflammation of protruding areas on the gingiva away from the margin. Ulceration often accompanies both forms (Gillette and van House 1980).

Gingival recession has been related separately and collectively to alveolar bone dehiscences, inflammation, malalignment of teeth, toothbrushing, fastidious injuries, muscle pull, orthodontic tooth movement, dental trauma and iatrogenesis (Källestal and Uhlin 1992). According to Gorman (1967) Miller stated in 1950 that gingival recession resulted from occlusal traumatism produced by overfunction and/or underfunction, improper toothbrushing and psychosomatic factors particularly associated with depression.

Gingival recession, predominantly on the vestibular tooth surfaces, is often attributed to incorrect toothbrushing technique (Sandholm *et al.* 1982). Findings that individuals with recession have lower mean plaque and mean gingival inflammation scores than individuals without recession support this hypothesis (Niemi 1987). Lesions are seldom seen on lingual and approximal surfaces; they tend to be more pronounced in the cervical regions of incisors, canines and premolars (Sangnes and Gjermo 1976). Furthermore, it has been observed that such defects are more prevalent in the maxilla than in the mandible.

In an adult population, subjects with thin gingival tissues may be more susceptible to gingival recession than subjects with thick gingival tissues (Olsson and Lindhe 1991). In older individuals, gingival recession is more prevalent and tends to show a generalized pattern, perhaps as the combined consequence of loss of attachment due to periodontal disease and the presence of calculus and toothbrushing trauma (Serino *et al.* 1994, van Palenstein Helderman *et al.* 1998). Kalsbeek *et al.* (1996), in a study on oral health in Dutch adults, found a positive relationship between age and mean number of roots exposed to the oral cavity. In the age category 45–54 years this number (8.6 surfaces) was approximately 2.5 times higher than for those 25–34 years of age (3.4 surfaces). In a study among a group of subjects aged 18–65 years Khocht *et al.* (1993) also observed that the proportion of subjects with recession increased with age. Recession was also found to be more pronounced for subjects with a history of hard toothbrush use. The association with age does not necessarily suggest a physiological effect of ageing on recession. It may just reflect the fact that older people have been subject to the force of brushing and irritant effects of plaque for a longer period (Joshipura *et al.* 1994). Paloheimo *et al.* (1987) observed in a Finnish adolescent population that recession was associated with the length of service life of the toothbrush and with the toothbrushing technique.

Predictions that the increase in recession due to toothbrushing would result in an increase in the incidence of root caries in countries such as Finland, Switzerland and the Netherlands have not come true (König 1990, Mierau 1992). The problem seems to be replaced by another problem, that of cervical and V-shaped abrasions (König 1990).

Electric toothbrushes and gingival abrasion

As most of the previously published studies regarding gingival abrasion due to toothbrushing and the resultant gingival lesions predate the introduction of electric toothbrushes, less is known about the abrasive potential of automated brushing. From related studies, however, it would appear that electric toothbrushes should be at least as safe as a manual toothbrush. Indeed it has been shown that the brushing force applied by users of an electric toothbrush is lower than that applied with a manual toothbrush (van der Weijden et al. 1996b, Boyd et al. 1997).

The old generation of powered toothbrushes was effective and generally did not cause gingival abrasion because of low power exerted on the handle and because of the stop mechanism when excessive force was applied. However, these brushes functioned for relatively short time periods and were generally not used after the initial 'novelty' had worn off. Studies have looked at the number of gingival abrasions that have occurred with the use of a conventional electric toothbrush and compared their occurrence to the potential damage caused by manual toothbrushing by means of visual scoring (Niemi et al. 1986). Results demonstrated a greater number of abrasions following use of the manual brush. Walsh et al. (1989) found no differences between electric and manual toothbrushes with respect to gingival abrasion. However, in their study, subjects brushed at home; therefore the brushing time, the brushing pressure and the brushing method may have differed.

In most studies, plaque removal by the new generation of powered toothbrushes is greater than that by manual brushes (Walmsley 1997). Some studies have found a reduction in gingival inflammation and most have found that gingival abrasion is usually not present or minimal. Nevertheless, long-term outcomes regarding gingival abrasion with modern electric toothbrushes require further investigation (Saxer and Yankell 1997).

A sonic brush, which has a high frequency action, has been subjected to safety testing in dogs (Engel et al. 1993). It appeared that after brushing for 7.5 min daily for 2 months, no damage was evident on clinical or histological examination.

Recently Danser et al. (1998a) conducted a study to establish the incidence of gingival abrasion as a result of toothbrushing, using a manual toothbrush and an oscillating/rotating electric toothbrush. In agreement with Walsh et al. (1989) the results showed no differences in the amount of gingival abrasion caused by either the electric or manual brushes using standardized brushing time and procedures.

Grossman et al. (1996), in a comparative clinical study of stain removal with two oscillating/rotating electric toothbrushes, also found no evidence of soft or hard tissue abrasion in either group. Similarly, Cronin et al. (1998), reporting on a 3-month clinical study with an oscillating/rotating reciprocating electric toothbrush and a manual toothbrush, found that soft tissue abrasion was negligible and clinically insignificant in both groups. In a study testing another oscillating electric toothbrush, none of the brushes – including a manual – exhibited any propensity for injury or harm to the subjects' oral tissues beyond that transiently associated with the use of new toothbrush filaments (Khocht et al. 1992).

In two longitudinal investigations using two different oscillating/rotating toothbrushes, the indirect effect on the gingival tissues was studied. Neither brush caused more gingival abrasion than was observed with a manual toothbrush (Wilson et al. 1993, van der Weijden et al. 1994). Wilson et al. (1993) also measured gingival recession. They observed that neither the manual nor electric toothbrush group developed significant changes in the level of gingival recession over the 1-year study period.

In a 1-year study with a rotating action electric toothbrush the participants lost 0.12 mm attachment level on the buccal sides, whereas the manual toothbrush lost only about 0.05 mm (Boyd et al. 1989). These differences were not statistically significant, although 0.1 mm attachment loss in 1 year was higher than the epidemiological average in patients in a prophylactic programme (Saxer and Yankell 1997).

Morphology and histology of gingival lesions

Baker and Seymour (1976) suggested a localized inflammatory process as an etiological factor for gingival recessions. They speculated that the inflammatory reaction causes breakdown of the connective tissue leading to proliferation of the epithelium into the site of connective tissue destruction. This process would involve tissue remodelling, leading to gingival recession. This remodelling process is particularly likely to occur where the tissue is thin. The histological evidence from sections taken from broad recession areas tends to confirm the hypothesis that destruction of the intervening connective tissue cores more easily permits penetration of a proliferating dento-gingival epithelium until such time as the dento-gingival and oral epithelia coalesce. Loss of proper nutrition to the enlarged epithelial layer enhances loss of adhesiveness and/or physical removal (Smuckler and Landsberg 1984).

Not all damage is found in one form. Puncture wounds are observed as microhemorrhagic lesions, usually localized on the buccal aspect of the free gingiva or the interdental papilla. Generally only the superficial epithelial cell layers are damaged. Scratches are erosive lesions, generally extending along the marginal gingiva, with no involvement of the subepithelial connective tissue. The abrasion lesion is superficial; sometimes only the most superficial layers of the keratin are torn from the underlying cellular layer. Ulceration is described as tissue damage extending beyond the superficial epithelium and involving the subepithelial connective tissue. When the total thickness of the gingiva is destroyed and the root is evident, the lesion is a fenestration. These lesions are significant clinically because of their esthetic component. The traumatic toothbrushing lesions that are superimposed on a pre-existing gingival recession may act as an exacerbating factor in the extension of tissue damage (Figure 20.6). Impacted foreign materials such as toothbrush bristles (Agudio *et al.* 1987) may cause acute abscesses in gingival tissues.

Gingival lesions can be restricted to the superficial epithelium, thus damaging only the keratinized superficial layer of the epithelium, or they may proceed more deeply to involve the basal layer and the underlying connective tissue (Figure 20.7).

Diagnosis of gingival abrasion

Systems for classification of lesions related to mechanical tooth cleansing procedures, with proper consideration of differential diagnostic problems, are scarce. Sangnes and Gjermo (1976) pointed out that pockets generally associated with gingival recession are shallow. Recessions in areas with pocket depths of ≤ 1 mm are considered to be related to habitual toothbrushing (Sangnes and Gjermo 1976).

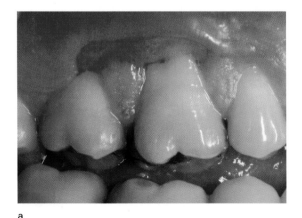 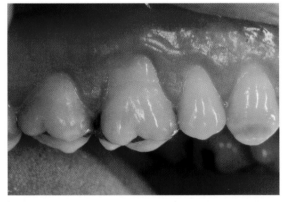

a   b

Figure 20.6

a An example of traumatic ulcerative gingival lesions.
b The same site shown after a period of 2 weeks of non-brushing but rinsing with chlorhexidine.

Diagnosis of toothbrushing recession is based on the localized nature. Usually on the facial surface and frequently V-shaped, recession often occurs in association with toothbrush abrasion of the tooth surface.

Gillette and van House (1980) have described a dental classification for injuries of this type which result from improper oral hygiene measures. Their classification is based upon source of injury, site of occurrence and potential side-effects. Gingival lesions, possibly caused by toothbrushing, may be classified in terms of three groups: laceration, gingival recession and hyperplasia, especially hyperkeratinization. Laceration

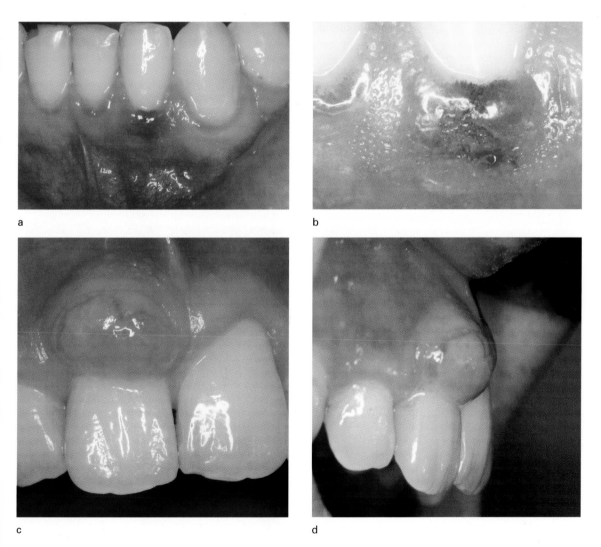

a

b

c

d

Figure 20.7

a and *b* Hematoma as a result of traumatic brushing. The patient presented as shown the morning after he had started brushing with a new toothbrush.
c and *d* Irritation fibroma as a result of traumatic brushing. The patient had a site with toothbrush trauma and continued brushing this site vigorously for 3 months to get rid of the irritation, which resulted in the situation illustrated here.

or ulceration of gingival tissues is usually recognized as an acute mechanical trauma, whereas gingival recession and hyperplasia are thought to be characteristics of chronic lesions.

Compared with clinical classification of gingival trauma, scanning electron microscopic (SEM) evaluation has been shown to be a more reliable method for further studying these lesions (Sandholm *et al*. 1982). A study by Sandholm *et al*. (1982) revealed that brushing may in many cases result in moderate to severe abrasion of the gingiva. All subjects participating in their study were brushed by one dental hygienist using hard and soft manual toothbrushes. Clinical evaluation (visual) and SEM findings were found to correlate significantly, although discrepancies between the two classification systems were observed. Niemi *et al*. (1986) investigated gingival injury caused by standardized brushing. One examiner scored the visible gingival abrasion and the consistency of this examiner was ascertained to be 90% compared with SEM analysis. For SEM assessment of gingival abrasion, replicas based on silicon rubber-based impressions are taken.

Three types of gingival lesions have been described using SEM and categorized as follows (Sandholm *et al*. 1982) (Figure 20.8):

- Type 1. Erosion of the epithelial surface at the gingival margin, with the appearance of a ribbon or a patch-like surface defect, or a diffuse border at the gingiva–tooth interface caused by bleeding or oozing of tissue fluid from the eroded area.
- Type 2. Epithelial; surface 'flap' turned or rolled up leaving the underlying tissue uncovered.
- Type 3. Rupture or fenestration of the surface epithelium in the middle of a prominent but otherwise healthy gingival area.

Breitenmoser *et al*. (1979) investigated the use of a disclosing agent for the identification of gingival abrasions. They found that a commercially obtained plaque disclosing solution could give excellent staining of the lesions and they could be distinguished easily from normal gingiva (Figure 20.9). In a recent study, it was found that before staining the gingiva small sites of abrasion were not visible with clinical evaluation (Danser *et al*. 1998b). A background incidence of toothbrush abrasion, which can be observed with a disclosing agent, is a normal response to brushing.

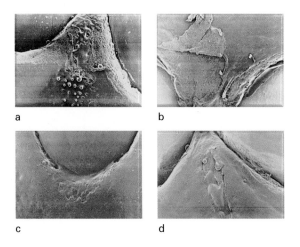

Figure 20.8

Gingival lesions (taken from Sandholm *et al*. 1982).

a Type 1 lesion.
b and *c* Type 2 lesions.
d Type 3 lesion.

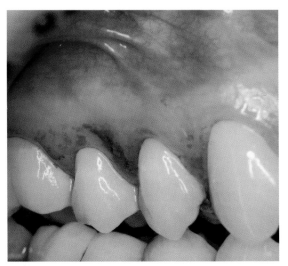

Figure 20.9

Example of sites with gingival abrasion after brushing by panellists, made visible after disclosing with Mira–2–Tone®. Small and large sites of abrasion can be seen.

In another study (Danser *et al.* 1998b), the incidence of abrasion after brushing with a manual and an electric brush and with two electric brushes with different bristle end-roundings was evaluated. In these two tests the incidence of sites of abrasion post-brushing was larger in the first phase (manual and electric brush) of the study than in the second phase (two electric brushes). However the pre-brushing scores in both parts were comparable. This indicates that the way the subject brushes is probably important and influences the observed effect.

Clinical investigations using staining

One of our first studies with a two-tone disclosing solution compared the number of gingival abrasions with oscillating/rotating and sonic electric toothbrushes (van der Weijden *et al.* 1996a).

The results with regard to abrasion are presented in Table 20.1. No difference in either large or small gingival abrasion sites was observed between the two brushes. Based on the results of this experiment two main questions arose:

- Is there a baseline level of abrasion after 24–48 h of non-brushing?
- What is the level of abrasion when brushing with a manual toothbrush?

To investigate these questions another study was carried out. One of the objectives was to establish the potential of manual and electric toothbrushes to cause gingival abrasion. Plaque and gingival abrasion were assessed by means

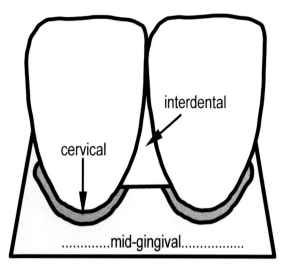

Figure 20.10

Diagram showing the division of the tooth-related soft tissues into three areas for the assessment of gingival abrasion: cervical, interdental and mid-gingival.

of a two-tone solution. The tooth-related soft tissues were divided into three areas: cervical, interdental and mid-gingival, as shown in Figure 20.10. The subjects brushed their teeth in a random split-mouth order with two electric brushes, using brush-heads of the same design. The gums were redisclosed and gingival abrasions were recorded. The mean gingival abrasion scores for the electric toothbrush and the manual brush at baseline for sites ≤5 mm were 2.67 and 2.43 respectively and for sites >5 mm it was 0.82 for the electric and 0.49 for the manual brush (Table 20.2). The difference between the brushes was not significant. No

Table 20.2 Gingival abrasion was scored as small ≤5 mm or large sites >5 mm (Danser *et al.* 1998a).

Sites	Manual brush	Significance	Electric brush
Small sites			
pre-brushing	2.43 (3.00)	NS	2.67 (2.69)
post-brushing	3.45 (3.10)	NS	3.55 (2.99)
Large sites			
pre-brushing	0.49 (0.94)	NS	0.82 (1.51)
post-brushing	0.20 (0.57)	NS	0.35 (0.80)

Standard deviation in parentheses.

Table 20.1 Gingival abrasion was scored as small ≤5 mm or large sites >5 mm.

Site	Oscillating/rotating brush	Significance	Sonic brush
Small sites	1.71 (2.86)	NS	2.00 (2.60)
Large sites	0.09 (0.37)	NS	0.06 (0.34)

Standard deviation in parentheses.

relationship between efficacy and the incidence of gingival abrasion was observed for both the manual versus electric brush. This suggests that within this study design, effective brushers are not more prone to gingival abrasion.

In a single-use study gingival abrasion with the oscillating/rotating was compared with the oscillating/rotating/reciprocating electric toothbrush. The mean number of small traumas increased from 2.57 at baseline to 4.04 after brushing with the oscillating/rotating brush and from 1.98 to 4.14 after brushing with the oscillating/rotating/reciprocating brush. There was no statistically significant difference between the two groups. For both toothbrushes, more small traumas were found in the upper jaw compared with the lower jaw. No increase in the number of large traumas was observed (Table 20.3).

Toothbrushing force

Several experimental and clinical studies support the assumption that excessive force in brushing is partly responsible for the origin of toothbrush trauma (Arnim and Blackburn 1961, Alexander et al. 1977, Niemi et al. 1987). Mierau and Spindler (1984) observed that in a group of subjects without recession the mean brushing force with a manual toothbrush was 2.12 N (± 0.31) whereas a group with multiple recession had a mean force of 3.75 N (± 0.47).

In the past a number of studies have assessed toothbrushing force and shown a significant variation in the magnitude of forces (e.g. Phaneuf et al. 1962, Fraleigh et al. 1967). Some of the differences appear to be related to the research method, brushing technique and variation in brushes. The 'average brushing force' has been reported to range from 92 to 175 g for electric toothbrushes and 318 to 471 g for manual brushes (Phaneuf et al. 1962, Fraleigh et al. 1967). Fraleigh et al. (1967) reported a mean force of 167 g with an electric toothbrush in the age group 16–25 years. More recently McLey and Zahradnik (1994) investigated brushing force with electric and manual brushes. They showed that less force was used with the electric brushes as compared with a manual toothbrush (N = 296 g). When a comparison was made between the habitual brushing force with two different oscillating/rotating toothbrushes (van der Weijden et al. 1995), the brushing forces were 173 g and 175 g respectively.

Burgett and Ash (1974) argued that the potential detrimental effect of brushing is related to the force applied at a particular point, which is actually pressure. As the forces are given as a total of the force over the entire brush, the unit pressure is less for smaller brush-heads.

Another study evaluated the habitual brushing force which individuals use with various toothbrushes (van der Weijden et al. 1996b). Besides a manual toothbrush, three electric toothbrushes were examined. The results showed that considerably more force is used with a manual brush than with the electric brushes, the difference being >100 g. Considering all these findings, there appears to be a range of forces used (e.g. 95–173 g), but they also show a specific trend that less force is used with electric toothbrushes as compared with manual toothbrushes. These results may have significance for the long-term integrity of oral hard and soft tissue exposed to various brushing devices.

Table 20.3 Gingival abrasion was scored as small ≤5 mm or large sites >5 mm. (Danser et al. 1998b).

Sites	Oscillating/rotating reciprocating brush	Significance	Oscillating/rotating brush
Small sites			
pre-brushing	1.98 (2.06)	NS	2.57 (2.59)
post-brushing	4.14 (3.24)	NS	4.04 (3.10)
Large sites			
pre-brushing	0.37 (0.81)	NS	0.43 (0.68)
post-brushing	0.39 (0.81)	NS	0.47 (0.77)

Standard deviation in parentheses.

Force and efficacy

A recent survey investigated the association between the efficacy of plaque removal and toothbrushing forces during a normal brushing regime (van der Weijden *et al*. 1998b). Brushing force has been measured using a computer set-up. A double strain gauge was glued to the handle of the toothbrush (Figure 20.11). The mean plaque reduction was 39% and the mean brushing force was 330 g. No correlation was observed between efficacy and brushing force. Multiple regression analysis entering squared values of force as an independent variable into the equation indicated that the relationship between efficacy and force was not linear. A curve could be fitted to the plot, demonstrating that up to a certain level of force an increase of force is associated with an increase in efficacy. Beyond this point, application of higher forces resulted in reduced efficacy. As was calculated in this particular test, this 'transition' level of force was 407.4 g.

Another study examined the relationship between brushing force and plaque removal efficacy comparing a regular manual toothbrush with an electric toothbrush. Different brushing forces were evaluated (100, 150, 200, 250 and 300 g). The results showed that when brushing force is increased, more plaque is removed with both of the two brushes (van der Weijden *et al*. 1996b).

Hasegawa *et al*. (1992) evaluated the effect of different toothbrushing forces on plaque reduction by brushing with 100 g intervals on a scale from 100 to 500 g. The results of their study corroborate the findings of the above study (van der Weijden *et al*. 1996b) and earlier studies (White 1983), that with increasing force more plaque is removed. In addition they observed that 300 g seems, for both children and adults, the most effective brushing force when using a manual toothbrush. Forces exceeding this 300 g caused pain and gingival bleeding.

Another investigation evaluated the habitual brushing force which individuals use with various toothbrushes (van der Weijden *et al*. 1996b). A manual toothbrush and three electric toothbrushes were examined. The results showed that considerably more force (273 g) is used with a manual brush than with the electric brushes (96–146 g). No significant relationship between brushing force and plaque removal was demonstrated for any of the brushes. This indicates that brushing force is not the sole factor in determining efficacy.

Force and gingival abrasion

Danser *et al*. (1998a) conducted a study in order to assess whether the brushing force used is correlated to the incidence of gingival abrasion. The mean force of brushing was 169 g. The mean maximum scores ranged between 54 and 304 g. Multiple regression analysis showed no correlations between toothbrushing force and the incidence of gingival abrasion. This indicates that other factors (e.g. brushing itself, tooth anatomy, bristle form, brush-head, brushing time and manual dexterity) appear to be more important than the force used with an electric brush. The results disagree with several experimental and clinical studies which support the assumption that excessive brushing force is partly responsible for the origin of toothbrush trauma (Arnim and Blackburn 1961, Alexander *et al*. 1977, Niemi *et al*. 1987). The average force used with the electric brush in this study was 169 g. There seems to be a specific trend that the average brushing force for powered brushing is significantly less than the force usually used in manual brushing (Phaneuf *et al*. 1962, Niemi *et al*. 1986, 1987, van der Weijden *et al*. 1996b).

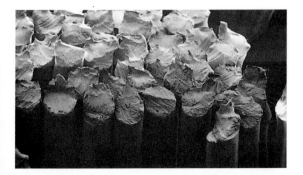

Figure 20.11

Non-end-rounded bristles (taken from Silverstone and Featherstone 1988).

Force control

Manual and electric toothbrush manufacturers have introduced toothbrush designs which would limit the amount of force used in order to reduce the chance of damage to soft and hard tissues (e.g. Soparker *et al.* 1991, van der Weijden *et al.* 1995). With the electric toothbrush, the level of force at which the feedback system should work has been debated. One brush manufacturer has set the level at 350 g (van der Weijden *et al.* 1995), which apparently did not reduce the mean force used while brushing. The results of a recent study (van der Weijden *et al.* 1998b) indicate that with the tested manual brush approximately 400 g was the optimal level. Applying more force would result, on average, in less effective brushing. A force indicator could therefore be set at such a level.

Filament stiffness and end-rounding

Tests in vitro using a variety of substrates including dentine suggest that the use of a toothbrush alone would have insignificant abrasive influences on dental hard tissues. Concerns over filament stiffness have therefore concentrated on potential damage to adjacent soft tissues, namely the attached gingiva and alveolar mucosa.

Toothbrushes are primarily designed to remove plaque from accessible tooth surfaces. To achieve this the filaments must have a degree of stiffness to create sufficient abrasion to dislodge plaque deposits. This stiffness has to be balanced against potential detrimental effects on dental hard and soft tissues. The determination of filament stiffness can be obtained mathematically using filament diameter and length, together with the modulus of elasticity of the filament material. Alternatively, an instrument has been designed to provide the grading of stiffness for brushes (Addy 1998).

Despite wide acceptance of the need for end-rounded bristles and the fact that grinding and polishing bristle tips is common practice, studies have found many differences in the bristle shapes (Adriaens *et al.* 1985, Silverstone and Featherstone 1988, Dellerman *et al.* 1994). Breitenmoser *et al.* (1979) evaluated the effect of bristle end form on the gingival surface. They found that manual toothbrushes with cut bristle ends (Figure 20.12) resulted in significantly greater gingival lesions than rounded ends using an average brushing force of 500 g. This is in agreement with other observations (Lange 1977).

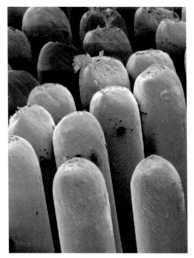 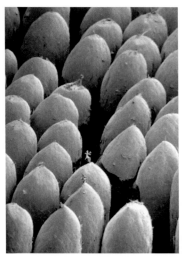

a   b

Figure 20.12

a 'Roman'-shaped end-rounding of toothbrush bristles.
b 'Gothic'-shaped end-rounding of toothbrush bristles.

A clinical trial that attempted to investigate the relative merits of cut-end and round-end bristles found no advantage in the round-end over the cut-end either in terms of keratinization or in the production of gingival abrasion and hyperemia (Breitenmoser *et al.* 1979). More recently, the end-rounding of the nylon bristles of widely used toothbrushes was compared and significant differences between the brands were reported (Mulry *et al.* 1992, Dellerman *et al.* 1994). The clinical relevance of these findings has yet to be substantiated.

In a recent study different levels of end-rounding were compared (Danser *et al.* 1998a). Both bristle types used in this study, had different styles of end-rounding (Figure 20.13). The 'roman'-shaped and the 'gothic'-shaped end-rounding are the two extreme end-roundings that can be produced. The gothic-shaped end-rounding resulted in more small sites of gingival abrasion than the roman-shaped end-rounding. For the toothbrushing exercise in this study a new brush-head was used every time. This implies that for the experiment a maximum possible abrasive effect was scored. However, it is questionable whether these types of end-rounding will remain when the brush is used daily. It has been found that sharp-edged bristle ends become rounded and less sharp with prolonged use. The results of a study by Kreifeldt *et al.* (1980) suggest that usage of a brush will change the original end-rounding due to wear. They observed that bristles of used toothbrushes in many instances show a tapering, proceeding from the insertion to the free end. Massassati and Frank (1982) observed that new synthetic bristles with some minor manufacturing defects improved with use, producing smooth rounded bristles. It appeared that bristle ends were in a better state of preservation for hard nylon as a function of use.

Dentifrice abrasiveness

It is generally agreed that the toothbrush alone does not have an abrasive effect on the tooth surfaces (Massassati and Frank 1982), but that abrasiveness depends mainly on the properties of the dentifrice. A large variety of dentifrices are available to the general public. These products

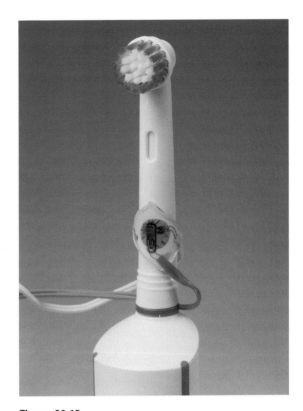

Figure 20.13

Brush-head equipped with a strain gauge.

contain a number of ingredients, but common to most are two ingredients which could cause tooth substance loss, namely detergents and abrasives. Dentine abrasion (RDA) and enamel abrasion (REA) values for commercial dentifrices vary widely from dentifrice to dentifrice (Barbakow *et al.* 1989). Adequate tooth cleansing can be achieved by brushing with a toothbrush only (Mooser 1959, Beyeler and Mooser 1960), but this does not prevent brown stain formation (Kitchin and Robinson 1948). A dentifrice containing adequate abrasives is needed to ensure faster removal of bacterial plaque and prevention of stain formation (Lobene 1968). Use of a dentifrice can also reduce the brushing time by 20–40% (Beyeler and Mooser 1960).

In assessing the safety of toothbrushes for hard tissues it would not seem unreasonable to consider this in the context of the interaction with dentifrice. For example, it might be expected that a hard brush tested with a standard paste would cause more abrasion of the substrate than a soft brush. Preliminary data, however, do not support this contention and filament stiffness appears not to be directly related to abrasion by a standard dentifrice. Consideration of this apparent anomaly in the light of polishing and abrasion of other surfaces makes the finding less surprising. Thus, polishing and/or abrasion of surfaces either employs materials of similar or greater hardness than the surface or a vehicle to carry a polishing agent.

One of the areas of concern has been the abrasiveness of the dentifrice. Miller conducted the earliest known study in 1907. His pioneer in-vitro work on the abrasive effect of dentifrices demonstrated the damage that dentifrices could cause to the enamel and dentine. By 'cross-brushing' the labial surfaces of extracted teeth with different dentifrices, he demonstrated an abrasive action on both enamel and dentine. Abrasives in dentifrice should preserve the tooth structure as much as possible (Baxter *et al.* 1981).

In studying dentifrices, it must be noted that the material is diluted to about 33% concentration by saliva (Manly 1944), and such allowance has to be made when evaluating abrasiveness of dentifrices in vivo. The amount of dentifrice applied to a particular brush may also contribute to the abrasion potential (Harte and Manly 1976). Beyeler and Mooser (1960), in a study of subjects with 'perfect' oral hygiene, showed that tooth abrasion and gingival injuries can be caused by the abrasive components of dentifrices.

Niemi *et al.* (1984) showed that a modest increase in plaque removing efficacy could be obtained with increasing stiffness of the tooth-brush bristles and with increasing abrasiveness of the dentifrice. However, this increase in efficacy is accompanied by increased damage caused to the gingival tissues. Especially highly abrasive tooth powder seemed to cause more abrasion.

Radentz *et al.* (1976) observed that cervical abrasion is related in some way to a factor or factors associated with the initial stages of the toothbrushing procedure. The evidence, furthermore, demonstrates that an excessive use of undiluted dentifrice, habitually placed in the same area of the mouth, may produce abrasion.

In view of this, it would seem prudent to advise patients to use decreased quantities of dentifrice and to initiate the brushing procedure on the occlusal surfaces of the teeth to effect a dilution of the dentifrice. The same effect might be accomplished by alternating the initial placement of the brush between the quadrants to distribute the abrasive effect more evenly.

Systemic effects

Bacteria may enter the bloodstream during certain oral hygiene measures, especially in patients with advanced chronic gingival disease. The rate of occurrence is unknown because conflicting results have been found in different studies. These bacteremias are of concern to patients who have rheumatic heart disease, prosthetic heart valves, prosthetic joints and renal dialysis shunts, or fistulas used in renal disease. The ability to predict bacteremia after toothbrushing, flossing, gingival stimulation and oral irrigation remains elusive (Gillette and van House 1980).

Final statements

There are numerous oral hygiene products, including toothbrushes, which reasonably should be evaluated for safety. However, the safety of brushes for hard and soft tissue in vivo is difficult to assess for many reasons. Firstly, tooth wear and gingival recession have multifactorial etiologies and are further complicated, almost certainly, by a variety of predisposing factors which may be anatomical, physiological or pathological. In addition, both conditions are slow to develop, and measurement techniques that could be applied in the mouth are in the main too imprecise to detect minor changes. This obviates short-term evaluations, where some attempt to control for other variables might be attempted.

Superficial cervical abrasion is so common in dentally aware subjects that it may be an inevitable minor side-effect of practising oral hygiene as recommended by the dental profession. Deep lesions or wedge-like defects, however, are undesirable. They probably reflect faulty toothbrushing habits, which may be not only ineffective for preventing disease, but also may cause damage to oral tissues. It seems fair to conclude that the possibility of developing such lesions on the teeth or the gingiva should not prevent dental professionals from recommending meticulous mechanical oral hygiene in the prevention of dental diseases. However, research on the specific aetiological factors involved in the development of the various lesions is desirable in order to reduce their frequency and severity.

If the unwanted effect of toothbrushing is unavoidable and concomitant with the efforts of maintaining oral health it may be regarded as acceptable. But, on the other hand, if abrasion lesions are the result of inadequate brushing habits, which also have unsatisfactory cleansing effects, this cannot be accepted and must be considered when recommending toothbrushing technique, so that people may be furnished with appropriate prophylactic measures that are effective for oral cleanliness but still harmless to oral tissues.

References

Abbas F, Voss S, Nijboer A et al. (1990) The effect of mechanical oral hygiene procedures on bleeding on probing. *J Clin Periodontol* **17**:199–203.

Addy M (1998) Measuring success in toothbrush design – an opinion and debate of the concepts. *Int Dent J* **48**(Suppl):509–18.

Adriaens PA, Seynhaeve TM, De Boever JA (1985) A morphologic and SEM investigation of 58 toothbrushes. *Clin Prev Dent* **7**:8–16.

Agudio G, Pini Prato G, Cortellini P, Parma S (1987) Gingival lesions caused by improper oral hygiene measures. *Int J Periodont Restor Dent* **1**:53–65.

Alexander JF, Saffir AJ, Gold W (1977) The measurement of the effect of toothbrushes on soft tissue abrasion. *J Dent Res* **56**:722–7.

Arnim S, Blackburn EM (1961) Dentifrice abrasion. Report of a case. *J Periodontol* **32**:43–8.

Attin T, Koidl U, Buchalla W et al (1997) Correlation of microhardness and wear of differently eroded bovine dental enamel. *Arch Oral Biol* **42**:243–50.

Baker DL, Seymour GJ (1976) The possible pathogenesis of gingival recession. A histological study of induced recession in the rat. *J Clin Periodontol* **3**:208–19.

Barbakow F, Imfeld T, Lutz F et al. (1989) Dentin abrasion (RDA), enamel abrasion (REA) and polishing scores of dentifrices sold in Switzerland. *Schweiz Monatsschr Zahnmed* **99**:408–13.

Baxter PM, Davis WB, Kackson J (1981) Toothpaste abrasive requirements to control naturally stained plaque. The relation of cleaning power to toothpaste abrasivity. *J Oral Rehabil* **8**:19–26.

Bergström J, Lavstedt S (1979) An epidemiologic approach to toothbrushing and dental abrasion. *Community Dent Oral Epidemiol* **7**:57–64.

Beyeler D, Mooser M (1960) Tooth abrasions, gingival injuries and daily oral hygiene. *Schweiz Monatsschr Zahnheilkunde* **70**:123–52.

Boyd RL, Murray P, Robertson PB (1989) Effect on periodontal status of rotary electric toothbrushes vs. manual toothbrushes during periodontal maintenance. I. Clinical results. *J Periodontol* **60**:390–5.

Boyd RL, McLey L, Zahradnik R (1997) Clinical and laboratory evaluation of powered electric toothbrushes: in vivo determination of average force for use of manual and powered toothbrushes. *J Clin Dent* **8**:72–5.

Breitenmoser J, Mörmann W, Mühlemann HR (1979) Damaging effects of toothbrush bristle end form on gingiva. *J Periodontol* **50**:212–16.

Bull WH, Callender RM, Pugh BR, Wood GD (1968) Abrasion and cleaning properties of dentifrices. *Br Dent J* **125**:331–7.

Burgett FG, Ash MM (1974) Comparative study of the pressure of brushing with three types of toothbrushes. *J Periodontol* **45**:410–13.

Cancro LP, Fishman SL (1995) The expected effect on oral health of dental plaque control through mechanical removal. *Periodontology 2000* **8**:60–74.

Cronin M, Dembling W, Warren PR (1998) A 3-month clinical investigation comparing the safety and efficacy of a novel electric toothbrush (Braun Oral-B 3D) with a manual toothbrush. *Am J Dent* **11** (Special issue):18–21.

Danser MM, Timmerman MF, IJzerman Y et al (1998a) Evaluation of the incidence of gingival abrasion as a result from toothbrushing. *J Clin Periodontol* **25**:701–6.

Danser MM, Timmerman MF, IJzerman Y et al (1998b) A comparison of electric toothbrushes in their potential to cause gingival abrasion of oral soft tissues. *Am J Dent* **11** (Special issue):35–9.

Dellerman PA, Burkett TA, Kreyling KM (1994) A comparative evaluation of the percent acceptable end-rounded bristles: Butler G.U.M., Colgate Plus, Crest Complete and Reach. *J Clin Dent* **5**:38–45.

Engel D, Nessly M, Morton T, Martin R (1993) Safety testing of a new electronic toothbrush. *J Periodontol* **64**:941–6.

Fraleigh CM, McElhaney JH, Heiser RA (1967) Toothbrushing force study. *J Dent Res* **46**:209–14.

Gillette WB, van House RL (1980) Ill effects of improper oral hygiene procedures. *J Am Dent Assoc* **101**:476–81.

Gorman WJ (1967) Prevalence and etiology of gingival recession. *J Periodontol* **38**:316–22.

Grossman E, Cronin M, Dembling W, Proskin H (1996) A comparative clinical study of extrinsic tooth stain removal with two electric toothbrushes (Braun D7 and D9) and a manual brush. *Am J Dent* **9**:25–9.

Hancock EB (1996) Prevention. In: Genco RJ, Newman MG, eds, *Annals of Periodontology*, 223–49. Illinois: American Academy of Periodontology.

Harrington JH, Terry IA (1964) Automatic and hand toothbrushing abrasion studies. *J Am Dent Assoc* **68**:343–50.

Harte DB, Manly RS (1976) Four variables affecting magnitude of dentifrice abrasiveness. *J Dent Res* **55**:322–7.

Hasegawa K, Machida Y, Matsuzaki K, Ichinohe S (1992) The most effective toothbrushing force. *Paediatr Dent J* **2**:139–43.

Hefferren JJ (1976) A laboratory method for assessment of dentifrice abrasivity. *J Dent Res* **55**:563–73.

Imfeldt T, Sener B (1998a) Relative dentin abrasion (RDA) by electric toothbrushes. *J Dent Res* **77**:1236 (abstract 233).

Imfeldt T, Sener B (1998b) In vitro evaluation of effects of electric toothbrushes on gingiva *J Dent Res* **77**:1262 (abstract 446).

Johnson BD, McInnes C (1994) Clinical evaluation of the efficacy and safety of a new sonic toothbrush. *J Periodontol* **65**:692–7.

Joshipura KJ, Kent RL, DePaola PF (1994) Gingival recession: intra-oral distribution and associated factors. *J Periodontol* **65**:864–71.

Kållestal C, Uhlin S (1992) Buccal attachment loss in Swedish adolescents. *J Clin Periodontol* **19**:485–91.

Kalsbeek H, van Rossum GMJM, Truin GJ et al (1996) *Tandheelkundige Verzorging Volwassenen 1983–1995*. Leiden, The Netherlands: TNO Preventie en Gezondheid.

Khocht A, Spindel L, Person P (1992) A comparative clinical study of the safety and efficacy of 3 toothbrushes. *J Periodontol* **63**:603–10.

Khocht A, Simon G, Person P, Denepitiya JL (1993) Gingival recession in relation to history of hard toothbrush use. *J Periodontol* **64**:900–5.

Kitchin PC, Robinson HBG (1948) The abrasiveness of dentifrices as measured on the cervical areas of extracted teeth. *J Dent Res* **27**:195–200.

König KG (1990) Changes in the prevalence of dental caries: how much can be attributed to changes in the diet? *Caries Res* **24**:16–18.

Kreifeldt JG, Hill PH, Calisti LJ (1980) A systematic study of the plaque removal efficiency of worn toothbrushes. *J Dent Res* **59**:2047–55.

Kuroiwa M, Kodaka T, Kuroiwa M (1993) Microstructural changes of human enamel surfaces by brushing with and without dentifrice containing abrasive. *Caries Res* **27**:1–8.

Lange DE (1977) Über den Einfluss verschiedener Zahnbürstentypen auf die gingivaoberfläche. *Zahnärztliche Mitteilungen* **67**:729–36, 747.

Lee WC, Eakle WS (1984) Possible role of tensile stress in the etiology of cervical erosive lesions of teeth. *J Prosthet Dent* **52**:374–80.

Listgarten MA (1988) The role of dental plaque in gingivitis and periodontitis. *J Clin Periodontol* **15**:485–7.

Lobene RR (1968) Effect of dentifrices on tooth stains with controlled brushing. *J Am Dent Assoc* **77**:843–5.

Löe H (1979) Mechanical and chemical control of dental plaque. *J Clin Periodontol* **6**:32–6.

Löe H, Kleinmann DV (1986) *Dental Plaque Control Measures and Oral Hygiene Practices*. IRL Press: Oxford.

Löe H, Anerud A, Boysen H (1992) The natural history of periodontal disease in man: prevalence, severity, and extent of gingival recession. *J Periodontol* **63**:489–95.

McLey L, Zahradnik R (1994) Clinical evaluation of brushing force for powered rotating brushing instruments. *J Dent Res* **73**:164 (abstract 500).

Manly RS (1944) Factors influencing tests on the abrasion of dentine by brushing by dentifrice. *J Dent Res* **23**:59–72.

Massassati A, Frank RM (1982) Scanning electron microscopy of unused and used manual toothbrushes. *J Clin Periodontol* **9**:148–61.

Mierau HD (1992) Der freiliegende Zahnhals. *Deutsche Zahnärztliche Zeitschrift* **47**:643–53.

Mierau HD, Spindler T (1984) Beitrag zur etiologie der Gingivarezessionen. *Deutsche Zahnärtzliche Zeitschrift* **39**:634–9.

Miller WG (1907) Experiments and observations on the wasting of tooth tissue. *Dental Cosmos* **49**:109–24.

Milosevic A, Lennon MA, Fear SC (1997) Risk factors associated with tooth wear in teenagers: a case control study *Community Dent Health* **14**:143–7.

Mooser M (1959) Abrasive action of toothbrushes with natural and synthetic bristles and of toothpastes. *Parodontologie* **13**:131–3.

Mulry CA, Dellerman PA, Ludwa R, White DJ (1992) A comparison of the end-rounding of nylon bristles in commercial toothbrushes: Crest Complete® and Oral-B®. *J Clin Dent* **3**:47–50.

Niemi M-L (1987) Gingival abrasion and plaque removal after toothbrushing with an electric and a manual toothbrush. *Acta Odontol Scand* **45**:367–70.

Niemi M-L, Sandholm L, Ainamo J (1984). Frequency of gingival lesions after standardized brushing as related to stiffness of toothbrush and abrasiveness of dentifrice. *J Clin Periodontol* **11**:254–61.

Niemi M-L, Ainamo J, Etemadzadeh H (1986). Gingival abrasion and plaque removal with manual versus electric toothbrushing. *J Clin Periodontol* **13**:709–13.

Niemi M-L, Ainamo J, Etemadzadeh H (1987) The effect of toothbrush grip on gingival abrasion and plaque removal during toothbrushing. *J Clin Periodontol* **14**:19–21.

Olsson M, Lindhe J (1991) Periodontal characteristics in individuals with varying form of the upper central incisors. *J Clin Periodontol* **18**:78–82.

Paloheimo L, Ainamo J, Niemi ML, Viikinkoski M (1987) Prevalence of and factors related to gingival recession in Finnish 15- to 20-year old subjects. *Community Dent Health* **4**:425–36.

Phaneuf EA, Harrington JH, Ashland AB et al. (1962) Automatic toothbrush: a new reciprocating action. *J Am Dent Assoc* **65**:12–25.

Plagmann H Ch, Goldkamp B, Lange DE, Morgenroth K (1978) Über die mechanische beeinflussung der alvealarmukosa und der gingiva durch verschieden zahnbürstentypen. *Deutsche Zahnärztlichen Zeitschrift* **33**:14–20.

Pilot T, Miyazaki H (1991) Periodontal conditions in Europe. *J Clin Periodontol* **18**:353–7.

Radentz WH, Barnes GP, Cutright DE (1976) A survey of factors possibly associated with cervical abrasion of tooth surfaces. *J Periodontol* **47**:148–55.

Reisstein J, Lustman I, Hershkovitz J, Gedalia I (1978) Abrasion of enamel and cementum in human teeth due to toothbrushing estimated by SEM. *J Dent Res* **57**:42.

Sandholm L, Niemi ML, Ainamo J (1982) Identification of soft tissue brushing lesions. A clinical and scanning electron microscopic study. *J Clin Periodontol* **9**:397–401.

Sangnes G, Gjermo P (1976). Prevalence of oral soft and hard tissue lesions related to mechanical tooth-cleansing procedures. *Community Dent Oral Epidemiol* **4**:77–83.

Saxer UP, Yankell SL (1997) Impact of improved toothbrushes on dental diseases. II. *Quint Int* **28**:573–93.

Schemehorn BR, Zwart AC (1996) The dentin abrasivity potential of a new electric toothbrush. *Am J Dent* **9**(Sp. iss.):S19–S20.

Schemehorn BR, Ball T, Bloom B (1993) A model to determine the relative abrasiveness of rotary toothbrushes. *J Dent Res* **72**:413 (abstract 2480).

Scutt JS, Swann CJ (1975) The first mechanical toothbrush? *Br Dent J* **139**:152.

Serino G, Wennstrom JL, Lindhe J, Eneroth L (1994) The prevalence and distribution of gingival recession in subjects with a high standard of oral hygiene. *J Clin Periodontol* **21**:57–63.

Silverstone LM, Featherstone MJ (1988) A scanning electron microscope study of the end rounding of bristles in eight toothbrush types. *Quint Int* **19**:87–107.

Slop D (1986) Abrasion of enamel by toothbrushing. Academic Thesis, University of Groningen, The Netherlands.

Smukler H, Landsberg J (1984) The toothbrush and gingival traumatic injury. *J Periodontol* **55**:713–19.

Soparker PM, Newman MB, De Pada PF (1991) The efficacy of novel toothbrush design. *J Clin Dent* **2**:107–10.

Stahl SS, Wachtel N, DeCastra C, Pelletier G (1953) The effect of toothbrushing on the keratinization of the gingiva. *J Periodontol* **24**:20–1.

Stookey GK, Muhler JC (1968) Laboratory studies concerning the enamel and dentin abrasion properties of common dentifrice polishing agents. *J Dent Res* **47**:524–32.

Van Palenstein Helderman WH, Lembariti BS, van der Weijden GA, van't Hof MA (1998) Gingival recession and its association with calculus in subjects deprived of prophylactic dental care. *J Clin Periodontol* **25**:106–11.

Van der Velden U, Timmerman MF, van der Weijden GA (1993) Abrasie, geen elektrisch probleem! *Nederlands Tandartsenblad* **48**:549.

Van der Weijden GA, Timmerman MF, Nijboer A, van der Velden U (1993) A comparative study of electric toothbrushes for the effectiveness of plaque removal in relation to toothbrushing duration. A timer study. *J Clin Periodontol* **20**:476–81.

Van der Weijden GA, Timmerman MF, Reijerse E et al (1994) The long term effect of an oscillating/rotating toothbrush. An 8 month clinical study. *J Clin Periodontol* **21**:139–45.

Van der Weijden GA, Timmerman MF, Reijerse E et al (1995) Comparison of two electric toothbrushes in plaque removing ability – professional and supervised brushing. *J Clin Periodontol* **22**:648–52.

Van der Weijden GA, Timmerman MF, Reijerse E et al (1996a) Comparison of an oscillating rotating electric toothbrush and a 'sonic' toothbrush in plaque-removing ability. *J Clin Periodontol* **24**:1–5.

Van der Weijden GA, Timmerman MF, Reijerse E et al (1996b) Toothbrushing force in relation to plaque removal. *J Clin Periodontol* **23**:724–9.

Van der Weijden GA, Timmerman MF, Danser MM, van der Velden U (1998a) The role of electric toothbrushes – advantages and limitations of electric toothbrushes.

In: Lang NP, Attström R, Löe H, eds, *Proceedings European Workshop on Mechanical Plaque Control*. Quintessence Publishing: Berlin.

Van der Weijden GA, Timmerman MF, Danser MM, van der Velden U (1998b) Relationship between the plaque removal efficacy of a manual toothbrush and brushing force. *J Clin Periodontol* **25**:413–16.

Vekalahti M (1989) Occurrence of gingival recession in adults. *J Periodontol* **60**:599–602.

Walmsley AD (1997) The electric toothbrush: a review. *Br Dent J* **182**:209–18.

Walsh M, Heckman B, Legott P et al (1989) Comparison of manual and power toothbrushing, with and without adjunctive oral irrigation, for controlling plaque and gingivitis. *J Clin Periodontol* **16**:419–27.

White L (1983) Toothbrush pressures of orthodontic patients. *Am J Orthod* **83**:109–13.

Wilson S, Levine D, Dequincey G, Killoy WJ (1993) Effects of two toothbrushes on plaque, gingivitis, gingival abrasion, and recession: a 1-year longitudinal study. *Compendium of Continuing Education in Dent* **16**:569–79.

PART III

Dentine Hypersensitivity

21

Dentine hypersensitivity: definition, prevalence, distribution and aetiology

Martin Addy

Introduction

The term dentine hypersensitivity has been used for many decades to describe a common painful condition of the teeth. Despite this there are many gaps in our knowledge concerning dentine hypersensitivity. It is perhaps not surprising therefore that one can still have sympathy with the statement made in 1982 by Johnson and co-workers that 'dentine hypersensitivity is an enigma, being frequently encountered yet ill understood'. Even the terminology for the condition can be inaccurate (Pashley 1990); dentine sensitivity may be a more correct descriptor (Dowell and Addy 1983, Flynn et al. 1985) – there being no evidence that the dentine is in any way different or the pulpal response exaggerated. Indeed, the histopathology of the dental pulp in dentine hypersensitivity has not been studied. What is now established, and consistent with the hydrodynamic theory of stimulus transmission (Gysi 1900, Brännström 1963) is that there are many more and wider open dentinal tubules at the surface in dentine hypersensitivity than in non-sensitive dentine (Ishikawa 1969, Absi et al. 1987, 1989). Alternative terms such as cervical dentinal sensitivity have been suggested (Chabanski and Gillam 1997), but not generally adopted. This is probably because, although dentine hypersensitivity has a predilection for buccal cervical sites, the condition can present at other tooth surfaces. Further and as a result of common usage, there appears to have been a consensus to keep the term dentine hypersensitivity to describe the condition (Holland et al. 1997) even though it may not be technically correct.

Most data concerning dentine hypersensitivity have been generated to compare treatments for the condition (Addy and Dowell 1983). The majority of these treatments, with the exception of potassium salts, have been based on the idea of directly or indirectly occluding tubules. This approach to management would appear to be seriously flawed (Dowell et al. 1985) for two reasons. Firstly, the aetiology of the condition is not considered and therefore recurrence could and does occur. A similarity in approach which could be drawn is with the earlier restorative plan for caries. Secondly, with a few exceptions, the actual effect of treatments on the dentine surface is not known with any degree of certainty. This makes it difficult to dissociate treatment effects from placebo responses or natural regression of the condition, both of which can be considerable (West et al. 1997, Yates et al. 1998a, 1998b). The aim of this chapter is to consider the prevalence, distribution and aetiology of dentine hypersensitivity, both individually and in their inter-relationships.

Definition of dentine hypersensitivity

In 1994 a committee of interested persons from academia and industry was convened to consider and prepare guidelines for the design and conduct of clinical trials on dentine hypersensitivity. A consensus report was published (Holland et al. 1997) in which the committee adopted a definition for dentine hypersensitivity. The definition was a minor modification of one suggested previously (Dowell *et al.* 1985, Orchardson and Collins 1987) namely: dentine hypersensitivity is characterized by short, sharp pain arising from exposed dentine in response to stimuli typically thermal, evaporative, tactile, osmotic or chemical and which cannot be ascribed to any other form of dental defect or pathology. Importantly, the definition has two parts. The first is a clinical descriptor of the most common presentation of the condition. However, it is acknowledged that occasionally there may be persistence of a dull ache in affected teeth. In these cases pulpal changes may be present (Dachi 1965) – possibly irreversible – and management options are therefore different from those applicable to uncomplicated lesions. The second part of the definition is important because it encourages consideration of a differential diagnosis (Dowell *et al.* 1985). Many other conditions exist where dentine is exposed and sensitivity, identical to that experienced with dentine hypersensitivity, occurs. Such conditions include chipped or fractured teeth, caries, marginal leakage of restorations, cracked cusps of teeth and even palatogingival grooves. For the most part the management of these related conditions is completely different to that of dentine hypersensitivity. Moreover, dual or multiple dental pathology can coexist in the dentition and this suggests that dentine hypersensitivity should be diagnosed by a process of elimination involving careful clinical and radiographic examinations.

Inherent in the definition of dentine hypersensitivity is exposure of dentine and, consistent with the hydrodynamic theory, dentinal tubules must be open at the dentine surface and patent to a vital pulp. Two processes must therefore occur to cause dentine hypersensitivity and these are probably inter-related. Firstly, dentine must be exposed by aetiological agents; lesion localization. Secondly, sensitivity must be induced by tubule exposure: lesion initiation. The latter can occur either through loss of cementum or a dentine smear layer, both of which appear to be very labile to a variety of mechanical or chemical agents (Addy *et al.* 1987a, Bevenius *et al.* 1994). In considering the localization and initiation of dentine hypersensitivity, it would seem reasonable to consider the prevalence and distribution of lesions to determine if there are associations with possible aetiological agents.

Prevalence of dentine hypersensitivity

Classical epidemiological studies to determine the prevalence of dentine hypersensitivity are few, if any, depending on the interpretation of the study designs. Some of the most recent studies relied only on self-reported sensitivity in response to questionnaires (Kanapka 1990, Murray and Roberts 1994). Other studies have shown differences between perceived and diagnosed dentine hypersensitivity prevalences (Flynn *et al.* 1985, Fischer *et al.* 1992). Surveys which examined for dentine hypersensitivity, however, provided surprisingly similar figures of between 15 and 18% of the study populations affected (Graf and Galasse 1977, Flynn *et al.* 1985, Fischer *et al.* 1992). This compares with the wider range of 8–30% when self-reporting or less precise diagnostic methods were used (Abel 1958, Jensen 1964, Graf and Galasse 1977, Flynn *et al.* 1985, Fischer *et al.* 1992). These data alone provide little insight into aetiological associations and perhaps more can be derived from age and to a lesser degree gender distributions.

The age range for dentine hypersensitivity is broad, spanning early teenage to more than 70 years (Fischer *et al.* 1992). However, peak incidence is between 20 and 40 years (Graf and Galasse 1977, Flynn *et al.* 1985), and slightly older if males are considered separately (Fischer *et al.* 1992). The common prevalence of the condition during the third and fourth decades would be consistent with the appearance and progression of gingival recession (Woofter 1969). The apparent paradoxical fall in prevalence in later decades probably reflects dentine and pulpal age/insult changes, reducing both dentine permeability and pulpal response – referred to in classical dental histopathology texts (Seltzer and Bender 1975).

Numerical gender differences are reported in some surveys with proportionately more females affected than males (Graf and Galasse 1977, Flynn *et al.* 1985, Addy *et al.* 1987b, Orchardson and Collins 1987). Such differences do not reach statistical significance, leaving a question as to whether no differences exist or the studies are insufficiently powered to detect differences. If differences between genders do indeed exist, it could be conjectured that these relate to the better oral hygiene of females compared with males, particularly at buccal sites (Buckley 1981, Dummer *et al.* 1987). Additionally, differences in diet – favouring 'healthy' but often acidic foods and drinks in females – may be relevant. Alternatively, the apparent gender difference may only reflect the greater dental attendance by females biasing surveys conducted in this environment.

Interestingly, recent questionnaire surveys of dentine hypersensitivity amongst patients referred to a specialist periodontology unit revealed much higher incidences (Chabanski *et al.* 1996), which confirmed a previous report (Collaert and Speelman 1991). There were no gender differences, but the peak incidence was in the fifth decade. The severity of the condition in this group was low and few sought treatment. The authors (Chabanski *et al.* 1996) concluded that either periodontal disease and/or periodontal treatment predisposed to dentine hypersensitivity, presumably through both having effects on dentine and gingival recession. An alternative interpretation could be that some of the sensitivity was not 'true' dentine hypersensitivity as defined in this chapter. It is known that in periodontal disease organisms penetrate dentinal tubules and to some considerable distance (Adriens *et al.* 1988). Pulpal responses to such bacteria could induce a sensitivity state which may be different from dentine hypersensitivity. This possible explanation is not too far removed from the reported bacteria-associated sensitivity induced when marginal leakage occurs around cavities and restorative materials (Brännström 1986).

Distribution of dentine hypersensitivity

The distribution of dentine hypersensitivity is most interesting and certain inferences can be drawn from the information available, albeit cautiously. The buccal cervical area of teeth is the site of predilection for dentine hypersensitivity (Jensen 1964, Graf and Galasse 1977, Flynn *et al.* 1985, Orchardson and Collins 1987). However, it is also the site of predilection for gingival recession (Watson 1984) and the area where enamel is the thinnest. Aetiological agents associated with enamel loss and gingival reces-

sion are therefore likely to be implicated in lesion localization if not lesion initiation.

Most studies on the site distribution of dentine hypersensitivity have reported the same order of predilection by tooth type. Most commonly affected are canines and first premolars, then incisors and second premolars and least often molars (Graf and Galasse 1977, Flynn *et al.* 1985, Fischer *et al.* 1992). Interestingly, one study reported most frequent sensitivity on molars (Chabanski *et al.* 1996). However, this study was concerned with periodontal patients where predisposition to dentine exposure by disease could favour molars. Alternatively as alluded to earlier, the sensitivity may have a different aetiology to true dentine hypersensitivity. The distribution of dentine hypersensitivity appears to show a negative correlation with plaque scores recorded by site in epidemiological studies (Alexander 1971, Addy *et al.* 1987a). Thus, buccal cervical plaque scores on canines and premolars tend to be lower than other buccal sites. A clinical trial (Addy *et al.* 1987b) involving 92 subjects with moderate to severe sensitivity showed not only the same tooth site frequency distribution, but also a pattern for a significantly greater proportion of left-sided tooth sensitivity compared with their right contralateral tooth types. Conversely, and consistent with epidemiological data (Addy *et al.* 1987c), the frequency of sensitivity was negatively correlated with plaque scores and again plaque scores were significantly reduced on left contralateral teeth. This would be consistent with the plaque distribution in populations where the majority of individuals are right-handed, cleaning left-sided buccal surfaces more effectively than right-sided teeth (Addy *et al.* 1987a). Interestingly, in a clinical study (Addy *et al.* 1987b) where 87 out of 92 subjects were right-handed, when plaque scores for only sensitive teeth were considered the tooth site and side distribution was lost, with all sensitive teeth exhibiting very low plaque scores. All these data implicate the role of toothbrushing with toothpaste as involved in at least the localization if not the initiation of dentine hypersensitivity. These points will be considered further under aetiology of the condition.

In conclusion, at this juncture epidemiological and clinical data on prevalence and distribution of dentine hypersensitivity permit only limited albeit interesting inferences to be drawn. Most of these suggest a role for oral hygiene practices in at least gingival recession if not dentine hypersensitivity itself. However, there is a need for information on socio-economic, occupational, dietary, gender, specific oral hygiene practices and other individual features of the condition as it affects population groups (Addy and Pearce 1994).

Aetiology of dentine hypersensitivity

To even begin to consider the aetiology of dentine hypersensitivity there is a need to understand the aetiology of dentine exposure. Logically dentine exposure can only occur by loss of periodontal tissue (gingival recession) or of enamel. Clearly the tissues are quite different; the periodontium has vital tissues which are both hard and soft, whereas enamel is a non-vital hard tissue. The aetiological factors and processes involved in their loss are likely to be different, although some causal factors could be common to both. Nevertheless, each will be considered separately and specifically as they might occur at the buccal cervical region of the dentition.

Gingival recession

Dentine hypersensitivity has been described as an enigmatic condition (Johnson et al. 1982) as has gingival recession (Smith 1997). This is not surprising, as the two conditions appear to be intimately related and perhaps more often so than enamel loss and dentine hypersensitivity. Gingival recession has been reviewed by both Watson (1984) and Smith (1997) with the authors reaching the same conclusions concerning the major predisposing and aetiological factors. These will be summarized here with additional comment from the present author. In any disease or condition predisposition may be dependent on anatomical, physiological, biochemical or pathological factors and all of these may have a genetic predisposition. In gingival recession, the most frequently cited predisposing factor is the anatomy of the alveolar bone and in particular

the labial plate (Aldritt 1968, Bernimoulan and Curilovie 1977, Löst 1984). Thus, thin, fenestrated or absent labial alveolar bone is considered the major predisposing factor to recession. Tooth anatomy (Olsson and Lindhe 1991) and tooth position (Gorman 1967, Modheer and Odenrick 1980) may in themselves influence alveolar bone thickness and therefore must also be considered as predisposing factors. In this respect orthodontic tooth movement could move teeth through the buccal plate to predispose to recession. Outside these anatomical factors it is difficult to clearly demarcate between predisposing and aetiological factors, a problem not peculiar to gingival recession.

Ageing is often cited as a physiological aetiological factor in gingival recession and, given the structure of the periodontium, is not outwith possibility. However, the more important aspect of age to recession is probably a dose response of the gingiva to other aetiological factors (for review see Watson 1984). Oral hygiene has been cited as a factor in recession and from opposite sides of the spectrum. Logically poor oral hygiene inevitably leads to gingivitis (Löe et al. 1965) and recession in chronically inflamed tissue may be expected. Clinical studies do not support this hypothesis (Ropner et al. 1972, Mazdyasma and Stoner 1980), with more recession found with good oral hygiene (Gorman 1967) or following improved oral hygiene (O'Leary et al. 1971). Indeed, it may be that prolonged chronic gingivitis could lead to fibrosis and even hypertrophy of tissues. Some acute gingival infections, notably acute necrotizing ulcerative gingivitis and more particularly acute necrotizing ulcerative periodontitis, certainly cause recession. Chronic periodontitis, presumably with the associated bone loss, appears to cause gingival recession, although the buccal area does not appear to be a site of predilection for periodontal lesions. As the lesions of periodontal disease progress the process of gingival recession may become more complex due to mobility and more particularly drifting of teeth.

Perhaps the factors most cited as aetiological agents in recession are acute and chronic trauma. Non-surgical (root planing) and surgical periodontal procedures are the most easy of those to prove. Impaction of foreign objects on the gingiva (Jenkins and Allan 1994) or factitious injury (Glenwright and Strahan 1994) by habits such as fingernail scratching also may cause recession. However, most attention has focused on the role of toothbrushing as an aetiological factor in gingival trauma and recession (Sandholm *et al*. 1982, Bergström and Eliasson 1988, Knocht *et al*. 1993). The surface and site distribution of recession relate to toothbrushing habits and plaque scores; the most brushed and cleanest tooth surfaces showing the most buccal recession (Addy *et al*. 1987b). Paradoxically, populations that practise little tooth cleaning also show considerable gingival recession (Baelum *et al*. 1986, Löe *et al*. 1992), although this may be due to periodontal breakdown and may also be at other sites.

The aspects of toothbrushing habits that influence recession have been a topic of conjecture rather than controlled clinical research. Thus, frequency, duration, method and force of brushing have been implicated in recession, as has filament stiffness (Hirschfeld 1939, Gorman 1967, O'Leary *et al*. 1971, Gillette and van House 1980). In vitro methods have been developed to simulate effects on soft tissues, including animal tissues (Imfeld and Sener 1998). However, as with clinical experiments (Sandholm *et al*. 1982), these only reveal surface excoriations and the relevance of these to gingival recession is unknown. Moreover, most studies in vitro and in vivo have not considered the variable of toothpaste, which could exert protective or detrimental effects when combined with a toothbrush. The mechanism by which recession occurs also has been a matter of hypothesis, with studies particularly concentrating on the establishment of a destructive chronic inflammatory response in the tissue (Baker and Seymour 1976). Again, it could be supposed that a chronic inflammatory response may result in fibrosis. Other aetiological agents in recession have included fraenal pull at the gingival margin (Mazdyasma and Stoner 1980, Powell and McEniery 1981), occlusal trauma (Parfitt and Mjor 1964, Trott and Love 1966) and even emotional stress (Stone 1948). None of these factors has received much research attention and often they were cited as particular authors' opinions.

In summary, gingival recession can be seen at a young age, although it is difficult to detect (Bevenius *et al*. 1994) and increases in prevalence and severity with age (for review see Watson 1984). It appears to have a multifactorial predis-

position and aetiology, and anatomical features and chronic trauma appear to be of considerable importance, particularly at buccal sites of recession. Depending on the aetiology of gingival recession it has been suggested that classification into different types may be appropriate (Bevenius *et al*. 1994). This is an interesting proposition, as the aetiological agent or agents may be relevant to the subsequent development of dentine hypersensitivity.

Enamel loss

Tooth wear in the absence of gingival recession begins with loss of enamel. This loss can be ascribed to three processes described in classic texts as attrition, abrasion and erosion. It is unlikely that a single process is involved at any one tooth surface, although one process could predominate in an individual. At buccal cervical sites, and with the exception of certain types of malocclusion, attrition cannot be involved and an interplay of erosion and abrasion are the more relevant processes. In developed countries, the most long-term abrasive influence is toothbrushing with a toothpaste. Studies in vitro have demonstrated that a toothbrush alone has no clinically significant effect on hard tissues (Absi *et al*. 1992). When toothbrushes are used with toothpaste measurable enamel loss occurs and this is primarily related to the abrasiveness of the toothpaste. Even so, the effects on enamel are very small compared with dentine (Davis and Winter 1980). Toothbrush variation – particularly in filament stiffness and configuration together with force, method, frequency and duration of brushing – may influence the toothpaste abrasiveness indirectly. But again, most data concern dentine and not enamel. Thus, brushes appear to vary in their ability to move and maintain toothpaste over surfaces; a similarity being drawn with polishing cloths and polish. Whether toothbrushing with toothpaste has significant effects on enamel in vivo is debatable (Addy 1997, van der Velden and Attstrom 1997).

Erosion is probably the most important phenomenon producing loss of enamel. Erosion can be caused by intrinsic or extrinsic agents (for review see Scheutzel 1996, Zero 1996), most of which are in the acid pH range. Intrinsic causes of erosion relate to acid regurgitation associated with a number of medical and psychological disorders (for review see Scheutzel 1996). Extrinsic erosion is considered to have a primary dietary aetiology (for review see Zero 1996), although occupational-associated dental erosion has been reported (Tuominen and Tuominen 1991, Peterson and Gormsen 1991). Evidence for acid erosion of enamel has been derived largely from studies in vitro (for reviews see Grenby 1996, Zero 1996) and animal studies (for review see Grenby 1996), and clinically from dental health surveys (O'Brien 1994) and case report data (Eccles and Jenkins 1974). The role of low pH carbonated and fruit drinks has received particular attention. Recently an in-situ method was developed to study erosion by fruit juices and drinks (West *et al.* 1998a). This was later employed to generate further data on fruit drinks and develop a virtually non-erosive fruit drink (Addy *et al.* 1998, Hughes *et al.* 1998, West *et al.* 1998b). Reports in the media also drew attention to the possibility of enamel erosion by some mouthwashes. Certainly, studies in vitro have shown erosion of dentine by some mouthrinses with some evidence for the same effect on enamel, albeit of much less magnitude (Hughes 1998). The combination of abrasion and erosion on mineral loss has also been considered. Studies in vitro have demonstrated that loss of enamel and dentine by toothpaste abrasion is markedly increased if there is prior exposure to low pH fluids such as orange juice (Davis and Winter 1980).

In summary, enamel loss at the cervical margin sufficient to expose dentine (i.e. lesion localization) could occur in relatively short periods of time under the combined actions of erosive and abrasive agents.

Initiation of the dentine hypersensitivity lesion

Once dentine is exposed by gingival recession or enamel loss, sensitivity can only be initiated if the tubules are opened at the dentine surface. Studies of early gingival recession indicate that the cementum layer is extremely labile (Bevenius *et al.* 1994) and therefore would appear to be of little relevance in offering protection against sensitivity. Non-sensitive dentine shows few tubules at the surface (Absi *et al.* 1987) and

presumably there is either a smear layer present or tubules are occluded by mineral deposits or other compounds. Studies to elucidate how dentinal tubules may be opened have almost entirely been conducted in vitro. Agents studied for effects on dentine can be categorized as either abrasive or erosive. In the abrasive category, toothbrushing and toothpastes have attracted the most attention. However, much of the attention has been more related to determining the relative abrasivity of different pastes or the potential for pastes to occlude tubules rather than to open tubules. As already stated, a toothbrush alone has clinically insignificant effects upon the dentine smear layer, although it can potentiate the erosive effects of dietary acids (Absi *et al.* 1992). Most toothpastes used as a slurry without brushing have no abrasive or erosive action on the dentine smear layer. Indeed, the abrasive systems may adhere to the dentine and occlude tubules (Addy and Mostafa 1989). However, when used with a brush, toothpastes could have several actions, i.e. (1) produce a smear layer by abrasion, (2) remove a smear layer by abrasion, (3) remove a smear layer by detergent action, (4) occlude tubules with toothpaste ingredients (for review see Adams *et al.* 1992). In view of the numerous toothpaste products and variability in toothbrushing times, it is almost impossible to reach a consensus as to the likely effects of toothbrushing with toothpaste on dentine in vitro let alone in vivo. Some permeability and observational studies support the idea that toothpastes would occlude tubules either by creating a smear layer or through abrasive particles or both (Pashley 1985, Addy and Mostafa 1989, Absi *et al.* 1992). However, other studies in vitro showed that in general toothpastes, their solid and liquid phases and toothpaste detergents, removed the smear layer to expose tubules (West *et al.* 1998c). One exception was an artificial silica abrasive, non-ionic detergent-based product which removed the smear layer but occluded tubules with particulate matter (West *et al.* 1998c), presumably abrasive material. Studies in situ also suggest that abrasive toothpastes will expose tubules whereas very low abrasion products will not (Kuriowa *et al.* 1994).

In the erosive agent category, more consistent data from studies in vitro have been obtained. Thus a number of studies have shown that a variety of acids and more interestingly acidic dietary fluids readily and rapidly remove the dentine smear layer to expose tubules (Absi *et al.* 1987). Saliva used in some experiments appeared to offer no protection (Absi *et al.* 1987). Again, erosion and tubule opening were enhanced by a short period of brushing with a nylon toothbrush and water (Absi *et al.* 1992). The erosion of dentine by drinks such as orange juice has been proven in situ, with losses of permanent and deciduous dentine being considerably greater than the enamel counterparts (Hunter 1998). Studies in vitro suggest that erosion of enamel and, of more relevance, dentine varies considerably depending on the type of drink consumed (Absi *et al.* 1987). Thus for example, colas are considerably less erosive than fruit drinks. For enamel erosion the same variability between drinks can be shown in situ (Addy *et al.* 1998, Hughes *et al.* 1998, West *et al.* 1998b). Although pH is a critical factor, other factors including the type of acid, acid titratability, buffering capacity and other ingredients, such as calcium, influence the amount of erosion that occurs. Furthermore, studies in situ have indicated that there is considerable individual variation in susceptibility to erosion (West *et al.* 1998a). Individual susceptibility to most diseases or conditions probably varies, but this factor appears to have received little attention with regard to erosion. Studies in this area should be considered, as susceptibility to erosion may be relevant to susceptibility to tooth wear in general and to dentine hypersensitivity. Finally, and of relevance to oral hygiene products, dentine erosion and tubule exposure can occur with some mouthrinses, most of which have pH values below 4.5 (Addy *et al.* 1991). This could have particular implications where such products are used or recommended as prebrushing rinses.

Conclusion

1. Dentine hypersensitivity can be defined as a distinct clinical entity, but requires differentiation from other dental conditions with similar symptoms.
2. Prevalence studies to date yield very limited associations with possible aetiological factors. However, distribution data suggest an association between tooth cleaning, gingival recession and dentine hypersensitivity. Bacterial plaque appears to be negatively associated with sensitivity and apparent plaque-induced sensitivity may be a different condition from dentine hypersensitivity.
3. Dentine exposure can occur by loss of enamel or by gingival recession. The localization of sites of dentine hypersensitivity appears to be more common by the latter process.
4. Cervical enamel loss probably occurs by a combination of abrasive and erosive influences, with toothbrushing with toothpaste and dietary acids being particularly involved.
5. Overall, gingival recession is poorly understood, but there is strong circumstantial evidence for the role of toothbrushing habits at buccal cervical sites. Major predisposing factors are anatomical relating to the presence and thickness of the buccal alveolar bony plate.
6. Initiation of sensitivity requires opening of dentinal tubules. Contrary to a previous conclusion reached by this author, studies in vitro suggest that most toothpastes remove the smear layer through abrasive and detergent actions. However, some can re-occlude tubules with abrasive particles. Erosive agents, particularly acid dietary fluids, readily expose tubules. pH is an important factor, but other characteristics of these solutions may be relevant to dentine erosion. Some low pH mouthrinses have the potential to cause dentine erosion. Combined abrasive and erosive insults to dentine readily open tubules and cause accelerated dentine loss.
7. There is a need to elucidate further the aetiological factors involved in localizing and initiating lesions of dentine hypersensitivity. These almost certainly will have to involve collecting clinical data, and performing controlled clinical trials or modelling studies in situ.

References

Absi EG, Addy M, Adams D (1987) Dentine hypersensitivity. A study of the patency of dentinal tubules in sensitive and non-sensitive cervical dentine. *J Clin Periodontol* **14**:280–4.

Absi EG, Addy M, Adams D (1989) Dentine hypersensitivity: the development and evaluation of a replica technique to study sensitive and nonsensitive cervical dentine. *J Clin Periodont* **16**:190–5.

Absi EG, Addy M, Adams D (1992) The effect of toothbrushing and dietary compounds on dentine *in vitro*. A SEM study. *J Oral Rehabil* **19**:101–10.

Adams D, Addy M, Absi EG (1992) Abrasive and chemical effects of dentifrices. In: Embery G, Rolla G, eds, *Clinical and Biological Aspects of Dentifrices*. Oxford: Oxford University Press.

Addy M (1997) Minority statement on consensus report of session 111. In: Lang NP, Karring T, Lindhe, eds, *Proceedings of the 2nd European Workshop on Periodontology*, 268. Quintessence: Berlin.

Addy M, Dowell P (1983) Dentine hypersensitivity – a review: clinical and *in vitro* evaluation of treatment agents. *J Clin Periodontol* **10**:351–63.

Addy M, Mostafa P (1989) Dentine hypersensitivity II. Effects produced by the uptake *in vitro* of toothpastes onto dentine. *J Oral Rehabil* **16**:35–48.

Addy M, Pearce N (1994) Dentine hypersensitivity: aetiology, predisposing and environmental factors in dentine hypersensitivity. *Arch Oral Biol* **39**(Suppl.):33S–38S.

Addy M, Absi EG, Adams D (1987a) Dental hypersensitivity: the effects *in vitro* of acids and dietary substances on root planed and burred dentine. *J Clin Periodontol* **14**:274–9.

Addy M, Mostafa P, Newcombe RG (1987b) Dentine hypersensitivity: the distribution of recession, sensitivity and plaque. *J Dent* **15**:242–8.

Addy M, Griffiths G, Dummer P et al (1987c) The distribution of plaque and gingivitis and the influence of brushing hand in a group of 11–12 year old school children. *J Clin Periodontol* **14**:564–72.

Addy M, Loyn T, Adams D (1991) Dentine hypersensitivity – effects of some proprietary mouthwashes on the dentine smear layer: a SEM study. *J Dent* **19**:145–52.

Addy M, Hughes JA, West NX et al (1998) Low erosive potential fruit drinks: Comparison with conventional products. *J Dent Res* **77**:845 (abstract 1710).

Adriens PA, De Boever JA, Loesche WS (1988) Bacterial invasion in rat cementum and radicular dentine of periodontally diseased teeth in humans. A reservoir of periodontopathic bacteria. *J Periodontol* **59**:222–9.

Aldritt WAS (1968) Abnormal gingival form. *Proc R Soc Med* **16**:137–42.

Alexander AG (1971) A study of the distribution of supra and subgingival calculus, bacterial plaque and gingival inflammation in the mouths of 400 individuals. *J Periodont* **42**:21–8.

Baelum V, Fejerskov O, Kerring T (1986) Oral hygiene, gingivitis and periodontal breakdown in adult Tanzanians. *J Periodont Res* **21**:221–32.

Baker DL, Seymour GJ (1976) The possible pathogenesis of gingival recession. *J Clin Periodont* **3**:208–12.

Bergström J, Eliasson S (1988) Cervical abrasion in relation to toothbrushing and periodontal health. *Scand J Dent Res* **96**:405–11.

Bernimoulin J, Curilovie Z (1977) Gingival recession and tooth mobility. *J Clin Periodontol* **4**:107–11.

Bevenius J, Lindskog S, Hultenby K (1994) The micromorphology in vivo of the buccocervical region of premolar teeth in young adults. A replica study by scanning electron microscopy. *Acta Odontol Scand* **52**:323–34.

Brännström M (1963) A hydrodynamic mechanism in the transmission of pain-producing stimuli through the dentine. In: Anderson DJ, ed, *Sensory Mechanisms in Dentine*, 73–9. Pergamon Press: London.

Brännström M (1986) The cause of post-restoration sensitivity and its prevention. *J Endodontics* **12**:475–81.

Buckley LA (1981)The relationships between malocclusion, gingival inflammation, plaque and calculus. *J Periodontol* **52**:35–40.

Chabanski MB, Gillam DG (1997) Aetiology, prevalence and features of cervical dentine sensitivity. *J Oral Rehabil* **24,** 15–19.

Chabanski MB, Gillam DG, Bulman JS, Newman HN (1996) Prevalence of cervical dentine sensitivity in a population of patients referred to a specialist periodontology department. *J Clin Periodontol* **23**:989–92.

Collaert B, Speelman J (1991) Traitement de l'hypersensibilité dentinaire. *Rev Belge Med Dent* **46**:63–73.

Dachi SF (1965) The relationship of pulpitis and hyperaemia to thermal sensitivity. *Oral Surg Oral Med Oral Pathol* **19**:776–85.

Davis WB, Winter PJ (1980) The effect of abrasion on enamel and dentine after exposure to dietary acid. *Br Dent J* **148**:253–6.

Dowell P, Addy M (1983) Dentine hypersensitivity – a review, aetiology, symptoms and theories of pain production. *J Clin Periodontol* **10**:341–50.

Dowell P, Addy M, Dummer P (1985) Dentine hypersensitivity: aetiology, differential diagnosis and management. *Br Dent J* **158**:92–6.

Dummer PMH, Addy M, Hicks R, Kingdon A (1987)

The effect of social class on the prevalence of caries, plaque, gingivitis and pocketing in 11–12 year old children in South Wales. *J Dent* **15**:185–90.

Eccles JD, Jenkins WG (1974) Dental erosion and diet. *J Dent* **2**:153–9.

Fischer C, Fischer RG, Wennberg A (1992) Prevalence and distribution of cervical dentine hypersensitivity in a population in Rio de Janeiro, Brazil. *J Dent* **20**:272–6.

Flynn J, Galloway R, Orchardson R (1985) The incidence of hypersensitive teeth in the West of Scotland. *J Dent* **13**:230–6.

Gillette WB, van House RL (1980) Effects of improper oral hygiene procedures. *J Am Dent Assoc* **10**:476–81.

Glenwright HD, Strahan JD (1994) *Self Assessment Picture Tests in Dentistry: Periodontology*, 38. Wolfe: London.

Gorman WJ (1967) Prevalence and etiology of gingival recession. *J Periodont* **38**:316–22.

Graf HE, Galasse R (1977) Morbidity, prevalence and intra-oral distribution of hypersensitive teeth. *J Dent Res* (Special issue A) **56**:abstract number 479.

Grenby TH (1996) Methods of assessing erosion and erosive potential. *Eur J Oral Sci* **104,** 221–9.

Gysi A (1900) An attempt to explain the sensitiveness of dentine. *Br J Dent Sci* **43**:865–8.

Hirschfeld I (1939) The toothbrush. Its use and abuse. In: *Dental Items of Interest*, 1–27, 262–27, 358–465, 484–95. Kimpton: London

Holland GR, Närhi MN, Addy M et al (1997) Guidelines for the design and conduct of clinical trials on dentine hypersensitivity. *J Clin Periodontol* **24**:808–13.

Hughes JA (1998) Enamel erosion in vitro by mouthrinses. Personal communication.

Hughes JA, West NX, Parker DM et al (1998) Erosion of enamel: compared to blackcurrant and orange drinks. *J Dent Res* **77**:794 (abstract 1303).

Hunter L (1998) The effect of orange juice on permanent and deciduous enamel and dentine *in situ*. Unpublished data.

Imfeld T, Sener B (1998) Brushing time, load, and speed of electric brushes and gingiva. *J Dent Res* **77**:664 (abstract 259).

Ishikawa S (1969) A clinico-histological study on the hypersensitivity of dentine. *J Japan Stomatol Soc* **36**:68–88.

Jenkins WMM, Allan CJ (1994) *Guide to Periodontics*, 3rd edn, 155–85. Wright: Oxford.

Jensen AI (1964) Hypersensitivity controlled by iontophoresis. Double blind clinical investigation. *J Am Dent Assoc* **68**:216–25.

Johnson RH, Zulgar-Nairn BJ, Koval JJ (1982) The effectiveness of an electro-ionising toothbrush in the control of dentinal hypersensitivity. *J Periodontol* **53**:353–9.

Kanapka JA (1990) Over the counter dentifrices in the treatment of tooth hypersensitivity: review of clinical studies. *Dent Clin North Am* **34**:545–60.

Knocht A, Simon G, Person P, Denepitiya JL (1993) Gingival recession in relation to history of hard toothbrush use. *J Periodontol* **64**:900–5.

Kuroiwa M, Kodaka T, Masayuki A (1994) Dentine hypersensitivity. Occlusion of dentinal tubules by brushing with and without an abrasive dentifrice. *J Periodontol* **65**:291–6.

Löe H, Theilade E, Jensen SB, Schiott CR (1965) Experimental gingivitis in man. *J Periodontoly* **36**:177–87.

Löe H, Anerud A, Boysen H (1992) The natural history of periodontal disease in man: prevalence, severity and extent of gingival recession. *J Periodontol* **63**:489–85.

Löst C (1984) Depth of alveolar bone dehiscences in relation to gingival recession. *J Clin Periodontol* **11**:583–9.

Mazdyasma S, Stoner JE (1980) Factors influencing gingival recession in the lower incisor region. *J Periodontol* **51**:74–8.

Modheer T, Odenrick L (1980) Post treatment periodontal status of labially erupted maxillary canines. *Acta Odontol Scand* **38**:253–7.

Murray LE, Roberts AJ (1994) The prevalence of self reported hypersensitive teeth. Hypersensitive dentine. *Arch Oral Biol* **39**(Suppl.):129S.

O'Brien M (1994) *Children's Dental Health in the United Kingdom 1993*. Office of Population Census and Surveys. HMSO: London.

O'Leary T, Drake RB, Crump PP (1971) The incidence of recession in young males. *J Periodontol* **42**:264–9.

Olsson M, Lindhe J (1991) Periodontal characteristics in individuals with varying form of upper central incisors. *J Clin Periodontol* **18**:78–82.

Orchardson R, Collins WJN (1987) Thresholds of hypersensitive teeth to two forms of controlled stimulation. *J Clin Periodontol* **14**:68–73.

Parfitt GJ, Mjor IA (1964) A clinical evaluation of local gingival recession in children. *J Dent Child* **31**:257–61.

Pashley DH (1985) Strategies for clinical evaluation of drugs and/or devices for the alleviation of hypersensitive dentine. In: Rowe, NH, ed, *Proceedings of*

Symposium on Hypersensitive Dentine. Origin and Management, 65. University of Michigan.

Pashley DH (1990) Mechanisms of dentine sensitivity. *Dent Clin North Am* **34**:449–74.

Petersen N, Gormsen C (1991) Oral conditions among German battery factory workers. *Community Dent Oral Epidemiol* **19**:104–6.

Powell RN, McEniery TM (1981) Disparities in gingival height in the mandibular central incisor region of children aged 6–12 years. *Community Dent Oral Epidemiol* **9**:32–5.

Ropner RE, Kineer GW, Gocka EF (1972) Periodontal disease in aged individuals. *J Periodontol* **32**:304–9.

Sandholm L, Niemi MI, Ainamo J (1982) Identification of soft tissue brushing lesion. A clinical and scanning electron microscopic study. *J Clin Periodontol* **9**:397–401.

Scheutzel P (1996) Etiology of dental erosion – intrinsic factors. *Eur J Oral Sci* **104**:178–90.

Seltzer S, Bender IB (1975) *The Dental Pulp: Biological Considerations in Dental Procedures*, 2nd edn, 306. Lippincott JB: Philadelphia and Toronto.

Smith RG (1997) Gingival recession. Reappraisal of an enigmatic condition and a new index for monitoring. *J Clin Periodontol* **24**:201–5.

Stone M (1948) Case report of psychosomatic factors in the etiology of gum recession. *NY University Dent J* **7**:33–5.

Trott JR, Love B (1966) An analysis of localised gingival recession in 766 Winnipeg High School students. *Dent Pract Dent Rec* **16**:209–13.

Tuominen M, Tuominen R (1991) Dental erosion and associated factors among factory workers exposed to inorganic acid fumes. *Proc Finn Dent Soc* **87**:359–64.

Van der Velden U, Attstrom R (1997) Consensus report of session III. In: Lang NP, Karring T, Lindhe J, eds, *Proceedings of the 2nd European Workshop on Periodontology*, 265–7. Quintessence: Berlin.

Watson PJC (1984) Gingival recession. *J Dent* **12**: 29–35.

West NX, Addy M, Jackson RJ, Ridge BD (1997) Dentine hypersensitivity: review and discussion of controls and the placebo response. A comparison of the effect of strontium acetate and potassium nitrate toothpastes on dentine hypersensitivity. *J Clin Periodontol* **24**:209–15.

West NX, Maxwell A, Hughes JA et al (1998a) A method to measure clinical erosion: the effect of orange juice consumption on erosion of enamel. *J Dent* **26**:329–36.

West NX, Hughes JA, Parker DM et al (1998b) Development of a low erosive drink: compared with orange juice. *J Dent Res* **77**:794 (abstract 1304).

West NX, Addy M, Hughes J (1998c) Dentine hypersensitivity: the effects of brushing desensitizing toothpastes, their solid and liquid phases, and detergents on dentine and acrylic: studies in vitro. *J Oral Rehabil* **25**:885–95.

Woofter C (1969) The prevalence and aetiology of gingival recession. *Periodontal Abstract* **17**:45–50.

Yates R, Owens J, Jackson RJ et al (1998a) A split mouth placebo controlled study to determine the effect of amorphous calcium phosphate in the treatment of dentine hypersensitivity. *J Clin Periodontol* **25**:687–92.

Yates R, West NX, Addy M, Marlow I (1998b) The effects of a potassium citrate, cetylpyridinium chloride, sodium fluoride mouthrinse on dentine hypersensitivity, plaque and gingivitis. A placebo controlled study. *J Clin Periodontol* **25**:813–20.

Zero DT (1996) Etiology of dental erosion – extrinsic factors. *Eur J Oral Sci* **104**:162–71.

22

Interaction of oral hygiene products with dentinal tubules: effects of stabilized stannous fluoride dentifrice on the permeability of in-situ brushed dentine and in-vitro chemical reactivity and solubility of apatite and dentine

Joop Arends, Toon Dykman, Jackie B Shaffer, Lori A Bacca, Anthony C Lanzalaco, Edward R Cox and Donald J White

Introduction

Research has demonstrated that dentine hypersensitivity results from three primary factors: exposure of root surfaces to the oral environment, development of surface porosity/permeability with exposure of patent dentinal tubules, and inherent susceptibility of pulpal nerve endings to changes in fluid transport within dentine (Pashley 1990, Addy and Pearce 1994, Kleinberg et al. 1994, Narhi et al. 1994). Technical approaches to the prevention or treatment of dentine hypersensitivity include reactivity of exposed dentine surfaces with chemical agents which either close up open dentinal tubules or make smear layer-covered surfaces resistant to tubule exposure (Ellingsen and Rölla 1987, Addy and Mostafa 1988, Dondi Dall'orologio et al. 1994, Gangarosa 1994, Goodis et al. 1994, Hack and Thompson 1994, Holborow 1994, Miller et al. 1994, Shono et al. 1994).

Anhydrous gel products containing 0.4% stannous fluoride have been shown clinically to reduce the pain associated with dentine hypersensitivity (Blong et al. 1985, Snyder et al. 1985). Available evidence suggests that the clinical effects of the anhydrous stannous fluoride gel products are the direct result of occlusion of

dentinal tubules with chemical precipitates formed from stannous fluoride (Ellingsen and Rölla 1987, Addy and Mostafa 1988, Miller et al. 1994). While anhydrous SnF_2 gels may provide significant and proven efficacy for treating caries, gingivitis and dentine hypersensitivity, the product form and added logistical requirements for application do not always meet patients' preferences. Recently, a commercial dentifrice has been developed using an improved combination of stabilized stannous fluoride within a conventional dentifrice vehicle (White 1995). This stabilized stannous fluoride dentifrice has proven to be effective for the prevention of both gingivitis and caries (Beiswanger et al. 1995, Faller et al. 1995, Perlich et al. 1995, McClanahan et al. 1997).

The objective of this study was to develop an improved understanding of the nature and mechanism of the chemical reactivity of dentine mineral with stabilized stannous fluoride dentifrice which may contribute to its specific efficacy in the prevention or treatment of dentine hypersensitivity and the prevention of root caries. These studies directly compared the reactivity and efficacy of stabilized stannous fluoride toothpastes and anhydrous stannous fluoride gels in vitro and in vivo.

Materials and methods

Reaction products of stannous fluoride with apatite mineral in vitro with pH cycling – chemical composition studies

Powdered synthetic hydroxyapatite mineral (Biogel HTP Hydroxyapatite; Biorad Laboratories, Richmond, CA, USA) samples (750 mg) were treated with aqueous solutions prepared from commercial dentifrice and gel preparations. Commercial and laboratory-prepared tooth-pastes, including a 0.243% NaF dentifrice (Procter and Gamble, Cincinatti, USA); an original formula 0.454% SnF_2, calcium pyrophosphate abrasive dentifrice (Procter and Gamble); a 0.454% SnF_2 dentifrice – stabilized with stannous gluconate – silica abrasive dentifrice (Procter and Gamble) and an anhydrous 0.4% SnF_2 gel (Colgate Palmolive, Piscataway, USA) were diluted 1:3 w/w with water and slurries were prepared with a rotary mixer. These slurries were centrifuged after preparation to remove particulate abrasives and supernate liquids were used to treat hydroxyapatite samples for 5 min with mixing at room temperature. Treated hydroxyapatite seeds were washed twice with distilled water and exposed to 7-day cycling demineralization conditions – including 20 h/day remineralization (Ca = 2.5 mM, P = 1.5 mM, 150 mM KCl, 20 mM cacodylate, pH 7.3) and 4 h/day demineralization (pH 4.5, 100 mM lactic acid). Treated cycled powders were dissolved in acid and analyzed for fluoride and tin uptake by ion-selective electrodes and atomic absorbance respectively.

Effect of topical fluoride reactivity on apatite and dentine susceptibility to acid demineralization in vitro

Powdered synthetic hydroxyapatite mineral (Biogel HTP Hydroxyapatite; Biorad Laboratories) samples were freshly treated with aqueous solutions prepared from commercial dentifrice and gel preparations as described above. Also included with these treatments were additional commercial toothpastes including a 0.243% NaF triclosan/copolymer dentifrice (Colgate Palmolive) and 0.243% NaF-pyrophosphate dentifrice (Procter and Gamble). Powdered samples of dentine were treated in a like set of limited experiments. Dentine powder was prepared by cutting dentine disks from molar teeth with a water-cooled saw. Enamel was removed by sectioning and dentine disks were ground into a powder by mortar and pestle. Following treatments with topical fluoride, apatite or dentine powders were inoculated into acid demineralization solution containing 100 mM lactic acid. Demineralization was followed by pH stat (0.01 M HCl titrant) using potentiometric control via an Orion combination pH electrode coupled to a PC-controlled Metrohm potentiostat. Apatite demineralization was produced in replicate for the following treatments: stabilized SnF_2, NaF/pyrophosphate, NaF/copolymer and NaF dentifrices. Dentine demineralization was preliminarily assessed following stabilized SnF_2 and NaF dentifrice treatments.

Comparison of stabilized stannous fluoride dentifrice and anhydrous stannous fluoride gel for reducing dentine permeability in vivo

General study design

Ten subjects participated in a four-part randomized cross-over design study. Subjects reviewed and signed an informed consent for participation and the protocol was reviewed and approved by the Institutional Review Board. Subjects were fitted with special dental prostheses holding four dentine samples each. The prostheses were fitted with two types of dentine samples (two each) including a polished and acid-etched sample (PAE) and a non-polished natural dentine (ND) surface. One of each specimen was included on each side of the mouth. Specimens were sterilized prior to use. A fresh set of dentine specimens was used for each cross-over treatment. Subjects in each treatment used test dentifrices for a period of 2 weeks, brushing twice per day (morning and evening) with the dentine samples inserted in the prostheses. Following treatment for 2 weeks, root sections were collected for iodide permeability assays to assess the porosity of dentine after treatment.

Dentine sample preparation

Roots from human teeth were cut longitudinally with a water-cooled saw and sections were first sterilized. PAE specimens were prepared by first embedding dentine specimens – except the surface – in PMMA. Surfaces were polished flat with 400 followed by 1200 grit wet silicon carbide sandpaper. Samples were kept moist throughout polishing. Dentinal smear layers on polished specimens were removed by treating roots with 0.5 M EDTA for 1 min. ND samples were prepared by embedding natural surfaces in PMMA, except for the curved natural surface. Samples were brushed with a non-fluoridated toothpaste prior to the start of the study.

Formulations tested and usage directions

SnF_2 dentifrice (0.454%), stabilized with stannous gluconate, was used twice per day for 2 min brushing ad libitum. A SnF_2-free non-fluoridated dentifrice was used twice per day for 2 min. In a SnF_2-free placebo gel treatment subjects brushed their teeth for 1 min twice per day with a 0.243% NaF dentifrice, followed by treatment for 2 min with topical gel. In the 0.40% SnF_2 active gel treatment, subjects brushed their teeth for 1 min twice per day with a 0.243% NaF dentifrice, followed by treatment for 2 min with topical gel.

Iodide permeability assays of dentine porosity

Rectangular windows measuring 3×3 mm were isolated using nail varnish. Samples were dipped in 0.5 M NaI solution for 5 min and blotted dry with tissue. Samples were placed in 3 ml of water and agitated for 5 min, after which 60 μl of ionic strength adjustment (ISA) solution was added to the solution and iodide content was measured with an iodide ion-specific electrode (Orion). Surface areas were checked by stereomicroscope and permeability was calculated as μg of iodide per square cm.

Results

Reaction products of stannous fluoride with apatite mineral in vitro – chemical composition studies

Fluoride and stannous ion uptake onto hydroxyapatite associated with topical application of stannous fluoride and control (NaF) formulations are shown in Table 22.1. Although fluoride uptake was similar for NaF and SnF_2 treatments, stannous uptake was also substantial for both the stabilized stannous fluoride dentifrice and the anhydrous stannous fluoride gel. Freshly made original formula SnF_2 dentifrice – a less stabilized form of SnF_2 in dentifrice – produced somewhat decreased fluoride and dramatically decreased stannous uptake.

Table 22.1 Fluoride and stannous uptake from topical treatments on apatite

Treatment	F uptake (ppm)	Sn^{2+} uptake (ppm)
NaF dentifrice	1521	...
Original formula SnF_2 dentifrice	1613	820
Stabilized SnF_2 dentifrice	1821	23,100
Anhydrous SnF_2 gel	2102	26,300

Effect of topical fluoride reactivity on apatite and dentine susceptibility to acid demineralization in vitro

The effects of topical treatments on acid demineralization of hydroxyapatite and powdered dentine are shown in Figures 22.1 and 22.2. In Figure 22.1, the effects of topical fluoride treatments on acid demineralization are shown by decreased levels of titrant acid to the demineralization media called for by calcium and phosphate release from dissolving mineral. Treatment with SnF_2 dentifrice and gels produced comparable acid demineralization

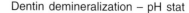

Apatite demineralization – pH stat

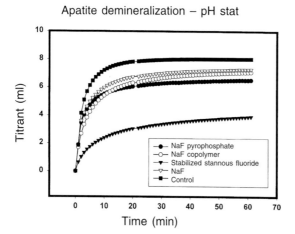

Figure 22.1

pH stat acid demineralization of synthetic hydroxyapatite following treatment with dentifrices.

Dentin demineralization – pH stat

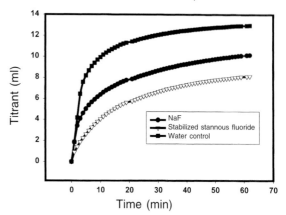

Figure 22.2

pH stat acid demineralization of dentine following treatment with dentifrices.

protection, both were superior to conventional NaF dentifrice pretreatment (demineralization profiles exhibit reproducibility of ±10%). Treatment with NaF-copolymer and NaF-pyrophosphate dentifrices provided enhanced protection versus NaF alone, but inferior to SnF_2 treatments. Treatment of dentine samples with the stabilized SnF_2 dentifrice likewise produced significant protection against acid solubilization as compared with NaF dentifrice treatment (Figure 22.2).

Comparison of stabilized stannous fluoride dentifrice and anhydrous stannous fluoride gel for reducing dentine permeability in vivo

Tables 22.2 and 22.3 show the results of iodide permeability assessments of PAE and ND specimens worn in vivo for 2 weeks with daily dentifrice or dentifrice plus gel treatments. For both PAE and ND substrates, in-vivo treatment with SnF_2-containing topical agents produced three-fold reductions in iodide permeability. The rank ordered effectiveness in reducing dentine sample permeability measured stabilized SnF_2 dentifrice = NaF dentifrice + SnF_2 gel > NaF dentifrice + placebo gel > placebo dentifrice.

Table 22.2 Iodide permeability PAE dentine treated in vivo

Treatment	Iodide permeability in $\mu g/cm^2$ (SD)
Stabilized SnF_2 dentifrice	51 (41) a
NaF dentifrice + SnF_2 gel	55 (10) a
NaF dentifrice + placebo gel	89 (41) b
Placebo toothpaste	162 (72) c

Treatment groups with different letter code designations are significantly different, i.e. a<b<c: P <0.05, Student's t test. Permeability starts at 150–250 $\mu g/cm^2$.

Table 22.3 Iodide permeability in ND dentine treated in vivo

Treatment	Iodide permeability in $\mu g/cm^2$ (SD)
Stabilized SnF_2 dentifrice	75 (46) a
NaF dentifrice + SnF_2 gel	68 (37) a
NaF dentifrice + placebo gel	115 (48) b
Placebo dentifrice	229 (90) c

Treatment groups with different letter code designations are significantly different, i.e. a<b<c: P <0.05, Student's t test. Permeability starts at 100–150 $\mu g/cm^2$.

Discussion

The hydrodynamic theory of dentine sensitivity is based upon the premise that sensitive dentine is permeable to fluid transport, which in turn excites pulpal nerves (Pashley 1990, 1994). Based upon this mechanism, a preferred approach to the topical desensitization of dentine has been the application of chemical agents which produce chemical obturation of open tubules or which produce decreased chemical reactivity of smear layer-covered dentine. The chemical closing of open tubules should be effective in hypersensitivity treatment, while the reactivity of smear layer-covered dentine to provide protection against environmental stress can contribute to the prevention of future hypersensitivity.

As described earlier, SnF_2 has been shown to produce tubule occlusion in in-vitro studies (Ellingsen and Rölla 1987, Addy and Mostafa 1988, Miller et al. 1994). Anhydrous gels containing SnF_2 have demonstrated chemical reactivity with dentine surfaces, producing strongly adherent layers containing both Sn^{2+} and F^- (Miller et al. 1994). These surface deposits decrease the permeability of dentine. This chemical reactivity is proposed as the mechanism behind the clinical effectiveness of anhydrous SnF_2 gels for treatment of sensitive dentine (Blong et al. 1985, Snyder et al. 1985).

The development of similarly effective forms of stannous fluoride in a dentifrice vehicle is worthwhile, as patient substitution for a new type of dentifrice is fairly easy to accomplish, as it is within established patterns of dental hygiene. Demonstration of hypersensitivity benefits for stabilized stannous fluoride dentifrice would expand the already proven benefits of this formulation in preventing both gingivitis and dental caries. Although one might naively expect a priori that high bioavailable SnF_2 dentifrice would provide efficacy in reducing dentinal hypersensitivity, a number of vehicle-related factors could also influence the efficacy of the dentifrice formulation. On the positive side, it might be anticipated that toothpaste abrasives could assist in enhancing SnF_2 dentifrice chemical actions, as abrasive components have been reported to contribute to tubule occlusion, providing possible desensitization actions (Pashley et al. 1984). On the other hand, chemical surfactants and humectants used in dentifrices could produce chemical

effects contraindicated for hypersensitivity prevention by dispersing developed smear layers (Absi et al. 1995). The objective of these preliminary experiments was to assess the chemical reactivity (fluoride and stannous uptake), acid protection and in-vivo permeability effects of a novel stabilized stannous fluoride dentifrice, to see if the anti-caries and anti-gingivitis effects of this dentifrice might be expected to be augmented with sensitivity protection benefits.

In in-vitro experiments, the chemical reactivity of SnF_2 as provided in stabilized dentifrice was compared with the reactivity provided by anhydrous SnF_2 gel and NaF dentifrice. The fluoride activity of the stabilized SnF_2 dentifrice was found to be similar to that of the SnF_2 gel and NaF dentifrice. Sn^{2+} uptake, probably important in the production of acid-resistant surface layers on dentine surfaces, was similar for SnF_2 dentifrice-treated and SnF_2 gel-treated samples.

Additional experiments examined the acid protective effects of the mineral precipitates formed by topical dentifrice and gel treatments. In these experiments, stabilized SnF_2 dentifrice provided superior acid protection benefits to conventional NaF-containing dentifrices – both with and without mineral reactive antitartar ingredients. Preliminary experiments with powdered dentine revealed a similar activity for stabilized SnF_2 dentifrice. The delivery of acid protective benefits to either developed (tubule blocking) or established smear layers may be vital to the provision of lasting dentine desensitization, as research continues to implicate acidic beverages as an important etiologic factor contributing to the development of dentine hypersensitivity (Addy et al. 1987, Absi et al. 1992).

The in-vivo study results demonstrated significant efficacy of stabilized SnF_2 dentifrice in reducing the permeability of dentine surfaces with open tubules, as well as in protecting natural dentinal surfaces from developing more permeability. Reductions in permeability matched those provided by direct treatment with SnF_2 gels – used as an adjunct to regular brushing regimens. It was interesting that during the study the etched and natural dentine surfaces progressed toward somewhat similar iodide permeability following in-vivo use for 2 weeks. This may reflect the equilibration of dentinal surfaces to a common endpoint produced through toothbrushing and dietary/plaque acid/remineralization cycles. While iodide permeability is a convenient marker for the study of in-situ specimens, it must be recognized that it is not necessarily equivalent to hydraulic conductance of dentine. On the other hand, it is reasonable to expect good correlations between substrate penetration into dentine and morphological and hydraulic conductance properties associated with hypersensitivity (Sena 1990).

These collective results are very positive for SnF_2 dentifrice, and suggest that this formulation would be expected to provide substantial efficacy in the treatment and prevention of dentinal hypersensitivity in the clinical situation. The strong chemical reactivity of stabilized SnF_2 dentifrice matches other fluoride topical agents and clinically proven anhydrous gel preparations. The reacted fluoride is extremely effective against acid demineralization, which is an equally important consideration. This chemical reactivity would be expected to contribute to lasting resistance of treated surfaces to the development of both subsequent and root caries (Faller et al. 1995). Complementing these in-vitro observations, in-vivo use of stabilized SnF_2 dentifrice resulted in significant reductions in permeability compared not only with placebo controls, but also with conventional NaF dentifrice treatments. This helped to confirm that the efficacy of the formulation was not restricted to simple effects of the toothpaste abrasive, but in fact was related to and enhanced by significant SnF_2 reactivity.

References

Absi EG, Addy M, Adams D (1992) Dentine hypersensitivity: the effect of toothbrushing and dietary compounds on dentine in vitro. J Oral Rehabil 19: 101–10.

Absi EG, Addy M, Adams D (1995) Dentine hypersensitivity: uptake of toothpastes onto dentine and effects of brushing, washing and dietary acid – SEM in vitro study. J Oral Rehabil 22: 175–82.

Addy M, Mostafa P (1988) Dentin hypersensitivity I: Effects produced by uptake in vitro of metal ions, fluoride and formaldehyde into dentin. J Oral Rehabil 15: 575–85.

Addy M, Pearce N (1994) Aetiological, predisposing and environmental factors in dentin hypersensitivity. Arch Oral Biol 39 (Suppl): S33–S38.

Addy M, Absi EG, Adams D (1987) Dental hypersensitivity: the effects in vitro of acids and dietary substances on root planed and burred dentine. J Clin Periodontol 14: 274–9.

Beiswanger BB, Doyle PM, Jackson RD et al (1995) The clinical effect of dentifrices containing stabilized stannous fluoride on plaque formation and gingivitis – a six month study with ad libitum brushing. J Clin Dent 6: 46–53.

Blong MA, Volding B, Thrash WJ, Jones DL (1985) Effects of a gel containing 0.4 percent stannous fluoride on dentinal hypersensitivity. Dent Hygiene 59: 489–92.

Dondi Dall'orologio G, Borghetti R, Caliceti C et al (1994) Clinical evaluation of Gluma and Gluma 2000 for treatment of hypersensitive dentin. Arch Oral Biol 39 (Suppl): S126.

Ellingsen JE, Rölla G (1987) Treatment of dentin with stannous fluoride – SEM and electron microprobe study. Scand J Dent Res 95: 281–6.

Faller RV, Best JM, Featherstone JDB (1995) Anticaries efficacy of an improved stannous fluoride toothpaste. J Clin Dent 6: 89–96.

Gangarosa LP Sr (1994) Current strategies for dentist-applied treatment in the management of hypersensitive dentin. Arch Oral Biol 39 (Suppl): S101–S106.

Goodis HE, White JM, Marshall SJ et al (1994) Measurement of fluid flow through laser treated dentin. Arch Oral Biol 39 (Suppl): S128.

Hack GD, Thompson VP (1994) Occlusion of dentinal tubules with cavity varnishes. Arch Oral Biol 39 (Suppl): S149.

Holborow DW (1994) A clinical trial of a potassium oxalate system in the treatment of sensitive root surfaces. Arch Oral Biol 39 (Suppl): S134.

Kleinberg I, Kaufman HW, Wolff M (1994) Measurement of tooth hypersensitivity and oral factors involved in its development. Arch Oral Biol 39 (Suppl): S63–S72.

McClanahan SF, Beiswanger BB, Bartizek RD et al (1997) A comparison of stabilized stannous fluoride dentifrice and triclosan/copolymer dentifrice for efficacy in the reduction of gingivitis and gingival bleeding: six-month study results. J Clin Dent 8: 38–45.

Miller S, Truong T, Heu R et al (1994) Effects on human dentin of treatment with an anhydrous stannous fluoride gel. Arch Oral Biol 39 (Suppl): S149.

Narhi M, Yamamoto H, Ngassapa D, Hivonen T (1994) The neurophysiological basis and the role of inflammatory reactions in dentine hypersensitivity. *Arch Oral Biol* **39** (Suppl): S23–S30.

Pashley DH (1990) Mechanisms of dentin sensitivity. *Dent Clin North Am* **34**: 449–73.

Pashley DH (1994) Dentine permeability and its role in the pathobiology of dentine sensitivity. *Arch Oral Biol* **39** (Suppl): S73–S80.

Pashley DH, O'Meara JA, Kepler EE et al (1984) Dentine permeability: effects of desensitizing dentifrices *in vitro*. *J Periodontol* **55**: 522–5.

Perlich MA, Bacca LA, Bollmer BW et al (1995) The clinical effect of a stabilized stannous fluoride dentifrice

on plaque formation, gingivitis and gingival bleeding: a six-month study. *J Clin Dent* **6**: 54–8.

Sena FJ (1990) Dentinal permeability in assessing therapeutic agents. *Dent Clin North Am* **34**: 475–90.

Shono YHH, Ogawa T, Terashita M, Pashley DH (1994) A new oxalate treatment for dentine tubule occlusion. *Arch Oral Biol* **39** (Suppl): S135.

Snyder RA, Beck FM, Horton JE (1985) The efficacy of a 0.4% SnFl solution on root surface hypersensitivity. *J Dent Res* **64**: 201.

White DJ (1995) A return to stannous fluoride dentifrices. *J Clin Dent* **6**: 29–38.

23

Responses of pulpal nociceptors to tissue injury and inflammation

Matti VO Närhi

Introduction

The dental pulp is richly innervated by both myelinated and unmyelinated axons (Byers 1984). A great majority of the fibres are sensory afferents and according to current knowledge they are mostly involved in pain mediation (Mumford and Bowsher 1976, Mumford 1982, McGrath et al. 1983, Virtanen et al. 1987, Närhi et al. 1992b). External irritation and tissue injury induce an inflammatory reaction in the pulp tissue and studies from the past few years indicate that the intradental sensory nerves play an active and significant role in the regulation of these responses (Taylor et al. 1988, Taylor and Byers 1990, Byers 1992, 1996, Byers and Taylor 1993). The morphological changes of the pulpal nociceptors in response to tissue injury include sprouting of the nerve endings and an increase in the neuropeptide immunoreactivity in the nerve fibres next to the inflamed area (Taylor et al. 1988; Taylor and Byers 1990, Byers and Taylor 1993, Byers 1996). However, little is known about the possible functional correlates of the morphological neural changes (Närhi et al. 1996).

Increased responses to external stimulation and ongoing activity have been recorded in intradental nerves in injured and inflamed teeth of experimental animals indicating sensitization of the pulpal nociceptors (Ahlberg 1978b, Närhi et al. 1996). It has also been shown that certain inflammatory mediators are able to activate pulp nerves and/or sensitize them to external stimuli (Olgart 1974, 1985, Närhi et al. 1992b, 1996, Olgart 1996b).

The sensitization of the pulpal nerves induced by tissue injury and inflammation in experimental animals corresponds to the clinical findings of increased pain responses induced from human teeth by external stimulation (Brännström 1981, Mumford 1982). It is well known that the pain symptoms connected with acute pulpal inflammation can sometimes be extremely intense, a condition known as 'hot tooth' (Brännström 1981, Mumford 1982). Also, the pain responses induced by stimulation of exposed hypersensitive human dentine can in many cases reach the maximum level of any pain scale (Närhi et al. 1992b, Kontturi-Närhi and Närhi 1993). However, the correlation between the histopathological pulpal changes and the intensity and type of the clinical pain symptoms in inflamed teeth seems to be poor (Seltzer et al. 1963, 1965, Brännström 1981, Mumford 1982). In fact, pulpitis may frequently proceed to total pulp necrosis with only minor symptoms or even without any symptoms at all (Brännström 1981, Olgart 1996a, 1996b, Närhi et al. 1996). Such a condition ('silent pulpitis') seems puzzling considering the dense nociceptive innervation of the pulp.

It has been proposed that pulpal inflammatory reactions and, consequently, nociceptor activation are controlled by effective local inhibitory mechanisms (Olgart and Gazelius 1977, Olgart 1996a, 1996b, Närhi et al. 1996). Also, regulation of the pain impulse transmission in the trigeminal pain pathways must be considered (Sessle 1978, 1987, Sigurdsson and Maixner 1994). The purpose of this chapter is to review the function of the pulp nerves, especially the pulpal neural responses to tissue injury and inflammation, and to discuss the role of such changes in the development of pulpal and dentinal pain.

Functional characteristics of pulpal nociceptors

Based on their conduction velocities, intradental nerve fibres can be classified as A and C type (Närhi *et al*. 1982d, Jyväsjärvi and Kniffki 1987, Närhi *et al*. 1992b) corresponding to the myelinated and unmyelinated fibres found in morphological studies (Beasley and Holland 1978, Reader and Foreman 1981, Holland and Robinson 1983, Byers 1984). Histological studies also show that a great majority (70–80%) of the axons entering the pulp are unmyelinated (Byers 1984). Electrophysiological recordings performed on experimental animals indicate that the two fibre groups differ in their functional characteristics, e.g. in their responses to various external stimuli (Närhi *et al*. 1982c, 1982d, Närhi 1985b, Jyväsjärvi and Kniffki 1987, Närhi *et al*. 1992b, Ikeda *et al*. 1997) and that A fibres are responsible for dentine sensitivity (Närhi 1985a, 1985b, Närhi *et al*. 1992a). Comparison of the function of single intradental nerve fibres to the sensory responses induced from human teeth and clinical cases of dental pain also indicates that the responses of the two fibre groups to tissue injury and inflammation may differ (Ahlquist *et al*. 1984, 1985, Närhi 1985b, Olgart 1985).

Most studies indicate that pain is the only sensation induced by external stimulation of human teeth. However, the quality of pain may be different in response to different stimuli (Hensel and Mann 1956, Ahlquist *et al*. 1984, 1985, Jyväsjärvi and Kniffki 1987, Kontturi-Närhi and Närhi 1993) and it is indicated that such variations are based on activation of different nerve fibre groups in addition to different patterns of nerve firing (Ahlquist *et al*. 1985, Närhi 1985a, Jyväsjärvi and Kniffki 1987, Närhi *et al*. 1992b). Non-painful (prepain) sensations can be induced by electrical stimulation at low intensities (Mumford and Bowsher 1976, Mumford 1982, McGrath *et al*. 1983, Virtanen *et al*. 1987). These sensations have been suggested to result from activation of low-threshold fastest conducting A-β-type pulpal afferents which have been proposed to respond to non-noxious mechanical stimulation of the tooth crown (Dong *et al*. 1985, 1993, Paphangkorakit and Osborn 1997, 1998). However, single fibre recordings in experimental animals indicate that the responses of pulpal A-β and A-δ fibres to external stimulation are similar and that the fibres belong to the same functional group (Närhi *et al*. 1982a, 1982b, Jyväsjärvi and Kniffki 1987, Närhi and Hirvonen 1987, Närhi *et al*. 1992b). Moreover, although A-β fibres have low electrical thresholds it should be noted that there is a considerable overlap between the thresholds of A-β and A-δ fibres and fibres of both groups are activated at the same low current intensities (Närhi *et al*. 1982d, Närhi *et al*. 1992b). Thus, both A-β and A-δ fibres may contribute to the prepain sensations. Virtanen *et al*. (1987) also showed that as a result of temporal summation induced by an increase in the stimulation frequency at prepain intensity level the perceived non-painful sensation changed to a painful one. This indicates that the same set of intradental afferents may mediate both prepain and pain sensations.

Intradental A fibres are responsible for the sensitivity of dentine and are activated by the hydrodynamic mechanism (see the section on Mechanisms of dentine sensitivity later in this chapter) as indicated by the results of both human and animal experiments (Gysi 1900, Brännström 1963, Brännström and Johnson 1970, Brännström 1981, Hirvonen *et al*. 1984, Närhi 1985a, 1985b, Vongsavan and Matthews 1994). The fibres which respond to dentinal stimulation can be regarded as high-threshold mechanoreceptors or mechanical nociceptors (Burgess and Perl 1967, Georgopoulos 1976), because the actual stimulus for their activation is probably mechanical distortion of the peripheral pulp tissue.

The functional characteristics of pulpal C fibres are clearly different from those of A fibres. According to the single fibre recordings they have high thresholds (Närhi *et al*. 1982c, 1982d) and their receptive fields are located in the pulp (Närhi *et al*. 1982c, Jyväsjärvi and Kniffki 1987). Intense stimuli which reach the pulp proper are needed for their activation. Dentinal (hydrodynamic) stimulation seems to be ineffective (Närhi *et al*. 1982c, Närhi and Haegerstam 1983, Närhi *et al*. 1992b). As already mentioned, C fibres respond to heat (Närhi *et al*. 1982c, Närhi, 1985a) and cold (Närhi 1985a, Jyväsjärvi and Kniffki 1987). They are also activated by certain inflammatory mediators (Närhi 1985a, Närhi *et al*. 1992b). Both bradykinin and histamine applied to the exposed pulp induce activation of the C fibres and so does capsaicin, which is known to be a selective irritant for small (nociceptive and neuropeptide-containing) afferents (Kenins 1982, Närhi 1985a, Närhi et al. 1992b, Ikeda et al. 1997). Considering the characteristics of the pulpal C fibre function it can be concluded that the dull pulpal inflammatory pain may be related to the activation of this fibre group.

Intense heat and cold stimuli applied to cat canine teeth are able to induce an immediate or short-latency activation of intradental A fibres (Närhi 1985a, Jyväsjärvi and Kniffki 1987, Närhi et al. 1992b), probably due to dentinal fluid flow induced by the rapid temperature change (Brännström 1963, 1981). Firing of C fibres can be evoked if the stimulation is continued (Närhi et al. 1982c, 1992b, Jyväsjärvi and Kniffki 1987). The C fibre responses are induced with considerably longer latencies than A fibre firing and are, most probably, caused by a direct effect of the stimuli on the nerve endings in the pulp. Similar thermal stimulation of human teeth is able to evoke an immediate sharp pain sensation followed by dull, radiating pain (Hensel and Mann 1956, Jyväsjärvi and Kniffki 1987). Moreover, it has been shown in human experiments that selective activation of pulpal A and C fibres can induce sharp and dull pain, respectively (Ahlquist et al. 1985). Altogether, comparison of the intradental nerve responses and the evoked sensations in human subjects suggests that intradental A and C fibres may mediate different components of dental pain, sharp and dull, respectively. In this context it is also worth noting that dentinal stimulation, which in a great majority of cases induces sharp pain from human teeth (Kontturi-Närhi and Närhi 1993), seems to activate only pulpal A fibres in experimental animals (see above). The results from animal experiments using osmotic stimulation (Närhi et al. 1982a, Närhi and Hirvonen 1987, Närhi et al. 1992b) also suggest that intradental A fibres are able to encode the intensity of the stimuli applied to dentine.

Mechanisms of dentine sensitivity

The concept that the sensitivity of dentine is based on the stimulus-induced fluid flow in the

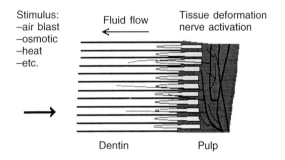

Figure 23.1

Hydrodynamic mechanism of pulp nerve activation. Any stimulus capable of removing fluid from the outer ends of the dentinal tubules induces a rapid outward fluid movement in the tubules due to high capillary forces. As a result the peripheral pulp tissue with the nerve endings is mechanically distorted and, consequently, the pulpal nociceptors are activated.

dentinal tubules and consequent nociceptor activation in the pulp/dentine border area (hydrodynamic mechanism; Figure 23.1) (Gysi 1900, Brännström 1963, 1981) is supported by a considerable amount of data from both human and animal experiments.

It has been shown in human studies that the patency of the dentinal tubules is a major characteristic of sensitive dentine (Brännström 1962, 1963, 1965, Absi et al. 1987, Närhi et al. 1992a). A significant positive correlation between the density of open dentinal tubules and the intensity of the pain responses induced from exposed cervical dentine surfaces has also been reported (Närhi and Kontturi-Närhi 1994). The condition of dentine with either open or blocked tubules is decisive regarding the hydraulic conductance of dentine (Pashley 1990, 1992) and thus stimulus-induced fluid flow in the dentinal tubules.

After drilling, the sensitivity of dentine can be significantly increased by acid-etching, which removes the smear layer that blocks the dentinal tubules (Brännström 1963, 1981). Correspondingly, the responsiveness of the intradental nerves to dentinal stimulation is significantly increased after acid-etching of drilled dentine surface, as shown in electrophysiological recordings performed on experimental animals (Närhi *et al.* 1982a, 1982b, Närhi and Haegerstam 1983, Panopoulos *et al.* 1983a, 1983b) and this change is related to the patency of the dentinal tubules as shown in scanning electron microscopic examination (Hirvonen *et al.* 1984). Blocking of the tubules with oxalates greatly reduces the sensitivity of the recorded nerve fibres (Hirvonen *et al.* 1984).

Further, in line with the hydrodynamic mechanism are the electrophysiological studies showing that the same individual intradental nerve fibres are activated by several different stimuli, such as probing and air-drying and hyperosmotic solutions applied to dentine (Närhi *et al.* 1982a, 1982b, Närhi 1985a, 1985b, Närhi and Hirvonen 1987, Närhi *et al.* 1992b), which are all able to induce fluid flow in the dentinal tubules as shown in vitro (Brännström 1963, Brännström and Johnson 1970, Horiuchi and Matthews 1973, Brännström 1981). Both electrophysiological recordings on experimental animals and human studies also indicate that in stimulation of dentine with hyperosmotic solutions, the intradental nerve activation is dependent on the osmotic pressure and ability to induce fluid flow in dentinal tubules rather than the chemical composition of the applied solutions (Anderson 1963, Anderson and Matthews 1967, Anderson *et al.* 1967, Närhi *et al.* 1982a, Närhi and Hirvonen 1987). Moreover, a direct relationship between the dentinal fluid flow and intradental nerve firing has been reported in electrophysiological studies (Vongsavan and Matthews 1994).

Therefore, it seems to be well established that the most important factor determining the sensitivity of dentine is the patency and, accordingly, the hydraulic conductance (Pashley 1990, 1992) of the dentinal tubules. Thus, blocking of the tubules should abolish dentinal pain symptoms effectively. In some cases, however, sensitivity may remain in spite of the tubule block (Närhi *et al.* 1992a). In such cases inflammatory reactions and consequent sensitization of the intradental nerves may be present. Knowledge about the effects of such reactions on the development of dentinal pain symptoms is limited. They may be especially significant when dentine with open tubules is chronically exposed, as in many clinical cases of dentine hypersensitivity (Närhi *et al.* 1992a).

Structural responses of pulp nerves to tissue injury and inflammation

As already mentioned, hydrodynamic stimulation of dentine activates intradental nerves as a result of fluid flow in the dentinal tubules and consequent mechanical distortion of the peripheral pulp tissue. The related morphological changes have been examined in studies on both human and animal teeth and they have shown that such stimulation may result in tissue injury in the pulp–dentine border area (Brännström 1963, 1981, Lilja *et al.* 1982, Hirvonen and Närhi 1986). The degree of the injury is dependent on the type and intensity of the applied stimuli and may include disruption of the odontoblast layer as a result of aspiration of the cells into the dentinal tubules (Brännström 1963, 1981, Lilja *et al.* 1982). Also, the nerve endings in the area seem to get injured (Närhi *et al.* 1987, Byers 1992). However, it has been shown in acute experiments on dog teeth that the responsiveness of the recorded intradental nerve fibres to dentinal stimulation may not be abolished in spite of the induced morphological changes (Hirvonen and Närhi 1986). Furthermore, in human studies considerable tissue damage and pronounced inflammatory changes can be found in the peripheral pulp under sensitive dentine (Brännström 1981, Lilja *et al.* 1982). These results indicate that the sensitivity of dentine is not dependent on the existence of odontoblasts and nerve fibres in the dentinal tubules. In fact, the tissue injury induced by hydrodynamic stimulation, together with the release of neuropeptides from the activated nerve endings, may be important for the initiation of pulpal inflammatory reactions and consequent nerve sensitization.

Recent studies also show that the intradental nociceptors can actively respond to injury, resulting in profound morphological changes. These changes include sprouting of the nerve endings and an increase in their neuropeptide content. These responses may be largely connected to the efferent functions of the pulpal nociceptive nerve fibres, i.e. to the regulation of the inflammatory reactions (Byers and Närhi 1999). Other studies indicate that the sensory nerves may be important for the defence and repair reactions of the pulp tissue (Byers 1992, 1996). In rats, tissue regeneration was shown to be impaired in denervated teeth as compared with the controls (Byers and Taylor 1993).

Intradental nerves contain numerous neuropeptides, including substance P (SP) and calcitonin gene-related peptide (CGRP) (Gazelius *et al*. 1981, Olgart 1985, Kimberly and Byers 1988, Byers 1992, 1996). After dentine exposure with pulp injury, sprouting of the CGRP immunoreactive nerve fibres has been shown to occur (Byers 1992, 1996). Also, the intensity of the CGRP immunolabelling is increased (Kimberly and Byers 1988, Byers 1992). The changes in the SP immunoreactivity seem to be less pronounced (Byers 1992). The morphological changes reflect the plasticity of the peripheral nociceptive innervation and its capability to respond to altered environmental conditions. In addition, the regional changes in the density of the innervation in the dentine and pulp might result in changes in the regional sensitivity of the affected tooth.

It can be seen that the morphological neural responses induced by pulpal tissue injury are well established. The changes in the nociceptor structure seem to be extensive and could have a significant effect on the sensory function of the pulpal nociceptors (Närhi *et al*. 1996). However, only a few electrophysiological recordings have tried to correlate the morphological changes to the nerve function and, thus, knowledge about the possible functional correlates of the morphological changes is limited.

The role of inflammatory reactions in pulpal and dentinal pain

As described earlier, several inflammatory mediators have been shown to either sensitize or activate intradental nociceptors in cat and dog teeth. The sensitivity of pulpal C fibres to histamine and bradykinin may be important for the development of pain symptoms in pulpal inflammation (Närhi 1985a, Närhi *et al*. 1992b). With regard to dentinal pain it is important to note that in acute experiments on cat and dog teeth serotonin has been shown both to activate intradental A fibres and to sensitize them to

external stimulation (Olgart 1974, Närhi *et al*. 1992b, Ngassapa *et al*. 1992). After local application of serotonin (5-HT) deep in dentine, close to the nerve endings the proportions of the nerve fibres responding to various hydrodynamic stimuli are significantly increased (Närhi *et al*. 1992b, Ngassapa *et al*. 1992). Prostaglandins seem to be active in heat-induced sensitization of the intradental nerves (Ahlberg 1978a). Thus, in addition to the condition of the dentine, inflammatory reactions in the pulp may be important in the aetiology of dentine hypersensitivity. It should also be noted that intense thermal stimulation may activate intradental nerves by a direct effect, in addition to the hydrodynamic mechanism (Matthews 1977, Närhi *et al*. 1994). Because of sensitization of the nociceptors such responses may be significant for induction of pain symptoms in inflamed teeth (Närhi *et al*. 1992a, Ngassapa *et al*. 1992).

Low-level release of neuropeptides from the sensory nerve endings can occur even in healthy teeth without any firing of action potentials (Olgart and Kerezoudis 1994, Olgart 1996a, 1996b) and it may be needed for the maintenance of the tissue homeostasis, e.g. sufficient blood flow under normal conditions. In response to external irritation and consequent nerve firing, sufficient amounts of sensory neuropeptides, CGRP and substance P are released to induce a neurogenic inflammatory reaction which may initiate the inflammation cascade (Olgart 1996a, 1996b). The released neuropeptides function in close interaction with the other inflammatory mediators (Olgart 1996a, 1996b). The neurogenic inflammatory responses can be induced in normal healthy teeth, but they may be even more pronounced in injured and inflamed pulps with nociceptor sprouting and increased neuropeptide activity.

Sensory neuropeptides have been localized especially in unmyelinated nerve fibres, but they are also present in some small-diameter myelinated afferents (Byers 1992, 1996). Thus, activation of these nerve fibre groups may be particularly significant for the initiation of the neurogenic inflammatory reactions in the pulp. C fibres may be especially important, but smaller-diameter slow-conducting A-δ fibres may also be involved. As regards the neurogenic inflammatory responses to hydrodynamic stimulation of dentine, it is interesting to note that single fibre recordings performed on cats and dogs indicate that only the faster conducting intradental nerve fibres can be activated by dentinal stimulation (Närhi *et al.* 1982a, 1982b, Närhi *et al.* 1992a, 1992b). However, according to Olgart (1996a, 1996b), dentinal stimulation results in pulpal blood flow responses which indicate that the activated (myelinated) nerve fibres are able to induce neurogenic vascular effects and, accordingly, these fibres may contain neuropeptides and release them in response to stimulation. It is also possible that some nerve fibres which are insensitive to hydrodynamic stimulation in healthy teeth become responsive when the pulp is injured and inflamed.

According to the results of single fibre recordings performed on experimental animals, a considerable proportion of pulpal A fibres does not respond to hydrodynamic stimulation of the coronal dentine in normal healthy teeth (Matthews 1977, Närhi *et al.* 1992a, 1992b, 1994, 1996). A majority of such fibres are of slow A-type according to the conduction velocities (Närhi *et al.* 1996). Their receptive fields are located in the pulp and they only respond to mechanical and intense thermal stimulation of the pulp proper (Närhi *et al.* 1994, Yamamoto and Närhi 1994). It seems that the function of this fibre group can be significantly affected by pulpal inflammation. In experiments on inflamed dog teeth it was found that the proportion of the fibres responding to dentinal stimulation was significantly higher compared with uninflamed controls (Närhi *et al.* 1996). The effect was most pronounced in the slow conducting A fibres (Närhi *et al.* 1996). Activation of such 'silent' nociceptors in inflamed teeth may have a significant effect on the development of dentinal and pulpal pain symptoms.

The receptive field of each single intradental A fibre which responds to hydrodynamic stimulation of dentine is usually composed of a small spot on the exposed dentine surface and can be localized and mapped by gentle probing (Närhi *et al.* 1992a, 1992b, Yamamoto and Närhi 1994, Närhi *et al.* 1994). A small proportion of the fibres have multiple receptive fields and in some cases an individual fibre may innervate both coronal and cervical dentine (Närhi *et al.* 1994, Yamamoto and Närhi 1994). The inflammation-induced sprouting of the pulpal nociceptors could result in an increase in the size of the

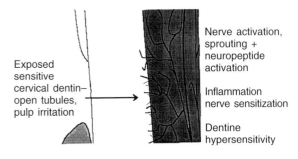

Exposed sensitive cervical dentin—open tubules, pulp irritation → Nerve activation, sprouting + neuropeptide activation / Inflammation nerve sensitization / Dentine hypersensitivity

Figure 23.2

The possible effects of pulp irritation and consequent inflammatory reactions on cervical dentine sensitivity. External irritation through the open dentinal tubules may result in nerve sensitization. Also sprouting of the nerve endings may take place resulting in an increase in the size of the receptive fields of individual fibres. This would result in spatial summation of the nerve activity and an increase in the sensitivity of dentine.

receptive fields of the fibres. In fact, results from studies with dog teeth indicate that such changes in the receptive fields of single fibres may occur (Närhi *et al.* 1996). Widening of the receptive fields of the individual fibres would result in increased overlap between the receptive areas and, consequently, spatial summation in the nerve activity and an increase in dentine sensitivity (Figure 23.2).

The branching nerve axons with receptive areas in both the tooth crown and the cervical dentine (Närhi *et al.* 1994, Yamamoto and Närhi 1994) may have significant effects in the spread of neurogenic inflammatory reactions in the pulp and in the development of cervical dentine hypersensitivity. Activation of their coronal endings could result in axon reflexes which would release neuropeptides in the pulp–dentine border in the cervical area of the tooth. This could induce neurogenic inflammation and thus have an effect on the sensitivity of the cervical dentine. For example, leaky fillings irritating the coronal pulp could modify the sensitivity of cervical dentine in human teeth. In fact, replacement of old fillings in hypersensitive teeth may significantly increase the efficacy of the treatment of cervical dentine hypersensitivity (Hovgaard *et al.* 1991).

In addition to the neural responses, both short- and long-term structural changes in dentine may significantly affect dentine sensitivity (Pashley 1990, 1992). Such changes include accumulation of material originating from the pulp, such as cellular debris and plasma proteins, into the dentinal tubules (Hirvonen *et al.* 1992). Also mineralization on the dentine surface, within the tubules and in the pulp plays a role (Pashley 1990, 1992). The rate and extent of these changes may also be affected by the pulpal inflammatory reactions.

As already mentioned, there is great variability in the occurrence and intensity of pain in connection with pulpal inflammation. The correlation between the actual pulpal histopathological changes and the clinical pain symptoms is poor (Seltzer *et al.* 1965, Brännström 1981, Mumford 1982). Several local factors in the pulp have been proposed to regulate the inflammatory reactions and also nociceptor activation (Olgart 1996b, Närhi *et al.* 1996). These include local opioids, somatostatin and noradrenaline. They may have multiple effects on the inflammatory reactions, e.g. reduction of the CGRP and substance P release from the afferent nerve endings (Olgart 1996b). Hirvonen *et al.* (1998) found that local application of a somatostatin antagonist in deep dentinal cavities significantly increased nerve activity in inflamed dog teeth. Preliminary results also indicate that naloxone may have similar effects (Närhi and Hirvonen, unpublished observations). The results indicate that somatostatin and local opioids may have a tonic inhibitory effect on the peripheral nociceptors in inflamed tissues. Such local mechanisms may partly explain the clinical finding that pulpitis may so frequently be almost or completely symptomless.

Changes in pain impulse transmission in the central nervous system

A number of studies have shown that injury and inflammation in the peripheral tissues may result in profound morphological and functional changes in the pain pathways in the central nervous system (CNS). These include both short- and long-term changes and they may play a significant role in the development of various chronic pain conditions. For example, it has been shown in acute experiments on human subjects that repeated painful stimulation may result in an increase in the intensity of the experienced pain responses (wind-up) and this change seems to be due to activation of certain cell membrane receptors, e.g. *N*-methyl-D-aspartate (NMDA) receptors of the second order neurons of the pain pathway (Price *et al.* 1994; see also Chapter 24). Also, noxious stimulation of the dental pulp results in discrete morphological changes in the trigeminal second order neurons (Coimbra and Coimbra 1994). Based on electrophysiological recordings it has been suggested that functional changes in the CNS induced by peripheral nerve injuries may be significant in the development of chronic orofacial pain (Sessle 1978, 1987). The extent to which chronic inflammatory conditions in the orofacial area may play a role in the development and maintenance of various pain conditions, including dentine hypersensitivity, is not known.

The pain symptoms related to exposed cervical dentine may be more or less persistent, extremely intense and continue for years (Närhi *et al.* 1992a). In this respect dentine hypersensitivity can be regarded as a chronic pain condition in which CNS mechanisms could be activated. It is also interesting to note that a considerable variation in the intensity of the pain symptoms over time has been reported in individual patients with dentine hypersensitivity (Pashley 1990, Närhi *et al.* 1992a). A number of peripheral factors have been proposed to explain such a variation, but it is possible that changes in the mechanisms of pain impulse transmission in the CNS may also be significant.

References

Absi EG, Addy M, Adams D (1987) Dentine hypersensitivity. A study of the patency of dentinal tubules in sensitive and non-sensitive cervical dentine. *J Clin Periodontol* **14**:280–4.

Ahlberg KF (1978a) Dose dependent inhibition of sensory nerve activity in the feline dental pulp by anti-inflammatory drugs. *Acta Physiol Scand* **102**:434–40.

Ahlberg KF (1978b) Influence of local noxious heat stimulation on sensory nerve activity in the feline dental pulp. *Acta Physiol Scand* **103**:71–80.

Ahlquist ML, Edwall LGA, Franzén OG, Haegerstam GAT (1984) Perception of pulpal pain as a function of intradental nerve activity. *Pain* **19**:353–66.

Ahlquist ML, Franzen OG, Edwall LGA et al (1985) Quality of pain sensations following local application of algogenic agents on the exposed human tooth pulp: a psychophysiological and electrophysiological study. In: Fields HL, ed, *Advances in Pain Research and Therapy*, Vol 9, 351–59. Raven Press: New York.

Anderson DJ (1963) Chemical and osmotic excitants of pain in human dentine. In: Anderson DJ, ed, *Sensory Mechanisms in Dentine*, 88–93. Pergamon Press: Oxford.

Anderson DJ, Matthews B (1967) Osmotic stimulation of human dentine and the distribution of dental pain thresholds. *Arch Oral Biol* **12**:417–26.

Anderson DJ, Matthews B, Shelton LE (1967) Variations in the sensitivity to osmotic stimulation of human dentine. *Arch Oral Biol* **12**:43–7.

Beasley WL, Holland GR (1978) A quantitative analysis of the innervation of the pulp of cat's canine tooth. *J Comp Neurol* **178**:487–94.

Brännström M (1962) Observations on exposed dentine and the corresponding pulp tissue. A preliminary study with replica and routine histology. *Odontologisk Revy* **13**:235–45.

Brännström M (1963) A hydrodynamic mechanism in the transmission of pain-producing stimuli through the dentine. In: Anderson DJ, ed, *Sensory Mechanisms in Dentine*, 73–9. Pergamon Press: Oxford.

Brännström M (1965) The surface of sensitive dentine. *Odontologisk Revy* **16**, 293–9.

Brännström M (1981) *Dentin and Pulp in Restorative Dentistry*. Dental Therapeutics AB: Nacka, Sweden.

Brännström M, Johnson G (1970) Movements of the dentine and pulp liquids on application of thermal stimuli. An in vitro study. *Acta Odontol Scand* **28**:59–70.

Burgess PR, Perl ER (1967) Myelinated afferent fibers responding specifically to noxious stimulation of the skin. *J Physiol* **190**:541–62.

Byers MR (1984) Dental sensory receptors. *Int Rev Neurobiol* **25**:39–94.

Byers MR (1992) Effect of inflammation on dental sensory nerves and vice versa. *Proc Finn Dent Soc* **88** (Suppl.1):459–506.

Byers MR (1996) Neuropeptide immunoreactivity in dental sensory nerves: variation related to primary odontoblast function and survival. In: Shimono M, Maeda T, Suda H, Takahashi K, eds, *Dentin/pulp Complex*, 124–9. Quintessence: Tokyo.

Byers MR, Närhi M (1999) Dental injury models: experimental tool for understanding neuroinflammatory interactions and polymodal nociceptor function. *Crit Rev Oral Biol Med* **10**:4–39.

Byers MR, Taylor PE (1993) Effect of sensory denervation on the response of rat molar pulp to exposure injury. *J Dent Res* **72**:613–18.

Coimbra F, Coimbra A (1994) Dental noxious input reaches the subnucleus caudalis of the trigeminal complex in the rat, as shown by c-fos expression upon thermal or mechanical stimulation. *Neurosci Lett* **173**:201–4.

Dong WK, Chudler EH, Martin RF (1985) Physiological properties of intradental mechanoreceptors. *Brain Res* **334**:389–95.

Dong WK, Shiwaku T, Kawakami Y, Chulder EH (1993) Static and dynamic responses of periodontal ligament mechanoreceptors and intradental mechanoreceptors. *J Neurophysiol* **69**:1567–82.

Gazelius B, Brodin E, Olgart L (1981) Depletion of substance P-like immunoreactivity in the cat dental pulp by antidromic nerve stimulation. *Acta Physiol Scand* **111**:319–27.

Georgopoulos AP (1976) Functional properties of primary afferent units probably related to pain mechanisms in primate glabrous skin. *J Neurophysiol* **39**:71–83.

Gysi A (1900) An attempt to explain the sensitiveness of dentin. *Br J Dent Sci* **43**:865–8.

Hensel H, Mann G (1956) Temperaturschmerz und Wärmeleitug im menschlichen Zahn. *Stoma* **9**:76–85.

Hirvonen T, Närhi M (1986) The effect of dentinal stimulation on pulp nerve function and pulp morphology in the dog. *J Dent Res* **65**:1290–3.

Hirvonen TJ, Närhi MVO, Hakumäki MOK (1984) The excitability of dog pulp nerves in relation to the condition of the dentin surface. *J Endodontics* **10**:294–8.

Hirvonen T, Ngassapa D, Närhi M (1992) Relation of dentin sensitivity to histological changes in dog teeth with exposed and stimulated dentin. *Proc Finn Dent Soc* **88** (Suppl 1):133–41.

Hirvonen T, Hippi P, Närhi M (1998) The effect of an opioid antagonist and a somatostatin antagonist on the nerve function in normal and inflamed dental pulps. *J Dent Res* **77**:1329 (abstract).

Holland GR, Robinson PP (1983) The number and size of axons at the apex of the cat's canine tooth. *Anat Rec* **205**:215–22.

Horiuchi H, Matthews B (1973) In vitro observations on fluid flow through human dentine caused by pain-producing stimuli. *Arch Oral Biol* **18**:275–94.

Hovgaard O, Larsen MJ, Fejerskov O (1991) Tooth hypersensitivity in relation to the quality of restorations. *J Dent Res* **70** (Special issue):abstract 1667.

Ikeda H, Tokita Y, Suda H (1997) Capsaicin-sensitive A-delta fibers in cat tooth pulp. *J Dent Res* **76**:1341–49.

Jyväsjärvi E, Kniffki K-D (1987) Cold stimulation of teeth: a comparison between the responses of cat intradental A and C fibres and human sensation. *J Physiol* **391**:193–207.

Kenins P (1982) Responses of single nerve fibres to capsaicin applied to the skin. *Neurosci Lett* **29**:83–8.

Kimberly CL, Byers MR (1988) Inflammation of rat molar pulp and periodontium causes increased calcitonin gene-related peptide and axonal sprouting. *Anat Rec* **222**:289–300.

Kontturi-Närhi V, Närhi M (1993) Testing sensitive dentine in man. *Int Endodontic J* **26**:4.

Lilja J, Nordenvall K-J, Brännström M (1982) Dentine sensitivity, odontoblasts and nerves under dessicated or infected experimental cavities. *Swed J Dent Res* **6**:93–103.

McGrath PA, Gracely RH, Dubner R, Heft MW (1983) Non-pain and pain sensations evoked by tooth pulp stimulation. *Pain* **15**:377–88.

Matthews B (1977) Responses of intradental nerves to electrical and thermal stimulation of teeth in dogs. *J Physiol* **264**:461–4.

Mumford JM (1982) *Orofacial Pain. Aetiology, Diagnosis and Treatment*, 3rd edn. Churchill Livingstone: Edinburgh.

Mumford JM, Bowsher D (1976) Pain and protopathic sensibility. A review with particular reference to teeth. *Pain* **2**:223–43.

Närhi MVO (1985a) The characteristics of intradental sensory units and their responses to stimulation. *J Dent Res* **64**:564–71.

Närhi MVO (1985b) Dentin sensitivity: a review. *J Biol Buccale* **13**:75–96.

Närhi M, Haegerstam G (1983) Intradental nerve activity induced by reduced pressure applied to exposed dentine in the cat. *Acta Physiol Scand* **119**:381–6.

Närhi MVO, Hirvonen T (1987) The response of dog intradental nerves to hypertonic solutions of $CaCl_2$ and NaCl, and other stimuli, applied to exposed dentine. *Arch Oral Biol* **32**:781–6.

Närhi M, Kontturi-Närhi V (1994) Sensitivity and surface condition of dentin – a SEM-replica study. *J Dent Res* **73**:122 (abstract).

Närhi MVO, Hirvonen TJ, Hakumäki MOK (1982a) Activation of intradental nerves in the dog to some stimuli applied to the dentine. *Arch Oral Biol* **27**:1053–8.

Närhi MVO, Hirvonen TJ, Hakumäki MOK (1982b) Responses of intradental nerve fibres to stimulation of dentine and pulp. *Acta Physiol Scand* **115**:173–8.

Närhi M, Jyväsjärvi E, Hirvonen T, Huopaniemi T (1982c) Activation of heat-sensitive nerve fibres in the dental pulp of the cat. *Pain* **14**:317–26.

Närhi M, Virtanen A, Huopaniemi T, Hirvonen T (1982d) Conduction velocities of single pulp nerve fibre units in the cat. *Acta Physiol Scand* **116**:209–13.

Närhi M, Byers MR, Hirvonen T, Dong WK (1987) The effect of external irritation on the morphology and function of pulpal and dentinal nerves. In: *Proceedings of the Workshop on Dentin and Dentinal Reactions in the Oral Cavity*, 77–84. IRL Press: London.

Närhi M, Kontturi-Närhi V, Hirvonen T, Ngassapa D (1992a) Neurophysiological mechanisms of dentin hypersensitivity. *Proc Finn Dent Soc* **88** (Suppl 1):15–22.

Närhi M, Jyväsjärvi E, Virtanen A et al. (1992b) Role of intradental A- and C-type nerve fibres in dental pain mechanisms. *Proc Finn Dent Soc* **88** (Suppl 1):507–16.

Närhi M, Yamamoto H, Ngassapa M, Hirvonen T (1994) Dentin hypersensitivity – the neurophysiological basis and the role of inflammatory reactions. *Arch Oral Biol* **39**(Suppl.):S23–S30.

Närhi M, Yamamoto H, Ngassapa D (1996) Function of intradental nociceptors in normal and inflamed teeth. In: Shimono M, Maeda T, Suda H, Takahashi K, eds, *Dentin/pulp Complex*, 136–40. Quintessence: Tokyo.

Ngassapa D, Närhi M, Hirvonen T (1992) Effect of serotonin (5-HT) and calcitonin gene-related peptide (CGRP) on the function of intradental nerves in the dog. *Proc Finn Dent Soc* **88** (Suppl 1):143–8.

Olgart L (1974) Excitation of intradental sensory units by pharmacological agents. *Acta Physiol Scand* **92**:48–55.

Olgart L (1985) The role of local factors in dentin and pulp in intradental pain mechanisms. *J Dent Res* **64** (Special issue):572–8.

Olgart L (1996a) Neural control of pulpal blood flow. *Crit Rev Oral Biol Med* **7**:159–71.

Olgart L (1996b) Neurogenic components of pulp inflammation. In: Shimono M, Maeda T, Suda H, Takahashi K, eds. *Dentin/pulp Complex*, 169–75. Quintessence: Tokyo.

Olgart L, Gazelius B (1977) Effects of adrenaline and felypressin (octapressin) on blood flow and sensory nerve activity in the tooth. *Acta Odontol Scand* **35**:69–75.

Olgart L, Kerezoudis N (1994) Nerve–pulp interactions. *Arch Oral Biol* **39**(Suppl.):S47–S54.

Panopoulos P, Gazelius B, Olgart L (1983a) Responses of feline intradental sensory nerves to hyperosmotic stimulation of dentine. *Acta Odontol Scand* **41**:369–75.

Panopoulos P, Mejare B, Edwall L (1983b) Effects of ammonia and organic acids on the intradental sensory nerve activity. *Acta Odontol Scand* **41**:209–15.

Paphangkorakit J, Osborn JW (1997) The effect of pressure on a maximum incisal bite force in man. *Arch Oral Biol* **42**:11–17.

Paphangkorakit J, Osborn JW (1998) Effects on human maximum bite force of biting on a softer or harder object. *Arch Oral Biol* **43**:833–9.

Pashley DH (1990) Mechanisms of dentin sensitivity. *Dent Clin North Am* **34**:449–73.

Pashley DH (1992) Dentin permeability and dentin sensitivity. *Proc Finn Dent Soc* **88** (Suppl 1):31–7.

Price DP, Mao J, Frenk H, Mayer DJ (1994) The N-methyl-D-aspartate receptor antagonist dextrometorphan selectively reduces temporal summation of second pain in man. *Pain* **59**:165–74.

Reader A, Foreman DW (1981) An ultrastructural quantitative investigation of human intradental innervation. *J Endodontics* **7**:493–9.

Seltzer S, Bender IB, Ziontz M (1963) The dynamics of pulp inflammation: correlations between diagnostic data and actual histopathological findings in the pulp. *Oral Surg Oral Med Oral Pathol* **16**: 969–77.

Seltzer S, Bender IB, Nazimov H (1965) Differential diagnosis of pulp conditions. *Oral Surg Oral Med Oral Pathol* **19**:383–91.

Sessle BJ (1978) Oral-facial pain: old puzzles, new postulates. *Int Dent J* **28**:28–42.

Sessle BJ (1987) The neurobiology of facial and dental pain: present knowledge, future directions. *J Dent Res* **66**:962–81.

Sigurdsson A, Maixner W (1994) Effects of experimental clinical noxious counterirritants on pain perception. *Pain* **57**:265–75.

Taylor PE, Byers MR (1990) An immunocytochemical study of the response of nerves containing calcitonin gene-related peptide to microabscess formation and healing in rat molars. *Arch Oral Biol* **33**:629–38.

Taylor PE, Byers MR, Redd PR (1988) Sprouting of CGRP nerve fibers in response to dentin injury in rat molars. *Brain Res* **461**:371–6.

Virtanen ASJ, Huopaniemi T, Närhi MVO et al. (1987) The effect of temporal parameters on subjective sensations evoked by electrical tooth stimulation. *Pain* **30**:361–71.

Vongsavan N, Matthews B (1994) The relationship between fluid flow in dentine and the discharge of intradental nerves. *Arch Oral Biol* **39**(Suppl.):S140.

Yamamoto H, Närhi M (1994) Function of nerve fibers innervating different parts of dentine. *Arch Oral Biol* **39**(Suppl.):S141.

24

Biochemical, physiological and psychological aspects of pain and pain assessment

John I Alexander

Introduction

Pain is an unpleasant sensory and emotional experience associated with actual or potential tissue damage, or described in terms of such damage (definition of the Taxonomy Group of the International Association for the Study of Pain). It can be described in terms of its site (angina pectoris, toothache, headache) or its cause (ischaemic pain, neuralgia, intermittent claudication). The best treatment is usually removal of the cause (although this is not always successful in relieving the pain) and, for this reason, analgesic drugs may be withheld until a diagnosis is made. However, untreated pain can itself cause serious effects and increase morbidity.

Afferent pain pathways from the periphery to the brain

Although the afferent pain pathways will be described from the periphery to the higher centres, these are an oversimplification. The pathways do not transmit pain, since, even if the perception of a noxious stimulus (nociception) is transmitted without facilitation or inhibition, the stimulus does not necessarily result in pain. Only some of these pathways respond solely to nociceptive impulses. Moreover, nociception is the product of stimulus, inhibition, facilitation and induction of responses which appeared not

to be present until after tissue damage (Wall 1994). Some of the inflammatory mediators of nociception – histamine, reactive oxygen species, protons, bradykinin – most probably enhance nociception; others such as serotonin, adenosine, even prostanoids, may sometimes inhibit it (Dray 1994).

Nociceptive nerve fibres

The axons of primary afferents end in the skin and other structures after branching profusely. Near the peripheral end, the perineural sheaths are missing and the Schwann cells are irregular.

The nerves vary in size and conduction velocity. The larger nerves have individual myelin sheaths which reduce the flow of charge laterally, thereby increasing it along the length of the nerve. The change in transmembrane potential, or impulse generation, moves quickly from one gap in the myelin sheath to the next (saltatory conduction). This is faster than solely cell membrane conduction. The larger the thickness of the myelin sheath, the less is the charge lost laterally, the further apart are the gaps in the myelin (nodes of Ranvier) and the faster is the conduction of impulses along the length of the nerve. The large myelinated nerves (A-α, A-β) therefore conduct impulses faster than the thinly myelinated nerves (A-δ) or the unmyelinated C nerve fibres which latter conduct impulses arriving from, although not exclusively, noxious or potentially noxious stimuli.

Receptors

The large myelinated nerve fibres end in specialized encapsulated structures which are transducers converting touch, distortion, deceleration, etc. to neuronal impulses. Conversely, most of the endings of A-δ or C fibres terminate as free nerve endings, the axon surrounded only by its basal lamina and a Schwann cell. In the tooth, both myelinated and unmyelinated endings lose their Schwann cell sheath in the pulp and the fibre components (about 1 μm diameter) respond to low intensity mechanical, chemical or thermal stimuli (see also Chapter 23).

In the human skin, about 75% of the A-δ fibre-related receptors and about 5% of the C fibre receptors respond to low threshold mechanical, thermal or chemical stimuli and the remainder to high threshold, i.e. tissue-threatening or tissue-damaging (noxious) stimuli, and are called nociceptors. These are subdivided into those which respond to mechanical stimuli (high threshold mechanoreceptors or HTM), those which respond to mechanical and thermal stimuli and those which respond to mechanical, thermal and chemical stimuli (polymodal nociceptors) (Lynn 1994).

Some nociceptors respond best to high threshold or noxious stimuli, but also respond to lower threshold, or only threatening, stimuli. About 20% of the afferent nerves with high threshold mechanoreceptors supply both skin and subcutaneous structures such as fascia. Although these mechanoreceptors do not normally respond to noxious heat or cold or chemicals, they may do so after the tissue is subjected to repeated heat stimuli. This is called *sensitization*.

Whereas small myelinated mechanoreceptors have small receptive fields of about 1–2 mm of differing densities in different parts of the body, the C-polymodal nociceptive afferents have receptive fields of up to 15 mm^2. The greatest sensitivity to thermal stimuli is around 45–51°C. The myelinated mechanothermal nociceptors (A-δ) have a greater sensitivity to noxious thermal stimuli than mechanical nociceptors and are sensitized by repeated heating. Cold receptors respond to noxious cold, but not to mechanical stimuli.

Verbal reports of pain correlate with C fibre discharge, but the threshold temperature for activating the nociceptors is lower than that of the thermal pain threshold, suggesting that temporal summation or inhibition of inhibitory neurones is necessary for pain perception.

A transient stimulus like a pin-prick produces firstly a pricking pain and secondly, after a short pain-free interval, a longer burning pain. This time gap is elicited only in the limbs and in the anterior trunk wall below the third thoracic dermatome.

Muscle pain is mainly due to stimulation of unmyelinated muscle afferents, is deep and aching in character and is diffuse and hard to locate. Joint nociceptors variously respond to innocuous joint movement, extreme joint movement or do not respond at all in normal joints. Inflammation increases the background and stimulation rates of impulses of these, and low threshold units may respond where previously they were unresponsive. Joint pain is characteristically dull and aching. The periosteum has a low nociceptive threshold via A-δ and C fibres. The nerves also run in the canals in the bone.

Visceral pain and nociception are different from the above. The autonomic afferents from the viscera are mainly associated with visceral reflexes but, under conditions such as inflammation, can initiate feelings of fullness, distension or pain. The ratio of small nerve fibres to large is much greater in the afferent nerves from the viscera than from those in the skin. There are also many fewer nerves with more branching and about 100% overlap in their receptor areas. There is therefore less localization of the stimulus, although the intensity can be at least as great.

The innervation of teeth is both intradental and periodontal. Non-pain sensation by just-threshold tooth stimulation demonstrates innervation by both A-δ, C and some A-β fibres. Most afferent C fibres are activated by heat, but A-δ fibres respond most to rapid movements of dentinal fluid caused by mechanical, chemical and cold stimuli. The application of cold (e.g. ethyl chloride spray) produces a sharp pain (similar to a prick in the skin), but heat causes a dull ache.

Indeed, teeth exemplify the distinction between the sharp sensation provoked by A-δ stimulation and the duller sensation by that of C fibres. Sensory fibres in teeth enter the root and coronal pulp. After branching, they form endings along the blood vessels, in a plexus near the periphery of the coronal pulp and in the pulp–dentine border, including the inner 0.2 mm of the dentinal tubules. The endings of the latter are free and uncovered. Dentinal innervation is found most (>50%) around the tip of the coronal pulp (pulp horn), less in the mid-crown and least in the roots. Stimulation of the dentine causes a sensation which is said to be most sharp in the tip of the crown, less sharp in the mid-crown and least sharp in the *normal* root.

Teeth also demonstrate the relative lack of localization of C fibre sensation. Pain from pulpitis tends not to be localized to one tooth, but is felt in adjacent teeth or teeth on the opposing arch. Dentinal pain from exposure of the tubules to oral fluids and thereafter heat, cold, highly osmotic or mechanical stimuli tends to cause localized pain.

Nociception from the nociceptor to the dorsal horn

The nociceptive C and A-δ fibres have their cell bodies in the dorsal root ganglion which, for most spinal nerves, lies in the intervertebral foramina. The trigeminal afferent ganglion serves nociception from the face and teeth. The proximal axon usually travels with the dorsal root, through Lissauer's tract, to synapse in the dorsal horn of the spinal cord. However, some of the smaller nerves, sometimes as many as 30%, reach the dorsal horn by the ventral root (Bonica 1990). The nociceptive fibres tend to be concentrated in the lateral part of the dorsal root. The morphology and physiology of the medullary dorsal horn (the trigeminal subnucleus caudalis) are very similar to that of the spinal dorsal horn.

Within the dorsal horn, there is a convergence of visceral and somatic neurones serving nociception, which is segmentally distributed, although some afferent fibres may travel a segment or two rostrally or caudally before synapsing. There is also marked branching of the fibres within segments and spread medially and laterally.

Morphology of dorsal horn (Bonica 1990, Dubner and Basbaum 1994)

The spinal cord grey matter is divided into several layers or laminae. Of these laminae I–VI

correspond to the dorsal horn. Lamina I is called the marginal zone. The substantia gelatinosa (SG) is variously ascribed to lamina II or to laminae II and III. If lamina II is described as the SG, it is usually subdivided into an inner (IIi) and an outer (IIo) part. Laminae III and IV are most usually called the nucleus proprius and lamina V the neck of the dorsal horn or the spinal nucleus.

The A-β fibres (which serve touch, proprioception, etc.) branch before entering the dorsal horn. Most fibres pass medially to enter the dorsal columns, either extending initially a short distance caudally or continuing rostrally to the medulla. Some collateral branches enter the dorsal horn, passing down to lamina V. Most of these reverse their direction and terminate in lamina III, but some end in laminae IV, V, VI, even VIII and IX, where they terminate directly on motor neurones – making monosynaptic reflexes such as the knee jerk possible.

A-δ fibres run from the lateral part of the dorsal rootlet into the medial part of Lissauer's tract. They terminate in laminae I, IIo, III, IV and V and some descend to lamina X around the central canal.

C fibres enter the dorsal horn from the medial Lissauer's tract and terminate in laminae I, IIo and V. The mediolateral dimension and terminal branching or arborization of C fibres is much less than that of A-δ collaterals and they form tangential or longitudinal slabs or bushy terminals.

Fine muscle afferents, both high threshold myelinated mechanoreceptors and C muscle afferents, terminate in laminae I and V.

Sympathetic A-δ and C fibres terminate mainly in laminae I and V, but some synapse in laminae IV, VI, VII and X. Visceral afferents also synapse on cells in laminae I and V that are excited by somatic afferents – which are therefore called viscerosomatic dorsal horn neurones.

The second–order neurones can also be differentiated by size and receptive field (Table 24.1).

Table 24.1 Size of dorsal horn nerve cells and their receptive fields

Lamina	Size (μm)	Receptor field	Dynamic range
I	8–10	Small	
II	7	Medium	
III	9	Medium	
IV	15–45	Medium	Narrow
V	20–40	Large	Narrow and wide
VI	25–50	Large	Wide

The substantia gelatinosa contains small neurones which lie rather superficially in lamina II and which receive input from small diameter C fibres. Although some of their axons ascend to higher centres, most synapse at the segment of entry or within one or two segments and appear to be involved in the spatial or modality convergence of information onto neurones in the deeper parts of the spinal cord. The larger sensory neurones are found either in lamina I or lamina V. They respond both to nociceptive and non-nociceptive stimuli, i.e. they show modality convergence. Those in lamina I receive input from relatively few C and A-δ fibres, have small receptive fields and may have a function in localizing the noxious stimulus. Those in lamina V receive input from many nociceptive nerve fibres, some relayed from the small neurones in other laminae. They are excited by noxious stimuli from a large area of body surface and probably code nociceptive intensity rather than localization. The axons of these neurones in laminae I and V cross over the midline and ascend in the anterolateral tract to the brainstem and, usually, the thalamus (Forrest 1998).

Dynamic range

Some cells in the dorsal horn respond only to innocuous stimuli, to high threshold mechanical stimuli or to noxious stimuli. These are said to have a narrow dynamic range. Others are multireceptive: they respond in a frequency-dependent way to stimuli of increasing intensity and receive convergent input from cutaneous, visceral and muscle afferents. They produce a sustained discharge in response to pressure, but are rapidly adapting in response to light touch. They also respond to noxious heat, cold and chemical stimuli. They constitute about 30% of the cells in the spinothalamic tract (Bonica 1990).

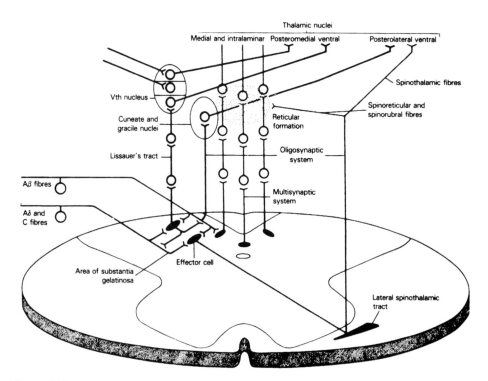

Figure 24.1

The spinal ascending pathways (reproduced with permission from Dr K Budd)

Spinothalamic and spinoreticular pathways (Figure 24.1)

The neurones of the dorsal horn project to the brain, either to the cortex or through the limbic system. The most important pathways are the spinothalamic and spinoreticular tracts, but the spinomesencephalic tract, dorsal column postsynaptic spinomedullary system and the propriospinal multisynaptic ascending systems are also involved. The spinothalamic and spinoreticular tracts lie in the anterolateral quadrant of the cord (although the precise site is variable), which is the section lesioned in cordotomy for intractable pain. This quadrant also contains the spinomesencephalic tract and these tracts are collectively known as the anterolateral fasciculus. At the rostral part of the mid-brain, the spinothalamic tract separates into a medial part of fine fibres that project to the medial and intralaminar thalamic region and a lateral part to the ventrobasal and posterior thalamus.

The spinoreticular pathway contains cell axons which are thinner on average than those of the spinothalamic tract. Some axons are contralateral and some ipsilateral to the cell bodies and project to the reticular formation. Excitation triggers arousal and contributes to the motivational or affective aspects of pain and mediates autonomic and somatic motor reflexes.

The trigeminal system is slightly different. The trigeminal mesencephalic nucleus is a collection of cell bodies of primary neurones which have migrated into the mid-brain and are associated with proprioception. The other afferents have their pseudo-unipolar cell bodies in the Gasserian (trigeminal) ganglion. The central processes project to the main sensory nucleus and the spinal trigeminal nucleus. This latter is in three parts, of which the subnucleus caudalis extends as far as the second or third cervical segment. The A and C fibres terminate in the subnucleus caudalis, whereas the large myelinated fibres terminate in the main sensory nucleus and give off collaterals which descend with decreasing calibre to the spinal nucleus. Although the myelinated fibres from the three divisions of the trigeminal nerve terminate in sharply defined sectors, the smaller diameter nociceptive afferents are found in the less defined subnucleus caudalis. Nevertheless, the neotrigeminothalamic tract (nTTT) is somatotropically organized and terminates in the ventroposteriomedial (VPM) thalamic nucleus. Other neurones in subnucleus caudalis project to the medial and intrathalamic nuclei, to the peri-aqueductal grey matter and to the hypothalamus.

The posterior and ventrobasal, medial and lateral, nuclei project to the somatosensory areas of the cortex in the postcentral gyrus and the parietal lobe. Axons from these cells project back to the same part of the thalamus and form part of the corticobulbar and corticospinal systems.

The smaller fibres of the spinothalamic tract (or nTTT) and those originating in the spinoreticular pathway terminate in the medial and intralaminar thalamic nuclei. These have diffuse connections and widespread cortical influences, in contrast to the discrete projections of the ventrobasal nuclei. These projections are involved in the motivational and affective (aversion and unpleasantness) features of pain. They activate or modify hypothalamic and limbic forebrain to alter autonomic reflex responses concerned with ventilation, circulation and neuroendocrine function.

Descending inhibitory influences

The synaptic transmission of afferent nociceptive neurones in the dorsal horn is inhibited by impulses that have their origin in the cortex, the peri-aqueductal or periventricular grey matter of the mid-brain, the locus coeruleus of the pons, the raphe nuclei of the medulla or the dorsolateral funiculus of the spinal cord. Endogenous opioids can act on the central grey matter and the nuclei raphe magnus as well as the substantia gelatinosa of the spinal cord to reduce afferent input (see below). Adrenergic cells which have their cell bodies in the locus coeruleus project to the spinal cord and have an inhibitory influence (usually) on nociception. Serotonergic cells in nuclei raphe magnus in the medulla project in the dorsolateral funiculus to inhibit directly or indirectly the nociceptive afferent terminals. Some of the cells in the nuclei raphe magnus contain noradrenaline and inhibit via alpha-2 receptors. These cells are separate from and independent of the noradrenergic cells in the locus coeruleus. The relevant alpha-2 receptors are sited post-synaptically and, when activated, hyperpolarize the second-order neurones. The nucleus paragigantocellularis in the ventromedial medulla receives a projection from the periaqueductal grey matter (which is sensitive to opioids) and projects to the spinal cord, the nuclei raphe magnus *and* to the locus coeruleus (Stamford 1994). Inhibitory interneurones release gamma-amino-butyric acid (GABA) or glycine which inhibits activation and may act on the nociceptive afferents. Descending inhibitory control may be initiated by cortical activity (suppression or distraction, hypnosis), by noxious stimuli in the same or other parts of the body (diffuse noxious inhibitory control) or by drugs (opioids, tricyclic antidepressants).

Gate control theory of pain

The gate control theory of pain was published by Melzack and Wall in 1965 (Figure 24.2). The transmission of impulses from afferent fibres to spinal cord transmission cells, which project towards the brain, is modulated by a spinal gating system in the dorsal horns. This is influenced by the relative amount of activity in the large (A-β) and small (A-δ and C) diameter fibres: the large fibres tend to inhibit transmission and the small fibres facilitate it. The gating mechanism is modified by impulses descending from the brain. These include cognitive processes which are triggered by fast-conducting fibres. When the activity of the spinal cord transmission cells exceeds a threshold, it triggers the action system, which initiates the sensory and emotional pattern of activity perceived as pain.

Neurotransmitters

The primary afferents influence the second-order neurones by the release of substances which excite or inhibit. The most abundant excitatory neurotransmitters are the amino acids aspartate and glutamate, found especially in larger primary nociceptive afferents. Peptides are also released, especially from the smaller fibres. These include:

* substance P
* neurokinin A (from fine afferents)
* vasoactive intestinal (poly)peptides (VIP)
* somatostatin (SRIF)(SS)
* cholecystokinin (CCK)
* gastrin-releasing peptide (GRP)
* calcitonin gene-related peptide (CGRP)
* dynorphin (DYN)
* enkephalin (ENK)
* angiotensin II
* bombesin (Fleetwood-Walker 1995)
* endomorphin 1 and 2 (Zadina *et al.* 1997)

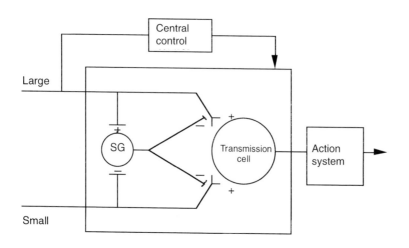

Figure 24.2

The concept of the gate control theory of pain (redrawn with permission from Melzack and Wall 1965).

The precursors of these peptides are synthesized in the cell bodies of the spinal and Gasserian ganglia, cleaved and transported to the central and peripheral terminals and stored in vesicles. Substance P may have a role in influencing the environment of the peripheral primary afferent terminals. Some peptides, such as galanin and neuropeptide Y, are induced in afferents after nerve damage (Dickenson 1995).

The monoamines, norepinephrine (noradrenaline), dopamine and serotonin (5-hydroxytryptamine, 5-HT) are also influential. These are synthesized in the terminals by enzymes, translated ribosomally in the cell bodies and transported to the terminals. At different sites, they may enhance or suppress nociception.

Norepinephrine (noradrenaline) acts on the alpha-2 receptors in a similar way to that in which opioids act on mu and delta receptors, to promote potassium efflux, inhibit cyclic AMP and reduce the rise of intracellular ionic calcium. The decreased intracellular potassium increases the polarity of the membrane inhibiting the depolarization and generation of impulse. The inhibition of rise in intracellular calcium reduces the release of transmitters such as substance P. GABA may act on GABA-B receptors to act in this way or on GABA-A receptors to increase conduction in chloride channels. This hyperpolarizes cells and opposes the change in total charge caused by sodium influx during depolarization.

The influence of these neurotransmitters or neuromodulators may depend on circumstances and other interacting substances. For example, under normal circumstances, primary afferent neurones do not have catecholamine sensitivity and their activity is unaffected by sympathetic outflow (Jänig et al. 1996). Yet, after nerve section or damage or inflammation, primary afferents acquire noradrenaline sensitivity either directly or via prostaglandin release (Baron 1998, Forrest 1998). Cholecystokinin 8 (CCK-8) is an abundant central nervous system (CNS) peptide and high concentrations are found in lamina II of the spinal cord and the ventral periventricular grey matter. Brief, intense nociception may be followed by attenuation of nociception because of the release of endogenous opioid. CCK-8 reduces this analgesic effect when it is associated with opioid release, but the nociception is unaffected by CCK-8 when not attenuated by opioids or attenuated by other factors (Faris et al. 1983).

Stages of pain

Tissue injury

1. Peripheral nerves are almost always damaged during trauma to the body and this causes bursts of afferent action potentials followed, within a few milliseconds, by sustained nociceptive impulses in afferent somatosensory and sympathetic neurones.
2. Following severe or sustained damage, the nociceptors become sensitized to further stimulation.
3. The cells that are injured by trauma or by chemical mediators will break down and release the phospholipids of the cell wall. These will be broken down and synthesized into arachidonic acid, leukotrienes and prostaglandins. The tissue mediators stimulate and sensitize nociceptors.
4. The damaged endothelium, smooth muscle and blood cells associated with bleeding release nociceptive mediators. These, too, stimulate afferent somatosensory and sympathetic neurones and perivascular mast cells which release histamine and serotonin. Bradykinin from platelets and extravasation of plasma proteins activates phospholipase A_2 which acts to produce arachidonic acid, prostaglandins and leukotrienes.

Primary hyperalgesia

Efferent sympathetic activity and local prostaglandins and neutrophil-dependent factors rapidly increase neuronal sensitivity at the site of injury. Hypersensitivity causes hyperalgesia (i.e. increased sensitivity to a stimulus which is normally painful). Following injury to the peripheral endings or the trunk of primary afferent neurones, there is increased sensitivity to norepinephrine (noradrenaline) because of a decrease in the threshold for stimulation in the sympathetic postganglionic neurones (SPGN)

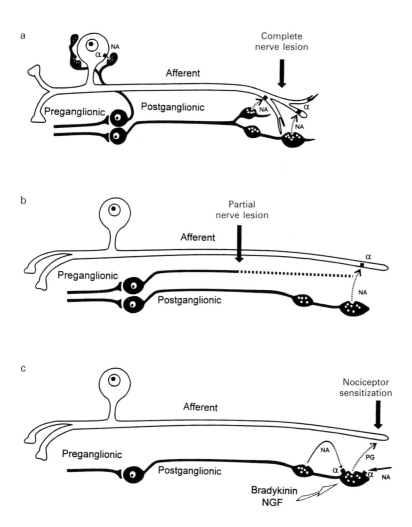

Figure 24.3

The effects of the postganglionic sympathetic neurones on the afferent nerves after complete nerve section, partial nerve damage and during nociception. (*a*) After complete nerve section, noradrenaline (NA) is released around the neuroma which forms at the site of damage and around the dorsal root ganglion. (*b*) After partial nerve damage, the sympathetic fibres which are intact release noradrenaline around the distal nerve. (*c*) During nociception and after tissue injury, the postganglionic sympathetic fibre releases noradrenaline onto the sympathetic fibre terminals which release prostaglandins, which in turn sensitize the afferent sensory nerve. Prostaglandin release from the postganglionic sympathetic fibres is also the mediator of the sensitization of the nociceptor by bradykinin and nerve growth factor (NGF). (Reproduced with permission from Baron 1998.)

along their length and at the terminal buds (Figure 24.3). Responses in these neurones are also increased. Norepinephrine (via alpha-2 receptors) and bradykinin induce production of prostaglandin by sympathetic postganglionic neurones and cause incremental increases in their sensitivity (wind-up) and hypersensitization of the primary afferent somatic neurones. Bradykinin may be increased during extravasation or by the breakdown of platelets. Prostaglandin alters the potassium efflux during repolarization of C fibre membranes and thereby increases the maximal frequency of firing.

Norepinephrine from the SPGN also affects the nociceptive afferents directly by acting on the alpha-1 receptors.

The release of chemotactic substances at the site of injury causes neutrophil leukocytes to migrate to that site and they are activated by leukotrienes (especially dihydroxy eicosotetraenoic acid (dHETE) and leukotriene B_4) and by prostaglandins, released by the breakdown of phospholipids.

Nerve growth factor, a neurotrophin, is increased during inflammation and alters the sensitivity of nociceptor neurones.

Secondary hyperalgesia

This is caused by the increased sensitivity of the N-methyl-D-aspartate (NMDA) receptor-linked channel, the expression of proto-oncogenes, the instability of the receptor fields and their expansion as a result of injury and the sympathetic responses. The NMDA receptor-linked cation channel is both ligand- and voltage-gated. In the resting state, with normal levels of polarization, calcium and magnesium, the receptor is activated only by strong or sustained stimuli. In practice, the neurotransmitters (aspartate and glutamate) released by these stimuli act on amino-3-hydroxy-5 methyl-4-isoxazole propionic acid (AMPA) channels, which allow the influx of sodium, thereby depolarizing part of the postsynaptic membrane. The affinity of magnesium for the channels of neighbouring NMDA receptors is reduced and the displacement of magnesium from this channel allows the passage of calcium associated with subsequent release of excitatory amino acids such as glutamate. The intracellular changes effected by calcium are of greater duration than those by sodium, so that depolarization in the secondary neurone can be maintained by less intense or less frequent stimuli than those required to initiate it.

The calcium influx directly or indirectly, in association with protein kinase C, promotes the synthesis of nitric oxide and the expression of the proto-oncogenes c-*fos* and c-*jun*. Nitric oxide may diffuse back across the synapse to increase the release of glutamate. Proto-oncogenes alter the messenger RNA and can cause further sensitivity and expand the receptor fields. A second neurotrophin (BDNF), acting on receptors on the dorsal horn neurones, generates nociceptive hypersensitivity at this site (Woolf 1998).

Receptor fields may also be expanded by the activation of silent nociceptors. These occur in healthy articular tissue, viscera and skin and have thresholds so high that they cannot be activated even by very intense mechanical stimuli. However, when the threshold is reduced by hypersensitization, these cause increasing neuronal activity at central terminals of primary afferent neurones (Dray 1994). These nociceptors contain many neuropeptides such as substance P, neurokinin, calcitonin gene-related peptide and somatostatin. The onset of their activity is typically 2–3 h after the initial release of tissue mediators.

Psychology (Chapman 1985)

Acute pain (Alexander and Gardner 1994, Salmon 1994)

In acute pain, the severity of the pain is approximately proportional to the strength of the stimulus, but is also related to the psychological state of the patient. A major influence in acute pain is anxiety, which increases the activity of the reticular activating system, the higher centres and the sympathetic system. Anxiety may be divided into two types – state and trait. State anxiety is the anxiety the victim feels as a result of the presenting circumstances or in anticipation of a forthcoming exciting or fearful event (context-based). Trait anxiety is the baseline or average anxiety level which accompanies all events or anticipations and which varies greatly from person to person. The increase in pain because of anxiety correlates well with state anxiety and poorly with trait anxiety.

However, sensitization can also occur with anxiety. Preparation of a child for hospitalization and surgery has been shown to reduce pre- and post-operative distress and pain. Such preparation involves hospital tours, modelling (rehearsals) in play or video films or explanations by similar children who have undergone the same experience. Modelling may be contraindicated in those who require frequent invasive procedures, because these may become sensitized such that their distress increases with viewing preparation. Distraction and comforting can reduce the overt distress and apparent pain perceived, especially in young children, who appear to tolerate uncomfortable or painful procedures when being cuddled or breast-fed.

Chronic pain

In chronic pain, the emotional part of pain has achieved a large but varying proportion of the total experience to the point where the relationship between the stimulus and the experience of pain may be difficult to discern. The approach to understanding, diagnosing, treating or managing this part of this experience of pain may appear to differ from one clinician to another, from one pain management programme to another and even from one psychologist to another. Differences of approach suggest differences of starting point or basic theory or the simplistic model of the emotion that the subject feels, the behaviour that it engenders, and the way that the subject thinks about and responds to the experience of pain. Although these theories or models appear to differ, when stated in simplistic forms, their applications show more similarities than differences when applied to any one type of subject. There are perhaps four principal approaches, theories or models, as outlined below.

The classic medical model

In this model pain is seen as a symptom of a psychiatric disorder, either as a neurosis such as a depressive neurosis, whereby the normal distribution of range of perceptions and emotions has developed a skew, or a psychosis in which the emotional reflexes are such that the normal perception cannot be regained spontaneously. A medical analogy might be that of cardiac decompensation in which activities, hormones and transmitters that previously increased the output of the heart now cause it to fail. As the perception by the subjects of nociception and their expression, either verbally or by behaviour, is distorted, the symptoms expressed by the subject require interpretation or translation by the therapist. However, Merskey (1965) has shown that the incidence of neurosis was higher in those subjects presenting with chronic pain to the psychiatric clinics than in those who presented with a range of other non-painful conditions. However, the comparative incidence of endogenous depression and psychosis was lower. It is also found that the incidence of hysterical reactions or tendency to hysterical somatization is greater than average in the chronic pain population, but that this tendency does not increase as the pain problem develops nor does it decrease as the problem resolves or is treated.

The illness behaviour approach

This approach also says that the perception and expression of pain is an interaction not only within the subject, but also between the subject and

society. The subjects' perception of worth may be changed by their inability to work or interact socially or by their dependence on, or value to, a carer. Social status may also be determined by the subject's inability to work because of illness compared to that because of inadequacy or redundancy. Financial rewards may also be enhanced by the label of illness. In this approach, the expression and behaviour of pain regains significance.

The behaviourism approach

As exemplified by Wilbert Fordyce (Fordyce *et al.* 1985, 1990), this approach says, simplistically, that although pain is fundamentally subjective, it gives rise to pain behaviour which can be quantified. When pain provokes a reward, it will be reinforced, whereas, if rewards, medication and sympathy are not dependent on pain, the reinforcement is less. An allied approach says that alteration of the behaviour associated with pain can reduce disability. Furthermore, if disabilities can be overcome, even by small amounts, despite the continued presence of pain, the satisfaction or reward that this engenders may itself alter the expression and experience of pain.

The neurophysiological approach

This approach suggests that stresses caused by the environment (such as nociception), by emotional tensions or by changes in hormonal and neurotransmitter expression can result in neurophysiological changes that produce pain. Autonomic reflexes and interactions, muscle contraction, reflexes and contractures are all influential and are seen to be altered in, for example, the complex regional pain syndromes. Stresses which may be helpful in reducing pain initially can be harmful when translated into anger, frustration, personal confrontations, muscle shortening, increased visceral reflexes and ischaemia. Nevertheless, the symptoms of stress can prove useful as a way of modulating the stress.

A flexible approach

Although there is a tendency for any clinician or therapist to favour one approach over another, the principle of having models is that they should fit the subject of the pain rather than the therapist. Since the symptom complex of the pain subject may alter with time, the duration of the pain, the changed social circumstances and physical disability, the psychological approach may also have to change.

Psychological approach

Such evaluation is important not only as a prelude to treatment by psychological methods, but also as a part of every pain assessment. The longer the duration of the pain, the greater is the chance that the pain experience is influenced by psychological factors. The success of physical methods of pain relief, especially the more invasive or long-term methods such as spinal cord stimulation, is improved by psychological evaluation (Gybels *et al.* 1998).

Pain assessment

Until recently, it was impossible to measure pain directly and objectively. Because pain is an emotional as well as sensory experience and subject to convergence of nociception, it may not be directly proportional to the severity of the stimulus, nor be perceived as coming from the site of its cause. The measurement of pain therefore depends upon the subjective assessment of the victim, the semi-subjective judgement of the victim's pain-related behaviour by an observer or the objective assessment of pain-related responses.

Pain is usually assessed clinically by the subject's own assessment of the site, severity, character and temporal nature of pain and the factors which aggravate and alleviate it. The diagnosis is refined by the subject's responses to stimuli; not so much in matching the severity of the pain by exogenous stimuli, but assessment of the responses to touch, pressure, heat, nociception, repeated stimuli, and thresholds and tolerance to innocuous and noxious stimuli.

The site of pain is best evaluated with a drawing of the extent of the pain within a diagram of the body. It is usual to specify whether the pain is felt to be on the surface or

deep within the body and whether the pain radiates to another site. The diagram of the painful part of the body must be large enough to distinguish the various structures, e.g. tongue, teeth, uvula, etc.

The severity of the pain can be assessed by a verbal rating – none, mild, moderate, severe, excruciating, a numerical rating scale of 0–10, or a visual analogue scale. The most common, sensitive and reliable of the latter is a horizontal 10-cm line with the words 'no pain' at one end and 'worst pain imaginable' at the other. The amount of pain is indicated by a mark. The distance along the line from the 'no pain' end gives the pain score. A refinement of this scale is that the line is on one side of a measuring device and the scale is on the other (Figure 24.4a) (Thomas and Griffiths 1982). For those unable to read or to understand the linear visual analogue scale, pictures of faces showing increasing distress can be used (Figure 24.4b).

The severity of pain can also be judged by the means necessary to effect its relief. The amount of pain is judged by an open-ended scale – somewhere between 'no pain' and an unknown 'worst pain imaginable'. The scale is elastic, depending upon previous experience or on pain more severe than that experienced previously requiring assessments at the upper end of the scale. When pain relief is measured, the scale has two known points – 'no pain' and 'previous pain'. Readings more probably lie on a scale which is constant in time and between individuals. These scales can be used for pain at any one moment in time, for worst or least pain or for the average pain over time. Serial assessments which can be plotted against time, such that the area under the curve represents the pain experience or total pain scores are more informative.

A popular and numerical method of measuring pain is by the amount of analgesic drug required to achieve satisfactory pain relief. A patient-controlled analgesic device is used. A syringe containing a potent and effective analgesic drug is connected to the patient, usually intravenously, such that the patient can make a demand of the device by a hand-held or breath-activating trigger. On each successful demand, an aliquot of analgesic is delivered. After each delivery, there is a pre-set lock-out time during which the trigger or demand apparatus is ineffective. Pain is assessed by the amount of analgesic

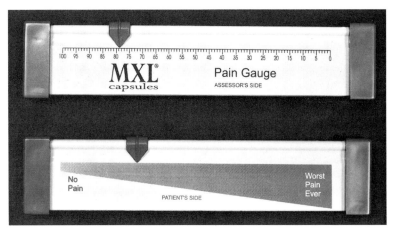

a

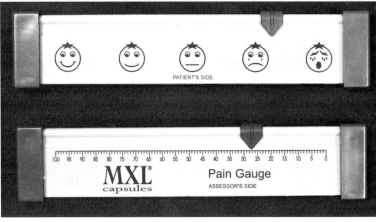

b

Figure 24.4

Commercially available pain slide rules. (a) On one side is a plain 10-cm line representing the pain experience from no pain to worst pain possible; the line is unmarked to prevent the congregation of choices to points on the line. The scores can be read on the reverse side. (b) The second slide rule is designed for those unable to read: the pictures show various degrees of happiness or unhappiness and the unhappiness score can be read from the reverse side.

consumed, the number of successful and unsuccessful demands made, the size of the aliquots (each dose) and the pain score and satisfaction rating. However, the patient rarely titrates to a state of 'no pain' and the reasons for failing to relieve all pain are many and varied.

However, pain is not a uni-dimensional experience, sensory or emotional, and, even at any one site, it may have different characters whose severities alter independently. The McGill Pain Questionnaire (Melzack 1975) seeks to assess different severities of the different characteristics of pain and to give a score that is reproducible and sensitive. Melzack and Torgerson (1971)

established that a sensory word such as 'stabbing' was more evocative of severe pain than 'pricking' or that 'scalding' is reckoned more severe than 'hot'. Affective words can be similarly graded: 'exhausting' is more severe than 'tiring' and 'vicious' more than 'punishing'. Each word has a value and the sum of the scores is called the 'present pain intensity'. A simpler form of this assessment is the short-form McGill pain questionnaire (Melzack 1987) in which the different characters of pain are graded from 'none' through 'mild' and 'moderate' to 'severe'. Many studies have shown this format to be capable of discriminating between the sensory, affective and evaluative elements of pain. This questionnaire has demonstrated that acute pain or recurrent but brief pain has high sensory scores, but that tonic (continuous, unremitting) pain has relatively higher affective scores (Chen and Treede 1985). It has shown, reliably and reproducibly, that hypnosis reduces both the affective and sensory elements of pain, but that the affective element is reduced more (Melzack and Perry 1975).

Objective but indirect assessments of pain depend upon the effect of pain on the subject. For example, thoracic and abdominal pain cause muscle spasm and guarding of the thoraco-abdominal cage and adversely affect ventilation. Tests of voluntary ventilatory function such as vital capacity or peak flow, or involuntary function such as pressure volume loops or functional residual capacity are an indication of this effect. Sympathetic tone usually, but not always, increases with pain, and this is shown by increasing pallor, tachycardia and blood pressure. Facial expressions such as the accentuation of the nasolabial folds, contraction of the corrugator muscle and the orbicularis orbis are usually indicative of pain. In infants the body responses (withdrawal, rigidity, flailing) and the noise spectrum of the cry have been taken as indicators or even measures of pain.

In chronic pain, objective but indirect measures include measures of physical performance such as distance on a bicycle, distance walked, press-ups, etc.; amount of time which is not spent resting or reclining (uptime); amount of drug use, use of other health resources. There are many questionnaires which are designed to evaluate these aspects of chronic pain and which are specific or nearly so for patients with chronic pain. These include the Sickness impact profile, Oswestry low back pain disability questionnaire, SF-36 (a 36-question version of the Medical Outcomes Study questionnaire) and the West Haven-Yale multidimensional pain inventory (Williams 1995).

Assessments of the mechanism or pathways of pain are reliant on the careful measurement of sensory thresholds, allodynia, hyperpathia, measurement of motor or autonomic dysfunction and the effects of blocking neural afferents.

More recently, Craig et al. (1996), contrary to the prediction of Professor Wall (1994), may have demonstrated a centre for pain itself.

Activity in the brain is shown by increases in regional blood flow. In the presence of pain, this is usually a compound of nociception localization, associated sensory activity, association areas, activation of the autonomic system and so on. Pain without nociception has been shown to be reflected in activity in the anterior superior cingulate gyrus, radiating to the amygdala and probably thence to the remainder of the limbic system as demonstrated by positron emission tomography, high frequency magnetic radio-imaging and the thermal grill. The thermal grill consists of two coils of tubes in which the tubes on the surface of the cylinder are alternately at 40°C and 20°C. Neither of these alone causes noxious stimulation, but touching both at the same time causes a pain which resembles the burn of noxious cold. It is well known that peripheral cold stimulation can inhibit pain processing centrally and an A fibre block that eliminates cold sensibility can cause cold allodynia in which an innocuous thermal stimulus up to 24°C can elicit burning pain, whereas the usual limit is 15°C. This is presumably caused by central disinhibition of a polymodal nociceptive spinothalamic channel by reduction of the activity in an innocuous cold-specific thermoreceptive spinothalamic channel in lamina I. In the thermal grill, the specific cold-sensitive cell activity is reduced by the presence of the interspersed warm bars, while the polymodal nociceptive C fibre activity is unaffected. The mid and anterior insula is the only part of the brain whose regional blood flow is increased by thermal stimuli, noxious or innocuous. However, blood flow in the anterior cingulate cortex is increased by noxious stimuli but not by innocuous warm or cold stimuli. It is possible that the allodynia which occurs after some cerebrovascular accidents or, more rarely, after dental trauma and temporomandibular dysfunction and nerve compression, may be accentuated by disruption of thermosensory and pain integration.

Summary

Pain is an emotional and sensory experience which is associated with actual or potential tissue damage.

It is perceived by receptors which are either specific for harmful stimuli or which respond to a range of stimuli which includes noxious stimuli.

Nociception is transmitted by small myelinated and unmyelinated fibres through oligosynaptic (fast) and multisynaptic (slow) pathways to the somatosensory areas of the brain and also to the cingulate cortex, the limbic system and the hypothalamus.

The perception of noxious stimuli and the perception of innocuous stimuli as noxious is enhanced by chemical substances which increase the activity of nociceptors and the frequency of impulse generation. It is enhanced by the activation of the sympathetic system and by wind-up within the spinal cord, at least in part by the dissociation of magnesium from the NMDA channel and the expression of proto-oncogenes.

The treatment of pain is dependent on assessment of its site, severity, cause and character, either directly or indirectly, subjectively or objectively. The effective treatment of the presently intractable pain problems must be subject to greater understanding of the mechanisms of the perceptions of pain and distress.

Acknowledgement

Although acknowledgement has been given to Professors Wall and Bonica where their publications have been directly and knowingly quoted, their writings and lectures have been so extensive and influential that it is possible that other statements in this text are similar to work already published.

References

Alexander JI, Gardner FV (1994) Prevention and management of postoperative pain. In: Gibson HB, ed, *Psychology, Pain and Anaesthesia*, 1–24. Chapman & Hall: London.

Baron R (1998) The influence of sympathetic nerve activity and catecholamines on primary afferent neurones. *International Association for the Study of Pain Newsletter* (May/June) 3–8.

Bonica JJ (1990) Anatomic and physiologic basis of pain. In: Bonica JJ, ed, *The Management of Pain*, 28–94. Lea and Febiger: Philadelphia.

Chapman CR (1985) Psychological factors in postoperative pain and their treatment. In: Smith G, Covino BG, eds, *Acute Pain*, 22–41. Butterworth: London.

Chen ACN, Treede RD (1985) McGill pain questionnaire in assessing the differentiation of phasic and tonic pain: behavioral evaluation of the 'pain inhibiting pain' effect. *Pain* **22**:67–79.

Craig AD, Reiman EM, Evans A, Bushnell MC (1996) Functional imaging of an illusion of pain. *Nature* **384**:258–60.

Dickenson A (1995) Novel pharmacological targets in the treatment of pain. *Pain Rev* **2**:1–12.

Dray A (1994) Inflammatory mediators of pain. *Br J Anaesth* **75**:125–31.

Dubner R, Basbaum AI (1994) Spinal dorsal horn plasticity following tissue or nerve injury. In: Wall PD, Melzack R, eds. *Textbook of Pain*, 3rd edn, 225–41. Churchill Livingstone: Edinburgh.

Faris PL, Komisaruk BR, Watkins LR, Mayer DJ (1983) Evidence for the neuropeptide cholecystokinin as an antagonist of opioid analgesia. *Science* **219**:310–12.

Fleetwood-Walker SM (1995) Nonopioid mediators and modulators of nociceptive processing in the spinal cord as targets for novel analgesics. *Pain Rev* **2**:153–73.

Fordyce WE (1990) Learned pain: pain as behavior. In: Bonica JJ, ed, *The Management of Pain*, 291–9. Lea and Febiger: Philadelphia.

Fordyce WE, Roberts AH, Sternbach RA (1985) The behavioral management of chronic pain: a response to critics. *Pain* **22**:113–25.

Forrest J (1998) *Acute Pain: Pathophysiology and Treatment*. Manticore: Grimsby, Ontario.

Gybels J, Erdine S, Maeyaert J et al. (1998) Neuromodulation of pain. *Eur J Pain* **2**:203–9.

Jänig W, Levine JD, Michaelis M (1996) Interactions of sympathetic and primary afferent neurones following nerve injury and tissue trauma. *Prog Brain Res* **113**:161–84.

Lynn B (1994) The fibre composition of cutaneous nerves and the classification and response properties of cutaneous afferents, with particular reference to nociception. *Pain Rev* **1**:172–83.

Melzack R (1975) The McGill Pain Questionnaire: major properties and scoring methods. *Pain* **1**:277–99.

Melzack R (1987) The short-form McGill Pain Questionnaire. *Pain* **30**:191–7.

Melzack R, Perry C (1975) Self-regulation of pain: the use of alpha-feedback and hypnotic training for the control of chronic pain. *Exp Neurol* **46**:452–69.

Melzack R, Torgerson WS (1971) On the language of pain. *Anesthesiology* **34**:50–9.

Melzack R, Wall PD (1965) Pain mechanisms: a new theory. *Science* **150**:971–9.

Merskey H (1965) The characteristics of persistent pain in psychological illness: psychiatric patients with persistent pain. *J Psychosom Res* **9**:291–9.

Salmon P (1994) Psychological factors in surgical recovery. In: Gibson HB, ed, *Psychology, Pain and Anaesthesia*, 229–58. Chapman & Hall: London.

Stamford JA (1994) Descending control of pain. *Br J Anaesth* **75**:217–27.

Thomas TA, Griffiths MJ (1982) A pain slide rule. *Anaesthesia* **37**:960–1.

Wall PD (1994) Inflammatory and neurogenic pain: new molecules, new mechanisms. *Br J Anaesth* **75**:123–4.

Williams AC de C (1995) Pain measurement in chronic pain management. *Pain Reviews* **2**:39–63.

Woolf CJ (1998) Neurotrophins and pain. In [no ed.]: *Novel Targets in the Treatment of Pain* (D & MD Reports). International Business Communications, Inc: Southborough, Mass.

Zadina JE, Hackler L, Ge L–J, Kastin AJ (1997) A potent and selective endogenous agonist for the mu–opiate receptor. *Nature* **386**:499–502

25

Present and future methods for the evaluation of pain associated with dentine hypersensitivity

David G Gillam, Robin Orchardson, Matti VO Närhi and
Vuokko Kontturi-Närhi

Introduction

Orchardson (1997) reported that Robert Burns' description of his toothache included words such as stinging, tortured, gnawing, tearing, bitter, shooting and twinge. These relate to the most severe word descriptors in their respective categories in the McGill Pain Questionnaire, although these words do not appear to relate to modern day evaluation of dentine hypersensitivity (Gillam *et al.* 1993). However, it is not easy to define pain, which has been described as a subjective and multi-dimensional experience (Melzack 1975, McGrath 1986). The diversity of the pain experience explains why it has been impossible to provide a satisfactory definition of the word. Melzack and Wall (1988) suggested that the reason for this is that 'pain' represents a category of experiences having different causes, and characterized by different qualities, varying along a number of sensory, affective and evaluative dimensions. The perception of pain is based on a number of variables, including the significance of a given pain, individual personality, psychological factors, cultural attitudes, anticipation and degree of anticipation (Mumford 1973).

Verbal and non-verbal (numerical) scales as well as questionnaires such as the McGill Pain Questionnaire (MPQ) (Clark and Troullos 1990) have been used to provide both qualitative and quantitative information about the subjective nature of dental pain following an evoked response from a painful stimulus. However, there is a need to discriminate between actual physiological neural activity, the sensory response to pain, the emotional response and the more long-term behaviour of the subject in coping with pain. Other studies have also explored diverse aspects of this phenomenon; for example, Zborowski (1952) postulated that an individual's ethnic origin influenced his or her perception and reaction to pain. In other words there would be a difference in the emotional response to pain in such individuals even though the memory response was probably similar. There is no doubt that patients self-report discomfort arising from various stimuli, but the highly subjective nature of dentine hypersensitivity makes it extremely difficult to evaluate objectively. This is particularly true when evaluating the efficacy of desensitizing agents in the clinical trial setting. Evaluation of the pain response in clinical trials designed to assess the efficacy of desensitizing products and techniques is problematic. This is due in part to the highly subjective nature of the problem as well as the influence of Hawthorne and placebo effects throughout the duration of the trial. Other factors such as lack of statistical power (small sample size) and lack of standardization of the methodology used in clinical trials to determine treatment outcomes can also influence the results.

Assessment of dentine hypersensitivity in clinical trials

Traditionally dentine hypersensitivity has been mainly (subjectively) evaluated on the basis of

Box 25.1 Examples of pain scores used in recent clinical studies: subjective evaluation following tactile and/or thermal stimulation

(a) Simple binary pain scale pain before treatment pain/no pain after treatment (Hansen 1992)

(b) 0 = No discomfort
     1 = Mild discomfort
     2 = Marked discomfort
     3 = Marked discomfort that lasted >10 s
     (Gillam and Newman 1993)

(c) 1 = No pain
     2 = Discomfort only
     3 = Pain
     4 = Severe pain
     5 = Unbearable pain
     (Gedalia et al. 1987)

(d) 0 = No significant discomfort, aware of the stimulus
     1 = Discomfort but no severe pain
     2 = Severe pain during application of stimulus
     3 = Severe pain during and continuing after application of stimulus
     (Lecointre et al. 1986, Thrash et al. 1992, Ayad et al. 1994, Schiff et al. 1998, Nagata et al. 1994)

(e) 0 = Tooth/subject does not respond to air stimulus
     1 = Tooth/subject responds to air stimulus but does not request discontinuation of stimulus
     2 = Tooth/subject responds to air stimulus and requests discontinuation or moves from stimulus
     3 = Tooth/subject responds to air stimulus considers stimulus to be painful and requests discontinuation of stimulus
     (Ayad et al. 1994, Schiff et al. 1998 [Schiff's cold air score])

Box 25.2 Stimuli used to assess dentine hypersensitivity in the clinical trial setting

Mechanical (tactile) stimuli
    Explorer probe
    Constant pressure probe (Yeaple)
    Mechanical pressure stimulators
    Scaling procedures
Chemical (osmotic) stimuli
    Hypertonic solutions, e.g. sodium chloride, glucose, sucrose and calcium chloride
Electrical stimulation
    Electrical pulp testers
    Dental pulp stethoscope
Evaporative stimuli
    Cold air blast
    Yeh air thermal system
    Air jet stimulator
    Temptronic device (microprocessor temperature-controlled air delivery system)
Thermal stimuli
    Electronic threshold measurement device
    Cold water testing
    Heat
    Thermo-electric devices (e.g. Biomat Thermal Probe)
    Ethyl chloride
    Ice-stick

NB Hydrostatic pressure evaluation has also been reported in the literature, but can be considered impractical for use in clinical studies

the individual patient's subjective response to the presenting stimulus (as described below), e.g. in the form of verbal rating and visual analogue scales and questionnaires (Box 25.1). According to recent recommendations by Holland et al. (1997), dentine hypersensitivity may be evaluated either in terms of the stimulus intensity required to evoke pain (stimulus-based assessment), or as the subjective evaluation of the pain produced by a stimulus (response-based assessment). Stimulus-based methods usually involve the measurement of a pain threshold; response-based methods involve the estimation of pain severity. The presenting stimuli can be grouped into five main categories: mechanical, chemical, electrical, evaporative and thermal (Box 25.2).

Subjective evaluation

Verbal rating scales

Keele (1948) described a four-point scale grading pain as slight, moderate, severe and agonizing. Verbal rating scales (VRS) offer a restrictive choice of words that may not represent the pain experience with significant precision for all patients (Huskisson 1974, Clark and Troullos 1990). More recently, modification of this type of pain scale has been reported (Box 25.1). However, the mathematical interpretation of the scoring system has been challenged, in that the scores are often arbitrarily assigned numerical values, and the assigned scores are then analysed as if these numbers reflected true quantitative differences in pain, rather than simple qualitative differences (McGrath 1986). This may be true for all pain score analysis.

Visual analogue scales

A visual analogue scale (VAS) is a line 10 cm in length, the extremes of the line representing the limits of pain a patient might experience from an external stimulus (no pain at one end and the most severe pain at the other end of the line). Patients are asked to place a mark on the 10-cm line which indicates the intensity of their current level of sensitivity or discomfort following application of test stimuli. VAS pain intensity can be shown either as an absolute score value or as a percentage of the maximum. The validity and reliability of the VAS measurement of both experimental and clinical pain has been demonstrated by several investigators. Clark and Troullos (1990) reported that once the VAS procedure is properly explained to patients, it is simple to understand and suitable for use in the evaluation of the stimulus response in dentine hypersensitivity dentifrice studies. Several investigators have compared the VAS with other pain scales and the results indicate that the VAS correlates well with these methods and appears to be more sensitive in discriminating between various treatments and changes in pain intensity (Ekowski et al. 1972, Joyce et al. 1975, Ohnhaus and Adler 1975). Downie et al. (1978) reported that numerical rating scales (0–10) performed better than both four-point descriptive scales and a continuous (visual analogue) scale. Scott and Huskisson (1976) demonstrated that graphic rating scales which are VAS, with descriptive terms placed at intervals along a 10-cm line, may have the advantage of helping patients to decide the position of their score. This is especially the case in the absence of previous experience of pain measurement procedures, as well as enabling different subjects to record the same degree of severity of pain in the same position. These investigators concluded that this type of rating provided the best available method for measuring pain or pain relief. One objection to the graphic rating scale is that the words underneath the scale may induce a higher density of clustering of responses close to them (Seymour 1982); although Seymour (1982) questioned the validity of any postulated advantage to be gained by using the graphic rating scale as opposed to the plain 10-cm VAS. It is apparent that the VAS can give only a one-dimensional assessment of pain, and as such cannot distinguish between the sensory, intensity and affective (unpleasantness) aspects of pain. However, the VAS is considered preferable to a numerical rating scale where the subject rates pain intensity on a scale comprising several distinct categories. Furthermore, the VAS offers the advantage of being a continuous scale, thereby providing quantitative measurements that are readily averaged and tested with parametric statistics (Holland et al. 1997).

Verbal descriptor checklists

According to Gracely et al. (1978), verbal descriptor checklists appear to allow quantitative assessment of both the sensory and affective dimensions of pain using a continuum across different pain conditions, instead of words intended to distinguish conditions (syndromes). The main disadvantage of rating scales is that pain is assumed to be a one-dimensional experience varying only in intensity, and as such a broad range of psychological experience is compressed into an artificially small continuum. Patients tend to spread their responses over the entire scale regardless of the magnitude of the actual sensations (Gracely 1980). Chapman et al. (1985) reported a tendency for investigators to treat scores from studies as interval or ratio level scaling in statistical analysis, without evidence that patients actually use the numbers in this way. Data interpreted in this manner suggest a ranking order and imply that interval differences between the individual values are equal in magnitude, which may not necessarily be true. Heft and Parker (1984) have shown that category scale values are not equally spaced when labelled with words commonly used to describe pain and they advocated the use of irregular spacing, which would reflect differences in word meaning. Price et al. (1983) modified VAS methodology to allow for separate assessment of both intensity and affective (unpleasantness) aspects of pain. Duncan et al. (1989) compared both verbal descriptor checklists and the multi-dimensional VAS methodology and concluded that both VAS and verbal descriptors successfully quantified sensory intensity and affective aspects of pain, but that verbal descriptors may provide the more sensitive tool for separating intensity and unpleasantness. However, caution should be exercised when interpreting results from dentine hypersensitivity studies using pain score data which are highly subjective. Recently, Gillam *et al.* (1997a) compared verbal descriptors, VAS and numerical rating VAS in order to quantify both the sensory and affective aspects of dentine hypersensitivity. These investigators reported that all methods of measurement clearly demonstrated that the subjective response to an evaporative stimulus was perceived to cause more discomfort than that from a tactile stimulus. In view of the highly subjective nature of the pain response these investigators advocated the use of a moving average technique to analyse data from pain studies (Figures 25.1–25.3). The use of verbal descriptors may also be restrictive in that they may not offer enough descriptions that can be placed in a continuous and ascending (or descending) order of severity of pain. Category scales are non-continuous and the averaging of responses is not always meaningful and sometimes may be misleading. VDS should usually be examined by non-parametric methods (Holland *et al.* 1997).

McGill word descriptors (MPQ)

Word descriptors from both the McGill questionnaire (MPQ) (Melzack 1975) and short form McGill questionnaire (SFMPQ) (Melzack 1987) have been used to determine the nature of the discomfort from dentine hypersensitivity and to monitor response to treatment. However, one of the main problems with word descriptors from these questionnaires is that there is reliance on the ability of the subject to understand the words presented to them. In other words it relies on the subject's vocabulary and consequently subjects who do not understand certain words in a subgroup will either ignore that group or choose a word which they understand (i.e. lacerating or cutting). Furthermore, it is also questionable whether the subject's choice of word descriptor

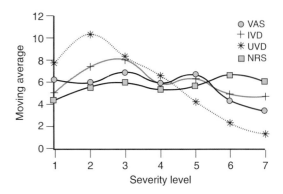

Figure 25.1

Comparison of overall sensitivity scores using an unweighted moving average technique of analysing pain scores (from Gillam *et al.* 1997a).

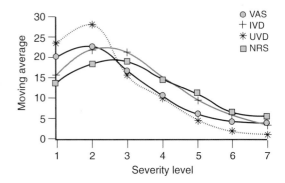

Figure 25.2

Comparison of tactile sensitivity (Yeaple probe) using an unweighted moving average technique of analysing pain scores (from Gillam *et al.* 1997a).

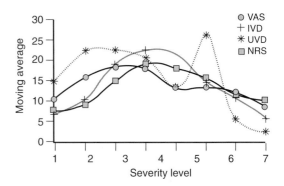

Figure 25.3

Comparison of evaporative sensitivity (cold air) using an unweighted moving average technique of analysing pain scores (from Gillam *et al.* 1997a).

is reproducible (Gillam *et al.* 1992c, 1994a). It may therefore be more practical to note how subjects express, in their own words, the perceived discomfort each time they are interviewed, rather than restrict them to a rigid framework of words which they may or may not understand (particularly in terms of severity). Several investigators (Hall *et al.* 1986, Zakrzewska and Feinmann 1990) have reported that the MPQ (complete questionnaire) was useful in diagnosis as well as monitoring treatment outcome, although Hansson *et al.* (1988) reported little correlation between the MPQ and other pain rating scales (VAS, VDS and NRS) when used to evaluate dentine hypersensitivity. Ide *et al.* (1998) reported mixed success in assessing dentine hypersensitivity with VAS and SFMPQ following tactile and thermal stimulation on selected sensitive teeth.

Hospital Anxiety and Depression scale (concept of well-being)

With clinical studies of this nature, the influence of the subject's state of well-being (mood) as well as other effects such as the placebo and Hawthorne effects cannot be ignored (Pearce *et al.* 1994, Gillam *et al.* 1996a, 1997b, West *et al.* 1997, Yates *et al.* 1998). Indeed, any claims of efficacy of the products tested must be statistically greater than what would be anticipated from results of the control group. The Hospital Anxiety and Depression scale (Zigmond and Snaith 1983) may be one way of determining whether well-being has an impact on the efficacy of a dentifrice during a study. To date, only a few published studies on dentine hypersensitivity (Gillam *et al.* 1994b, 1995a) have looked at the influence of well-being (mood) on dentifrice efficacy. It is evident from these studies that this scale is not sensitive enough to detect such changes from low grade levels of pain (Figure 25.4)

Objective assessment

Mechanical stimulation

Probing of dentine with a sharp dental explorer (Carlo *et al.* 1982, Collins and Perkins 1984) has been used for mechanical (tactile) stimulation. In

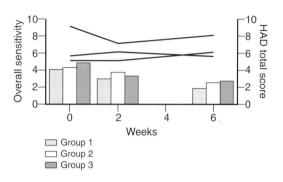

Figure 25.4

Comparison of mean overall sensitivity (bars) and median total HAD (Hospital and Anxiety Depression scale), scores (lines) over time

order to make tactile stimulation more accurate, pressure-sensitive probes with quantifiable and reproducible forces have been developed (Green *et al.* 1977, Silverman 1985, McFall and Hamrick 1987, Minkoff and Axelrod 1987, Orchardson and Collins 1987b, Chesters *et al.* 1992, Gillam *et al.* 1994c, 1996a, 1996b, 1997b, Chabanski *et al.* 1997, Yates *et al.* 1998). While most of these studies have not adopted a threshold approach, several investigators (Orchardson and Collins 1987b, Leight *et al.* 1991, Gillam, unpublished data) have evaluated the tactile response in this manner. While this approach is laudable it is very time consuming for both investigator and subject. A limitation of tactile stimulation, however, is that in many cases the sensitivity of dentine is limited to a small area which is not necessarily reached by the stimulating probe. It is evident from this observation that not all hypersensitive teeth are sensitive to tactile stimulation (Flynn *et al.* 1985). In animal experiments reproducible intradental nerve responses to probing of dentine can be recorded even with rather short intervals (a few seconds) between mechanical stimulus applications (Närhi and Hirvonen 1987, Ngassapa 1991). Furthermore, prolonged testing with one form of stimulus may interfere with the next one and consequently there may be an altered subjective response from the subject. Conditioning of the tooth may also be a problem. Repeated probing may result in the occlusion of the dentine tubules which can affect dentine hypersensitivity (Brännström 1981, Gillam and Newman 1993).

Chemical (osmotic) stimulation

Osmotic stimuli, such as hypertonic solutions of sucrose or $CaCl_2$, have been used to test the sensitivity of dentine (Anderson and Matthews 1967, Clark et al. 1987, McFall and Hamrick 1987, Ong and Strahan 1989). The use of hyperosmotic solutions is complicated, because the solute in solution diffuses into the dentine fluid. Thus, on repeated applications, the osmotic pressure difference between the tubular fluid and the applied fluid will decrease and reduce the effect of the solution as an osmotic stimulus (Pashley 1986). To avoid this effect, long time intervals must be allowed between the applications of the solutions. Thus, osmotic stimuli have not been recommended as clinical tests of dentine hypersensitivity (Pashley 1986, 1990). In animal experiments time intervals of several minutes are needed between stimulus applications and dentine must be washed thoroughly with water in order to get reproducible responses from intradental nerve fibres (Närhi and Hirvonen 1987, Ngassapa 1991).

Electrical stimulation

In assessing dentine hypersensitivity it is imperative to have a measurable and controlled stimulus (Ash 1986). Electrical stimulation is convenient in this regard, because the stimulus intensity needed to evoke a sensory response can be determined accurately. Electric pulp testers have been used in clinical trials, and some studies indicate that electrical thresholds of teeth are inversely correlated to the degree of dentine hypersensitivity (Stark et al. 1977, Tarbet et al. 1982, Kanapka and Colucci 1986, Kleinberg et al. 1990). In the instruments used in these studies, the output readings were proportional to voltage, not to the stimulation current (Stark et al. 1977, Tarbet et al. 1979, 1982, Kanapka and Colucci 1986, Kleinberg et al. 1990) and the stimulators were not of the constant current type. Any changes in the impedance of the stimulation circuit would have resulted in a change in the effective (stimulating) current intensity in the pulp. The current density in the area of the nerve fibres is decisive for their activation (Mumford 1982). The current reading is thus a more valid measure of the sensory

threshold than the voltage. In studies reported by Närhi et al. (1991) using a constant current stimulator, there was no correlation between the electrical thresholds measured in microamps and the VAS pain ratings to air blasts and cold stimulation applied to the same teeth (Närhi et al. 1991, Kontturi-Närhi 1993, Kontturi-Närhi and Närhi 1993). These results indicate that the electrical threshold is not a valid measure of dentine hypersensitivity. The effectiveness of an electrical stimulus in stimulating a tooth does not depend on the presence of receptors at the pulp–dentine junction. Activation probably occurs on more central components of the axons in the dental pulp (Mumford 1982, Närhi 1985b). Thus, electrical threshold determination does not give much, if any, information on receptor sensitivity. Teeth with hyperaemia or acute pulpitis do not have lower electrical thresholds than healthy teeth (Mumford 1982). The results of studies on teeth with hypersensitive dentine (Kontturi-Närhi 1993, Kontturi-Närhi and Närhi 1993) are in agreement with these earlier findings (Närhi et al. 1991). It is possible that the reported changes in electrical thresholds related to the changes in dentine hypersensitivity, measured in voltage (Tarbet et al. 1979, Kanapka and Colucci 1986, Kleinberg et al. 1990), could in fact be due to changes in the impedance of the tooth. However, it is possible that functional changes in the central nervous system could affect the dental pain perception (Sessle 1987) and, thus, also the thresholds to electrical stimulation. Such changes may occur in connection with painful conditions, especially chronic pain (Sessle 1987). It would be important to know whether long-lasting cases of dentine hypersensitivity have any features of chronic pain. Little is known about the general psycho-physiological characteristics of dentine hypersensitivity as compared to other pain conditions. The results of a recent questionnaire study indicate that the subjects with other pain conditions report more intense dental pain in connection with the listed external stimuli (Kontturi-Närhi 1993).

Dehydrating (evaporative) stimuli

Air blasts have been used in most studies on hypersensitive dentine (Kleinberg et al. 1990). An air blast may be considered a combined thermal and evaporative stimulus. Which of the effects is more pronounced is probably dependent on the duration and temperature of the air stream (Pashley 1990, Närhi et al. 1992). The initial wetness of the stimulated surface may also have an effect. In most studies, room temperature (20°C) air blasts have been used (Collins and Perkins 1984, Addy et al. 1987, Orchardson and Collins 1987a, 1987b, Ong and Strahan 1989, Gillam et al. 1992a, 1992b, 1994c, 1996a, 1996b, 1997, Ayad et al. 1994, Schiff et al. 1998, Ide et al. 1998). In other studies the degree of dentine hypersensitivity has been related to a change in the tooth surface temperature needed to induce a pain response (Thrash et al. 1983). However, in this way the evaporative effect of the air blasts is not taken into account. Short (1 s) air blasts have been recommended (Pashley 1990) in order to avoid excess evaporation and consequent changes in dentine hypersensitivity (Brännström 1963, 1981, Pashley et al. 1984) as well as undesirable pulpal effects. Several recent studies (Gillam 1992, Kontturi-Närhi 1993, Kontturi-Närhi and Närhi 1993, Gillam et al. 1994c) reported that air blasts at 20°C were more effective than contact cold (thermal probe) at 20°C and as effective as contact cold at lower temperatures in inducing pain. This difference may be due to the evaporative effect of the air blasts. Air blasts also affect a wider area of dentine, which could have contributed to the more intense pain responses in comparison with contact cold at 20°C. The evaporative effect and consequent activation of the hydrodynamic forces in dentine tubules (Brännström 1981) are difficult to control. The intensity of pain induced by air blasts as estimated by VAS measurement is correlated to the intensity of the pain responses induced by contact cold stimulation and to the density of open dentinal tubules as observed in SEM-replica studies (Närhi et al. 1991, Kontturi-Närhi 1993, Kontturi-Närhi and Närhi 1993). Stimulation with air blasts is a valid stimulus for estimation of dentine sensitivity. However, the pain responses are due to the evaporative, rather than the thermal, effects of the air blasts as also suggested by Pashley (1990).

Thermal stimulation

In studies on dentine hypersensitivity, cold water of different temperatures (Johnson et al. 1982, Brough et al. 1985, Muzzin and Johnson 1989, Lawson et al. 1991), cold air (Minkoff and Axelrod 1987, Person et al. 1989), ethyl chloride (Absi et al. 1987) and various types of contact cold probes (Naylor 1961, Smith and Ash 1964, Green et al. 1977, Thrash et al. 1983, 1992, McFall and Morgan 1985, Ong and Strahan 1989, Närhi et al. 1991, Gillam et al. 1994c, 1994d [threshold evaluation], Orro et al. 1994, Smart et al. 1998) have been applied. Cold seems to be the most potent stimulus to induce pain from hypersensitive dentine (Brännström 1981, Dowell et al. 1985, Flynn et al. 1985, Orchardson and Collins 1987a, 1987b, Närhi et al. 1991, Gillam 1992, Kontturi-Närhi 1993, Kontturi-Närhi and Närhi 1993). Thus, cold is probably a most valid stimulus for determination of the degree of dentine hypersensitivity. Most hypersensitive teeth respond to cold and the sensation is typical for hypersensitive dentine: fast, sharp and transient (Närhi et al. 1991, Kontturi-Närhi and Närhi 1993). Heat stimulation is much less effective than cold (Gillam 1992, Kontturi-Närhi and Närhi 1993). Patients tolerate cold stimuli better than hot stimuli and there is less danger of causing pulp damage (Pashley 1990). Responses to cold stimulation in clinical tests have a good correlation to the hypersensitivity symptoms encountered in everyday life (Kontturi-Närhi 1993). Heat seems to be rather ineffective in inducing pain from hypersensitive teeth in clinical tests (Närhi et al. 1991, Gillam 1992, Kontturi-Närhi 1993, Kontturi-Närhi and Närhi 1993). This correlates with the results of several questionnaire studies, i.e. that hot fluids and foods or hot air were rarely reported as inducing pain (Kontturi-Närhi 1993, Gillam et al. 1995b, 1996c, 1997c). Heat can induce strong pain in teeth with pulpitis (Brännström 1981, Mumford 1982). It is known to activate mostly intradental C fibres which are not involved in dentine hypersensitivity (Närhi 1985a, 1985b, 1990). Heat stimulation thus seems to be of limited value in the clinical testing of dentine hypersensitivity but could be useful in discriminating teeth with acute pulpitis. Warm air has been used as a heat stimulus applied to exposed dentine. Responses have been induced from sensitive dentine at temperatures below 45°C (Person et al. 1989). However, it is evident – as demonstrated in other studies – that evaporation of fluid on the dentine surface is probably the most effective stimulus (Kontturi-Närhi 1993,

Kontturi-Närhi and Närhi 1993). It is important to point out that both thermal probes and water bath evaluation have limitations (Holland *et al.* 1997).

Hydrostatic pressure

Stimulation with elevated or reduced hydrostatic pressure has been used in animal experiments (Närhi and Haegerstam 1983, Vongsavan and Matthews 1992). Ahlquist *et al.* (1988) induced sharp pain sensations by hydrostatic pressure stimulation in humans. Fluid filtration, which would be an ideal stimulus, has not been used clinically because of technical difficulties (Pashley 1990), although the method was applied successfully in cat teeth in vivo (Vongsavan and Matthews 1992). For these reasons hydrostatic pressure evaluation has not been recommended for the assessment of dentine hypersensitivity.

Outcome measures

According to Holland *et al.* (1997) the minimum requirements for the clinical trial assessment of improvements in dentine hypersensitivity trials (with the appropriate objective methodology preferably two hydrodynamic stimuli) should be two evaluations, one made at baseline and the second at the end of the study. Additional time points may also be beneficial during trials of longer duration (e.g. 2–3 months). The subject's overall (global) assessment of the treatment may be completed either by VAS or questionnaire at each time period throughout a longitudinal study and, if required, to evaluate any longevity effects of a particular product following cessation of the study. Treatment evaluations should also include a subjective evaluation of changes in individual overall sensitivity to 'everyday' stimuli. It is recognized that this particular outcome is difficult to assess, but nevertheless it may be the most important from the subject's perspective (Holland *et al.* 1997).

The collection of data obtained from such outcome measurements during a trial, however, should be in a form that is amenable to statistical analysis and interpretation. Moreover, clinical measurement procedures, together with the data collected, should be in accordance with FDA and European Guidelines for Good Clinical Practice. As a general comment, hard and fast rules cannot be laid down about which statistical technique should be used for every study, and pragmatically the study design and outcome measures should dictate the statistical interpretation. Obviously statistical advice is essential when establishing a trial design, but analysis and interpretation of the data are dependent on whether they are, for example, normally distributed or not. This may be particularly true in interpreting results from pain studies that may yield highly subjective data and are subsequently analysed by complex (mathematical) statistical packages in order to demonstrate statistical significance. From previous experience of conducting clinical trials comparing the efficacy of desensitizing products, this particular problem may compound rather than help to determine whether there is a true effect of a given product over placebo. On reviewing the literature, most randomized trials (parallel arm) of this nature have utilized two-sample t tests, Wilcoxon/Mann-Whitney tests, Kruskal-Wallis test and one-way analysis of variance (these may be weighted if the study is taking into account the variability of the numbers of test/control sites per subject). In trials of desensitizing products, most investigators have reported on teeth which test sensitive to the objective stimulus and monitored outcome measures throughout the trial period (non-sensitive teeth are generally not included). However, Chesters *et al.* (1992) have advocated the use of logit analysis for the assessment of the efficacy of desensitizing products. This procedure analyses the reported treatment effects in terms of the proportion of teeth (both sensitive and non-sensitive) improving or worsening throughout the trial. However, this technique of analysis fails to take into account any changes in severity of the reported response. For example, it does not distinguish between a change in a tooth being severely uncomfortable to uncomfortable. Furthermore, inclusion of non-sensitive as well as sensitive teeth may actually complicate the analysis of the results. Testing should therefore be restricted to teeth that have evidence of exposed (root) dentine. Teeth that do not respond to the test stimuli, at the agreed levels of response at baseline, should not be included in the study. It should also be acknowledged that the individual subject should be the unit of analysis and the multiple measures need to be summarized with a summary statistic (e.g. mean values). Alternatively a statistical analysis method could be employed that can take into account tooth-specific measurements while maintaining the subject as the unit of analysis. The use of meta-analysis in multi-centred trials has also been advocated, as this prevents undeserved weight been given to trials with poor compliance.

Discussion

Pain is the principal and primary clinical outcome of dentine hypersensitivity, although it should be acknowledged that pain arising from hypersensitive dentine is not continuous, but occurs in response to a stimulus and as such may complicate any perceived treatment effects during a clinical trial. Nevertheless, clinical success or failure is generally judged (by both subject and investigator) in terms of pain reduction. The ideal goal for any desensitizing agent or product is to abolish the symptoms of pain or discomfort, if the subject is to be satisfied with the outcome of treatment. Currently, pain measurement intrinsically requires the assessment of a subject parameter. Assessment of pain is inherently subjective; various methodologies are utilized in a variety of clinical fields (e.g. analgesics) to assess pain. Only widely accepted methodologies should be utilized in clinical trials of chemotherapeutic agents, as it is the latter that should be tested, not the assessment technique itself. Furthermore, the perception of pain is not always directly proportional to the extent of tissue damage or physical trauma that is produced by a defined stimulus. Because of this, visual analogue scales (VAS) are among the better assessment techniques, as they allow the individual patients to define for themselves the limits of acceptable pain (the ultimate clinical end-point). Furthermore, these scales tend to be less influenced by bias introduced from more precise scale descriptors.

While more objective means of assessing dentine hypersensitivity may be desirable, future work towards this goal must ensure that new measures are highly and directly correlated with patient-perceived pain. For clinical trials, the pain stimulus must be controlled. To this end, the stimulus should be applied to the patient by a trained, qualified (by experience), treatment-blinded clinician. Stimulation of the tooth should occur only at the site of exposed dentine. The type and degree of the stimulus must be reproducible and documented. Various types of stimuli are acceptable and have been discussed in this chapter. Those that are (1) quantifiable, (2) reproducible and (3) of clinical relevance are preferred. Mechanical/tactile and thermal stimuli tend to meet these criteria more often than other types, such as electrical and chemical stimuli. Scratching dentine should be avoided because of potential damage to the tooth surface. Controlled pressure probes with blunt probe tips meet these criteria for providing a stimulus to specific sites with exposed dentine and are reproducible in the intensity of the stimulus. Prolonged testing, however, may produce fatigue in both the subject and the investigator. Testing should be conducted in a relaxed environment (testing should not be rushed) and be pragmatic in its approach. Allowances for such an approach should be incorporated into study protocols; screening and testing teeth is very time-consuming, particularly if threshold measurements are incorporated into the study. Sufficient time intervals between repeated stimulation should be agreed, where possible on the basis of scientific data. Such an approach should be flexible and practical, to enable the investigator to complete all measurements within a reasonable time frame. Holland et al. (1997) recommended that at least two hydrodynamic stimuli should be used in view of the evidence from previous studies (Närhi 1985a, 1985b, Orchardson and Collins 1987a, 1987b) that the dentine hypersensitivity response may be different for different stimuli. The sequence of application, however, is important. Tactile stimuli appear to be less damaging than thermal and as such should be used first (Gillam and Newman 1993). Repeated multiple stimulus application and threshold evaluation may also be time-consuming and this could limit the number of teeth tested during the study. Furthermore, anticipation of pain as well as repeated painful stimulation may also influence outcome measurements (Holland et al. 1997).

It is evident that some stimuli (e.g. electrical and thermal) can cause pain even in healthy teeth, and with these stimuli, a suitable criterion of success might be to restore sensitivity to 'normal' levels evident in symptom-free and/or comparable control teeth. Evaporative, chemical, osmotic and mechanical stimuli do not tend to cause pain from 'normal' or non-sensitive teeth, and if these stimuli are used the criterion for success is no pain on stimulation (i.e. thresholds off the scale, or subjective pain intensity reduced to zero). However, the absolute magnitude of the degree of change (in thresholds and/or subjective ratings) that can be achieved with these stimuli should be sufficiently wide to permit adequate measurement of effect and allow discrimination between agents. Nevertheless, mechanical, thermal, electrical and osmotic stimuli can be quantified, which is necessary for measuring the degree of dentine hypersensitivity (Närhi 1985b, Kleinberg et al. 1990).

Air blasts are more difficult to quantify, mainly because the effect is dependent on several factors, including the wetness of the dentine surface. The stimulus effect starts whenever the evaporation of dentinal fluid occurs. This will increase outward fluid flow in dentine tubules and activate dentinal nerve terminals (Närhi 1985a). Air blasts, mechanical, thermal, hydrostatic pressure and osmotic stimuli most probably activate intradental nerves through a hydrodynamic mechanism (Närhi 1985a). These stimuli exert their effect by activating the receptors in the pulp–dentine border area and the induced pain responses are dependent on the sensitivity of these receptors. As subjects' naturally occurring responses are also initiated by hydrodynamic stimuli (Orchardson and Collins, 1987a, 1987b), these hydrodynamic stimuli may be considered valid tests of dentine hypersensitivity. However, from a practical standpoint, hydrostatic pressure and osmotic stimuli are probably the least suitable for routine clinical use. Hydrostatic pressure stimuli are technically difficult to apply. Chemical and osmotic stimuli will alter the osmolarity of the dentinal fluids and hence require lengthy intervals between tests. Relatively few patients complain of pain with hot stimuli, and in clinical testing, cold stimuli are generally found to be more effective than heat stimuli (Gillam and Newman 1993). Thus tactile, cold and evaporative (air-jet) stimuli appear to be the most suitable models of hydrodynamic stimulation for clinical testing.

In contrast to hydrodynamic stimuli, electric current, if of sufficient magnitude, causes pain by directly generating action potentials in axons in the most central parts of the dental pulp (Mumford 1982, Närhi 1985a). Current opinion is divided on the usefulness of electrical stimuli in assessing dentine hypersensitivity. Most electrical stimulators deliver voltage pulses, and do not directly measure the current that is the adequate stimulus for action potential generation. However, Kleinberg et al. (1990, 1994) and other investigators report that changes in the electrical threshold of hypersensitive teeth measured by voltage variation are consistent with measurement of changes in sensitivity to tactile and air stimuli. However, Kontturi-Närhi and Närhi (1993) failed to demonstrate any correlation between electrical current threshold of hypersensitive teeth and subjective ratings of pain to cold stimuli when measured by current variation. This apparent discrepancy can be resolved by the fact that current variation measurement is not affected by impedance differences in the tooth and is designed to determine the current threshold needed to cause a pulpal neural response. If there is little or no damage to pulpal nerve fibres, which is believed to be the case in dentine hypersensitivity, no or poor correlation of electrical stimulation and tooth sensitivity would be expected, as reported by Kontturi-Närhi (1993). On the other hand, voltage pulses would more easily cause a pulpal neural response at a lower threshold should the electrical impedance of the tooth tissues decrease. This would appear to be the situation when the dentine tubules are patent and would explain the observations by Kleinberg et al. (1994), who used voltage measurements and reported a correlation between electrical measurements and dentine hypersensitivity.

With tactile and air stimuli, there is a clear distinction between thresholds of hypersensitive and non-sensitive teeth (Orchardson and Collins, 1987b, Kleinberg et al. 1994, Gillam et al. 1994c, 1994d, Smart et al. 1998). In contrast, voltage thresholds of hypersensitive and non-sensitive teeth show considerable overlap (Kleinberg et al. 1994). For this reason, electrical stimuli should not be used to identify teeth that are sensitive during screening for hypersensitive teeth.

However, this does not appear to be an issue during a clinical trial, as each tooth acts as its own control.

Currently, no single method of eliciting and assessing dentine hypersensitivity may be considered ideal. The plethora of devices used would also suggest that no one device is universally accepted as the ideal method for assessing dentine hypersensitivity. The absence of suitably objective methodology for assessing dentine hypersensitivity and the lack of standardized measurement of the subjective response following application of stimuli, therefore, still gives cause for concern (Gillam and Newman 1993). Several comments may be valid in this context. Stimuli used for testing the subjective response should represent real life and be hydrodynamic in nature. At least two stimuli should be used, the least severe first, and there should be little or no interaction between stimuli. Intervals between testing should be sufficient to prevent this interaction. There are still few published data on recommended intervals between testing. Methodology used in clinical trials should be recognized as having validity, e.g. details and specifications published in refereed journals or accepted by a regulatory body. Measurement tools should also conform to recent cross-infection control and safety specifications. However, one of the problems encountered in evaluating dentine hypersensitivity is the highly subjective nature of the pain response despite so-called objective methodology. Indeed, problems still exist because of investigators' inability to observe patients' responses to external stimuli objectively (Dayton *et al.* 1974). Threshold measurements alone are insufficient because of variability in individual pain threshold as discussed previously, and because they are expressed in terms of stimulus rather than perception of pain (McGrath 1986). Complete absence of pain from dentine hypersensitivity, therefore, is probably the only true end-point measurement rather than attempting to quantify objective measures of tactile and thermal thresholds.

Conclusion

A review of the current literature would indicate that there are problems in evaluating patients' subjective responses to the various stimuli used in the assessment and treatment of dentine hypersensitivity. Opinions still vary as to the reliability of some of these methods of assessment, although more recently efforts have been made to develop controlled reproducible stimuli more suited to the evaluation of dentine hypersensitivity. The ideal goal for any dentine desensitizing agent/product is to abolish the symptoms of pain or discomfort. However, a more realistic expectation might be for OTC/in-office treatments to reduce tooth sensitivity to levels that are acceptable to the patient, or at least to reduce sensitivity to the levels evident in symptom-free teeth. The main objective should be to produce a clinically significant reduction in symptoms rather than a small but statistically significant reduction. Indeed, it could be argued that despite the so-called objective methodology used to evaluate dentine hypersensitivity in terms of centimetres or grams, etc. the final arbiter is the subject (absence/presence of pain). Treatment effects may be expressed in terms of the degree of reduction produced in the clinical symptoms, but the wisdom of setting arbitrary percentage changes is questionable, especially if non-linear sensory scales are employed. The degree of treatment effect that can be achieved will be influenced by the baseline sensitivity levels, which should be neither too modest nor too severe. The magnitude of the anticipated treatment effects should be established at the outset. The expected end-point (e.g. the anticipated level of therapeutic effect) will influence the trial design. Trial design will also be affected by whether the study is intended to establish efficacy or equivalency/superiority of the test agent compared with a placebo or standard agent and the intention of the study must be declared at the outset. Statistical methods of analysis should be developed in concert with trial design, preferably in consultation with a competent statistician, and objectives should be clearly stated in the study protocols prior to the start of the study. Finally, it must be concluded that despite the information discussed throughout this chapter, the evaluation of treatment for dentine hypersensitivity, particularly in the clinical trial environment, is difficult (and will remain so in the future) regardless of the methodology employed.

References

Absi EG, Addy M, Adams D (1987) Dentine hypersensitivity. A study of the patency of dentinal tubules in sensitive and non-sensitive cervical dentine. *J Clin Periodont* **14**:280–4.

Addy M, Mostafa P, Newcombe R (1987) Dentine hypersensitivity. A comparison of five toothpastes used during a 6-week treatment period. *Br Dent J* **163**:45–51.

Ahlquist ML, Coffey JP, Franzen OB, Pashley DH (1988) Sharp dental pain selectively induced by positive and negative exogenous hydrostatic pressure changes. *Eur J Neurosci* **12** (Suppl):S176.

Anderson DJ, Matthews B (1967) Osmotic stimulation of human dentine and the distribution of pain thresholds. *Arch Oral Biol* **12**:417–26.

Ash MM (1986) Quantification of stimuli. *Endodontics Dent Traumatol* **2**:153–6.

Ayad F, De Vizio W, McCool J et al (1994) Comparative efficacy of two dentifrices containing 5% potassium nitrate on dentinal sensitivity: a twelve week clinical study. *J Clin Dent* **5** (Sp. iss.):97–101.

Brännström M (1963) A hydrodynamic mechanism in the transmission of pain-producing stimuli through the dentine. In: Anderson DJ, ed, *Sensory Mechanism in Dentine*, 73–9. Pergamon Press: Tokyo.

Brännström M (1981) *Dentin and Pulp in Restorative Dentistry*. Dental Therapeutics AB: Nacka, Sweden.

Brough KM, Anderson DM, Love J, Overman PR (1985) The effectiveness of iontophoresis in reducing dentin hypersensitivity. *J Am Dent Assoc* **111**:761–5.

Carlo GT, Ciancio SC, Seyrek SK (1982) An evaluation of iontophoretic application of fluoride for tooth desensitization. *J Am Dent Assoc* **105**:452–4.

Chabanski MB, Gillam DG, Bulman JS, Newman HN (1997) Clinical evaluation of cervical dentine sensitivity in a population of patients referred to a Specialist Periodontology Department. *J Oral Rehabil* **24**:666–72.

Chapman CR, Casey KL, Dubner R et al (1985) Pain measurement. An overview. *Pain* **22**:1–31.

Chesters R, Kaufman HW, Huntington E, Kleinberg I (1992) Use of multiple sensitivity measurements and logit statistical analysis to assess the effectiveness of a potassium citrate-containing dentifrice in reducing dentinal hypersensitivity. *J Clin Periodontol* **19**:256–61.

Clark GE, Troullos ES (1990) Designing hypersensitivity clinical studies. *Dent Clin North Am* **34**:531–44.

Clark DC, Al-Joburi W, Chan EC (1987) The efficacy of a new dentifrice in treating dentin sensitivity: effects of sodium citrate and sodium fluoride as active ingredients. *J Periodontal Res* **22**:89–93.

Collins JF, Perkins L (1984) Clinical evaluation of the effectiveness of three dentifrices in relieving dentin sensitivity. *J Periodontol* **55**:720–5.

Dayton RE, DeMarco TJ, Swedlow D (1974) Treatment of hypersensitive root surfaces with dental adhesive materials. *J Periodontol* **45**:873–8.

Dowell P, Addy M, Dummer P (1985) Dentine hypersensitivity: a review. Etiology, differential diagnosis and management. *Br Dent J* **158**:92–6.

Downie WW. Leatham PA, Rhind VM et al (1978) Studies with pain rating scales. *Ann Rheum Dis* **37**:378–81.

Duncan GH, Bushnell MC, Lavigne GJ (1989) Comparison of verbal and visual analogue scales for measuring the intensity and unpleasantness of experimental pain. *Pain* **37**:295–303.

Ekowski C, Hrubes V, Joyce CRB et al (1972) An experimental study of two methodological problems in clinical evaluation. Different types of scales and the availability of patients' previous judgments. *Psychopharmacology* **26** (Suppl):70.

Flynn J, Galloway R, Orchardson R (1985) The incidence of hypersensitive teeth in the West of Scotland. *J Dent* **13**:230–6.

Gedalia I, Brayer L, Stabholtz A, Shapiro L (1987) Clinical evaluation of the effectiveness of aminfluoride fluid, aminfluoride gelee and strontium chloride paste in relieving dentine sensitivity. *Pharm Acta Helv* **62**:188–90.

Gillam DG (1992) The assessment and treatment of cervical dentinal sensitivity. DDS Thesis, Edinburgh.

Gillam DG, Newman HN (1993) Assessment of pain in cervical dentinal sensitivity studies. *J Clin Periodontol* **20**:383–94.

Gillam DG, Newman HN, Davies EH, Bulman JS (1992a) Clinical efficacy of a low abrasive dentifrice for the relief of cervical dentinal hypersensitivity. *J Clin Periodontol* **19**:197–201.

Gillam DG, Newman HN, Bulman JS, Davies EH (1992b) Dentifrice abrasivity and cervical dentinal hypersensitivity. Results 12 weeks following cessation of 8 weeks' supervised use. *J Periodontol* **63**:7–12.

Gillam DG, Bulman JS, Newman HN (1992c) Quantification of pain in cervical dentinal sensitivity (CDS) studies. *J Dent Res* **71**:628 (abstract 902).

Gillam DG, Bulman JS, Newman HN (1993) Use of word descriptors in cervical dentinal sensitivity (CDS) studies. *J Dent Res* **72**:740 (abstract 430).

Gillam DG, Bulman JS, Newman HN (1994a) Reliability of word descriptors in cervical dentinal sensitivity (CDS) studies. *J Dent Res* **73**:826 (abstract 320).

Gillam DG, Bulman JS, Newman HN (1994b) The effect of wellbeing in patients participating in clinical trials. *J Dent Res* **73**:835 (abstract 390).

Gillam DG, Davies EH, Newman HN, Bulman JS (1994c) Clinical evaluation of the Biomat Thermal Probe. *Arch Oral Biol* **39** (Suppl):127S.

Gillam DG, Newman HN, Davies EH, Bulman JS (1994d) Determination of TST values in 'non-sensitive' teeth. *J Dent Res* **73**:826 (abstract 319).

Gillam DG, Bulman JS, Newman HN (1995a) The influence of well being in subjects participating in cervical dentinal sensitivity (CDS) studies. *J Dent Res* **74**:864 (abstract 340).

Gillam DG, Chabanski MB, Bulman JS, Newman HN (1995b) Self-reporting of tooth sensitivity in a selected population of patients. *J Dent Res* **74**:448 (abstract 383).

Gillam DG, Bulman JS, Jackson RJ, Newman HN (1996a) Comparison of two desensitizing dentifrices with a commercially available fluoride dentifrice in alleviating cervical dentinal sensitivity (CDS). *J Periodontol* **67**:737–42.

Gillam DG, Bulman JS, Jackson RJ, Newman HN (1996b) Efficacy of a potassium nitrate-based mouthwash in alleviating cervical dentinal sensitivity (CDS). *J Clin Periodontol* **23**:993–7.

Gillam DG, Bulman JS, Jackson RJ, Newman HN (1996c) Prevalence of dentine hypersensitivity in a general practice population. *J Dent Res* **75**:321 (abstract 2429).

Gillam DG, Bulman JS, Newman HN (1997a) An assessment of alternative methods of quantifying dental pain with particular reference to dentine hypersensitivity. *Community Dent Health* **14**:92–6.

Gillam DG, Coventry J, Manning R et al (1997b) Comparison of two desensitizing agents for the treatment of dentine hypersensitivity. *Endodontics Dent Traumatol* **13**:36–9.

Gillam DG, Seo HS, Newman HN (1997c) Comparison of dentine hypersensitivity in selected occidental and oriental populations. *J Dent Res* **76**:351 (abstract 2702).

Gracely RH (1980) Pain measurement in man. In: Ng LKY, Bonica JJ, eds, *Pain Discomfort and Humanitarian Care*, 111-38. Elsevier North Holland: New York.

Gracely RH, McGrath P, Dubner R (1978) Ratio scales of sensory and affective verbal pain descriptors. *Pain* **5**:5–18.

Green BL, Green ML, McFall WT (1977) Calcium hydroxide and potassium nitrate as desensitizing agents for hypersensitive root surfaces. *J Periodontol* **48**:667–72.

Hall EH, Terezhalmy GT, Pelleu GB (1986) A set of descriptors for the diagnosis of dental pain syndromes. *Oral Surg Oral Med Oral Pathol* **61**:153–7.

Hansen EK (1992) Dentine hypersensitivity tested with a fluoride-containing varnish or a light-cured glass-ionomer liner. *Scand J Dent Res* **100**:305–9.

Hansson RE, Bye FL, Smith BA (1988) Four different pain rating scales used to evaluate dentin hypersensitivity. *J Dent Res* **67** (Special issue):292 (abstract 1433).

Heft MW, Parker SR (1984) An experimental basis for revising the category rating scale for pain. *Pain* **19**:153–61.

Holland GR, Närhi MN, Addy M et al (1997) Guidelines for the design and conduct of clinical trials on dentine hypersensitivity. *J Clin Periodontol* **24**:808–13.

Huskisson EC (1974) Measurement of pain. *Lancet* **2**:1127–31.

Ide M, Morel AD, Wilson RF, Ashley FP (1998) The role of a dentine bonding agent in reducing cervical dentine sensitivity. *J Clin Periodontol* **25**:286–90.

Johnson RH, Zulqar-Nain BJ, Koval JJ (1982) The effectiveness of an electro-ionizing toothbrush in the control of dentinal hypersensitivity. *J Periodontol* **53**:353–9.

Joyce CRB, Zutshi DW, Hrubes V, Mason RM (1975) Comparison of fixed interval and visual analogue scales for rating chronic pain. *Eur J Clin Pharmacol* **8**:415–20.

Kanapka JA, Colucci SV (1986) Clinical evaluation of dentinal hypersensitivity: a comparison of methods. *Endodontics Dent Traumatol* **2**:157–64.

Keele KD (1948) The pain chart. *Lancet* **11**:6–8.

Kleinberg I, Kaufman HW, Confessore F (1990) Methods in measuring tooth hypersensitivity. *Dent Clin North Am* **34**:515–29.

Kleinberg I, Kaufman HW, Wolff M (1994). Methods of measuring tooth sensitivity and oral factors in its development. *Arch Oral Biol* **39** (Suppl):S63–S71.

Kontturi-Närhi V (1993) Dentin hypersensitivity – factors related to the occurrence of the pain symptoms. PhD Thesis, Kuopio. University Publications, Series B. Dental Sciences.

Kontturi-Närhi V, Närhi M (1993) Testing sensitive dentin in man. *Int J Endodontics* **26**:4.

Lawson K, Gross KBW, Overman PR, Anderson D (1991) Effectiveness of chlorhexidine and sodium fluoride in reducing dentin hypersensitivity. *J Dent Hyg* **65**:340–44.

Lecointre C, Apiou J, Marty P, Poitou P (1986) Controlled trial of the action of a toothpaste containing nicomethanol hydrofluoride in the treatment of dentine hypersensitivity. *J Int Med Res* **14**:217–22.

Leight RS, Troullos ES, Ryan P (1991) A new method of quantifying dentinal tactile hypersensitivity. *J Dent Res* **70**:474 (abstract 1668).

McFall WT, Hamrick SW (1987) Clinical effectiveness of a dentifrice containing fluoride and a citrate buffer system for the treatment of dentinal sensitivity. *J Periodontol* **58**:701–5.

McFall WT, Morgan WC (1985) Effectiveness of a dentifrice containing formalin and sodium monophosphate. *J Periodontol* **56**:288–92.

McGrath PA (1986) The measurement of human pain. *Endodontics Dent Traumatol* **2**:124–9.

Melzack R (1975) The McGill Pain Questionnaire: major properties and scoring methods. *Pain* **1**:277–99.

Melzack R (1987) The short form McGill Pain Questionnaire. *Pain* **30**:191–7.

Melzack R, Wall P (1988) *The Challenge of Pain*, 34–46. Penguin Books: London.

Minkoff S, Axelrod S (1987) Efficacy of strontium chloride in dental hypersensitivity. *J Periodontol* **58**:470–4.

Mumford JM (1973) *Toothache and Related Pain*, 57–107. Churchill Livingstone: Edinburgh.

Mumford JM (1982) Orofacial pain. *Aetiology, Diagnosis and Treatment*, 3rd edn. Churchill Livingstone: Edinburgh.

Muzzin KB, Johnson R (1989) Effects of potassium oxalate on dentin hypersensitivity in vivo. *J Periodontol* **60**:151–8.

Nagata T, Ishida H, Shinohara H *et al* (1994). Clinical evaluation of a potassium nitrate dentifrice for the treatment of dentinal hypersensitivity. *J Clin Periodontol* **21**:217–21.

Närhi MVO (1985a) The characteristics of intradental sensory units and their response to stimulation. *J Dent Res* **64**:564–71.

Närhi MVO (1985b) Dentin sensitivity: a review. *J Biol Buccale* **13**:75–96.

Närhi MVO (1990) The neurophysiology of the teeth. *Dent Clin North Am* **34**:439–48.

Närhi M, Haegerstam G (1983) Intradental nerve activity induced by reduced pressure applied to exposed dentine in the cat. *Acta Physiol Scand* **119**:381–6.

Närhi MVO, Hirvonen T (1987) The response of dog intradental nerves to hypertonic solutions of $CaCl_2$ and NaCl, and other stimuli, applied to exposed dentine. *Arch Oral Biol* **32**:781–6.

Närhi M, Kontturi-Närhi V, Markkanen H (1991) Sensitivity of teeth with exposed dentine to air blasts, cold and electrical stimulation. *J Dent Res* **70**:488.

Närhi M, Kontturi-Närhi V, Hirvonen T, Ngassapa D (1992) Neurophysiological mechanism of dentin hypersensitivity. *Proc Finn Dent Soc* **88** (Suppl I):15–22.

Naylor MN (1961) A thermo-electric tooth stimulator. *Br Dent J* **110**:228–30.

Ngassapa D (1991) Dentine sensitivity: factors influencing intradental nerve activation in dog teeth. PhD Thesis. *Publications of the University of Kuopio*, Kuopio, Finland. Medicine 1–107.

Ohnhaus EE, Adler R (1975) Methodological problems in the measurement of pain. A comparison between the verbal rating scale and the visual analogue scale. *Pain* **1**:379–84.

Ong G, Strahan JD (1989) Effects of a desensitizing dentifrice on dentinal hypersensitivity. *Endodontics Dent Traumatol* **5**:213–18.

Orchardson R (1997) Toothache – the 'hell of all diseases'. *Br Dent J* **182**:71–3.

Orchardson R, Collins WJN (1987a) Clinical features of hypersensitive teeth. *Br Dent J* **162**:253–6.

Orchardson R, Collins WJN (1987b) Thresholds of hypersensitive teeth. *J Clin Periodontol* **14**:68–73.

Orro M, Truong T, de Vizio W et al (1994) Thermodontic stimulator – a new technology for assessment of thermal dentinal hypersensitivity. *J Clin Dent* **5** (Special issue):83–6.

Pashley DH (1986) Sensitivity of dentin to chemical stimuli. *Endodontics Dent Traumatol* **2**:130–7.

Pashley DH (1990) Mechanisms of dentin sensitivity. *Dent Clin North Am* **34**:449–73.

Pashley DH, O'Meara JA, Kepler EE et al (1984) Dentin permeability. Effects of desensitizing dentifrices in vitro. *J Periodontol* **55**:522–5.

Pearce N, Addy M, Newcombe RG (1994) Dentine hypersensitivity: a clinical trial to compare 2 strontium desensitising toothpastes with a conventional fluoride toothpaste. *J Periodontol* **65**:113–19.

Person P, Demand EE, Koltun L, Spindel M (1989) A microprocessor temperature-controlled air delivery system for dentinal hypersensitivity testing. *Clin Prev Dent* **11**:3–9.

Price DD, McGrath PA, Raffi A, Buckingham B (1983) The validation of visual analogue scales as ratio measurements of experimental and chronic pain. *Pain* **17**:45–56.

Schiff T, Santos MD, Laffi S et al (1998) Efficacy of a dentifrice containing 5% potassium nitrate and 1500 ppm sodium mono-fluorophosphate in a precipitated calcium carbonate base on dentine hypersensitivity. *J Clin Dent* **9**:22–5.

Scott J, Huskisson EC (1976) Graphic representation of pain. *Pain* **2**:175–84.

Sessle BJ (1987) The neurobiology of facial and dental pain: present knowledge, future directions. *J Dent Res* **66**:962–81

Seymour RA (1982) The use of pain scales in assessing the efficacy of analgesics in post-op dental pain. *Eur J Clin Pharmacol* **23**:441–4.

Silverman G (1985) The sensitivity-reducing effect of brushing with a potassium nitrate–sodium monofluorophosphate dentifrice. *Compendium of Continuing Education in Dentistry* **6**:131–6.

Smart G, Riches M, Young K et al (1998) Thermal probe evaluation of sensitive and non-sensitive teeth. *J Dent Res* **77**:746 (abstract 916).

Smith B, Ash MM (1964) A study of a desensitizing dentifrice and cervical hypersensitivity. *J Periodontol* **35**:222–31.

Stark MM, Pelzner RB, Leung RL (1977) Rationalization of electric pulp-testing methods. *Oral Surg Oral Med Oral Pathol* **43**:598–606.

Tarbet WJ, Silverman G, Stolman JM, Fratarcangelo PA (1979) An evaluation of two methods for the quantification of dentinal hypersensitivity. *J Am Dent Assoc* **98**:914–18.

Tarbet WJ, Silverman G, Fratarcangelo PA, Kanapka JA (1982) Home treatment for dentinal hypersensitivity. A comparative study. *J Am Dent Assoc* **105**:227–30.

Thrash WJ, Dorman HL, Smith FD (1983) A method to measure pain associated with hypersensitive dentin. *J Periodontol* **54**:160–2.

Thrash WJ. Jones DL, Dodds WJM (1992) Effect of a fluoride solution on dentinal hypersensitivity. *Am J Dent* **5**:299–302.

Vongsavan N, Matthews B (1992). Fluid flow through cat dentine in vivo. *Arch Oral Biol* **37**:175–85.

West NX, Addy M, Jackson RJ, Ridge DB (1997) Dentine hypersensitivity and the placebo response. A comparison of the effect of strontium acetate, potassium nitrate and fluoride toothpastes. *J Clin Periodontol* **24**:209–15.

Yates R, West N, Addy M, Marlow I (1998) The effects of a potassium chloride, sodium fluoride mouthrinse on dentine hypersensitivity, plaque and gingivitis. A placebo-controlled study. *J Clin Periodontol* **25**:813–20.

Zakrzewska JM, Feinmann C (1990) A standard way to measure pain and psychological morbidity in dental practice. *Br Dent J* **169**:337–9.

Zborowski M (1952) Cultural components in response to pain. *J Social Issues* **8**:16–30.

Zigmond AS, Snaith RP (1983) The Hospital Anxiety and Depression Scale. *Acta Psychol Scand* **67**:361–70.

26

Design and conduct of clinical trials on dentine hypersensitivity

Frederick A Curro, Michael Friedman and Ronald S Leight

Introduction

Dentifrices, over the years, have assumed a product identity much greater than their original intent of a cosmetic cleansing agent for teeth. They can now consist of a number of active agents addressing not only the cleansing and whitening of teeth but also contain agents that affect clinical therapeutic end-points such as caries, gingivitis and hypersensitivity. These clinical end-points establish the regulatory category for a dentifrice as an over-the-counter (OTC) drug product directed toward the consumer.

The clinical end-points for a dentifrice that has a number of therapeutic indications can be established for each indication. The mechanism of action of the active or pharmacological agents in the treatment of dentinal hypersensitivity is described in Chapter 27. Briefly, there are currently two clinical approaches, one is to occlude the dentinal tubules and the other is to depress the nerve action potential of the odontoblastic cell body. The target end-point for dentinal hypersensitivity can be varied both by treatment and by the physiology of the pulpal response. The condition describes little distinction between treatment and management. This may explain why the condition is so prevalent and why the clinical impression suggests that recurrence is common (Yates *et al.* 1998).

Additionally, clinical outcomes for dentinal hypersensitivity studies suggest a wide assortment of possible effective treatment modalities, with some studies demonstrating limited benefits of the active formulation against a placebo control. Explanations of this response may include a lack of understanding of the effects produced on the dentine surface by the active agent, phenomena associated with clinical trials on hypersensitive teeth and the subjects' natural temporal improvement with symptoms exhibiting a regression to the mean (Yates *et al.* 1998). In a recent study (West *et al.* 1997), the placebo effects were shown to be as high as 40%, thereby minimizing the symptom range available to show significance for the test agent.

Dentinal hypersensitivity studies can be viewed in the larger context of the art and science of clinical pharmacology. This viewpoint reveals that many of the issues or confounding factors confronted in conducting a clinical dentinal hypersensitivity study are not unique to dentistry. However, demonstrating drug action is complex given the nature of the condition, and any investigator who has conducted a clinical dentinal hypersensitivity study can attest to its high degree of difficulty. This chapter will attempt to explain the difficulties encountered in conducting clinical dentinal hypersensitivity studies by applying pharmacological principles of drug action. Additionally, physiological limitations of the target site, concurrent with changes of the cell body mediating the response and its environment and an understanding of the chronicity of the condition can offer further insight and explanations for the sometimes variable outcome of clinical dentinal hypersensitivity studies. Finally, the methodological issues surrounding the measurement and interpretation of tactile pain thresholds and the magnitude, time course and variability of the placebo response will be discussed.

Pharmacodynamic considerations affecting the clinical outcome of dental hypersensitivity studies

Dentifrices containing an active agent in a complex vehicle and directed toward alleviating the discomfort of dentinal hypersensitivity have pharmacodynamic considerations which uniquely affect their ability to have an effect on the tooth. Drug distribution depends upon how much active agent reaches the area of dentinal erosion and its degree of substantivity to the dentinal surface. Studies utilizing dentifrices as drug vehicles are unique to the target organ, with the disadvantages outweighing the advantages (Table 26.1). Distribution, mainly by diffusion, of the active agent to the target site, requires a high enough concentration gradient of the active agent to get into the tubule to affect the odontoblastic fibril or the fluid within to elicit an effect at the level of the odontoblast by depolarization and/or suppression.

The traditional treatment of dentinal hypersensitivity currently consists of two modalities, one is by direct consumer use, usually in the form of a toothpaste, the other is by professional application in the dental office. The active agent or drug is part of a complex formulation designed for other purposes, such as cleansing, but can be viewed as a drug delivery system or vehicle for the active agent directed towards hypersensitivity. The body system most directly affected by the application of a toothpaste is the mouth, particularly the teeth, which can be used as a port of entry for drug delivery for systemic purposes. Drugs can be swallowed (oral), placed under the tongue (sublingual) or placed in the cheek pouch (buccal) for eventual systemic dissemination. With very few exceptions, systemic drugs have a targeted site of action affecting a bodily system, tissue or cell or having a molecular target. The target site for the treatment of dentinal hypersensitivity is currently thought to be the dentinal tubule or its contents: the fibril from the odontoblast within the tubule or the odontoblastic cell body itself.

Pharmacodynamically, the active agent must be delivered onto or into a dentinal tubule for an effect to occur. For an active agent to be evaluated for its effect on the teeth, the delivery of the active agent poses difficulties unique to the target organ. The active agent as part of a complex drug delivery system (dentifrice) must be applied by a device, i.e. a toothbrush (to first remove the biofilm), within a constantly diluted and buffered system within the oral cavity. The amount of dentifrice applied is not always consistent nor is the time of application. The size of the toothbrush head and its bristle density and stiffness can also vary. After patients have applied the active agent they further dilute the effect by thoroughly rinsing their mouths out with water. Thus, the whole operation of applying the active agent with a device, to the tooth, is in opposition to traditional pharmacological principles whereby the accumulation effect at the target site may not be maximized or may be limited by a ceiling effect (Figure 26.1). Medical conditions such as gastro-esophageal reflux and the patient's daily food and drink, partly related to the pH, may also be confounding variables on drug efficacy (Bartlett 1997). To further complicate matters, known drug reservoirs are not available at the site of action. It appears that the drug must be delivered to the target site at the time of application, and accumulation with daily use must be assumed. Additionally, defense mechanisms of the pulpal tissue to stimuli and inflammation due to exposed dentine are continually operative, affecting the subject's response and further accentuating the self-limiting nature of the condition (Linde and Goldberg 1993).

The systemic pharmacodynamics of drug action (considered with as many compartments as one wants to apply) has, as a common basis, the blood system to act as a reservoir and carrier of the drug to the site of action. More impor-

Table 26.1 Studies utilizing dentifrices as drug vehicles

Advantages	Disadvantages
Schedule of application	Schedule may vary
	Amount of dentifrice varies
Compliance of use	Time of brushing varies
	Force applied to brush varies
	Condition of mouth varies
	Condition of toothbrush varies
	Rinsing of mouth varies
	No drug reservoirs

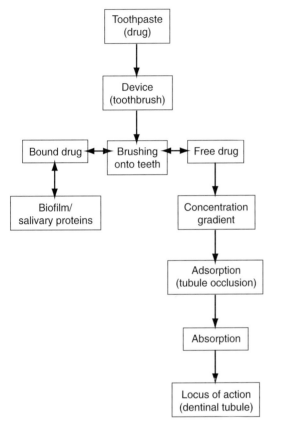

Figure 26.1

Toothpastes as drug vehicles. Active agent or drug utilizing a toothpaste formula can most likely have a direct effect at the site of action (dentinal tubule) without the traditional concerns required of the transport of drugs across cell membranes, i.e. charge, lipid solubility, etc.

tantly, the concentration of the drug within the blood can be measured to explain the temporal or pharmacodynamic effect of the drug's action.

Concentration effect curves for active agents applied to dentinal hypersensitivity studies have yet to be devised considering the complex nature of their application. Thus, the complexity of the active agent getting onto or into the dentinal tubule site to elicit its effect is pharmacodynamically more complex than the traditionally viewed pharmacokinetic drug profile. Given these factors, drug effect variability and a considerable 'lag time' for the drug's effect (weeks) is not

surprising. In addition to the placebo effect, the dentinal tubule may be affected by the multiple ingredients of the toothpaste, particularly the abrasive system (Addy *et al.* 1987), and by the effect of brushing/burnishing. The latter may change the landscape of the number of open tubules within the area of dentinal erosion. This creates a difficult pharmacological target, whereby the traditional law of mass action may not be applicable. Although other studies have shown that the abrasivity of a dentifrice does not affect the desensitizing activity (Gillam *et al.* 1992a, Gillam *et al.* 1992b), the tooth remains a challenging target for drug action.

The tooth, it appears, is a rather specific target or site of action, requiring some form of direct application of an active agent either by rinsing, brushing or chewing.

Additionally, paradoxical anatomical, pharmacological and physiological circumstances, such as extensive neuronal convergence of teeth allowing pulpo-dentinal pain to be poorly localized (clinically manifested as diagnosing two or three teeth adjacent to the affected tooth), the fact that local anesthetics applied topically to the dentine are not effective and the unknown contribution of the periodontal ligament to the augmentation of the dentinal response to the evoked stimulus, add to the complexity of conducting a dentinal hypersensitivity study (Curro 1990).

Therapeutic range

A particular challenge for clinical research directed towards over-the-counter products is to occasionally be able to evaluate and assess the efficacy of a naturally active or synthetic pharmacological agent in comparison to one that is already on the market and perceived to be efficacious by the consumer. Clinical design, controls and the appropriate population are paramount to success. Clinical success is usually defined by achieving statistical significance ($P < 0.05$) with respect to some previously agreed clinical endpoints or parameters. Statistical significance, depending upon the indication or use of the active agent, may or may not include clinical significance. Clinical significance can vary according to the therapeutic range and endpoints assigned to it.

Prescription drugs are usually more potent and are designed to treat serious medical conditions that would have a therapeutic end-point that is both clinically and statistically significant. Prescription drugs may be used to treat a symptom of a serious medical condition (e.g. depression or anxiety) which, having a wide therapeutic range, could differ in clinical and statistical significance as clinical end-points. That is, a study could show a statistically significant difference between active agent and placebo, but the result could be clinically irrelevant because it is too far down on the therapeutic scale to have a meaningful effect on the symptoms. Drugs used to treat symptoms, such as pain, hypersensitivity, anxiety or sleep, and having a wide therapeutic range with an increasing level of response, along with a high therapeutic index, are usually good candidates for OTC use or for a prescription-only (Rx) to OTC switch.

Consumer-directed agents or OTC products usually, but not always, treat symptoms of a condition and the dose as a rule is lower (one-half) than the prescribed dose. Like many OTC indications, dentine hypersensitivity is a symptom, further complicated by being a self-limiting condition and having a rather narrow therapeutic range, where the magnitude and nature of the response (nerve action potential) are relatively close together. This may confound the interpretation between what is clinically and statistically relevant. It is this small therapeutic range that produces controversy in the literature, as well as in conducting clinical studies. Since thermal and tactile responses may be mediated by different receptors, our database suggests that the use of a single, well-defined stimulus would simplify the interpretation of the clinical outcome. It would also be expected that there would be a higher placebo effect with an OTC product in a well-controlled, randomized, double-blind study compared with actual consumer use of the product where there is no prescriber–patient interaction.

The clinical efficacy of current products tested in dentinal hypersensitivity studies appears to be performing at the lower end of the therapeutic range. This could be a function either of the potency of the active agent itself or problems in reaching the target site, or could be due to limitations in the sensitivity of the clinical design, i.e. the nature and difficulty of evoking and evaluating both the stimulus and the patient response. Additionally, the clinical responses can be affected by the investigator technique as well as the doctor–patient relationship. Furthermore, teeth may vary in their individual responses to thermal and tactile changes. A true comparison of clinical studies can only be assured if the responses can be matched up to the same teeth.

Given the difficulty and nature of such studies it is not surprising that the literature includes both positive and negative clinical studies on the same active agent. It is for the discerning clinician to scrutinize and assess the spectrum of data

Table 26.2 Requirements for conducting a dentinal hypersensitivity clinical study; proper design controls must be incorporated to minimize clinical outcome variability

Variable factor	Design control
Doctor–patient interactions	Double-blind conditions
Investigator and patient bias	
Placebo responses	Placebo control group
Chance outcomes	Properly powered study
Subjective assessment of pain	Response quantified
Fluctuation in symptoms	Random allocation of patients
Clinical outcome	Statistical analysis of results
Evaluation criteria	Defined parameters
Fluctuation of control group	Positive control
Non-responders	Screening and baseline visits
Evoked stimulus (thermal)	Direct, reproducible, repeatable
Evoked stimulus fluctuation (tactile)	Calibration
Drug delivery/device	Control of amount and time of application/standard toothbrush
Confidence of clinical outcome	Use of well-defined stimuli

and draw a conclusion based on the evidence as to whether an agent is efficacious or not.

Dentinal hypersensitivity studies must be designed with the proper controls (Table 26.2) and guidelines as described under good clinical practice (below). This ensures a level of confidence that the data are meaningful and within the limits of the sensitivity of the clinical study. Good clinical practice is defined as a standard for the design, conduct, performance, monitoring, auditing, recording, analysis and reporting of clinical trials that provides assurance that the data and reported results are credible and accurate, and that the rights, integrity and confidentiality of trial subjects are protected (Code of Federal Regulations 1998).

Eliciting a response

Tooth erosion or abrasion of either enamel or cementum leading to tooth hypersensitivity – or more accurately, dentinal sensitivity or hypersensitivity – is described clinically as an exaggerated response to a non-noxious sensory stimulus. The sensory stimuli usually applied to a tooth to elicit a response are thermal/evaporative – the application of a burst of air to the tooth – and tactile – running a metal dental instrument, sometimes attached to a force transducer, across the hypersensitive region of the tooth.

Dentine sensitivity presents clinically as a sharp, transient, well-localized pain that does not occur spontaneously and does not persist after the removal of the stimulus. It is a self-limiting condition. The dentifrice is marketed directly to the consumer with a focused indication. Eliciting a response from an area of exposed dentine does not require actual tissue damage in the acute sense, but can involve potential tissue damage with constant erosion of the enamel or cementum along with the concomitant pulpal response. The present subjective evaluation of tooth hypersensitivity uses current pain questionnaires and visual analog pain scales and is thus described in such terms. Dentinal hypersensitivity is a response to a non-noxious stimulus and a chronic condition with acute episodes when the area is further challenged; whereas tooth pain – originating from the dentine and expressed as a pulpal response – is a response to a noxious stimulus and usually an acute condition unless the pulp is undergoing pathological changes. This temporal difference in the two conditions may affect higher central nervous system centers, producing psychological and physiological differences similar to those described for acute and chronic pain (Table 26.3). In addition, these differences may alter the subject's affective state, possibly causing variability in the subjective response or description due to the evoked stimulus (Capra and Dessein 1992).

Dentinal hypersensitivity clinical studies satisfy the criteria from the temporal behavioral aspect of pain suggesting a direct clinical pathway (Figure 26.2). In assessing a subject for a dentinal hypersensitivity clinical study, particular attention

Table 26.3 Relationship of dentinal hypersensitivity to acute and chronic pain

Variable	Acute pain	Chronic pain	Dentinal hypersensitivity
Conduction pathways	Rapid	Slow	Rapid
Response	Mild/severe	Mild/severe	Sharp, transient
	Localized	Diffuse	Localized
Tissue injury	Clearly causal	Minor or absent	Clearly causal
Autonomic response	Present	Absent	Present
Biological value	High	Low	High
Mood	Anxiety	Depression, anxiety	Anxiety
Social effects	Slight	Marked	Slight
Effective treatment	Analgesics	Variable, sometimes none	Variable, sometimes none
Dysfunction	Possible	Present	Possible
Learned behavior	No	Yes	Yes
Somatization	No	Can be present	Can be present
Hypochondriasis	No	Can be present	Can be present

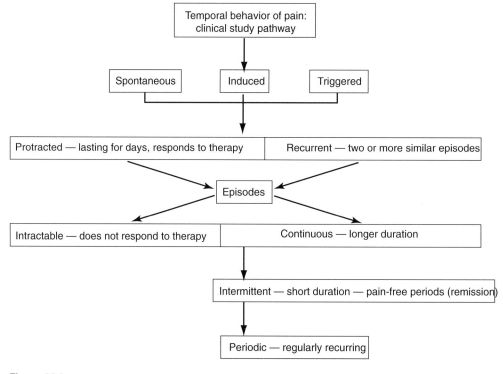

Figure 26.2

Clinical study pathway for pain should be the most direct, reproducible, and repeatable minimizing effects from both the peripheral and autonomic nervous system. Dentinal hypersensitivity can be induced, is episodic (recurrent), intermittent, and can be periodic.

should be given to parameters that may possibly contribute to variability in the manner in which the patient may describe the response to a stimulus. Thus, the subject's medical history, emotional state, habits of use, traumatic incidents, and the condition of the dentition and supporting structures are important attributes in patient selection for dentinal hypersensitivity clinical studies. Periodontal influences producing anachoresis may contribute to the variability of the response and should be an exclusion criterion. Conducting a clinical study which requires a stimulus to evoke a response from a subject, as in a dentinal hypersensitivity study, raises some interesting confounding issues in quantifying a patient's response and mirrors the complexity of a pain study. Pain is considered a multidimensional experience consisting of motivational, cognitive, affective and discriminative components (Melzack 1975). The motivational compo-

nent concerns itself with the escape mechanism, such as turning away from the source of the painful stimuli. The cognitive component is the past memory of the painful experience, i.e. knowing that the stimulus will cause pain. The affective component is concerned with the anxiety and stress associated with the painful experience, and the discriminative component is concerned with the onset, duration, intensity and location of the pain. Stress and anxiety can adversely affect several physiological processes and increase symptom reporting (Turner *et al.* 1994). All too often, dentists may focus more on the discriminative component while patients focus more on the other three components, especially the affective component rendering the painful event as a private experience. A dental patient who has had an initially good experience in the dental office would have a very low motivational component; that is, he or she would not want to leave the office. This patient would have a low affective component, i.e. a decrease in anxiety and apprehension. This patient would also have a very low cognitive component of negative experiences of past dental visits and thus would be able to describe pain in a more objective manner. This would allow the doctor a clearer picture with which to assess the patient's pain response. Conversely, a patient who has had negative experiences in the dental office would be very eager to leave and would have a high motivational component, would be very apprehensive, and thus would have a high affective component. He or she would remember a bad experience or response and therefore would have a high cognitive component.

These components would cloud the objective presentation of the discriminative component, posing a problem for the doctor in treatment and management of the patient and particularly in the assessment of the evoked response during a clinical study. Thus, the interaction between the patient and dentist or any past negative or positive experiences may affect the outcome of the study. Additionally, placebos seem to be most effective for highly anxious subjects, and placebo effects are often attributed to anxiety reduction and associated decreased suffering (Evans 1985). Placebos have been shown to decrease anticipatory anxiety; however, it is not clear whether anxiety reduction is a cause of the placebo effect, or a component of it (Wall 1993).

Tactile pain thresholds

Pain is a complex sensation. Its measurement requires a cognitive response to an external stimulus that has been detected by bio-organic sensors and relayed to the brain by an electrochemical transmission system. Electrophysiologists have discovered that it is a noisy system; one which, even when not stimulated, will spontaneously fire at random intervals. Witness the phenomena of flashing lights observed by individuals who have spent long periods of time in absolute darkness or the well-known phenomenon of phantom limb pain. Like all sensory systems, each human sensory system can be characterized by a threshold, a working range and a saturation limit. Measurement of the

tactile pain threshold as a clinical end-point is of interest in dentinal hypersensitivity studies.

The simplest definition of a threshold would be the minimum stimulus intensity or frequency that triggers a measurable response in the detector. However, this definition is incomplete. It leaves out the often unspoken limitation: under well-defined operating conditions. For example, the response threshold of an electronic detector minimally depends on its operating temperature and voltage. These are factors that can be controlled or at least independently measured. Once known, their effect on the limits of detection (the threshold) can be predicted, either theoretically or from an existing calibration curve.

In the realm of physiological detectors, the situation is not so straightforward. The threshold of a physiological detector can be influenced by the hydration state of the surrounding tissues, the overall nutritional state of the organism, the overall fatigue state of the organism, influence from higher centers within the central nervous system, the current local environment, etc. Investigators have little or no control over any of these, and they can and do vary from instant to instant.

In the realm of human sensory response, there is an additional layer of complication. If individuals had to consciously attend to every signal from every sensory receptor in their bodies, they would be overwhelmed by the flood of information. Therefore, at both a physiological level and at a cognitive level, the human sensory system only responds to changes to the sensory inputs. Not only does a stimulus have to exceed the physiological threshold of the receptor, but it must also exceed the cognitive threshold of 'important change' from current background.

These factors and over 100 years of empirical data have led sensory specialists to define sensory thresholds in a probabilistic fashion. It has also led them to define two different types of thresholds: detection threshold and recognition threshold. The distinction is the difference between being able to say 'I see someone coming this way' and 'I see my friend Max coming this way'. With respect to dentinal hypersensitivity, it is the difference between the patient noticing that something is touching a tooth and deciding that the touch is painful. The former would be the detection threshold and the latter the pain recognition threshold. It is the recognition threshold that is of interest in hypersensitivity studies.

The recognition threshold for a sensory stimulus can be defined as 'the minimum physical intensity of a stimulus for which there is a specified probability (most frequently 0.50) that an assessor will assign the same descriptor each time it is presented' (ASTM Committee 1997). This type of definition is common in the life sciences. Consider, for example, the widely used concepts of LD_{50} (median lethal dose) and ED_{50} (median effective dose). While these two examples represent population statistics, the principles apply just as strongly in the determination of pain thresholds for individual teeth. As a probability cannot be calculated from a single response, a tactile pain threshold *cannot be determined by a single positive response*.

Many methods have been developed to determine sensory thresholds. The 'up and down' method has generally been considered to be the most efficient in that, for a given degree of precision, it requires fewer stimulus presentations than most other methods (Bi and Ennis 1998). A simple variant of this method can produce stable tactile pain thresholds (Leight *et al.* 1991). However, both ethical and practical concerns lead us to question the necessity of employing methods that require multiple painful stimuli. Thus, this group has recently employed a method which meets what are considered to be the minimum requirements for determining a parameter which has a probabilistic definition. It starts from a minimum force value and increases in a step-wise fashion until a value is reached which produces two consecutive 'pain'

Table 26.4 Summary of clinical studies on hypersensitivity

Study	Product type	Number of subjects	Tactile threshold	Air blast	Subjective score	Active agent
I	Toothpaste	105	Yes	VDS	VDS	$SrCl_2$
II	Gum	58	Yes	VAS	VAS	KCl
III	Toothpaste	118	Yes	VAS	VAS	Amine F, NaF
IV	Rinse	108	Yes	VAS	VAS	0.5% KCl, 1.0% KCl
V	Toothpaste	106	Yes	VDS	VDS	KNO_3
VI	Toothpaste	142	Yes	VAS	VAS	KNO_3/other
VII	Toothpaste	101	Yes	VAS	VAS	KCl
VIII	Toothpaste	132	No	VAS	VAS	Other
IX	Toothpaste	118	Yes	VAS	VAS	KNO_3/other
X	Toothpaste	95	Yes	VAS	VAS	KNO_3/other

Gum, chewing gum; Rinse, mouth rinse; VAS, 100 mm visual analog scale (line scale); VDS, 9-point verbal descriptor scale; none, extremely weak, very weak, weak, mild, moderate, slightly intense, intense, extremely intense.
The raw data from 10 recent studies by Block Drug Company were combined to evaluate the false positive rate within studies. All studies consisted of two or three parallel groups which were followed over periods ranging from 4 to 12 weeks. One group in each study received a placebo treatment. Nine of the 10 studies measured tactile pain threshold. Eight of the 10 studies measured air blast and subjective response using 100-mm line scales; the two remaining studies used a 9–point verbal descriptor scale.

Table 26.5 False positive rate by study

	n	Mean	SD	Range
False positive rate by study	9	4.80%	6.40	0, 20.90%
Overall (all sequences)	11 253	5.02%	–	–

The false positive rate is real and highly variable. Some investigators/sites have extremely low false positive rates, but others have rates as high as 20%.

Table 26.6 False positive rate by visit

	Qualifying visit	Base	Week 1	Week 2	Week 4	Week 6	Week 8	Week 12
Rate (%)	7.39	4.18	0	2.80	4.53	3.64	3.32	2.48
n	3383	2509	193	1499	1698	659	1203	109

n = number of sequences. False positives are almost twice as common at the qualifying visit as at subsequent visits. This is most likely a learning effect on the part of both the subjects and the examiners.

Table 26.7 Difference in grams between the first 'yes' response and the confirmed threshold

	0 g	+5 g	+10 g	>10 g
Percentage of thresholds under-estimated by this amount	0.35	52.04	24.78	22.83

When false positives occur, the response will be at least 10 g too low almost 48% of the time. An average of the 565 differences yields an expected under-estimate of the threshold of 9.86 g. Therefore, the 5% false positive rate will result in threshold estimates which are ~0.5 g too low. In the worst case of a 20% false positive rate, the mean threshold estimates will be almost 2 g too low.

Table 26.8 Percentage of false positives occurring at each force level

	10 g	15 g	20 g	25 g	30 g	>30 g
% of false positives occurring at each level	30.09	26.37	17.88	8.14	8.32	9.20
% of stimuli at each level	22.6	21.5	19.4	10.8	8.0	17.6

False positives are more likely to occur at low force levels. Proportionately, this could increase the placebo response more than the treatment response. This in turn would reduce the size of the treatment effect.

responses. The practical necessity of using this procedure is illustrated in Tables 26.4–26.7.

In any diagnostic procedure, there is a probability of a false positive response. To evaluate the false positive rate, 10 clinical studies on dentinal hypersensitivity conducted by the Block Drug Company have been reviewed (Table 26.4). In the procedure for determining thresholds described above, a false positive occurs any time a response of 'pain' is followed by a response of 'no pain' at the same force setting. In the nine studies reviewed here, there are a total of 11 253 tactile testing sequences in which a confirmed threshold was recorded, i.e. the patient responded 'pain' to two consecutive stimulations at the same force. In 565 (5.02%) of these sequences a false positive response was recorded (Table 26.5). Across studies, the false positive rate ranged from 0% to a high of 20.9%. The rate at the 'qualifying visit' (7.39%) is almost twice the mean rate of all other visits (3.9%) (Table 26.6). When a false positive response occurs the confirmed threshold will be ≥10 g higher than the first 'pain' response in 47.96% of cases (Table 26.7). That is, in almost one-half of the cases an error of ≥10 g can occur. There is an apparent tendency for false positives to occur more frequently than expected at lower force values (Table 26.8), i.e. false positive responses do not occur at random, but are more likely to occur at the lower gram forces.

Assessment of the placebo response

A clinical dentinal hypersensitivity study should be conducted under the same aegis and concern as any clinical pain study (Clark and Troullos, 1990). Difficulties in patient recruitment, the changing landscape of the exposed dentinal area, continuation of the underlying physiological process and the inherent shortcomings and difficulty in evaluating the subjects' response require that a placebo cell be considered in the design of a dental hypersensitivity study. Theoretically, a placebo control group provides a baseline against which the effectiveness of an active agent can be measured, i.e. to demonstrate that the active agent is better than no treatment. However, the placebo effect has repeatedly been shown to be something 'other' than merely having no effect and different from the 'no-treatment' group; yet why and how it works remains largely unknown. Even the magnitude of the placebo effect in a clinical study is hard to determine. In part, this is because normal spontaneous remission of a disease that may be self-limiting cannot be distinguished from the placebo effect unless there is a control group that has received no treatment at all. No-treatment controls are not common, although they have been used in alcohol studies, often employing the 'balanced placebo design'. In the four cells of such a design, participants: a) are told they will get a drug, and do get it, b) are told they will get a drug, but receive placebo, c) are told they will get placebo, and do get it, or d) are told they will get placebo, but get a drug. In a number of dentinal hypersensitivity studies it has been observed that there is an increasing degree of difficulty in patient recruitment to reach the required sample size of 50 subjects per group. This is partly because modern restorative dental techniques (such as bonding agents) have made an impact on subject recruitment for dentinal hypersensitivity studies over the last 10 years or so. Dentinal hypersensitivity studies are taking longer to complete and incorporation of additional groups to evaluate the placebo response can only complicate already difficult studies.

To evaluate and compare an active agent in the clinical development stage this group normally runs a three cell study consisting of: a) an active agent, b) a positive control, and c) a placebo control. The placebo control is evaluated within the study and compared to the database of placebo controls. Tables 26.9 and 26.10 compare baseline and post-baseline placebo effects at weeks two, four and eight from an existing database of clinical studies with a published study conducted by Silverman et al (1996) and with summary data on file for strontium chloride, a purported tubule occluding agent. The actual potential therapeutic effect for the percentage subjective and thermal sensitivity reduction is depicted in Table 26.11.

Table 26.9 Characteristics of mean efficacy scale measurements at baseline for placebo treatment groups

Efficacy scale	Subjective sensitivity (mm)	Thermal sensitivity (mm)	Tactile sensitivity (g)
Mean score at baseline			
n	8	8	9
Mean	47.7	50.9	20.5
Median	46.9	51.8	20.2
SD	2.4	3.1	5.7
Range	45.3, 52.7	46.0, 54.8	10.0, 31.7

Subjective and thermal scales are summarized in this table only for studies where sensitivity was measured in mm on a 100 mm visual analog scale (VAS) anchored at 0 (no pain) and 100 (intense pain). Two other studies used a 9-point verbal descriptor scale anchored at 0 (no pain) and 8 (extremely intense pain). Tactile sensitivity was measured as a threshold in grams. n = number of studies.

Table 26.10 Post-baseline placebo effects

Efficacy scale	Placebo effect from baseline		
	2 weeks	4 weeks	8 weeks
Subjective sensitivity reduction (%)			
n	8	10	8
Mean	15.9	24.2	37.3
Median	12.1	21.6	34.4
SD	8.8	7.7	9.1
Range	9.6, 34.0	16.8, 37.2	28.0, 51.9
Silverman study[1]	5.3	16.2	29.4
SrCl$_2$ study[2]	8.5	13.5	17.5
Thermal sensitivity reduction (%)			
n	8	10	8
Mean	14.1	24.3	37.6
Median	13.7	24.5	36.8
SD	4.6	6.2	7.0
Range	6.1, 22.5	14.1, 36.8	28.7, 49.1
Silverman study	6.2	14.3	30.4
SrCl$_2$ study	10.8	15.3	24.1
Tactile threshold improvement (g)			
n	7	9	7
Mean	4.8	9.0	13.6
Median	4.6	6.8	10.3
SD	3.5	5.5	7.7
Range	−0.9, 9.3	1.7, 17.1	4.3, 22.1
Silverman study	5.3	9.0	13.3
SrCl$_2$ study	1.4	7.4	12.0

Both studies using the VAS scale and studies using the verbal descriptor scale for subjective and thermal sensitivity are included in this table.
[1]Silverman *et al.* (1996) (see Reference section for details).
[2]Block Drug Company data on file.

Table 26.11 Potential therapeutic range

Efficacy scale	Time from baseline		
	2 weeks	4 weeks	8 weeks
Subjective sensitivity reduction (%)	84.1	75.8	62.7
Thermal sensitivity reduction (%)	85.9	75.7	62.4

Therapeutic range calculated as 100% minus the placebo effect.

Figure 26.3 describes the mean percentage sensitivity reduction from baseline comparing potassium nitrate (a putative neuronal suppressant) with strontium chloride. The placebo responses from the two studies are both directional, crossing each other approximately at week four. A difference of approximately 10% between the two agents exists at Week 8. The mean active and placebo treatment effects for tactile sensitivity are depicted in Figure 26.4. The profiles of tactile improvement for the two agents are very similar. The close relationship of the two studies may suggest more of a common basis for similar mechanisms than previously

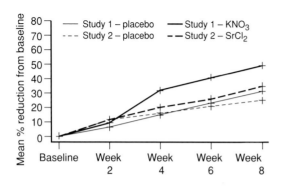

Figure 26.3

Comparison of mean active and placebo treatment effects on thermal sensitivity of two different agents in two clinical hypersensitivity studies. Study 1: Silverman *et al.* 1996 (see Reference section for details); $P < 0.05$ after 4 and 8 weeks. Study 2: Block Drug Company 1994; $P < 0.05$ after 8 weeks.

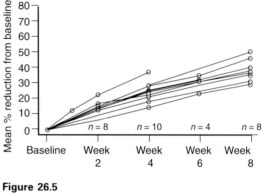

Figure 26.5

Comparison of placebo responses in a number of dentinal hypersensitivity studies on thermal sensitivity. n = number of studies conducted by the Block Drug Company.

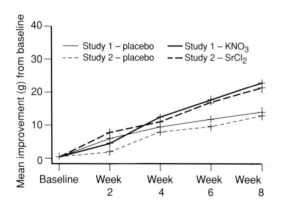

Figure 26.4

Comparison of mean active and placebo treatment effects on tactile sensitivity of two different agents in two clinical hypersensitivity studies. Study 1: Silverman *et al.* 1996 (see Reference section for details); $P < 0.05$ after 4 and 8 weeks. Study 2: Block Drug Company 1994; $P < 0.05$ after 2, 6, and 8 weeks.

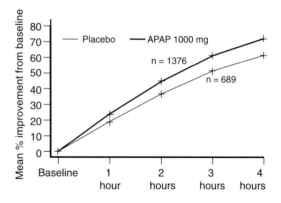

Figure 26.6

Comparison of mean APAP (*N*-acetyl-*p*-aminophenol, acetaminophen) 1000 mg and placebo treatment effects for pain intensity in Bristol-Myers muscle contraction headache studies (Bristol-Myers Products 1988; see Reference section for details). Combined data from four studies; $P < 0.001$ after 1, 2, 3, and 4 hours.

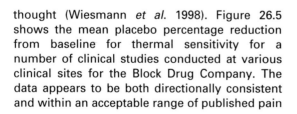

thought (Wiesmann *et al.* 1998). Figure 26.5 shows the mean placebo percentage reduction from baseline for thermal sensitivity for a number of clinical studies conducted at various clinical sites for the Block Drug Company. The data appears to be both directionally consistent and within an acceptable range of published pain

studies for the placebo response. Beecher (1955) reviewed 15 studies of patients suffering from a variety of conditions including postoperative pain, cough, angina pectoris, headache, drug-induced mood changes, seasickness, anxiety and tension, and the common cold, and concluded that on average, symptoms were 'satisfactorily

Table 26.12 Percentage improvement from baseline for placebo and acetaminophen (Tylenol) in four muscle contraction headache studies

Percent reduction from baseline (%)	Treatment effect on pain intensity from baseline			
	1 hour	2 hours	3 hours	4 hours
Placebo (n = 689)	19.3	36.9	51.9	61.4
APAP 1000 mg (n = 1376)	24.0	44.6	61.4	72.1
APAP placebo	4.7	7.7	9.5	10.7

Pain intensity was scored on a 0–3 scale. Combined data from four studies submitted to the FDA (1988) by Bristol-Myers Products, comparing Extra-Strength Excedrin, Tylenol and placebo.

relieved' by the placebo in 35% of patients in these studies, but the placebo response rate ranged from 15 to 58%.

Comparison of the placebo effect in dentinal hypersensitivity studies and in submitted data supporting the analgesic adjuvancy of caffeine in combination with acetaminophen (APAP) using the muscle contraction headache pain model is shown in Table 26.12 and Figure 26.6. The combination of a weak analgesic agent utilizing a subjective model of pain is overcome by the large number of subjects used in the study. The difference between the acetaminophen and the placebo group is statistically significant for improvement of pain. However, the small percentage difference between the active agent and placebo groups suggests that statistical significance reflects the OTC nature and use of acetaminophen. Looked at differently, the analgesic efficacy is at the low end of the therapeutic scale. Further comparison of the differences between the active agent and the placebo effect across a number of different products is depicted in Table 26.13. Dentinal hypersensitivity studies do not appear to be unusual in their placebo response when compared to other studies requiring a subjective evaluation of a stimulus that is rather poorly controlled for an outcome measure that is difficult to quantify.

The treatment of dentinal hypersensitivity by a dentifrice over time should have the effect of lowering the sensitivity while raising the threshold of the tooth (Figure 26.7). The cumulative effect of using a dentifrice (tubule occluder) is depicted by e1, e2 and e3 and could be representative of the percentage difference between an active agent versus placebo over, for example, a 2-, 4- and 8-week period of a hyper-

sensitivity clinical study. If the furthest curve to the right represents the normal time course of a sensitive tooth, it is known from clinical experience that eventually the tooth becomes nonresponsive and loses its vitality. It is postulated that by lowering the level of sensitivity while raising the threshold of the tooth a beneficial effect beyond patient comfort should be prolongation of the tooth's vitality.

Patient recruitment for a clinical study can also vary with their degree of dentinal sensitivity. Tooth sensitivity is greatest at the cementoenamel junction, usually where the earliest signs

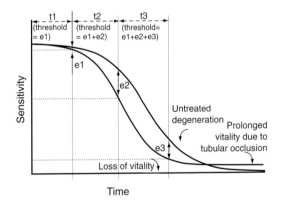

Figure 26.7

Treatment of dentinal hypersensitivity by tubular occlusion studies. The postulation that the effect of using a dentifrice in unit dose (e) should increase the tooth's threshold while lowering its sensitivity is compared with an untreated tooth over time. t1, t2, t3 = time intervals; e1, e2, e3 = cumulative effect of unit doses.

Table 26.13 Comparison of placebo effects across OTC product lines

Indication	Active agent (A)	Placebo effect (B)	Difference (A – B)
[1]Plaque reduction	Triclosan dentifrice	Dentifrice vehicle	
3 months	33%	27%	6%
6 months	60%	31%	30%
[1]Gingivitis reduction			
3 months	26%	13%	13%
6 months	27%	9%	18%
[2]Sleep latency	Diphenhydramine	Placebo tablet	
	2.07	1.68	0.39 (23% improvement relative to placebo)
[3]Duration of RAU lesion	Pencyclovir	Placebo	
	4.5 days	5 days	0.5 (10% improvement relative to placebo)
[4]RAU pain reduction	Amlexanox	Vehicle	
Day 3	39%	28%	11%
Day 4	60%	48%	12%
Day 5	74%	63%	11%
[5]Chronic constipation (number of bowel movements/day)	PEG-EL solution 5.81	Water 4.36	1.45 (33% improvement relative to placebo)

[1]Mankodi *et al.* (1992); [2]Rickels *et al.* (1983); [3]PDR, 52nd edn, (1998); [4]Khandwala *et al.* (1997); [5]Andorsky and Goldner (1990) (see Reference section for details). RAU, recurrent aphthous ulcers; PEG-EL, polyethylene glycol electrolyte lavage.

of erosion are seen. The appropriateness of recruiting subjects with very sensitive teeth has yet to be determined, as it would be difficult to establish a threshold or baseline response. Our database on file suggests that for both tactile and thermal sensitivity, the teeth with greater baseline sensitivity show a greater measured change. However, the current goal of a study would be to demonstrate that an efficacious agent should have an effect in raising the threshold within a shorter time frame than those presently available on the market. A weaker agent would be ineffective. Moving further along the curve could be a problem, as the tooth would be less sensitive and result in weak agents appearing to be efficacious. The ideal level of sensitivity for patient recruitment requires further study. Some standardization of achieving tactile pain thresholds should be agreed upon for comparison of clinical studies. In particular, the method of mapping the area of dentinal erosion,

for tactile response, should include the greatest area possible while being consistent with the technique throughout the course of the study.

A dentinal hypersensitivity study as outlined in Table 26.2 is designed to achieve minimum variability and consistency in the placebo response. However, the very nature of the clinical study incorporates some variability that cannot be 'designed out'. Studies such as dentinal hypersensitivity, that place limitations on patient selection, can add another dimension to the apparent placebo effect. Thus, the total placebo effect can be viewed as consisting of the underlying physiological improvement plus the brushing effect (if any) and the apparent improvement consisting of the Hawthorne effect, a regression to the mean and possibly other effects. Regression to the mean in dentinal hypersensitivity studies is caused by random variation in patient symptoms over time and can result in an apparent placebo effect. The more challenging and error-prone the measurement is, the greater the effect will be. Most acute and some chronic pain problems resolve on their own irrespective of treatment. Many individuals can have recurrent episodes of pain interspersed with no or minimal pain – as in dentinal hypersensitivity, headache or low back pain. Patients with chronic conditions typically have fluctuating symptoms and when they are participating in a clinical study the change in their symptoms is likely to be one of improvement. This tendency of extreme symptoms or findings to return to the individual's more typical state is exemplified by the condition seen in dentinal hypersensitivity.

It has been both widely theorized and demonstrated that expectations represent an important mechanism underlying the placebo (i.e. non-specific treatment) effects (Swartzman and Burkell 1998). That is, people may selectively attend to and report events (e.g. symptomatic improvement or side-effects) that are consistent with their expectations (Pennebaker 1982). In fact, some investigators have equated the 'expectancy effect' with the placebo effect (Eisenberg et al. 1993).

The balanced placebo design provides a powerful method for teasing out the relative effects of expectancy and pharmacology (as well as their interactions). The balanced placebo design has not, to our knowledge, been used in hypersensitivity clinical trials. Moreover, ethical considerations (i.e. the deception inherent in the expectancy manipulation) arguably preclude its use in clinical trials.

That is not to say, however, that patients' expectations are not influenced (intentionally or unintentionally) in clinical trials (Swartzman and Burkell 1998). For example, Kleijnen et al. (1994), in a review article addressing the placebo effect and expectancy in double-blind clinical trials, point out that the informed consent procedure itself can serve as an expectancy manipulation that can, in turn, affect the reports of subjective improvement and of side-effects. Kirsch and Rosadino (1993) employed a variation of the balanced placebo design to assess the effects of caffeine. The results showed that only subjects who knowingly received caffeine registered physiological and subjective increases in tension. In other words, only expectation of receiving the drug, coupled with actually receiving it, produced the tension effect.

Additionally, Kirsch and Sapirstein (1998) challenged the standard design in a meta-analysis examining 19 double-blind, placebo-controlled trials of various antidepressants involving 2318 patients. They came to the surprising conclusion that only 25% of the response to any drug was actually the effect of the drug and not the placebo effects, and that a 25% response is large if the antidepressants are actually responsible for that effect. It is also possible that the apparent response to the drug really may be an 'active placebo' effect, i.e. the placebo effect may have a physiological basis for its action.

The placebo effect may vary greatly in degree and in size, frequently involving many more people than the often-cited one-third of a given study group (Turner et al. 1994). It also varies in strength and scope, depending on the disorder, but because very few studies on the effect itself have been done, little is known about which disorders (including dentinal hypersensitivity) are more susceptible to it.

Much work remains to be done to determine whether biochemical and neural pathways are activated by the psychological mechanisms involved, to produce physiological changes that affect dentinal hypersensitivity itself. What is known is that placebos seem capable, in some instances, of relieving the pain and discomfort that can attend disease as well as pain due to dentinal hypersensitivity and may be more aptly described in a clinical study as a 'lower boundary limit' of the response. Furthermore, the magnitude of the placebo effect in dentinal hypersensitivity studies appears to be consistent with, and is no greater than, that of other clinical studies in the OTC and Rx drug categories.

References

Addy M, Mostafa P, Newcombe R (1987) Dentine hypersensitivity: a comparison of five toothpastes used during a 6-week treatment period. *Br Dent J* **163**:45–51.

Andorsky RI, Foldner F (1990) Colonic lavage solution (polyethylene glycol electrolyte lavage solution) as a treatment for chronic constipation. A double-blind, placebo-controlled study. *Am J Gastroenterol* **85**:261–5.

ASTM Committee E-253 (1997). Standard terminology relating to sensory evaluation of materials and products. In: *Annual Book of ASTM Standards* (American Society for Testing and Materials, Philadelphia:15.07, (16).

Bartlett DW (1997) The causes of dental erosion. *Oral Dis* **3**:209–11.

Beecher HK (1955) The powerful placebo. *J Am Med Assoc* **159**:1602–6.

Bi J, Ennis DM (1998) Sensory thresholds concepts and methods. *J Sensory Studies* **13**:133–48.

Bristol-Myers Products (1988) The analgesic efficacy of EXCEDRIN Extra-Strength: demonstration of the analgesic efficacy of caffeine. Submission by Bristol-Myers Products to FDA Docket No. 77N-0094.

Capra NF, Dessein D (1992) Central connections of trigeminal primary afferent neurons: topographical and functional considerations. *Crit Rev Oral Biol Med* **4**:1–52.

Clark GE, Troullos ES (1990) Designing hyper-sensitivity clinical studies. *Dent Clin North Am* **34**:531–44.

Code of Federal Regulations, Food and Drug Administration (1998). Institutional Review Boards, Title 21, part 56.

Curro FA (1990) Tooth hypersensitivity in the spectrum of pain. *Dent Clin North Am* **34**:429–37.

Eisenberg DM, Delbanco TL, Berkey CS et al (1993) Cognitive behavioral techniques for hypertension: are they effective? *Ann Intern Med* **118**:964–72.

Evans FJ (1985) Expectancy, therapeutic instructions, and the placebo response. In: White L, Tursky B, Schwartz GE, eds. *Placebo: theory, research and mechanisms*, 215–28. Guilford Press: New York.

Gillam DG, Newman HN, Bulman JS, Davies EH (1992a) Dentifrice abrasivity and cervical dental hyper-sensitivity. Results 12 weeks following cessation of 8 weeks supervised use. *J Periodontol* **63**:7–12.

Gillam DG, Newman HN, Davies EH, Bulman JS (1992b) Clinical efficacy of a low abrasive dentifrice for the relief of cervical dental hypersensitivity. *J Clin Periodontol* **19**:197–201.

Khandwala A, van Omwegen RG, Alfano MC (1997) 5% Amlexanox oral paste, a new treatment for recurrent minor aphthous ulcers. I. Clinical demonstration of acceleration of healing and resolution of pain. *Oral Surg Oral Med Oral Pathol* **83**:222–30.

Kirsch I, Rosadino MJ (1993) Do double-blind studies with informed consent yield externally valid results? An empirical test. *Psychopharmacology (Berl)* **110**:437–42.

Kirsch I, Sapirstein G (1998) Listening to Prozac but hearing placebo: a meta-analysis of antidepressant medication. *Prevention & Treatment I*: article 00029 posted June 26, 1998.

Kleijnen J, deCraen AJM, Everdingen J, Krol L (1994) Placebo effect in double-blind clinical trials: a review of interactions with medications. *Lancet* **344**:1347–9.

Leight RS, Troullos ES, Ryan P (1991) A new method for quantifying dentinal tactile hypersensitivity. *J Dent Res* **70** (Special issue):474.

Linde A, Goldberg M (1993) Dentinogenesis. *Crit Rev Oral Biol Med* **4**:679–728.

Mankodi S, Walker C, Conforti N et al (1992) Clinical effect of a Triclosan-containing dentifrice on plaque and gingivitis: a six month study. *Clin Prev Dent* **14**:4–10.

Melzack R (1975) The McGill Pain Questionnaire: major properties and scoring methods. *Pain* **I**:277–99.

Pennebaker JW (1982) *The Psychology of Physical Symptoms*. Springer-Verlag: New York.

Physicians' Desk Reference, 52nd edn (1998) Medical Economics Company: Montvale, NJ.

Rickels K, Morris R, Newman RH et al (1983) Diphen-hydramine in insomniac family practice patients: a double-blind study. *J Clin Pharmacol* **23**:235–42.

Silverman G, Berman E, Hanna CB et al (1996) Assessing the efficacy of three dentifrices in the treatment of dental hypersensitivity. *J Am Dent Assoc* **127**:191–201.

Swartzman LC, Burkell J (1998) Expectations and the placebo effect in clinical drug trials: why we should not turn a blind to unblinding, and other cautionary notes. *Clin Pharmacol Ther* **64**:1–7.

Turner JA, Deyo RA, Loeser JD et al (1994) The importance of placebo effects in pain treatment and research. *J Am Med Assoc* **271**:1609–14.

Wall PD (1993) Pain and the placebo response. *Ciba Found Symp* **174**:187–211.

West N, Addy M, Jackson RJ, Ridge DB (1997) Dentine hypersensitivity and the placebo response. A comparison of the effect of strontium acetate, potassium nitrate and fluoride toothpastes. *J Clin Periodontol* **24**:209–15.

Wiesmann HP, Plate U, Zierold K, Höhling HJ (1998) Potassium is involved in apatite biomineralization. *J Dent Res* **77**:1654–7.

Yates R, Owens J, Jackson RJ et al (1998) A split-mouth placebo-controlled study to determine the effect of amorphous calcium phosphate in the treatment of dentine hypersensitivity. *J Clin Periodontol* **25**:687–92.

27

Strategies for the management of dentine hypersensitivity

Robin Orchardson

Introduction

Effective management of a clinical condition is based ideally on an understanding of the aetiology and underlying biological mechanisms. A correct diagnosis is the first step along this path. Dentine hypersensitivity is characterized by short, sharp pains arising typically when thermal, evaporative, mechanical or osmotic stimuli are applied to exposed dentine, that cannot be explained by any other form of dental defect or pathology (Addy 1992, Addy and Pearce 1994). There are other possible causes of dentinal pain and these must be eliminated by thorough examination before a diagnosis of dentine hypersensitivity is made (Dowell *et al.* 1985). Other chapters will cover the clinical features of this troublesome condition and the current methods of treatment (see Chapters 21 and 28–30). The purpose of this chapter is to review the overall basis of current strategies for managing dentine hypersensitivity and also to consider possible future trends in this area.

Mechanisms of dentine sensitivity

It is now generally accepted that most dentinal stimuli cause pain by generating action potentials in intradental nerves through a hydrodynamic mechanism (Brännström 1963, Anderson *et al.* 1972). Stimuli applied to dentine increase the rate of fluid flow in dentinal tubules (Figure 27.1). The fluid flow in turn excites nerve terminals at the inner ends of the tubules or in the outer layers of the pulp. Exceptions to this are

electric current and intense cold, which can stimulate pulpal nerves directly (Närhi 1985, Närhi *et al.* 1994). The basic principles of the hydrodynamic mechanism have been established for a long time, but some of the details have been confirmed only recently. Painstaking experiments have shown that individual intradental sensory units can be excited by a range of dentinal stimuli (Hirvonen *et al.* 1984, Närhi and Hirvonen 1987). Vongsavan and Matthews (1992) developed a technique for measuring dentinal fluid flow in vivo. The methodology enabled Matthews and Vongsavan

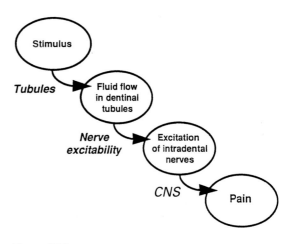

Figure 27.1

Hydrodynamic mechanism: the basic sequence of events (circled) by which stimuli applied to dentine excite intradental nerves and cause pain. The points at which desensitizing treatments may act are also indicated.

(1994) to demonstrate that tubular fluid flow, generated by hydrostatic pressure stimuli, was correlated with intradental nerve discharge. Intradental nerves could be activated by stimuli that generated both outward and inward fluid flow. The greater the fluid flow, the greater the nerve impulse discharge. One unexpected observation was that intradental nerves were more responsive to stimuli that caused fluid flow away from the pulp. The mechanism by which the increased fluid flow activates nerves has not been identified. However, Matthews and Vongsavan (1994) suggested that the nerve terminals are mechano-nociceptors with stretch-sensitive channels. These channels could be activated by shearing forces produced by the relatively rapid fluid flow in the narrow periodontoblastic space at the inner ends of the tubules. This information has been derived from animal experiments and as yet the entire causal chain linking the stimulus, increased tubular fluid flow, increased intradental nerve discharge and the resultant pain has not been demonstrated in humans. However, the hydrodynamic hypothesis remains the most plausible explanation for dentine sensitivity.

The traditional approaches for treating hypersensitive dentine are based on the hydrodynamic mechanism (Figure 27.1). Treatments for dentine hypersensitivity aim to interrupt this sequence of events by (a) preventing the stimulus-evoked increase in tubular fluid flow, or (b) reducing the excitability of intradental nerves. A third possibility could be to block nerve activity in peripheral nerves or in the central nervous system. Current treatments, which may be professionally applied in the dental office, or self-applied by patients at home, tend to focus on making the dentine less sensitive, rather than on why it became sensitive.

Dentine hypersensitivity

The clinical features and characteristics of hypersensitive teeth are well documented (Flynn *et al.* 1985, Addy *et al.* 1987, Orchardson and Collins 1987a, Fischer *et al.* 1992). However, further epidemiological studies are required in order to identify potential contributory and/or predisposing factors.

Morphology

The morphology of hypersensitive dentine has been reviewed by Holland (1994). Scanning electron microscopic studies of hypersensitive dentine surfaces reveal that they have more patent tubules per unit area than non-sensitive dentine (Absi *et al.* 1987, Yoshiyama *et al.* 1989). Also, tubules in superficial parts of hypersensitive dentine are on average twice as wide as tubules in non-sensitive dentine (Absi *et al.* 1987). Yoshiyama *et al.* (1989) reported that in naturally desensitized dentine, most of the tubules were occluded. On the basis of transmission electron microscopic studies Yoshiyama *et al.* (1990) reported that tubular occlusions could be due to extension of the intratubular dentine layer or deposition of substances in the tubules. Some of the occlusions were crystals of inorganic salts, but some may be organic in origin. However, the nature of the occluding layer is important. Some surfaces where the tubules were observed to be occluded with a 'dense pellicle', were found to very sensitive (Brännström 1992). Pashley and Carvalho (1997) noted that tubules apparently occluded with a smear plug are permeable to both solvent and solute. Thus, surface appearance alone may not correlate with sensitivity or permeability.

Sensitivity

Pain is the only consistent symptom of dentine hypersensitivity (Addy and Pearce 1994). However, it is not known whether hypersensitive teeth lie at one extreme of a normal distribution of dentine sensitivity (Figure 27.2a), or if they represent a separate population of teeth that are abnormally sensitive – or 'hypersensitive' (Figure 27.2b). Not all areas of exposed dentine are sensitive and hypersensitive surfaces can vary in their sensitivity to different stimuli. Table 27.1 shows how sensitivity to probe and air-jet stimuli varied in three different investigations. In spite of the investigations being carried out in different parts of the world, the percentages of teeth sensitive to the various stimuli were very similar. In addition, it was found that teeth that were sensitive to more than one stimulus had significantly lower pain thresholds than teeth that were

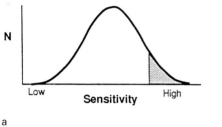

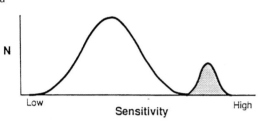

Figure 27.2

Representations of dentine hypersensitivity (hatched area).

a One extreme of a normal distribution.
b A separate population of abnormally sensitive ('hypersensitive') teeth.

sensitive to one stimulus only (Orchardson and Collins 1987b). There is some evidence that initial sensitivity patterns can affect treatment outcome (Orchardson 1985). One of the challenges facing the hydrodynamic mechanism is to explain why there can be so much variation in the sensitivity of dentine to different stimuli. There may be variations in the way in which different stimulus energies are converted into fluid flow. The direction of fluid flow is impor-

tant. Air stimuli increase outward tubular fluid flow, while probing increases inward flow. Intradental nerves are more responsive to outward fluid flow (Matthews and Vongsavan 1994) and this is consistent with clinical observations that air-jet stimuli are more effective than probing in eliciting pain (Table 27.1). Another source of variability is the state of the pulp (Brännström 1992). It is known that mild pulpal inflammation can increase dentine sensitivity to osmotic (Anderson and Matthews 1966) and other stimuli (Närhi *et al.* 1994).

Clinical presentation.

The majority (>90%) of hypersensitive areas occur on root dentine exposed at the cervical margins, usually on the vestibular surfaces (Orchardson and Collins 1987a) (Figure 27.3a). Of these, the majority of sensitive surfaces are found on canine and premolar teeth (Flynn *et al.* 1985, Orchardson and Collins 1987a, Addy *et al.* 1987, Fischer *et al.* 1992). When hypersensitivity occurs after periodontal treatment, a different distribution may be evident (DG Gillam, personal communication). However, sensitive dentine can be found in any tooth and at other sites. Dentine may be exposed by removal of enamel at tips of cusps or incisal edges by mechanical trauma, such as attrition or abrasion (Figure 27.3b). Dentine can also be exposed when enamel is eroded, e.g. with acid of exogenous or endogenous origin (Figure 27.3c). The cases shown in Figure 27.3 (a–c) differ, both in presentation and likely aetiology; the only common feature was the pain associated with dentine hypersensitivity. In view of these differences it is unreasonable to suppose that the clinical management of these

Table 27.1 Percentages of hypersensitive teeth that were sensitive to tactile (probe) and air-jet stimuli in three independent studies

	Country	Probe only	Air-jet only	Probe and air
Orchardson and Collins 1987b	Scotland	16	33	51
Fischer *et al.* 1992	Brazil	5	28	67
Kleinberg *et al.* 1994	USA	16	33	51

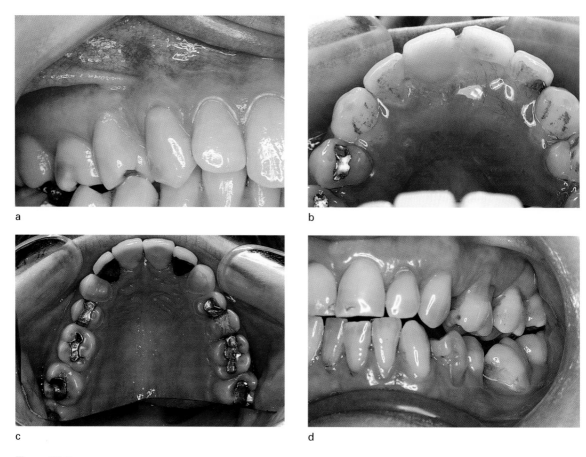

Figure 27.3

Hypersensitive areas (photographs by courtesy of the Photographic Unit, Glasgow Dental Hospital and School, Glasgow, UK).

a Typical presentation of hypersensitive cervical dentine. Note the localized gingival recession and exposed root dentine on tooth 13.
b Hypersensitive dentine associated with cuspal wear on teeth 13 and 23, possibly due to attrition.
c Hypersensitive dentine associated with extensive acid erosion of palatal surfaces. In this case, regions on the palatal surfaces of teeth 14, 16, 24, 25 and 26 were hypersensitive to probe or air-jet stimulus.
d Extensive exposure of root dentine due to periodontal disease. Of the teeth shown, only tooth 26 was sensitive to probe or air-jet stimuli.

cases should be the same. It is also important to remember that not all exposed dentine is sensitive (Figure 27.3d). Regardless of how it is exposed, dentine sensitivity tends to decrease with time due to a combination of environmental factors and physiological desensitizing processes.

Origins of hypersensitive dentine

The aetiology of dentine hypersensitivity has been the subject of several recent reviews (Addy 1992, Brännström 1992, Addy and Pearce 1994, Addy and West 1994). The reader is also referred to Chapter 2 on this subject. However, a brief

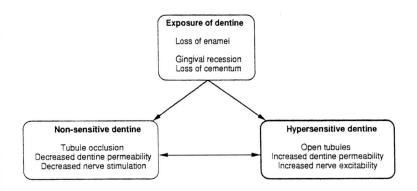

Figure 27.4

Origins of dentine hypersensitivity.

summary is appropriate, as clinical management must take account of aetiology.

Freshly exposed dentine is sensitive by virtue of its relationship with the pulp (Anderson *et al.* 1972). However, there seems to be relatively little information on the sensitivity of 'normal' dentine, possibly because it is usually exposed under local anaesthetic. The sensitivity of dentine generally correlates well with tubule patency (Cuenin *et al.* 1991, Närhi *et al.* 1992). Although dentine is usually sensitive when it is first exposed, it tends to become less sensitive over time (Figure 27.4). However, dentine sensitivity is subject to spontaneous fluctuations (Zappa 1994) so that previously non-sensitive dentine may become hypersensitive. There is very little quantitative information on these spontaneous variations in dentine sensitivity and this is an area where further research is necessary.

A range of factors may contribute to the development of dentine hypersensitivity after the

Table 27.2 Dentine hypersensitivity: associated and predisposing factors and their possible consequences (each factor may be related to several consequences)

Factor	Possible consequence
Abrasive trauma	Dentine exposure
Oral hygiene methods	Loss of smear layer
Erosive factors	Increased tubule patency
Saliva	Less intratubular dentine
Dentine–pulp response	Less tertiary dentine
Neurogenic pulp inflammation	Increased intradental nerve excitability

initial exposure of dentine (Table 27.2). Dentine may be exposed by removal of enamel or cementum, and the mode of exposure may be important in determining sensitivity. Once dentine has been exposed, the state of the dentinal tubules will be determined by complex interactions between the occluding effects of brushing with dentifrice and the unblocking actions of erosive agents (Table 27.2). Erosive agents can be exogenous – including environmental, dietary and lifestyle factors and medications (Zero 1996), or endogenous – such as reflux of gastric acid (Scheutzel 1996).

The protective effect of endogenous factors such as saliva is uncertain. Saliva is unable to combat repeated erosive challenges, which will overwhelm its limited buffering capacity (Imfeld 1996). However, saliva is present all the time, and may be able to influence the state of dentine and its sensitivity due to its buffers, mineral ions and protein content. There are reported differences in salivary pH and $[Ca^{2+}]$ in caries-prone and caries-resistant people (Kleinberg *et al.* 1994). Differences in salivary flow or composition could contribute to the development of hypersensitive dentine by affecting the formation of a surface layer (Kerns *et al.* 1991) or even by deposition of intratubular dentine.

Finally, there is no reliable information about the state of the pulp in hypersensitive teeth. It is often assumed that hypersensitive teeth have normal pulps, but there is no definite information about this, as teeth are not extracted merely because they are hypersensitive. However, it is possible that there is some degree of inflammation in the pulps of hypersensitive teeth, and this could account for the increased sensitivity

(Brännström 1992). Also, resultant alterations in pulpal haemodynamics and dentinal fluid flow may be responsible for the variations in dentine sensitivity that occur over time. This is another area where further research is needed.

Management of dentine hypersensitivity

Having examined the basic mechanisms of dentine sensitivity, we can now consider how this information may be utilized for making dentine less sensitive.

Prevention

'Prevention is better than cure' and one role of dental health education should be to prevent dentine hypersensitivity from occurring (Addy and West 1994). It is interesting to note that many of the preventive methods that have been suggested for dealing with dental erosion (Imfeld 1996) also seem suitable for managing dentinal hypersensitivity. In cases of established dentine hypersensitivity, it is necessary to remove any causative or predisposing factors. Basic approaches could include preventing exposure of root dentine by reducing the incidence of gingival recession and identification and elimination of any intrinsic or extrinsic erosive factors. The latter requires careful examination and questioning about potential predisposing factors. A dietary log may prove useful to identify erosive factors. Another way to improve host resistance might be to enhance salivary flow; for example, gum chewing will tend to increase flow rate and oral pH. The buffering effects of bicarbonate toothpastes have been suggested as possible ways to combat acid erosion (Imfeld 1996) and this might prove beneficial for dentine hypersensitivity.

Tubule occlusion

Current evidence implicates patent dentinal tubules in hypersensitive dentine and it follows that one way to reduce dentine sensitivity is to occlude the tubules. In principle it should be possible to occlude tubules anywhere along their length. Tubule occlusion may occur naturally or by means of externally applied desensitizing agents.

Endogenous desensitization

The surface layer

Clinically hypersensitive surfaces have wider and more numerous tubules than non-sensitive dentine, which displays few patent tubules (Absi et al. 1987, Yoshiyama et al. 1989). One treatment objective would be to promote formation of smear layers or impermeable surface deposits and to prevent their removal. Surface coverings could include deposition of salivary minerals, as in calculus formation. Would it be possible to induce calculus deposition within tubules rather than on the tooth surface?

Intratubular dentine

Transmission electron microscopy of non-sensitive dentine reveals that the dentinal tubules are occluded by electron-dense material (Yoshiyama et al. 1990), which could be intratubular (or peritubular) dentine. The mode of formation of intratubular dentine is uncertain, but it appears to require the presence of viable odontoblast processes (Linde and Goldberg 1993). Sites of formation of intratubular dentine vary with age and with the site in the tooth (Holland 1994). There is some evidence that its composition may differ between root and coronal dentine. In coronal dentine, intratubular crystalline deposits may be of salivary origin (Eda et al. 1996), while sclerosis of root dentine may be due to deposition of material from the pulp (Kawakami et al. 1996).

Tertiary dentine

Dead tract dentine is insensitive to stimulation (Thomas 1944). Dead tracts are formed when atubular tertiary dentine is rapidly laid down, effectively isolating the tubules from the pulp. Two types of tertiary dentine are distinguished

(D'Souza and Litz 1996). *Reactionary dentine* is laid down by primary odontoblasts, in response to a mild dentinal stimulus. *Reparative dentine* is produced by a new generation of (secondary) odontoblasts, derived from pulp cells, in response to a more intense stimulus. This type contains fewer tubules than primary or secondary dentine (see Chapter 5). Both forms of tertiary dentine can be induced by the presence of non-collagenous dentine matrix proteins applied to the exposed pulp or to deep cavities in dentine (Smith *et al.* 1990, 1994, Rutherford *et al.* 1995, Rutherford 1996). These reactions are specific and dose-dependent. The amount of tertiary dentine laid down decreases with increasing thickness of dentine remaining over the pulp. At present, the responses to trans-dentinal stimulation are effective only at thicknesses of 100–200 μm.

There is considerable interest in the notion that the key events in hard tissue formation are also instrumental in repair (D'Souza and Litz 1996). It may become possible to switch on the genes regulating the expression of dentine matrix proteins and so perhaps harness reparative dentinogenesis as a means of reducing dentine hypersensitivity (see Combe and Douglas 1998).

Exogenous materials

The most direct approach to desensitizing dentine is to block tubule orifices with a barrier (Ling and Gillam 1996). As with erosion defects (Lambrechts *et al.* 1996), surface barriers can be created from toothpaste constituents or by application of topical agents or a range of restorative materials, including varnishes, dentine bonding agents, composite resins, glass–ionomer cements and compomers. Surface barriers tend to be effective as long as they remain in place. However, once the covering is removed, sensitivity usually returns to starting levels (Orchardson *et al.* 1993). To provide effective desensitization, one would suppose that materials need to be sufficiently retentive and robust. Desensitizing effectiveness should be improved if the material can enter the tubules to form 'tags', as can be the case with some resins (Brännström *et al.* 1979). However, the quality of resin–dentine bonds is an extremely complex issue (Pashley and Carvalho 1997). While bond strength may determine retention of the material, the extent of intratubular 'tags' may be more important in providing an effective seal. Many of the materials used for treating hypersensitive dentine are 'borrowed' from restorative dentistry. These materials, especially adhesives, are perhaps best suited for dealing with isolated regions of hypersensitivity where there is loss of tooth substance due to abrasion or erosion. There is a need to develop materials that are specifically designed to penetrate dentinal tubules and adhere to the intratubular dentine, and in effect become part of the dentine. One exciting area of future development will be biomimetic materials, that are structurally similar to the dental hard tissues (Combe and Douglas 1998).

Tubule contents.

The fluid within the dentinal tubules is an important link in the hydrodynamic mechanism (Figure 27.1). It is believed that the stimulus-induced fluid flow is responsible for intradental nerve activation. It might therefore be possible somehow to increase the viscosity of tubular fluid so that a given stimulus generates less fluid flow. Viscosity of tubular fluid could be raised by increasing its macromolecular protein content. Exogenous materials applied to the dentine surface would tend to be washed out of the tubules by the continuous outward flow of dentinal fluid. However, dentinal fluid contains plasma proteins such as fibrinogen (Pashley *et al.* 1984) and albumin (Bergenholtz *et al.* 1996), derived from the pulpal blood vessels. These proteins probably form part of the pulpal defence reaction and may contribute to natural desensitization mechanisms. At present, it is difficult to envisage how the viscosity of tubular fluid can be altered as a therapeutic measure.

Modifying nerve excitability

Diffusion in dentinal tubules

Some desensitizing agents, such as potassium ions, are intended to reduce intradental nerve excitability. Markowitz *et al.* (1991) suggested that potassium ions applied to the outer dentine surface might diffuse along the tubules and block intradental nerve function by raising the local extracellular potassium ion concentration. This hypothesis is based on animal experiments, but has never been confirmed in human teeth, where diffusion distances are greater (Peacock and Orchardson 1995).

It is technically difficult to measure the [K^+] at the inner ends of dentinal tubules in vivo. However, Pashley and his colleagues (Pashley *et al.* 1977, Pashley *et al.* 1981, Pashley and Matthews 1993) have studied the diffusion of radioactive iodide (^{131}I) through dentine in vitro and in vivo. Diffusion along a dentinal tubule was shown to depend on the concentration gradient, the length of the tubule and the diffusion coefficient of the substance.

Stead *et al.* (1996) used a mathematical approach to model K^+ diffusion in dentine. The model revealed that when the [K^+] at the outer ends of the tubules is raised to 500 mM to simulate the action of a desensitizing toothpaste, the [K^+] at the inner end of the tubules could exceed the minimum [K^+] necessary to block nerve conduction (Peacock and Orchardson 1995). However, the effects were transient, and the actual [K^+] achieved depended on the velocity of tubular fluid flow and the permeability of the diffusion barrier between the tubule and the pulp. McCormack and Davies (1996) suggested that the odontoblasts could be involved in mediating the desensitizing actions of K^+, through a second messenger system involving release of nitric oxide (NO). It is proposed that K^+ might somehow act on the peripheral end of the odontoblast processes, with NO being released in the pulp to modulate intradental nerve excitability. However, to date this hypothesis has not been tested experimentally.

Dentinal fluid flow

In open dentinal tubules, there is a steady outward flow of dentinal fluid (Vongsavan and Matthews 1992), which will tend to oppose any inward diffusion (Pashley and Matthews 1993, Stead *et al.* 1996). Pashley and Matthews (1993) showed that inward diffusion of ^{131}I across dentine in vitro against a forced outward flow of

fluid was greater in the presence of an intact smear layer. Intuitively, it might be expected that diffusion would be greater where dentinal tubules had wider openings. However, for a given fluid pressure gradient across dentine (effectively the pulpal blood pressure), dentinal tubular flow will be reduced by a narrowed tubule opening. As bulk flow varies with the fourth power of the tubule radius, while diffusion varies with the square of the radius, a given decrease in tubule radius will cause a proportionately greater reduction in fluid flow than in diffusion. However, fluid flow through dentine is not uniform. Using scanning electrochemical microscopy, Macpherson *et al.* (1995) found that fluid flow through dentine varies considerably between tubules even within an area of dentine 500 µm square. These regional differences in dentine permeability, where fluid flow may be concentrated in a few tubules, may be related to variations in tubule density and in the pattern of branching between tubules (Mjör and Nordahl 1996).

Pulpal pressure

A positive pressure could be applied to overcome the pulpal pressure, or the pulpal pressure could be reduced. The pressure driving dentinal tubular fluid is derived from the pulpal blood vessels. The pulpal blood flow is reduced following infiltration of 2% lignocaine plus 1:100 000 adrenaline (Kim *et al.* 1984). This was due partly to the action of the vasoconstrictor, as well as blockade of the sensory nerves, which are known to exert a tonic vasodilator action (Jacobsen and Heyeraas 1997).

Inward diffusion of applied substances can be increased by increasing the concentration gradient. This has proved effective with local anaesthetic solutions topically applied to dentine (Amess and Matthews 1996). Diffusion of charged particles may also be enhanced with iontophoresis (Gangarosa 1983). However, although it is possible to overcome the problems of getting agents along the dentinal tubules towards the pulp, it is more difficult to retain the material in the tooth for any significant period of time, without the material being washed away from its intended site of action. Leakage of material from the tubular space to the pulp is not merely a theoretical possibility. Pashley *et al.* (1981) reported that radioactive iodide (^{131}I) placed on to the dentine surface in anaesthetized dogs was rapidly absorbed into the systemic circulation via the pulpal blood vessels. Thus, although the barrier between the pulp extracellular fluid and the tubular space is impermeable to substances such as lanthanum (Bishop 1992), it is permeable to iodide ions.

Inflammation

A final question concerns the pulpal environment of hypersensitive teeth. Trauma to dentine provokes reactions in the pulp, which depend on the severity of the injury. These reactions include changes in the morphology of intradental nerves such as localized sprouting (Byers 1992, 1994) and alterations in the local neurochemistry (Närhi *et al.* 1994). Even relatively minor interventions such as drilling the tooth surface or ultrasonic scaling can trigger neurogenic inflammation in the pulp (Olgart *et al.* 1991). At present, there is insufficient information to confirm or refute the possibility that similar changes are present in the pulps of hypersensitive teeth.

Summary

Successful management of dentine hypersensitivity in the future may depend as much on prevention as on the development of new agents and treatments. While it may not be feasible to prevent dentine exposure, it should be possible to prevent exposed dentine from becoming unduly sensitive. This will require identification and elimination of the various factors predisposing to persistent tubule patency. This will require more research into the factors associated with dentine hypersensitivity, such as diet, lifestyle and salivary flow or content. It is desirable to develop novel agents that are capable of more effective and lasting tubule occlusion. It may even be possible to develop methods that mimic or harness the natural defence reactions of the dentine–pulp complex. One day it might even be possible to deal with hypersensitive or worn teeth by growing new dental tissue to replace that which has been lost.

References

Absi E, Addy M, Adams D (1987) Dentine hypersensitivity: a study of the patency of dentinal tubules in sensitive and non-sensitive cervical dentine. *J Clin Periodontol* **14**:280–4.

Addy M (1992) Clinical aspects of dentine hypersensitivity. *Proc Finn Dent Soc* **88** (Suppl 1):23–30.

Addy M, Pearce N (1994) Aetiological, predisposing and environmental factors in dentine hypersensitivity. *Arch Oral Biol* **39** (Suppl):S33–S38.

Addy M, West N (1994) Etiology, mechanisms, and management of dentine hypersensitivity. *Curr Opin Periodontol* **1994**:71–7.

Addy M, Mostafa P, Newcombe RG (1987) Dentine hypersensitivity: the distribution of recession, sensitivity and plaque. *J Dent* **15**:242–8.

Amess TR, Matthews B (1996) The effects of topical applications of lignocaine to dentin in the cat on the response of intradental nerves to mechanical stimuli. In: Shimono M, Maeda T, Suda H, Takahashi K, eds, *Proceedings of International Conference on Dentin/Pulp Complex*, 272–3. Quintessence: Tokyo.

Anderson DJ, Matthews B (1966) An investigation into the reputed desensitising effect of applying silver nitrate and strontium chloride to human dentine. *Arch Oral Biol* **11**:1129–35.

Anderson DJ, Hannam AG, Matthews B (1972) Sensory mechanisms in mammalian teeth and their supporting structures. *Physiol Rev* **50**:171–95.

Bergenholtz G, Knutsson G, Jontell M, Okiji T (1996) Albumin flux across dentin of young human premolars following temporary exposure to the oral environment. In: Shimono M, Maeda T, Suda H, Takahashi K, eds, *Proceedings of International Conference on Dentin/Pulp Complex*, 51–7. Quintessence: Tokyo.

Bishop MA (1992) Extracellular fluid movement in the pulp; the pulp/dentin permeability barrier. *Proc Finn Dent Soc* **88** (Suppl 1):331–5.

Brännström M (1963) A hydrodynamic mechanism in the transmission of pain-producing stimuli through the dentine. In: Anderson DJ, ed, *Sensory Mechanisms in Dentine*, 73–9. Pergamon: Oxford.

Brännström M (1992) Etiology of dentin hypersensitivity. *Proc of the Finn Dent Soc* **88**(Suppl 1) 7–13.

Brännström M, Johnson G, Nordenvall K-J (1979) Transmission and control of dentinal pain: resin impregnation for the desensitisation of dentin. *J Am Dent Assoc* **99**:612–18.

Byers MR (1992) Effects of inflammation on dental sensory nerves and vice versa. *Proc Finn Dent Soc* **88** (Suppl 1):499–506.

Byers MR (1994) Dynamic plasticity of dental sensory nerve structure and cytochemistry. *Arch Oral Biol* **39** (Suppl):S13–S21.

Combe EC, Douglas WH (1998) The future of dental materials. *Dent Update* **25**:411–417.

Cuenin MF, Scheidt MJ, O'Neal RB et al (1991) An in vivo study of dentin sensitivity: the relation of dentin sensitivity and the patency of dentinal tubules. *J Periodontol* **62**:668–73.

Dowell P, Addy M, Dummer P (1985) Dentine hypersensitivity: aetiology, differential diagnosis and management. *Br Dent J* **158**:92–6.

D'Souza RN, Litz M (1996) Odontoblast gene regulation during development and repair. In: Shimono M, Maeda T, Suda H, Takahashi K, eds, *Proceedings of International Conference on Dentin/Pulp Complex*, 99–104. Quintessence: Tokyo.

Eda S, Hasegawa H, Kawakami T (1996) Crystals closing tubules in sclerosed root dentin of the aged. In: Shimono M, Maeda T, Suda H, Takahashi K, eds, *Proceedings of International Conference on Dentin/Pulp Complex*, 283–4. Quintessence: Tokyo.

Fischer C, Fischer RG, Wennberg A (1992) Prevalence and distribution of cervical dentine hypersensitivity in a population in Rio de Janeiro, Brazil. *J Dent* **20**:272–6.

Flynn J, Galloway R, Orchardson R (1985) The incidence of hypersensitive teeth in the West of Scotland. *J Dent* **13**:230–6.

Gangarosa LP (1983) *Iontophoresis in Dental Practice*. Quintessence: Chicago.

Hirvonen TJ, Närhi MVO, Hakumäki MOK (1984) The excitation of dog pulp nerves in relation to the condition of dentine surface. *J Endodontics* **10**:294–8.

Holland GR (1994) Morphological features of dentine and pulp related to dentine sensitivity. *Arch Oral Biol* **39** (Suppl):S3–S11.

Imfeld T (1996) Prevention of progression of dental erosion by professional and individual prophylactic measures. *Eur J Oral Sci* **104**:215–20.

Jacobsen EB, Heyeraas KJ (1997) Pulp interstitial fluid pressure and blood flow after denervation and electrical tooth stimulation in the ferret. *Arch Oral Biol* **42**:407–15.

Kawakami T, Takei N, Eda S (1996) Crystals closing tubules in sclerosed coronal dentin of the aged. In: Shimono M, Maeda T, Suda H, Takahashi K, eds, *Proceedings of International Conference on Dentin/Pulp Complex*, 285–6. Quintessence: Tokyo.

Kerns DG, Scheidt MJ, Pashley DH et al (1991) Dentinal tubule occlusion and root hypersensitivity. *J Periodontol* **62**:421–8.

Kim S, Edwall L, Trowbridge H, Chein S (1984) Effects of local anesthetics on pulpal blood flow in dogs. *J Dent Res* **63**:650–2.

Kleinberg I, Kaufman HW, Wolff M (1994) Measurement of tooth hypersensitivity and oral factors involved in its development. *Arch Oral Biol* **39** (Suppl):S63–S71.

Lambrechts P, Van Meerbeek B, Perdigão J et al (1996) Restorative therapy for erosive lesions. *Eur J Oral Sci* **104**:229–40.

Linde A, Goldberg M (1993) Dentinogenesis. *Crit Rev Oral Med Biol* **4**:679–728.

Ling TYY, Gillam DG (1996) The effectiveness of desensitising agents for the treatment of cervical dentine sensitivity (CDS) – a review. *Periodontal Abstracts* **44**:5–12.

McCormack K, Davies R (1996) The enigma of potassium ion in the management of dentine hypersensitivity: is nitric oxide the elusive second messenger? *Pain* **68**:5–11.

Macpherson JV, Beeston MA, Unwin P et al (1995) Scanning electrochemical microscopy as a probe for local fluid flow through porous solids. *J Chem Soc Faraday Trans* **91**:1407–10.

Markowitz K, Bilotto G, Kim S (1991) Decreasing intradental nerve activity in the cat with potassium and divalent cations. *Arch Oral Biol* **36**:1–7.

Matthews B, Vongsavan N (1994) Interactions between neural and hydrodynamic mechanisms in dentine and pulp. *Arch Oral Biol* **39** (Suppl):S87–S95.

Mjör IA, Nordahl I (1996) The density and branching of dentinal tubules in human teeth. *Arch Oral Biol* **41**:401–12.

Närhi MVO (1985) The characteristics of intradental sensory units and their responses to stimulation. *J Dent Res* **64** (Special issue):564–71.

Närhi MVO, Hirvonen T (1987) The response of dog intradental nerves to hypertonic solutions of $CaCl_2$ and NaCl, and other stimuli applied to exposed dentine. *Arch Oral Biol* **32**:781–6.

Närhi M, Kontturi-Närhi V, Hirvonen T, Ngassapa D (1992) Neurophysiological mechanisms of dentine hypersensitivity. *Proc Finn Dent Soc* **88** (Suppl 1):15–22.

Närhi M, Yamamoto H, Ngassapa D, Hirvonen T (1994) The neurophysiological basis and the role of inflammatory reactions in dentine hypersensitivity. *Arch Oral Biol* **39** (Suppl):S23–S30.

Olgart L, Edwall L, Gazelius B (1991) Involvement of afferent nerves in pulpal blood-flow reactions in response to clinical and experimental procedures in the cat. *Arch Oral Biol* **36**:575–81.

Orchardson R (1985) Is calcium more effective than strontium as a desensitising agent for dentine? In: Lisney SJW, Matthews B, eds, *Current Topics in Oral Biology*, 205–15. University of Bristol Press: Bristol.

Orchardson R, Collins WJN (1987a) Clinical features of hypersensitive teeth. *Br Dent J* **162**:253–6.

Orchardson R, Collins WJN (1987b) Thresholds of hypersensitive teeth to two forms of controlled stimulation. *J Clin Periodontol* **14**:68–73.

Orchardson R, Collins WJN, Gilmour WH (1993) Pilot study of a fluoride resin and conditioning paste for desensitising dentine. *J Clin Periodontol* **20**:509–13.

Pashley DH, Carvalho RM (1997) Dentine permeability and dentine adhesion. *J Dent* **25**:355–72.

Pashley DH, Matthews WG (1993) The effects of outward forced convective flow on inward diffusion in human dentine in vitro. *Arch Oral Biol* **38**:577–82.

Pashley DH, Livingston MJ, Outhwaite WC (1977) Rate of permeation of isotopes through human dentin, in vitro. *J Dent Res* **56**:83–8.

Pashley DH, Kehl T, Pashley E, Palmer P (1981) Comparison of in vitro and in vivo dog dentin permeability. *J Dent Res* **60**:763–8.

Pashley DH, Galloway SE, Stewart FP (1984) Effects of fibrinogen on dentin permeability, in vivo. *Arch Oral Biol* **29**:725–8.

Peacock JM, Orchardson R (1995) Effects of potassium ions on action potential conduction in A- and C-fibers of rat spinal nerves. *J Dent Res* **74**:634–41.

Rutherford B (1996) Role of osteogenic protein in reparative and reactionary dentin. In: Shimono M, Maeda T, Suda H, Takahashi K, eds, *Proceedings of International Conference on Dentin/Pulp Complex*, 112–15. Quintessence: Tokyo.

Rutherford B, Spangberg L, Tucker M, Charette M (1995) Transdentinal stimulation of reparative dentine formation by osteogenic protein-1 in monkeys. *Arch Oral Biol* **40**:681–3.

Scheutzel P (1996) Etiology of dental erosion – intrinsic factors. *Eur J Oral Sci* **104**:178–90.

Smith AJ, Tobias RS, Plant CG et al (1990) In vivo morphogenetic activity of dentine matrix proteins. *J Biol Buccale* **18**:123–9.

Smith AJ, Tobias RS, Cassidy N et al (1994) Odontoblast stimulation in ferrets by dentine matrix components. *Arch Oral Biol* **39**:13–22.

Stead WJ, Orchardson R, Warren PB (1996) A mathematical model of potassium ion diffusion in dentinal tubules. *Arch Oral Biol* **41**:679–87.

Thomas BOA (1944) Protective metamorphosis of the dentine: its relationship to pain. *J Am Dent Assoc* **31**:459–63.

Vongsavan N, Matthews B (1992) Fluid flow through cat dentine in vivo. *Arch Oral Biol* **37**:175–85.

Yoshiyama M, Masada A, Uchida A, Ishida H (1989) Scanning electron microscopic characterization of sensitive v. insensitive human radicular dentin. *J Dent Res* **68**:1498–502.

Yoshiyama M, Noire Y, Azoic K et al (1990) Transmission electron microscopic characterization of hypersensitive human radicular dentin. *J Dent Res* **69**:1293–7.

Zappa U (1994) Self-applied treatments in the management of dentine hypersensitivity. *Arch Oral Biol* **39** (Suppl):S107–S112.

Zero DT (1996) Etiology of dental erosion – extrinsic factors. *Eur J Oral Sci* **104**:162–77.

28

Potential treatment modalities for dentine hypersensitivity: home use products

Robert J Jackson

Introduction

The incidence of dentine hypersensitivity has been reported to range from 8 to 35% in 'normal' populations (Addy 1990, Gillam 1992, Fischer *et al*. 1992, Murray and Roberts 1994). The condition is much more frequently encountered in certain specific populations, e.g. in those patients attending periodontal clinics (Gillam *et al*. 1994, Chabanski *et al*. 1996). A wide range of commercial products is available for self-treatment. The products include agents such as potassium salts, strontium salts and fluoride salts in toothpaste, mouthwash and gel formulations.

These agents are believed to reduce the symptoms of dentine hypersensitivity by either occluding dentine tubules and thus blocking the neural stimulus and response (Pashley *et al*. 1978a, 1978b), and/or intercepting the neural response by chemical intervention (Bilotto *et al*. 1978, 1988, Markowitz *et al*. 1991). Toothbrushing rarely lasts more than a minute (Duke and Forward 1982), neither does a mouthwash treatment: therefore, the effect of the agent in a toothpaste or mouthwash must either be rapid or else the agent must be substantive to the teeth and mucosa. Alternatively the effect of an agent could build up over the period of use of the product.

The effectiveness of self-applied products for the treatment of dentine hypersensitivity is often reduced by the lifestyle of the patient. Acid foods and drinks have been shown to soften dentine and may remove deposits on the dentine surface (Absi 1989). Brushing has been shown to exacerbate the removal of any surface deposits (Absi *et al*. 1995). These deposits may be performing the desirable function of blocking tubules and reducing dentine hypersensitivity. The effectiveness of these self-treatment products that occlude dentine tubules could perhaps be improved by counselling patients on their diet and brushing habits.

It is postulated that agents that intercept the neural response are effective because potassium ions from the applied products diffuse inwards and block the response by chemical intervention. For effective diffusion the ion concentration at the tubule orifice must be as high as possible; the longer the ion sink is retained, the greater the flow of ions. Diffusion is reduced by the outward flow of dentinal fluid (Sena 1990, Stead *et al*. 1994), and if this is too great, inward diffusion will be negligible. The effectiveness of these products may possibly be improved by increasing the concentration of the active agent in the product (i.e. the potassium salt content) or advising patients to brush or rinse with the product for a longer period of time.

Neither of these mechanisms could be expected to produce a permanent effect, indeed, the effect of self-applied treatments in reducing the symptoms of dentine hypersensitivity is not generally noticed immediately by patients; it may take some time and many treatments to become apparent. The effect may also have a short lifetime following the cessation of treatment.

Up to 90% of individuals suffering from dentine hypersensitivity report that the effect of a thermal stimulus, particularly a cold stimulus such as breathing through the mouth on a cold day or consuming a cold drink, causes the painful sensation associated with sensitive teeth (Orchardson and Collins 1984, Gillam 1992, Chabanski *et al.* 1996). A tactile stimulus, such as brushing the teeth, has been reported to affect up to 10% of the population who suffer from dentine hypersensitivity (Murray and Roberts 1994, Chabanski *et al.* 1996).

To relieve the symptoms of dentine hypersensitivity most patients suffering from sensitive teeth choose either self-help (Schuurs *et al.* 1995, Irwin and McCusker 1997), or some choose professional treatment (Murray and Roberts 1994). Irwin and McCusker (1997) have reported that of those who chose self-help (the use of a commercially available sensitive-teeth product), almost 75% reported a beneficial effect. Although the patient's perception of the efficacy of a particular treatment is probably the single most important factor in the choice of a self-applied treatment, the objective, clinical assessment of these treatments is still of major importance.

The evaluation of treatments for the relief of pain has long been recognized as extremely difficult. The criterion for success of a treatment is the subjective opinion of the patient. Pain perception is dependent on many variables, including the personality of the patient, psychological factors, cultural attitudes, anticipation of pain and the degree of apprehension (Mumford 1965). These aspects, along with other factors such as study design and the use of different stimuli, have led to contradictory results from studies. To overcome discrepancies in methodology the American Dental Association (ADA 1986) recommended specific guidelines for the evaluation of products for the relief of dentine hypersensitivity. More detailed guidelines have since been published (Holland *et al.* 1997).

Two different approaches to the evaluation of such products are taken: stimulus-related techniques involve assessment of the pain threshold to a variable stimulus and response-based methods involve eliciting patient response to a fixed, consistent stimulus. Almost all studies reported over the last few years have used response-based techniques; many of these have included stimulus-related measurements.

The most common pain-provoking stimuli used in studies have been those considered to be physiologically and clinically relevant, i.e. thermal and tactile stimuli. Variable pressure probes, e.g. the Yeaple probe (Yeaple, Vine Valley Research, Middlesex, NY, USA) or a standard dental explorer, are used to produce a tactile stimulus. They invariably have a metal tip. It may be hypothesized that the pain induced by this stimulus could be the result of tactile pressure, or the formation of a weak electrolytic cell, or a combination of both. A tactile stimulator should perhaps use a non-conductive tip, which if invoking pain would indicate a true tactile response. Similarly, the pain induced by a thermal stimulator or probe may be considered to be a tactile response, and furthermore, as the tips must be good thermal conductors and therefore good electrical conductors, the effect could be electrolytic, or indeed a combination of thermal, tactile and electrolytic stimuli. The response to cold air, often cited as the most common stimulus for inducing dental pain, may also not be a true response to temperature alone. It may be the result of pressure on the dentinal fluid, or an evaporative effect.

In studies to determine the effect of agents on dentine hypersensitivity, not only should the effect of the stimuli be questioned, but also the response to these stimuli. The ADA guidelines recommend that if more than one stimulus is used, interference between them must be minimized. If two or more stimuli are applied, it is probable that there is a patient expectation response (Mumford 1965). Many studies also report the effect of the application of stimuli to many teeth (Chesters *et al.* 1992), although none report on the possible effect of patients anticipation or apprehension, or the possible interaction between the neural transmissions from different teeth.

To improve the reliability of studies, in addition to considering the stimuli and subsequent patient responses, the selection of test teeth sites and patient volunteers should be considered in greater detail. It has long been recognized, particularly for analgesic studies using a dental pain model, that the response to the extraction of teeth from the maxilla is greater than that to teeth extracted from the lower jaw. Although many studies designed to assess the effect of products on dentine hypersensitivity report that the groups of different treatment regimes are balanced for sensitivity, it is seldom reported whether the groups are balanced for the responses of both the upper and lower jaw. As most studies are performed on both males and females the effect of the menstrual cycle in females should be considered; or alternatively studies could be performed only on male subjects! Perhaps the most important outcome of these clinical studies is the patient response – does the patient feel that

the treatment has yielded benefit? A 'quality of life' assessment may reveal an important quantifiable benefit to the patient.

Possible confounding factors make the evaluation and comparison of different treatments very difficult, and perhaps unreliable. A review by Zappa (1994) which summarized the effect of self-applied treatments concluded that, of the most commonly used agents, toothpastes containing

Table 28.1 Effect of toothpastes containing strontium salts on dentine hypersensitivity: change in mean subjective response

Reference	Stimulus	Time (weeks)	Placebo/control	Test product 1	Test product 2	Comments
			Change in mean subjective response			
Gillam et al. (1992)	Tactile	8	–	3.51→1.88 (n=20) 46.4%[‡]	3.46→1.78 (n=20) 48.6%[‡]	Test 1: silica base + SrCl$_2$
	Cold air	8	–	5.28→2.73 48.3%[‡]	5.11→2.85 44.2%[‡]	Test 2: diatomaceous earth + SrCl$_2$
	Subjective	8	–	4.15→1.94 53.3%[‡]	4.44→2.16 51.4%[‡]	Inter-group NS
Pearce et al. (1994)	Tactile	1	2.44→1.39 (n=41) 43.0%	3.24→1.78 (n=37) 54.9%	1.80→1.22 (n=41) 39.2%	Test 1: silica base + SrAc+ NaF
		4	2.44→0.72 70.5%	3.24→1.03 68.2%	1.80→0.80 55.6%	
		8	2.44→0.39 84.0%	3.24→0.31 90.4%	1.80→0.60 66.7%	Test 2: diatomaceous earth base + SrCl$_2$
		12	2.44→0.20 91.8%	3.24→0.32 90.1%	1.80→0.62 65.6%	
	Cold air	1	14.83→12.29 17.1%	15.27→13.50 11.6%	12.00→10.00 16.7%	Control: conventional fluoride (NaMFP) toothpaste
		4	14.83→8.85 40.3%	15.27→10.38 32.0%	12.00→6.59 45.1%	
		8	14.83→8.15 45.0%	15.27→6.83 55.3%	12.00→5.43 54.8%	
		12	14.83→6.34 57.2%	15.27→8.19 46.4%	12.00→5.15 57.1%	Inter-group NS
	Subjective	1	48.3→43.0 11.0%	56.4→49.4 12.4%	56.4→44.6 20.9%	Changes from baseline not analysed
		4	48.4→39.7 18.0%	56.4→44.2 21.6%	56.4→38.5 31.7%	
		8	48.3→31.3 35.2%	56.4→39.5 30.0%	56.4→39.3 30.3%	
		12	48.3→29.6 38.7%	56.4→36.9 34.6%	56.4→32.8 41.8%	
Gillam et al. (1996a)	Tactile	2	3.57→2.91 (n=19) 18.5% NS	2.60→2.36 (n=19) 9.2% NS		Test 1: silica base + SrAc + NaF
		6	3.57→1.93 45.9%[†]	2.60→1.30 50.0%[†]	–	
	Cold air	2	5.33→4.2 21.2%*	5.47→4.34 20.7%[†]	–	Control: conventional fluoride (NaMFP) toothpaste
		6	5.33→2.77 48.0%[‡]	5.47→2.92 46.6%[‡]	–	
	Subjective	2	4.86→3.36 30.9%*	4.32→3.78 12.5% NS	–	
		6	4.86→2.75 43.4%[†]	4.32→2.57 40.5%*		

Table 28.1 *Continued*

Reference	Stimulus	Time (weeks)	Placebo/control	Test product 1	Test product 2	Comments
			Change in mean subjective response			
Silverman *et al.* (1996)	Cold air	2	56.57→53.06 (*n*=61) 5.6%	54.77→51.33 (*n*=62) 6.2%		Test 1: silica base + SrCl$_2$
		4	56.57→48.46 (*n*=60) 13.9%	54.77→41.14 (*n*=61) 25.0%	–	Control: no active agents
		8	56.57→39.35 (*n*=60) 30.2%	54.77→34.81 (*n*=60) 36.4%		
	Subjective	2	52.85→50.04 (*n*=62) 5.5%	53.08→48.48 (*n*=62) 9.9%		Differences from baseline not reported
		4	52.85→44.29 (*n*=61) 16.5%	53.08→40.06 (*n*=61) 23.3%	–	
		8	52.85→37.33 (*n*=60) 35.3%	53.08→34.17 (*n*=60) 36.0%		
West *et al.* (1997)	Tactile	2	0.62→0.34 45.2%	0.86→0.52 39.5%		Test 1: silica base + SrAc + NaF
		6	0.62→0.30 51.6%	0.86→0.37 57.0%	–	
	Cold air	2	2.26→1.53 32.3%	3.18→2.08 34.5%	–	Control: conventional fluoride (NaMFP) toothpaste
		6	2.26→1.07 52.7%	3.18→1.71 46.2%		
	Subjective	2	3.7→3.0 18.9%	4.3→3.9 9.3%	–	Differences from baseline not reported
		6	3.7→3.0 18.9%	4.3→3.6 16.3%		

*P <0.05; †P <0.01; ‡P <0.001; NS, not significant; NaMFP, sodium monofluorophosphate.

Table 28.2 Effect of toothpastes containing strontium salts on dentine hypersensitivity: change in mean stimulus response

Reference	Stimulus	Time (weeks)	Placebo/control	Test product 1	Test product 2	Comments
			Change in mean stimulus response			
Gillam *et al.* (1992b)	Tactile	8	–	1.142→1.399 (*n*=20) 22.6%*	1.132→1.413 (*n*=20) 24.8%*	Test 1: silica base + SrCl$_2$ Test 2: diatomaceous earth base + SrCl$_2$
Gillam *et al.* (1996a)	Tactile	2	10.00→12.50 25.0% NS	10.00→15.00 50.0%*		Test 1: silica base + SrAC + NaF
		6	10.00→17.50 75.0%†	10.00→17.50 75.0%†	–	Control: fluoride (NaMFP) toothpaste
Silverman *et al.* (1996)	Tactile	2	18.81→24.14 28.3%	20.32→23.67 16.5%		Test 1: silica base + SrCl$_2$
		4	18.81→27.84 48.0%	20.32→29.82 46.8%	–	Control: no active agents
		8	18.81→32.11 70.7%	20.32→38.83 91.1%		Differences from baseline not reported

*P <0.05; †P <0.01; NS, not significant.

strontium salts seemed to be effective in relieving the pain of tooth sensitivity. It also concluded
that overall, the clinical evidence supported the
efficacy of potassium-containing toothpastes for
reducing tooth hypersensitivity.

The studies on self-applied treatment for the
relief of dentine hypersensitivity reported in the
literature since 1992 are summarized and

compared in Tables 28.1–28.8. Tables 28.1, 28.3,
28.5 and 28.7 summarize the change in the mean
subjective response to a given stimulus following
the use of the product for a specified period. The
mean baseline response to a fixed stimulus is
reported together with the mean response to that
stimulus after the specified period of application
of the product. The number of subjects in the

Table 28.3 Effect of toothpastes containing potassium salts on dentine hypersensitivity: change in mean subjective response

Reference	Stimulus	Time (weeks)	Placebo/control	Test product 1	Test product 2	Comments
			Change in mean subjective response			
Salvato et al. (1992)	Cold air	4	5.3→4.4 (n=21) 17.0%	5.4→3.4 (n=20) 37.0%		Test 1: DCP base + KCl + NaMFP Control: DCP base minus active agents
		8	5.3→4.2 20.8%	5.4→2.2 59.3%	–	
		12	5.3→3.7 30.2%	5.4→1.7 68.5%		
	Subjective	4	5.1→4.7 7.8%	5.0→3.2 36.0%		
		8	5.1→4.3 15.7%	5.0→2.1 58.0%	–	
		12	5.1→3.8 25.5%	5.0→1.7 66.0%		
Nagata et al. (1994)	Tactile	2	1.39→1.18 (n=13) 15.1% NS	1.80→1.45 (n=13) 19.4% NS		Test 1: DCP base + KNO$_3$ Control: DCP base minus active agents
		4	1.39→1.03 25.9% NS	1.80→0.80 55.5%*	–	
		8	1.39→1.03 25.9% NS	1.80→0.38 78.9%*		
		12	1.39→1.09 21.6% NS	1.80→0.33 81.7%*		
	Cold air	2	1.85→1.57 (n=18) 15.1% NS	1.82→1.30 (n=18) 28.6%*		
		4	1.85→1.41 23.8%*	1.82→0.80 56.0%*	–	
		8	1.85→1.35 27.0%*	1.82→0.49 73.1%*		
		12	1.85→1.36 26.5%*	1.82→0.36 80.2%*		
	Subjective	2	2.00→1.83 8.5%	2.00→1.47 26.5%		
		4	2.00→1.67 16.5%	2.00→1.06 47.0%	–	
		8	2.00→1.50 25.0%	2.00→0.56 72.0%		
		12	2.00→1.44 28.0%	2.00→0.44 78.0%		
Silverman et al. (1994)	Cold air	4	2.2→1.72 21.8%	2.3→1.30 43.5%	2.1→1.27 39.5%	Test 1: DCP base + KCl + NaMFP Test 2: DCP base + KCl Control: DCP base minus active agents
		8	2.2→1.59 27.7%	2.3→0.79 65.7%	2.1→0.83 60.5%	
	Subjective	4	2.2→1.76 20.0%	2.2→1.40 36.4%	2.2→1.48 32.7%	
		8	2.2→1.48 32.7%	2.2→0.85 61.4%	2.2→1.05 52.3%	

Table 28.3 *Continued*

Reference	Stimulus	Time (weeks)	Placebo/control	Test product 1	Test product 2	Comments
			Change in mean subjective response			
Schiff *et al.* (1994)	Cold air	6	2.3→2.4 5.0%	2.3→1.1 52.2%	–	Test 1: silica base + KNO_3 + soluble pyrophosphate + PVA/MA polymer + NaF
		12	2.3→2.3 0.0%	2.3→1.1 52.2%		
	Subjective	6	4.9→3.4 30.6%	5.2→3.6 30.8%		Control: silica base without KNO_3
		12	4.9→3.4 30.6%	5.2→2.5 51.9%	–	
Ayad *et al.* (1994)	Cold air	6		2.7→1.6 40.7%*	2.7→1.7 37.0%*	Test 1: silica base + KNO_3 + soluble pyrophosphate + PVA/MA polymer + NaF
		12	–	2.7→1.2 55.6%*	2.7→1.2 55.6%*	
	Subjective	6		5.7→4.7 17.5%*	6.1→4.9 19.7%*	Test 2: DCP base + KNO_3 + NaMFP
		12	–	5.7→3.9 31.6%*	6.0→3.6 40.0%*	
Silverman *et al.* (1996)	Cold air	2	56.57→53.06 (*n*=61) 5.6%	55.68→51.07 (*n*=52) 8.3%	55.12→49.36 (*n*=53) 10.4%	Test 1: base + KNO_3 + NaF
		4	56.57→48.46 (*n*=60) 13.9%	55.68→38.52 (*n*=51) 30.8%	55.12→38.19 (*n*=53) 30.7%	Test 2: base + KNO_3
		8	56.57→39.35 (*n*=60) 30.2%	55.68→28.93 (*n*=50) 48.0%	55.12→25.37 (*n*=50) 54.0%	
	Subjective	2	52.85→49.92 5.5%	55.77→47.79 14.3%	55.83→48.37 13.4%	Control: a toothpaste without active agents
		4	52.85→44.12 16.5%	55.77→38.46 31.0%	55.83→38.13 31.7%	
		8	52.85→37.17 35.3%	55.77→25.22 29.7%	55.83→25.47 54.4%	
Gillam *et al.* (1996a)	Tactile	2	3.57→2.91 (*n*=19) 18.5%	3.23→2.26 (*n*=18) 30.0%	–	Test 1: base + KCl + NaMFP
		6	3.57→1.93 45.9%	3.23→1.68 48.0%		
	Cold air	2	5.33→4.20 21.2%	4.91→3.77 23.2%	–	Control: conventional fluoride (NaMFP) toothpaste
		6	5.33→2.77 45.0%	4.91→2.39 51.3%		
	Subjective	2	4.86→3.36 30.9%	4.09→3.01 26.4%	–	
		6	4.86→2.75 43.4%	4.09→1.89 53.8%		
West *et al.* (1997)	Tactile	2	0.62→0.34 45.2%	0.49→0.37 24.4%	–	Test 1: silica base + KNO_3 + NaMFP
		6	0.62→0.30 51.6%	0.49→0.21 57.1%		
	Cold air	2	2.26→1.53 32.3%	2.67→1.76 34.1%	–	Control: conventional fluoride (NaMFP) toothpaste
		6	2.26→1.07 52.7%	2.67→1.40 47.6%		
	Subjective	2	3.7→3.0 18.9%	4.7→3.6 23.4%	–	Differences from baseline not reported
		6	3.7→3.0 18.9%	4.7→3.3 29.8%		

*P <0.05; DCP, di-calcium phosphate; NS, not significant.

Table 28.4 Effect of toothpastes containing potassium salts on dentine hypersensitivity: change in mean stimulus response

Reference	Stimulus	Time (weeks)	Placebo/control	Test product 1	Test product 2	Comments
				Change in mean stimulus response		
Salvato et al. (1992)	Tactile	8	26.5→38.1 43.8%	27→47.2 74.8%		Test 1: DCP base + KCl + NaMFP
		12	26.5→45.3 70.9%	27→56.5 109.3%	–	
Silverman et al. (1994)	Tactile	4	26→31.86 22.5%	26→41.28 58.8%	26→44.64 71.7%	Test 1: DCP base + KCl + NaMFP
		8	26→34.93 34.3%	26→51.78 99.0%	26→50.95 96.0%	Test 2: DCP base + KCl
Schiff et al. 1994	Tactile	6	12.2→15.3 25.4%	11.6→23.0 98.3%		Test 1: silica base + KNO_3 + soluble pyrophosphate
		12	12.3→15.0 22.0%	11.4→27.9 144.7%	–	PVA/MA polymer + NaF
	Thermal	6	29.6→34.6 16.9%	30.2→27.2 9.9%		Control: silica base without KNO_3
		12	29.7→35.7 20.2%	29.9→23.5 21.4%	–	
Ayad et al. (1994)	Tactile	6	–	12.7→23.9 88.2%	12.8→22.7 77.3%	Test 1: silica base + KNO_3 + NaF
		12	–	12.8→25.0 95.3%	12.9→27.2 110.9%	Test 2: DCP base + KNO_3 + NaMFP
Silverman et al. (1996)	Tactile	2	18.81→24.14 28.4%	22.88→26.98 17.9%	20.75→29.02 39.9%	Test 1: a base + KNO_3 + NaF
		4	18.81→27.84 48.0%	22.88→34.63 51.4%	20.75→38.01 83.2%	Test 2: base + KNO_3
		8	18.81→32.11 70.7%	22.88→44.95 96.5%	20.75→43.81 111.1%	
Gillam et al. (1996b)*	Tactile	2	10.0→12.5 25.0%	11.25→17.5 55.5%	–	Test 1: base + KCl + NaMFP
		6	10.0→17.5 75.0%	11.25→16.25 44.4%		

group is also given. The percentage change in the subject's response to each stimulus following the use of the product has been calculated to determine the effectiveness of the treatment and to allow a qualitative comparison to be made between treatments. The data presented in Tables 28.2, 28.4, 28.6 and 28.8 summarize the values of variable stimuli that elicit a painful response. The mean values of the stimulus that elicited a painful response both initially and after a specified period of use are reported, together with the number of subjects per group. The percentage change in the value of the stimulus has been calculated.

Strontium salts

Five studies have been reported since the review by Zappa (1994) that examined the effect of toothpastes containing strontium salts, either as the chloride or the acetate, on patients with dentine hypersensitivity. The results of the response-related parameters of these studies are summarized in Table 28.1 and the results of the stimulus-based techniques presented in Table 28.2. It is not possible to make an exact comparison of the results of these studies because the period of use of the toothpastes was not consis-

Table 28.5 Effect of mouthwashes containing potassium salts on dentine hypersensitivity: change in mean subjective response

Reference	Stimulus	Time (weeks)	Placebo/control	Test product 1	Test product 2	Comments
			Change in mean subjective response			
Gillam *et al.* (1996b)	Tactile	2	4.1→2.7 (*n*=23) 34.1%	3.7→2.0 (*n*=24) 45.9%		Test 1: mouthwash + silica + KNO_3 + NaF
		6	4.1→2.0 51.2%	3.7→1.5 59.5%	–	
	Cold air	2	5.4→4.3 20.4%	4.8→3.2 33.3%		Control: mouthwash + silica + NaF NaF
		6	5.4→2.0 63.0%	4.8→2.3 52.1%	–	
	Subjective	2	5.1→3.6 29.4%	5.0→3.2 36.0%	–	
		6	5.1→2.8 45.1%	5.0→2.9 42.0%		
Yates *et al.* (1998)	Cold air	4	2.56→1.75 (*n*=44) 31.6%	2.57→1.74 (*n*=44) 32.3%		Test 1: mouthwash + K citrate + CPC + NaF
		8	2.56→1.45 43.4%	2.57→1.31 49.0%	–	
	Subjective	4	2→2 0.0%	2→2 0.0%		Control: same formulation minus K citrate, CPC and NaF
		8	2→2 0.0%	2→2 0.0%		

CPC, cetyl pyridinium chloride.

Table 28.6 Effect of mouthwashes containing potassium salts on dentine hypersensitivity: change in mean stimulus response

Reference	Stimulus	Time (weeks)	Placebo/control	Test product 1	Test product 2	Comments
			Change in mean stimulus response			
Gillam *et al.* (1996b)	Tactile	2	10.00→11.25 12.5%[†]	10.00→17.5 75.0%[†]		Test 1: mouthwash + silica + KNO_3 + NaF
		6	10.00→13.75 37.5%[†]	10.00→26.25 162.5%[†]	–	
Yates *et al.* (1998)	Tactile	4	39.6→50.0 (*n*=39) 26.3%	40.1→57.7 (*n*=42) 43.4%		Test 1: mouthwash + K citrate + CPC + NaF
		8	39.6→57.3 44.7%	40.1→63.9 59.4%	–	

[†]*P* <0.01.

tent, the placebo or control toothpastes were not the same in all of the studies and the formulations of the test products were also different. However, a number of generalizations can be made.

All the studies demonstrated an improvement in patients' perception of their dentine hypersensitivity. The effectiveness of the toothpastes in reducing the symptoms increased with the period of use of the products. One study (Gillam *et al.* 1992) reported no difference in the effect on dentine hypersensitivity of two toothpastes both of which contained strontium chloride but with different silica abrasive systems. A later study (Pearce *et al.* 1994) reported that toothpastes containing either strontium chloride or

Table 28.7 Effect of various agents on dentine hypersensitivity: change in mean subjective response

Reference	Stimulus	Time (weeks)	Placebo/control	Test product 1	Test product 2	Comments
			Change in mean subjective response			
Plagmann et al. (1997)	Cold air	2	46.3→40.2 (n=16) 13.2%	47.5→43.8 (n=19) 7.8%	49.8→42.5 (n=13) 14.7%	Test 1: silica base + NaF (1400 ppm)
		4	46.3→37.6 18.8%	47.5→39.5 16.8%	49.8→36.6 26.5%	Test 2: silica base + amine F
		6	46.3→33.7 27.2%	47.5→36.8 22.5%	49.8→31.9 35.9%	(1400 ppm)
		8	46.3→30.3 34.6%	47.5→34.1 28.2%	49.8→29.7 40.4%	
	Subjective	2	45.8→42.1 8.1%	46.3→43.7 5.6%	46.7→42.6 8.8%	Control: silica base without
		4	45.8→38.0 17.0%	46.3→40.6 12.3%	46.7→37.5 19.7%	fluoride
		6	45.8→33.8 26.2%	46.3→37.1 19.9%	46.7→33.8 27.6%	Differences from baseline not
		8	45.8→32.7 28.6%	46.3→35.5 23.3%	46.7→30.5 34.7%	reported
Higuchi et al. (1996)	Tactile	4	1.25→0.68 (n=29) 45.6%	0.93→0.38 (n=27) 59.1%		Test 1: a mouthwash
		6	1.25→0.45 64.0%	0.93→0.21 77.4%	–	containing aluminium lactate
	Cold air	4	1.72→1.00 41.9%	1.79→0.72 59.8%		Control: same formulation
		6	1.72→0.85 50.6%	1.79→0.59 67.0%	–	mouthwash minus aluminium lactate

Table 28.8 Effect of other salts on dentine hypersensitivity: change in mean stimulus response

Reference	Stimulus	Time (weeks)	Placebo/control	Test product 1	Test product 2	Comments
			Change in mean stimulus response			
Plagmann et al. (1997)	Tactile	2	21.2→23.2 (n=16) 9.4%	20.8→23.2 (n=19) 11.5%	21.7→22.9 (n=13) 5.5%	Test 1: silica base + NaF (1400 ppm)
		4	21.2→25.2 18.9%	20.8→28.9 38.9%	21.7→26.5 22.1%	Test 2: silica base + amine F
		6	21.2→24.6 16.0%	20.8→30.4 46.2%	21.7→28.9 33.2%	(1400 ppm) Control: silica
		8	21.2→26.6 25.5%	20.8→28.8 38.5%	21.7→31.2 43.8%	base without fluoride

strontium acetate provided comparable benefits for the relief of dentine hypersensitivity. In the latter study (Pearce et al. 1994) and also a number of others (Gillam et al. 1996, Silverman et al. 1996, West et al. 1997), the negative control toothpaste reduced the symptoms of dentine hypersensitivity; this effect also increased with the duration of the treatment. In none of these studies was a consistent, significant improvement in patients' symptoms of dentine hypersensitivity observed for the strontium-containing products compared with the negative control toothpaste. It may therefore be concluded that strontium salts appear to have only a minimal effect in reducing the symptoms of dentine hypersensitivity.

Potassium salts

Potassium salts are now the most commonly used agents incorporated into toothpastes and mouthwashes for the self-applied treatment of dentine hypersensitivity. Tables 28.3–28.6 summarize the results of 10 studies that compared the effect on dentine hypersensitivity of toothpastes or mouthwashes containing potassium salts with that of a control product. The results of the response-related parameters of these studies are summarized in Tables 28.3 and 28.5 and the results of the stimulus-based techniques in Tables 28.4 and 28.6. All these studies demonstrated an improvement in the patients' perceived symptoms of dentine hypersensitivity after use of the products containing either potassium nitrate or potassium chloride. The effect of the product increased with time. The placebo effect (Yates et al. 1998) is also very apparent in these studies, with the beneficial effect of the control toothpaste or mouthwash also increasing with time. Studies on toothpastes reported by a number of authors (Salvato et al. 1992, Ayad et al. 1994, Nagata et al. 1994, Silverman et al. 1994, 1996, Schiff et al. 1994) all demonstrated a significant benefit for the toothpaste containing a potassium salt compared with the control toothpaste. However, other studies (Gillam et al. 1996, West et al. 1997) failed to show any benefit for a toothpaste containing the potassium salt compared with a conventional fluoride toothpaste.

Only two studies (Gillam et al. 1996b, Yates et al. 1998) have been reported which evaluated the effect of mouthwashes on dentine hypersensitivity. The results of these studies are summarized in Tables 28.5 and 28.6. Both of these studies showed an improvement in subjects' perception of their symptoms, but neither demonstrated a benefit for the product containing the potassium salt over the control mouthwash.

Other agents

The effects of different fluorides and of a mouthrinse containing aluminium lactate on dentine hypersensitivity have been reported in two studies (Higuchi et al. 1996, Plagmann et al. 1997); results are shown in Tables 28.7 and 28.8.

Plagmann et al. (1997) concluded that both sodium fluoride and amine fluoride reduced dentine hypersensitivity over a period of 8 weeks, although neither agent was more effective than a control toothpaste. Higuchi et al. (1996) reported that the daily use of a mouthrinse containing aluminium lactate significantly reduced the symptoms of dentine hypersensitivity compared with a control rinse. No other recent studies have been reported which confirm these results.

Conclusion

There appears to be little doubt that, under the controlled conditions of a clinical trial, toothpastes, whether or not they contain potential active agents such as strontium salts or potassium salts, appear to reduce the symptoms of dentine hypersensitivity. The reason for this effect is not clear. The effect could be attributed to a 'placebo' or 'Hawthorne' effect (Yates et al. 1998) which has been observed in many clinical studies. Alternatively, the control products may have activity in their own right. Many toothpastes contain silica, either as a polishing agent or as a thickener. It is well documented that these particles can effectively occlude dentine tubules and that the deposit is resistant to mild abrasion or an erosive challenge (Jackson et al. 1990, Absi et al. 1995). Sodium monofluorophosphate has also been reported in the past to reduce dentine hypersensitivity (Bolden et al. 1968, Hazen et al. 1968, Kanouse and Ash 1969) and this may also contribute to the activity of conventional toothpastes.

There is little convincing clinical evidence for the activity of strontium salts. Deposits from toothpastes that contain strontium salts consist mainly of the polishing agent or thickener, which are often insoluble silicas, or a combination of these. There is no reported evidence for strontium salts enhancing the deposition of material or increasing the longevity of the deposit. The evidence for the activity of potassium salts is also inconclusive. If the effect of potassium ions in reducing dentine hypersensitivity is dependent on the diffusion of the ions along the dentine tubules to the neural receptors, the probability of this occurring during the short period of use of a toothpaste or mouthwash is very low (Stead *et al.* 1994, Vongsavan and Matthews 1992). This may mean that some other mechanism must exist.

If any of these agents – strontium or potassium salts – are effective in reducing dentine hypersensitivity, then studies on simple aqueous solutions should be sufficient to demonstrate their activity. No studies have been reported in the literature that have evaluated the effect of such simple treatments.

References

Absi EG (1989) Studies on the aetiology, appearance and treatment of hypersensitive dentine. PhD Thesis, University of Wales College of Medicine.

Absi EG, Addy M, Adams D (1995) Dentine hypersensitivity: uptake of toothpastes onto dentine and effects of brushing, washing and dietary acid – SEM *in vitro* study. *J Oral Rehabil* **22**:175–82.

ADA ad hoc Advisory Committee (1986) Recommendations for evaluating agents for the reduction of dentinal hypersensitivity. *Endodontics Dent Traumatol* **2**:172–4.

Addy M (1990) Etiology and clinical implications of dentine hypersensitivity. *Dent Clin North Am* **34**:503–14.

Ayad F, Berta R, De Vizio W et al (1994) Comparative efficacy of two dentifrices containing 5% potassium nitrate on dentinal sensitivity: a twelve-week clinical study. *J Clin Dent* **5** (Special issue):97–101.

Bilotto G, Markowitz K, Kim S (1978) Experimental procedures to test the efficacy of chemical agents on intradental nerve activity. *J Endodontics* **13**:458–65.

Bilotto G, Markowitz K, Kim S (1988) Effects of ionic and non-ionic solutions on intradent nerve activity. *Pain* **32**:231–8.

Bolden TE, Volpe AR, King WJ (1968) The desensitizing effect of a sodium monofluorophosphate dentifrice. *Periodontics* **6**:112–14.

Chabanski MB, Gillam DG, Bulman JS, Newman HN (1996) Prevalence of cervical dentine sensitivity in a population of patients referred to a specialist Periodontology Department. *J Clin Periodontol* **23**: 989–92.

Chesters R, Kaufman HW, Wolff MS et al (1992) Use of multiple sensitivity measurements and logit statistical analysis to assess the effectiveness of a potassium-citrate-containing dentifrice in reducing dentinal sensitivity. *J Clin Periodontol* **19**:256–61.

Duke SA, Forward GC (1982) The condition occurring in vivo when brushing with toothpastes. *Br Dent J* **152**:952–4

Fischer C, Fischer RG, Wennberg A (1992) Prevalence and distribution of cervical dentine hypersensitivity in a population in Rio de Janeiro, Brazil. *J Dent* **20**:272–6.

Gillam DG (1992) The assessment and treatment of cervical dentinal sensitivity. DDS Thesis, University of Edinburgh.

Gillam DG, Newman HN, Bulman JS, Davies EH (1992) Dentifrice abrasivity and cervical dentinal hypersensitivity. Results 12 weeks following cessation of 8 weeks' supervised use. *J Periodontol* **63**:7–12.

Gillam DG, Jackson RJ, Newman HN, Bulman JS (1994) Prevalence of dentine hypersensitivity in patients recruited for clinical trials. *J Parodontol d'Implantol Orale* **1**:66.

Gillam DG, Bulman JS, Jackson RJ, Newman HN (1996a) Comparison of 2 desensitizing dentifrices with a commercially available fluoride dentifrice in alleviating cervical dentine sensitivity. *J Periodontol* **67**:737–42.

Gillam DG, Bulman JS, Jackson RJ, Newman HN (1996b) Efficacy of a potassium nitrate mouthwash in alleviating cervical dentine sensitivity (CDS). *J Clin Periodontol* **23**:993–7.

Hazen SP, Volpe AR, King WJ (1968) Comparative desensitizing effect of dentifrices containing sodium monofluorophosphate, stannous fluoride and formalin. *Periodontics* **6**:230–2.

Higuchi Y, Kurihara H, Nishimura F et al (1996) Clinical evaluation of a dental rinse containing aluminium lactate for treatment of dentinal hypersensitivity. *J Clin Dent* **7**:9–12.

Holland GR, Närhi MN, Addy M (1997) Guidelines for the design and conduct of clinical trials on dentine hypersensitivity. *J Clin Periodontol* **24**:808–13.

Irwin CR, McCusker P (1997) Prevalence of dentine hypersensitivity in a general dental population. *J Irish Dent Assoc* **43**:7–9.

Jackson RJ, Duke SA, Wicks MA, McDonald FE (1990) The effects of antisensitivity dentifrices on subjects consuming acid diets. *J Dent Res* **69**:988 (abstract 268).

Kanouse MC, Ash MM (1969) The effectiveness of a sodium monofluorophosphate dentifrice on dental hypersensitivity. *J Periodontol* **40**:38–40.

Markowitz K, Bilotto G, Kim S (1991) Decreasing intradental nerve activity in the cat with potassium and divalent ions. *Arch Oral Biol* **36**:1–7.

Mumford JM (1965) Pain perception threshold and adaptation of normal human teeth. *Arch Oral Biol* **10**:957–68.

Murray LE, Roberts AJ (1994) The prevalence of self-reported hypersensitive teeth. *Arch Oral Biol* **39**(Suppl.):S29.

Nagata T, Ishida H, Shinohara H et al (1994) Clinical evaluation of a potassium nitrate dentifrice for the treatment of dentinal hypersensitivity. *J Clin Periodontol* **21**:217–21.

Orchardson R, Collins WJN (1984) Dentine sensitivity. *Hygienists Forum* **34**:6–14.

Pashley DH, Livingston MJ, Greenhill JD (1978a) Regional resistances to fluid flow in human dentine *in vitro*. *Arch Oral Biol* **23**:807–10.

Pashley DH, Livingston MJ, Reeder OW, Horner J (1978b) Effects of the degree of tubule occlusion on the permeability of human dentine *in vitro*. *Arch Oral Biol* **23**:1127–33.

Pearce NX, Addy M, Newcombe RG (1994) Dentine hypersensitivity: a clinical trial to compare 2 strontium desensitizing toothpastes with a conventional fluoride toothpaste. *J Periodontol* **65**:113–19.

Plagmann H-C, Konig J, Bernimoulin J-P et al (1997) A clinical study comparing two high-fluoride dentifrices for the treatment of dentinal hypersensitivity. *Quint Int* **28**:403–8.

Salvato AR, Clark GE, Gingold J, Curro FA (1992) Clinical effectiveness of a dentifrice containing potassium chloride as a desensitizing agent. *Am J Dent* **5**:303–6.

Schiff T, Dotson M, Cohen S et al (1994) Efficacy of a dentifrice containing potassium nitrate, soluble pyrophosphate, PVM/MA copolymer, and sodium fluoride on dentinal hypersensitivity: a twelve-week clinical study. *J Clin Dent* **5** (Special issue):87–92.

Schuurs AH, Wesselink PR, Eijkman MA, Duivenvoorden HJ (1995) Dentists' views on cervical hypersensitivity and their knowledge of its treatment. *Endodontics Dent Traumatol* **11**:240–4.

Sena FJ (1990) Dentinal permeability in assessing therapeutic agents. *Dent Clin North Am* **34**:475–90.

Silverman G, Gingold J, Curro FA (1994) Desensitizing effect of a potassium chloride dentifrice. *Am J Dent* **7**:9–12.

Silverman G, Berman E, Hanna CB et al (1996) Assessing the efficacy of three dentifrices in the treatment of dentinal hypersensitivity. *J Am Dent Assoc* **127**:191–201.

Stead WJ, Warren PB, Orchardson R, Roberts AJ (1994) A mathematical model for potassium diffusion in dentinal tubules. *Arch Oral Biol* **39**(Suppl.):S145.

Vongsavan N, Matthews B (1992) Fluid flow through cat dentine *in vivo*. *Arch Oral Biol* **37**:175–85.

West NX, Addy M, Jackson RJ, Ridge DB (1997) Dentine hypersensitivity and the placebo response. A comparison of the effect of strontium acetate, potassium nitrate and fluoride toothpastes. *J Clin Periodontol* **24**:209–15.

Yates R, West NX, Addy M, Marlow I (1998) The effects of a potassium citrate, cetylpyridinium chloride, sodium fluoride mouthrinse on dentine hypersensitivity, plaque and gingivitis. *J Clin Periodontol* **25**:813–20.

Zappa U (1994) Self-applied treatments in the management of dentine hypersensitivity. *Arch Oral Biol* **39**(Suppl.):S107–S112.

29

Studies with the next generation of home care products for dentine hypersensitivity

Malcolm Williams, William Moffat, Anthony Moskwa, Michael Stranick and Abdul Gaffar

Introduction

Tooth hypersensitivity, or more precisely dentine hypersensitivity, is one of the oldest recorded complaints of discomfort to mankind. The problem results when the protective gingiva and cementum layers of the teeth are removed, thereby exposing the underlying innervated dentine to the oral environment. Improper tooth brushing, oral prophylaxis and periodontal surgery are the major causes of the erosion of these protective layers. When the exposed dentine comes in contact with certain stimuli such as hot or cold liquids, an acute, transient, localized tooth pain results. This is defined as dentine hypersensitivity. The hydrodynamic theory, initially proposed by Gysi (1900) and subsequently modified (Brännström 1963, Brännström et al. 1967), is the most widely accepted explanation of this condition. According to this theory, the movement of fluids or semi-fluid materials in the dentine tubules transmits peripheral stimuli by deforming sensory nerves in the pulp, which in turn causes pain. The mean prevalence of sensitive teeth was recently reported as being 14.8% in six countries around the world (Murray and Roberts 1994), with the degree of sensitivity peaking at 25–30 years of age (Pashley 1994).

Over the years, a number of topical therapies and procedures has been introduced to treat dentine hypersensitivity. All therapies operate by at least one of the mechanisms described by Kleinberg (1986). Treatments ranged from simple salt formulations that provide an effect weeks after continuous usage to varnishes that provide immediate sensitivity pain relief (Rosenthal 1990). One of the more popular early in-office treatments of hypersensitivity was the use of fluoride-containing medicaments. These treatments provided some degree of relief compared with a non-fluoride placebo (Bolden et al. 1968), but the effect was not robust enough even at 1400 ppm to warrant the use of fluoride as an effective tooth desensitizer (Federal Register 1982, Plaggman et al. 1997). With the availability of professional and over-the-counter dentifrices containing fluoride, it was fitting to combine fluoride with other known desensitizing agents, such as potassium nitrate, to take advantage of the anti-caries efficacy of fluoride. Such an approach was the basis of a dentifrice that prevents and treats sensitivity pain (Figure 29.1).

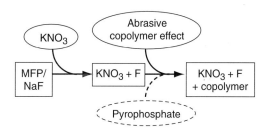

Figure 29.1

Evolution of a dentifrice that treats and prevents dentine hypersensitivity.

A dentifrice containing potassium nitrate in combination with fluoride, a copolymer and tartar-control ingredients, was reported to occlude dentine tubules and clinically reduce the pain associated with dentine hypersensitivity (Ayad *et al*. 1994, Bolden 1994, Miller *et al*. 1994, Schiff *et al*. 1994). This dentifrice was also shown to inhibit dental calculus formation (Cohen *et al*. 1994). The tartar-control component of the dentifrice has also been shown to clinically inhibit gingival recession (Rustogi *et al*. 1991, Triratana *et al*. 1991), a condition known to cause tooth sensitivity. The abrasive system and a copolymer were shown to be effective in coating and occluding the dentine tubules (Miller *et al*. 1994).

Various experimental methods have been developed to assess therapeutic agents for the treatment of dentine hypersensitivity. Some methods were designed mainly to assess dentine permeability, while others were designed to measure pulpal sensory nerve activity. One important permeability model, the dentine disk model, was developed by Outhwaite *et al*. (1974) and Pashley *et al*. (1988). In this model, thin slices of coronal dentine from extracted human molars were used as test substrates. Because this technique provided the ability to standardize variables in dentine disks, such as surface area, thickness and applied pressure, its use significantly advanced the understanding of dentine permeability. More importantly, a simple yet effective model was now available to measure the effects of agents on dentine hypersensitivity.

Absi *et al*. (1987) combined scanning electron microscopy (SEM) and classic dye penetration techniques to quantify the patency of dentine tubules. This technique provided a means of categorizing sensitive and non-sensitive teeth as to the number of tubular openings and their role in the hydrodynamic mechanism of hypersensitivity. SEM, along with other surface characterizing techniques such as electron spectroscopy for chemical analysis (ESCA), and X-ray analysis, has been used to fully characterize dentine surfaces and also to analyze the composition of materials deposited on the dentine surface during treatment (Miller *et al*. 1994, Pooman *et al*. 1997). These analytical techniques are now proven complements to other permeability measurements.

Alternative techniques used for the evaluation of desensitizing agents involve the pulpal sensory nerve activity (SNA) models. One such model is the multi-unit intradental recording method initially developed by Edwall and Scott (1971), Edwall and Olgart (1977) and later modified by Kim (1986). Briefly, two deep dentine cavities were prepared on the buccal surface of a canine tooth of anesthetized cats or dogs. These two cavities, one cut over the incisal pulp horn and the other within the gingival part of the crown, served as electronic recording cavities. A third deep-cut cavity was prepared on the lingual surface and was used to deliver solutions of therapeutic agents. The recording cavities, which contained low-impedance platinum or silver/silver chloride electrodes, were filled with isotonic saline. Silicone paste was used as insulation to prevent salt bridging, and the electrical potential was amplified for recording purposes. The effect of desensitizing agents on nerve activity was assessed via the potential drop across the recording cavities after application of a 3 M hypertonic sodium chloride solution before and after application of each test agent. Using this model, potassium ion was determined to be the active portion of potassium nitrate and other potassium compounds (Kim 1986). When this recording technique was used in human volunteers, it was found that the recorded nerve spike activity correlated well with the sensation of pain (Fors *et al*. 1984). The sensation that accompanied the sensory nerve activity evoked by hot, cold or ionic stimulation was described as a sharp pricking pain typical of A-δ fiber activity, the type of sensation associated with sensitive teeth.

Another method for studying sensory nerve activity involves dissection of intradental nerve fibers from the terminal branches of either the maxillary or mandibular nerve before they enter the apical foramen of the test tooth (Närhi 1985). This method has an advantage over the multi-unit intradental recording model in that the action potential of intradental C fibers can also be recorded. In the multi-unit intradental recording model, only part of the pulp nerve units (the myelinated A fibers) can be recorded (Haegerstam 1976, Lisney 1978). However, there are enough data to support both SNA models as suitable for studying nerve activity changes associated with desensitizing agents.

Clinically, dentine hypersensitivity has been evaluated on the basis of the individual patient's subjective response to any of the traditionally employed stimuli. Sensitivity to thermal stimuli, especially cold (air or water), seem to be the most troublesome for sufferers (Orchardson and Collins 1987). Therefore, the cold stimulus should be included as a measurement of sensitive levels in any clinical study. The two most commonly used techniques to stimulate a response to cold include application of a 1-s air blast (Tarbet *et al.* 1979, Silverman 1985) or application of cold water or ice to the involved tooth (Johnson *et al.* 1982, Brough *et al.* 1985). However, there are limitations to the accuracy of these two techniques (Clark and Troullos 1990, Orro *et al.* 1994, Gillam 1997). The rate of cooling is dependent on the surface area contacted, which does not remain constant when either of these techniques is employed. In addition, the use of ice or cold water causes an osmotic gradient to be established through the patent tubules in exposed dentine.

Tactile stimulation is another frequently used technique for evaluating dentine hypersensitivity. An explorer is scratched across the exposed dentine with sufficient pressure to deform the dentine. The amount of pressure required to elicit a pain response may be quantified by incorporating a calibrated strain gauge in the explorer (Orchardson and Collins 1987) or by using a Yeaple probe (Minkoff and Axelrod 1987). This method is simple but effective and when combined with other stimuli (such as a thermal stimulus) provides an adequate means of assessing most desensitizing agents.

In-vitro and clinical techniques, respectively, were used to (i) demonstrate the ability of a dentifrice containing 5% potassium nitrate/1500 ppm fluoride as sodium monofluorophosphate (MFP) in a precipitated calcium carbonate (PCC) base to occlude dentine tubules, and (ii) document the ability of this dentifrice to reduce dentine hypersensitivity. The findings of these studies are presented in the remainder of this chapter.

Methods

In-vitro study

In vitro, the occlusion of dentine tubules by a test formula was assessed quantitatively by measuring the flow rate of an aqueous solution under a fixed pressure before and after treatment of the dentine sample. The preparation of dentine disks was recently described by Miller *et al.* (1994). Briefly, dentine disks (~800 μm thick) were prepared from the crown of human molars and then etched for 2 min in 6% citric acid to remove the smear layer. Treatment was performed by manually brushing the coronal side of each disk 12 times for 60 s with a 1" ribbon of the test product. There was at least a 30-min interval between treatments. Disks were stored in phosphate buffer (2.6 mM PO_4, 0.1 M NaCl, pH 7.0) at room temperature.

Following treatments, the hydraulic conductance or fluid movement across the disks was measured by a modification of the procedure devised by Pashley *et al.* (1988). A dentine disk was placed in a custom-made Pashley cell (Biomedical Engineering Department, Medical College of Georgia) and equilibrated to atmospheric pressure. The amount of fluid flowing through the disk was determined gravimetrically under 70 cm of hydrostatic water pressure. An analytical balance was connected via an output data unit to a computer for collecting the weight of the flow solution (± 0.0005 g) every 30 s for 20 min. The flow solution was an aqueous phosphate buffer containing 1.48 mM PO_4, 0.1 M NaCl, pH 7.0. The hydraulic conductance of human dentine varies considerably from disk to disk, thus each disk was used as its own control. Hydraulic conductance was expressed as $mg(cm^2min.cmH_2O)^{-1}$.

The material occluding the dentine after treatment was characterized by SEM and ESCA. SEM provides a visual examination of the gross morphology of the treated surfaces, while ESCA provides an elemental analysis of the material coating the dentine.

Clinical study

The design and outline (Figure 29.2) of the study have been described by Schiff *et al.* (1998). Briefly, the study was a parallel, double-blind, stratified two treatment design. Adult male and female subjects who satisfied specific inclusion criteria were enrolled into the study; for example, those in good health and who had teeth with

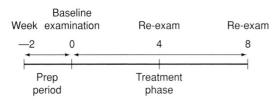

Figure 29.2

Outline of clinical trial. 48 subjects brushed for 2 weeks with a commercially available dentifrice. At the baseline examination, thermal and tactile stimulations were performed and recorded. Each subject used assigned dentifrice between weeks 0 and 8 (treatment phase).

exposed root-surface dentine. Subjects were excluded if they were pregnant or lactating, had any underlying medical condition, allergies to dental products, any dental condition that may affect the outcome of the study, recent oral surgery or scaling, or used desensitizing products within 3 months of the study. Forty-eight subjects who met the inclusion criteria and signed an informed consent form entered into the study. The protocol was approved by the appropriate Institutional Review Board. The study was conducted in accordance with the US Food and Drug Association's Good Clinical Practice regulations.

An initial examination to assess qualification for entry into the study was conducted 2 weeks prior to baseline examination. Subjects were asked to refrain from all oral hygiene practices and chewing gum for 8 h and from eating or drinking 2 h prior to their scheduled visit to the clinical facilities. The examination included a medical history, a thorough oral examination and evaluation for sensitive teeth. Sensitive teeth were assessed by means of a positive response to tactile stimulation with a dental explorer or a 1-s blast of cold air from a dental air/water syringe.

Qualified subjects were assigned to use a commercially available dentifrice and a soft-bristled toothbrush in place of their normally used oral hygiene products for 2 weeks. Subjects were instructed to continue their normal oral hygiene regimen with the exception of the substituted toothpaste and toothbrush.

Two weeks after the initial examination, subjects returned for a baseline examination, at which time tactile and thermal stimulations were

performed and recorded. The same restrictions imposed at the initial examination applied for the baseline and subsequent examinations. Tactile and thermal sensitivity were assessed as described previously by Schiff *et al.* (1994) and Ayad *et al.* (1994).

A Model 200A Yeaple Electronic Force Sensing Probe (Yeaple Research, Pittsford, NY, USA), calibrated prior to use, was used to assess tactile sensitivity. This probe was found to be consistent and provided the necessary type of test response (Pashley 1990). Tactile sensitivity was reported in terms of grams of force (Clark and Troullos 1990).

Thermal sensitivity was assessed by delivering a puff of air from a dental syringe at 60 psi (± 5 psi) and 70°F (± 3°F) to the sensitive tooth. Sensitivity was scored according to the 0–3 Schiff scale (Schiff *et al.* 1994). Evaluations were performed by the same dental examiner at the different examination points.

Subjects were stratified on a rolling basis, being randomly assigned to one of the two test groups on the basis of their mean pain ratings from tactile and air-blast stimulation. They were given their assigned product and a new tooth-brush and were informed of dosage and instructions to be practiced. Subjects were instructed to avoid any professional dental treatments during the 8-week treatment period, except in the case of emergencies. Visits for dental treatments during the study could disqualify the subject at the discretion of the principal investigator.

Subjects returned to the clinical facility after use of the assigned dentifrice for 4 weeks and 8 weeks. The same sensitivity scoring procedures and restrictions employed at baseline were repeated for these examinations.

The study was conducted according to the 1986 ADA 'Recommendations for Evaluating Agents for the Reduction of Dentine Hypersensitivity' (Ad Hoc Advisory Committee on Dentine Hypersensitivity 1986).

Data analysis

The data were analyzed using conventional parametric methods – analysis of variance (ANOVA). Treatment differences were declared statistically significant if the *P* value of the two-sided test was ≤0.05.

Results

In-vitro results

Hydraulic conductance

Figure 29.3 shows the average change in hydraulic conductance or fluid flow after 12 1-min brushings with water, and dentifrices containing 5% potassium nitrate in a PCC and dicalcium phosphate (DICAL) base. There was little change in fluid flow after treating with water. The small change was likely due to the redistribution of collagen protein and the formation of a smear layer. After 12 brushings with the KNO_3/DICAL dentifrice, fluid flow was reduced by an average of about 75%; whereas with the KNO_3/PCC dentifrice, the average reduction in fluid flow approached 90%. The primary occluding material in the KNO_3/PCC dentifrice was the abrasive, since potassium nitrate and the other dentifrice components are not known to occlude dentine.

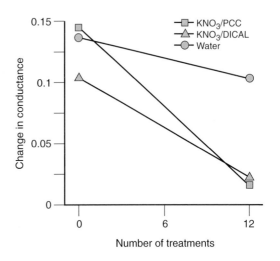

Figure 29.3

Change in hydraulic conductance of dentine after 12 × 1-min in-vitro treatments with water and dentifrices containing 5% KNO_3 in a PCC and DICAL base (average of three disks). Units are mg/(cm²min.cm H_2O).

SEM results

The electron micrographs of representative dentine disks treated with water, a commercially available KNO_3/DICAL dentifrice, and the KNO_3/PCC dentifrice are shown in Figures 29.4–29.8. The dentine surfaces treated with water showed that essentially all the tubules were open (Figure 29.4), consistent with dentine treated with water and similar to untreated dentine (Miller *et al.* 1994). Electron micrographs of dentine treated with a commercially available KNO_3/DICAL dentifrice revealed that most of the dentine tubules were open (Figure 29.5). A

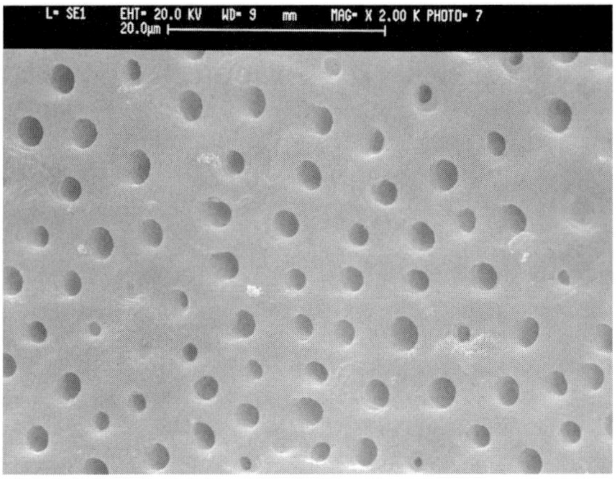

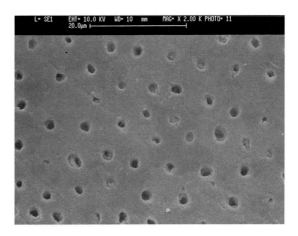

Figure 29.4

SEM of dentine surface after 12 × 1-min brushings with water (×2000).

Figure 29.5

SEM of dentine surface after 12 × 1-min brushings with 5% KNO_3/DICAL dentifrice (×2000).

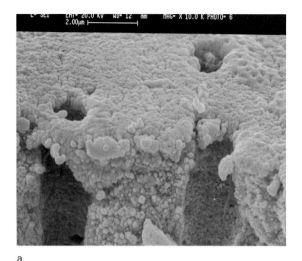

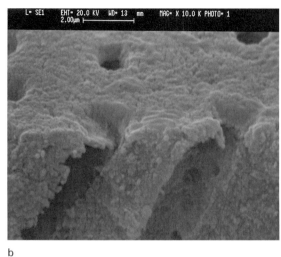

a   b

Figure 29.6

a and *b* SEM of cross-section of dentine after 12 × 1-min brushings with 5% KNO$_3$/DICAL dentifrice (×10 000).

cross-section of the disk showed a thin coating (~0.07 μm) of deposited material and particles lodged in the tubules. The lodged particles did not form a complete plug (Figures 29.6a, b). The thin deposit and the partially plugged tubules likely caused the reduction in hydraulic conductance observed in Figure 29.3. For dentine samples treated with the KNO$_3$/PCC dentifrice, electron micrographs revealed that about 100% of the dentine tubules were visibly occluded (Figure 29.7). A cross-section of the disks showed that occlusion was the result of particles lodged in the tubules or a 0.2-μm thick coating covering the tubules (Figure 29.8a, b). The particles lodged in the dentine tubules appear to completely plug the tubules. From SEM analysis, the apparent complete coating and plugging of dentine tubules would be expected to cause nearly 100% occlusion of the tubules. Poiseuille's law states that the filtration of fluid across dentine varies with the fourth power of the radius of the tubules, thus approximately 55% occlusion should theoretically cause about 100% reduction in fluid flow. However, from the hydraulic conductance data in Figure 29.3, occlusion was not 100%, suggesting the formation of a permeable deposit.

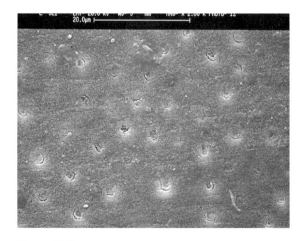

Figure 29.7

SEM of dentine surface after 12 × 1-min brushings with 5% KNO$_3$/PCC dentifrice (×2000).

ESCA results

The surface analysis data for water, KNO$_3$/DICAL dentifrice- and KNO$_3$/PCC dentifrice-treated dentine disks are shown in Table 29.1. Two 800-μm areas were analyzed for each disk – the

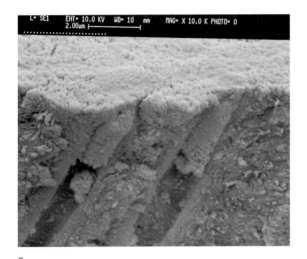
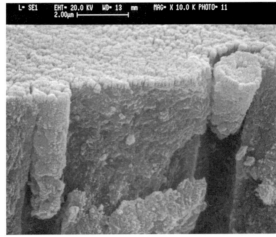

a b

Figure 29.8

a and *b* SEM of cross-section of dentine after 12 × 1-min brushings with 5% KNO$_3$/PCC dentifrice (×10 000).

average percent composition is reported. The surface compositions were reproducible for each area of each disk, indicating minimal surface heterogeneity. The composition of deposited materials was similar for both non-treated and water-treated disks (Table 29.1). The major changes in surface composition observed for the dentifrices versus water were a decrease in the nitrogen levels, an increase in calcium and phosphorus levels, and a decrease in the carbon/oxygen ratio. The atomic percentage of nitrogen (%N) may be used as a measure of the

level of dentine surface coating, i.e. the lower the %N, the more coating. A %N of about 14 is normally observed for acid-etched, non-treated disks. Here, the %N for the KNO$_3$/DICAL and KNO$_3$/PCC dentifrice-treated surfaces was 12.02 and 6.88, respectively. This indicates that the PCC-based dentifrice coated dentine surfaces more effectively than the DICAL-based dentifrice. The increased levels of Ca and P and the decrease in C/O ratio after treatment with the KNO$_3$/PCC dentifrice versus the KNO$_3$/DICAL dentifrice are also evidence of the greater coating

Table 29.1 ESCA results of dentine brushed 12 times for 1 min with water and dentifrices containing 5% potassium nitrate in a PCC or DICAL base (values reported are for the average of three disks)

Sample	Atomic percent					
	C	O	N	Ca	P	F
No treatment	64.83	20.76	13.59	0.29	0.38	0.00
Water	62.35	21.43	14.00	0.32	0.30	0.00
KNO$_3$/DICAL dentifrice*	49.46	30.17	12.01	4.48	3.75	0.00
KNO$_3$/PCC dentifrice	40.25	36.79	6.88	8.42	6.83	0.04

*Commercially available dicalcium phosphate dentifrice.

of dentine tubules by the PCC dentifrice. The relative proportions of these elements are indicative of a mixed calcium-phosphate-carbonate deposit. Interestingly, the level of phosphate in PCC abrasive is very low; therefore, the likely source of phosphate in the surface deposit was the buffer. The buffer used in the permeability studies and for disk storage between treatments contained 2.6 and 1.48 mM phosphate, respectively. The ESCA results suggest that occlusion of dentine tubules by KNO_3/PCC dentifrice observed in Figure 29.3 is due to a mixed calcium-phosphate-carbonate deposit.

Clinical results

A clinical study comparing the KNO_3/PCC dentifrice and a placebo dentifrice without potassium nitrate for the reduction of dentine hypersensitivity after 4 and 8 weeks was completed (Schiff *et al.* 1998). Changes in sensitivity, measured at baseline (week 0), 4 and 8 weeks, were assessed using an air-blast from a standard dental air syringe and a Yeaple probe for determining pain threshold. Subjects with strong to severe sensitivity (Schiff score >1 and tactile score between 10 and 50 gm.force) were selected at baseline to allow clinical detection of potential decreases in sensitivity. Subjects brushed twice daily with the assigned toothpaste. Of the 48 subjects who started the study, 43 completed 4 weeks of the study, while 39 completed the 8 weeks. There were no obvious or reported side-effects attributed to using the dentifrices. Those subjects who did not complete the study did so for reasons unrelated to dentifrice use.

Comparison of mean tactile sensitivity scores

The mean tactile sensitivity scores at baseline and after 4 weeks of dentifrice home use are shown in Table 29.2. Baseline mean scores are reported for subjects who returned for the 4-week examination. The mean baseline tactile sensitivity score for the placebo dentifrice group was 11.7 g.force, while the KNO_3/PCC group had a mean tactile score of 11.8 g.force. There was no significant difference between the dentifrice groups. After 4 weeks of dentifrice home use, the mean tactile sensitivity score for the placebo group was

Table 29.2 Comparison of mean tactile sensitivity scores (grams of force) of 5% potassium nitrate/PCC and placebo dentifrice groups

Examination	Dentifrice group	n	Mean tactile scores (g.force) ± SD	Percent* improvement (vs placebo)	Statistical significance
Baseline	Placebo	21	11.7 ± 3.0	–	
	Potassium nitrate/PCC	22	11.8 ± 3.3	–	NS
4 weeks	Placebo	21	18.3 ± 9.1	–	
	Potassium nitrate/PCC	22	32.7 ± 14.2	40.0%	P <0.01
Baseline	Placebo	18	11.9 ± 3.9	–	
	Potassium nitrate/PCC	21	11.9 ± 3.4	–	NS
8 weeks	Placebo	18	25.0 ± 14.3	–	
	Potassium nitrate/PCC	21	42.1 ± 11.0	40.6%	P <0.01

Taken from Schiff *et al.* (1998).
*A positive number represents an improvement.

18.3 g.force, versus 32.7 g.force for the KNO₃/PCC group. This difference represents a 40% reduction in tactile sensitivity pain scores for those subjects using the KNO₃/PCC dentifrice compared with the placebo group. An analysis of variance confirmed that this difference in tactile sensitivity scores after 4 weeks of continuous use of the two dentifrices was statistically significant at $P <0.01$.

The mean tactile sensitivity scores at baseline and after 8 weeks of dentifrice home use are also shown in Table 29.2. Baseline mean scores are reported for subjects who returned for the 8-week examination. The mean baseline tactile sensitivity score for the placebo dentifrice group and the KNO₃/PCC group was 11.9 g.force. After 8 weeks of dentifrice home use, the mean tactile sensitivity score for the placebo group was 25.0 g.force, compared with 42.1 g.force for the KNO₃/PCC group. This difference represents a 40.6% reduction in tactile sensitivity pain scores for those subjects using the KNO₃/PCC dentifrice compared to the placebo group. An analysis of variance confirmed that this difference in tactile sensitivity scores after 8 weeks of continuous use of the two dentifrices was statistically significant at $P <0.01$.

Air blast sensitivity examination (Schiff cold air sensitivity score)

The mean air blast sensitivity scores at baseline and after 4 weeks of dentifrice home use are shown in Table 29.3. Baseline mean scores are reported for subjects who returned for the 4-week examination. The mean baseline air blast sensitivity score for the placebo dentifrice group was 2.3, while the KNO₃/PCC group had a mean air blast score of 2.2. There was no significant difference between the dentifrice groups. After 4 weeks of dentifrice home use, the mean air blast sensitivity score for the placebo group was 2.0, versus 0.8 for the KNO₃/PCC group. This difference represents a 60% reduction in air blast sensitivity pain scores for those subjects using the KNO₃/PCC dentifrice compared with the placebo group. An analysis of variance confirmed that this difference in air blast sensitivity scores after 4 weeks of continuous use of the two dentifrices was statistically significant at $P <0.01$.

The mean air blast sensitivity scores at baseline and after 8 weeks of dentifrice home use are also shown in Table 29.3. Baseline mean scores are reported for subjects who returned for the 8-week

Table 29.3 Comparison of air blast sensitivity scores (Schiff Scale) of 5% potassium nitrate/PCC and placebo dentifrice groups

Examination	Dentifrice group	n	Mean tactile scores (g.force) ± SD	Percent* improvement (vs placebo)	Statistical significance
Baseline	Placebo	21	2.3 ± 0.5	–	
	Potassium nitrate/PCC	22	2.2 ± 0.5	–	NS
4 Weeks	Placebo	21	2.0 ± 0.7	–	
	Potassium nitrate/PCC	22	0.8 ± 0.5	60.0%	$P <0.01$
Baseline	Placebo	18	2.3 ± 0.5	–	
	Potassium nitrate/PCC	21	2.2 ± 0.5	–	NS
8 Weeks	Placebo	18	1.4 ± 0.8	–	
	Potassium nitrate/PCC	21	0.3 ± 0.4	60.9%	$P <0.01$

Taken from Schiff *et al* (1998).
*A positive number represents an improvement.

examination. The mean baseline air blast sensitivity score for the placebo dentifrice group was 2.3, while the KNO$_3$/PCC group had a mean air blast score of 2.2. There was no significant difference between the dentifrice groups. After 8 weeks of dentifrice home use, the mean air blast sensitivity score for the placebo group was 1.4, compared with 0.3 for the KNO$_3$/PCC group. This difference represents a 60.9% reduction in air blast sensitivity pain scores for those subjects using the KNO$_3$/PCC dentifrice compared with the placebo group. An analysis of variance confirmed that this difference in air blast sensitivity scores after 8 weeks of continuous use of the two dentifrices was statistically significant at $P < 0.01$.

Discussion

A precipitated calcium carbonate (PCC)-based dentifrice containing agents clinically proven to reduce dentine hypersensitivity (5% potassium nitrate) and prevent dental caries (1500 ppm fluoride as sodium monofluorophosphate) was evaluated for its ability to occlude dentine tubules and reduce the pain associated with tooth sensitivity. The data from in-vitro surface analysis indicate that the PCC-based dentifrice effectively coated and occluded dentine tubules with a deposit rich in calcium-phosphate-carbonate. The deposited material may be similar to a carbonato-apatite such as Ca$_{18}$[(PO$_4$)$_9$(CO$_3$)$_3$](OH)$_3$ described by Driessens and Verbeeck (1990). The KNO$_3$/PCC dentifrice was more effective in coating dentine surfaces than a commercially available dentifrice containing potassium nitrate and MFP in a DICAL base. Although PCC abrasive has only trace amounts of phosphate, the level of phosphate in the surface deposits after treatment with the PCC-based dentifrice was two-fold higher than that of the DICAL-base dentifrice. The source of the phosphate was most likely the buffer solutions, and would also be present in saliva. Under the pH conditions of the experiments, crystals containing calcium, carbonate and phosphate precipitated onto dentine disk surfaces. Such crystals also became lodged into the tubules, forming a plug. This was not evident for the KNO$_3$/DICAL-treated dentine. A similar reaction between the calcium carbonate of the KNO$_3$/PCC dentifrice and salivary phosphate is likely to occur in vivo, where phosphate in saliva is at saturating concentrations. Also, the presence of salivary proteins may further enhance the precipitation of the protective carbonato-apatite onto dentine.

The efficacy of the KNO$_3$/PCC-based dentifrice in alleviating dentine hypersensitivity was demonstrated in a recently concluded 8-week clinical study (Schiff et al. 1998). Compared with a potassium nitrate-free dentifrice, the active dentifrice significantly reduced tooth sensitivity in both efficacy comparisons, i.e. tactile sensitivity and thermal sensitivity. Both dentifrices gradually decreased sensitivity pain over the 8-week period. The KNO$_3$/PCC dentifrice was more effective in reducing sensitivity pain due to air blast than sensitivity pain caused by tactile stimulation. The data were consistent with in-vitro brushing study data which showed the test dentifrice to occlude dentine tubules. The placebo dentifrice (containing no potassium nitrate, but 1500 ppm fluoride as sodium monofluorophosphate) also reduced dentine hypersensitivity over the 8-week test period: a reduction of 52% compared with baseline. The likely mechanism of action for this observed placebo effect was the occlusion of dentine tubules by abrasive (calcium-phosphate-carbonate deposit) as observed in in-vitro studies. As shown in Figure 29.3, dentine occlusion increased with increased brushings.

A PCC-based dentifrice containing 1450 ppm fluoride as MFP was equivalent to a silica-based dentifrice containing 1100 ppm fluoride as NaF and 1450 ppm fluoride as MFP in preventing dental caries (Zhang et al. 1998). A drawback for dentifrices used in the treatment of dentine hypersensitivity is the taste. Because therapeutic agents are incorporated into these dentifrices, the taste may be adversely affected, especially when compared with conventional non-therapeutic dentifrices. Taste is one of the most important factors related to the continuous use of a particular dentifrice (Volpe 1982). The 1500 ppm F$^-$MFP/PCC dentifrice, with proven tooth sensitivity and anti-caries efficacy and no unpleasant taste, may be used daily as a means of building tolerance to thermal- and tactile-stimulated tooth sensitivity. However, the addition of potassium nitrate to this dentifrice provides a clinically proven and effective treatment for dentine hypersensitivity.

Conclusion

A dentifrice containing 5% potassium nitrate and 1500 ppm fluoride as sodium monofluorophosphate in a PCC base has been developed. Treatment of dentine with this dentifrice occludes dentine tubules with a mixed surface deposit of calcium-phosphate-carbonate. In addition, this dentifrice provides protection against dental caries, as it contains sodium monofluorophosphate – a clinically proven anti-caries agent. In an independent, double-blind and controlled clinical study, the dentifrice containing potassium nitrate and monofluorophosphate in a PCC base significantly reduced dentine hypersensitivity to tactile and thermal stimuli over an 8-week period, compared with a matching placebo dentifrice without potassium nitrate. Therefore, the results of in-vitro and clinical studies reported here demonstrate that a dentifrice containing potassium nitrate and sodium monofluorophosphate in a PCC base effectively reduces the pain associated with dentine hypersensitivity.

Acknowledgments

The authors would like to thank Eric Baines and Machiko Yoshioka for providing the test dentifrices, and Drs Robert Gambogi and Richard Robinson for critically reviewing the manuscript.

References

Absi EG, Addy M, Adams D (1987) Dentine hypersensitivity: a study of the patency of dentinal tubules in sensitive and nonsensitive cervical dentine. *J Clin Periodontol* **14**:280–4.

Ad Hoc Advisory Committee on Dentinal Hypersensitivity, ADA Council on Dental Therapeutics (1986) Recommendations for evaluating agents for the reduction of dentinal hypersensitivity. *J Am Dent Assoc* **112**:709–10.

Ayad F, Berta R, De Vizio W et al (1994) Comparative efficacy of two dentifrices containing 5% potassium nitrate on dentinal sensitivity: a twelve-week clinical study. *J Clin Dent* **5**:97–101.

Bolden TE (1994) A desensitizing dentifrice with multiple oral health benefits formulation for daily use. *J Clin Dent* **5**:68–70.

Bolden TE, Volpe AR, King WJ (1968) The desensitizing effect of a sodium monofluorophosphate dentifrice. *Periodontics* **3**:112–14.

Brännström M (1963) A hydrodynamic mechanism in the transmission of pain-producing stimuli through the dentine. In: Anderson DJ, ed, *Sensory Mechanisms in Dentine*, 73–9. Pergamon Press: Oxford.

Brännström M, Linden LA, Astrom A (1967) The hydrodynamics of the dental tubule and pulp fluid: a discussion of its significance in relation to dentinal sensitivity. *Caries Res* **1**:310–17.

Brough KM, Anderson DM, Love J, Overman PR (1985) The effectiveness of iontophoresis in reducing dentine hypersensitivity. *J Am Dent Assoc* **111**:761–3.

Clark GE, Troullos ES (1990) Designing hypersensitive clinical studies. *Dent Clin North Am* **34**:531–44.

Cohen S, Schiff T, McCool J et al (1994) Anticalculus efficacy of a dentifrice potassium nitrate, soluble pyrophosphate, PVM/MA copolymer, and sodium fluoride in a silica base: a twelve-week clinical study. *J Clin Dent* **5**:93–6.

Driessens FCM, Verbeeck MH (1990) The mineral in tooth enamel and dental caries. In: Driessens FCM, Verbeeck MH, eds, *Biomaterials*, 105–43. CRC Press: Boca Raton.

Edwall L, Olgart L (1977) A new technique for recording of intradental sensory nerve activity in man. *Pain* **3**:121–6.

Edwall L, Scott D (1971) Influence of changes in microcirculation of the excitability of the sensory unit in the tooth of the cat. *Acta Physiol Scand* **82**:555–66.

Federal Register (25 May 1982) **24**:22752.

Fors U, Ahlquist ML, Skagerwall R et al (1984) Relationship between intradental nerve activity and estimated pain in man – a mathematical model. *Pain* **18**:397–408.

Gillam DG (1997) Clinical trial designed for testing of products for dentine hypersensitivity – a review. *Periodontology Abstracts* **45**:37–46.

Gysi A (1900) An attempt to explain the sensitiveness of dentine. *Br J Dent Sci* **43**:865–8.

Haegerstam G (1976) The origin of impulses recorded from dentinal cavities in the tooth of the cat. *Acta Physiol Scand* **97**:121–8.

Johnson RH, Zulgar-Nain BJ, Koval JJ (1982) The effectiveness of an electro-ionizing toothbrush in the control of dentine hypersensitivity. *J Periodont Res* **53**:353–9.

Kim S (1986) Hypersensitive teeth: desensitization of pulpal sensory nerves. *J Endodontol* **12**:482–5.

Kleinberg I (1986) Dentinal hypersensitivity. Part II: Treatment of sensitive dentine. *Comp Con Ed Dent* **6**:280–4.

Lisney SJW (1978) Some anatomical and electrophysiological properties of tooth-pulp afferents in the cat. *J Physiol* **284**:19–36.

Miller S, Gaffar A, Sullivan R et al (1994) Evaluation of a new dentifrice for the treatment of sensitive teeth. *J Clin Dent* **5**:71–9.

Minkoff S, Axelrod S (1987) Efficacy of strontium chloride in dental hypersensitivity. *J Periodontol* **58**:470–5.

Murray LE, Roberts AJ (1994) The prevalence of self reported hypersensitive teeth. *Arch Oral Biol* **39**(Suppl.):S129.

Närhi MVO (1985) The characteristics of intradental sensory units and their responses to stimulation. *J Dent Res* **64**:564–71.

Orchardson R, Collins WJN (1987) Clinical features of hypersensitive teeth. *Br Dent J* **162**:253–6.

Orro M, Truong T, De Vizio W et al (1994) Thermodontic stimulator – a new technology for assessment of thermal dentinal hypersensitivity. *J Clin Dent* **5**:83–6.

Outhwaite WS, McKenzie DM, Pashley DH (1974) A versatile split-chamber device for studying dentine permeability. *J Dent Res* **53**:1503.

Pashley DH (1990) Mechanisms of dentine sensitivity. *Dent Clin North Am* **34**:449–73.

Pashley DH (1994) Theory of dentine sensitivity. *J Clin Dent* **5**:65–7.

Pashley DH, Dickson GD, Tao L et al (1988) The effect of a multistep dentine bonding system on dentine permeability. *Dent Mat* **4**:60–3.

Plagmann H-C, König J, Bernimoulin J-P et al (1997) A clinical study comparing two high-fluoride dentifrices for the treatment of dentinal hypersensitivity. *Quint Int* **28**:403–8.

Pooman J, Marcos AV, Gerald ED, Boyer DB (1997) Dentine desensitizing agents: SEM and x-ray microanalysis assessment. *Am J Dent* **10**:21–7.

Rosenthal WM (1990) Historic review of the management of tooth hypersensitivity. *Dent Clin North Am* **34**:403–28.

Rustogi KN, Triratana T, Timpawat S et al (1991) The effect of an anticalculus dentifrice on calculus formation and gingival recession in Thai children and teenagers: one year study. Study #2: an anticalculus dentifrice containing 1.3% soluble pyrophosphate and 1.5% of a copolymer. *J Clin Dent* **3**:B31–B36.

Schiff T, Dotson M, Cohen S et al (1994) Efficacy of a dentifrice containing potassium nitrate, soluble pyrophosphate, PVM/MA copolymer, and sodium fluoride on dentinal hypersensitivity: a twelve-week clinical study. *J Clin Dent* **5**:87–92.

Schiff T, Dos Santos M, Laffi S et al (1998) Efficacy of a dentifrice containing 5% potassium nitrate and 1500 ppm sodium monofluorophosphate in a precipitated calcium carbonate base on dentinal hypersensitivity. *J Clin Dent* **9**:22–5.

Silverman G (1985) The sensitivity-reducing effect of brushing with a potassium nitrate-sodium monofluorophosphate dentifrice. *Comp Cont Ed Dent* **6**:131–3, 136.

Tarbet WJ, Silverman G, Stolman JM, Fratarcangelo PA (1979) Evaluation of two methods for the quantitation of dentinal hypersensitivity. *J Am Dent Assoc* **98**:914–18.

Triratana T, Rustogi KN, Volpe AR (1991) The effect of an anticalculus dentifrice on calculus formation and gingival recession in Thai adults: one year study. Study #3: an anticalculus dentifrice containing 1.3% soluble pyrophosphate and 1.5% of a copolymer. *J Clin Dent* **3**:22–6.

Volpe AR (1982) Dentifrice and mouth rinses. In: Stallard RE, ed, *A Textbook of Preventive Dentistry*, 2nd edn, 182. WB Saunders: Philadelphia.

Zhang YP, Din CS, Schimid R, Gaffar A.(1998) Improved anti-caries efficacy in vivo of a stabilized MFP/PCC dentifrice. *Revista da Associação Brasileira de Odontologia* **6**:159–62.

30

Potential treatment modalities for dentine hypersensitivity: in-office products

David H Pashley

Introduction

The prevalence of dentine hypersensitivity is high enough (Chabanski *et al.* 1996) to warrant the development of effective in-office treatments. Patients who suffer from dentine hypersensitivity expect their dentists to have an effective treatment. Indeed, if the treatment is not effective, the patients may question the professional competence of their dentists. This chapter will attempt to survey the wide range of materials that has become available for the in-office treatment of hypersensitive dentine in recent years (Trowbridge and Silver 1990, Gangarosa 1994).

After diagnosing dentine hypersensitivity, it is important to explain the multi-faceted causes of the condition to patients. Dietary evaluation should be carried out as well as instruction and demonstrated proficiency in proper toothbrushing. Patients should be provided with an ultra-soft toothbrush and perhaps encouraged to brush without a dentifrice (Kuroiwa *et al.* 1994). Patients need to become involved in the resolution of their condition.

The treatment of dentine hypersensitivity must match its severity. For instance, advising a patient to use a desensitizing toothpaste twice a day is appropriate for patients with slight to mild hypersensitivity, but is inappropriate for patients with severe dentine hypersensitivity. In-office treatment of dentine hypersensitivity should be performed in all cases of severe hypersensitivity, especially if the condition has changed the patients' lifestyle (e.g. they cannot jog in cold air, must avoid cold drinks even in a hot climate, etc.). The treatment options are often dictated by

the clinical condition. If there is a loss of cervical tooth structure (e.g. presence of a wedge-shaped or grooved defect), then there is sufficient space for restorative treatments. The most difficult sites to treat are those where there is no loss of tooth structure, or insufficient loss of tooth structure to permit the use of restorative materials without over-contouring them and risking poor gingival health. Before treating regions of cervical dentine hypersensitivity, it is crucial that the exact region of hypersensitivity be identified. Although air blasts are useful as a screening tool, they cannot identify the exact site(s) of hypersensitivity. Commonly, less than 5–10% of exposed cervical dentine is sensitive. The buccal/labial surfaces should be gently evaluated with a dental explorer, in a raster-like pattern across the exposed surface. A 'map' of the exposed area should be drawn on the patient's chart and the location of the most sensitive sites indicated. This permits longitudinal evaluation of the specific sites before and after treatment.

All treatments should be done on unanesthetized patients so that they can provide immediate feedback regarding the effectiveness of a particular treatment. Some treatments will cause patient discomfort, but it will be transient and is generally a 'stinging' sensation caused by the hypertonicity of most dental medicaments. The treatments should be directed primarily at the hypersensitive sites. Treatment of the entire exposed dentine, while desirable for esthetic and preventive reasons, can be done after demonstration of the efficacy of a treatment in eliminating the dentine hypersensitivity of the most sensitive sites. Indeed, the goal should be the elimination of hypersensitivity. After that has been achieved, then the practitioner can focus on secondary issues such as esthetics.

The evaporation of water from dentinal tubules by an air stream, while it can occur if patients deliberately draw outside air across a sensitive quadrant or if they breathe cold air while jogging, is seldom a typical painful stimulus in patients with hypersensitive dentine. Thus, there is a danger in over-estimating dentine sensitivity clinically by the use of strong air blasts. It is not uncommon, when examining the hypersensitive region with an explorer, to find much less sensitivity. This is due, in part, to the fact that tactile stimuli are not as strong as air blasts (Pashley *et al.* 1996) and to the fact that only a very small area of dentine is being stimulated at any time with an explorer. Thus, the use of a strong air blast might induce fluid movement across dentine that is normally not sensitive, or is not sensitive to an explorer (Matthews *et al.* 1993).

What is needed is a weaker air stimulus that is as convenient as a standard dental syringe. Coleman and Kinderknecht have developed a simple air restrictor wheel that inserts between the body of the air syringe and the tip (personal communication) (Figure 30.1). By rotating a disk, a small hole can be placed within the air stream to greatly reduce the air flow when using the air syringe to test dentine sensitivity. For normal operation, the disk is rotated to the second unrestricted position

The method of air restriction was first reported by Orchardson and Collins (1987). The air syringe was modified to decrease the air flow from the normal 20 l/min down to 3 l/min. It had a number of additional improvements including a clear perspex shield that not only limited the air to the test tooth, but automatically maintained the distance of the tip of the air syringe from the tooth. Although a number of additional improvements have been made that are not easily adaptable to routine clinical practice, the items mentioned above are simple and should improve evaluations of dentine hypersensitivity.

There are disadvantages to using a dental explorer to evaluate post-treatment hypersensitivity. If a thin layer of unfilled adhesive resin was used to occlude dentine, it can be lacerated by a dental explorer (Hirvonen *et al.* 1984). Similarly, thin layers of resin-modified glass

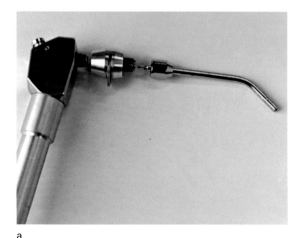

a

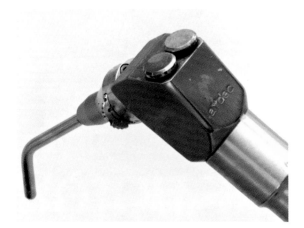

b

Figure 30.1

Modification of three-way dental syringe by placement of an air restriction hole between the syringe body and the tip. This can be rotated in or our of the air stream. (Courtesy of Dr Thomas Coleman, Shaftbury, VT, USA.)

ionomer cements could be torn by a dental explorer. In such cases, the use of an air stream or the placement of 0.05 ml of cold (4–10°C) water on the surface would be a better choice for the evaluation of post-treatment hypersensitivity. Both these stimuli must be avoided with freshly placed conventional glass ionomer cements (GIC) because of the danger of dehydrating or over-hydrating the GICs, respectively.

Box 30.1 In-office treatments for hypersensitive dentine

I   Treatment agents that do not polymerize
   A   Varnishes/precipitants
       1. Shellacs
       2. 5% sodium fluoride varnish
       3. 1% NaF, 0.4% SnF_2, 0.14% HF solutions
       4. 3% mono-potassium-monohydrogen oxalate
       5. 6% acidic ferric oxalate
       6. Calcium phosphate preparations
       7. Calcium hydroxide
   B   Primers containing HEMA
       1. 5% glutaraldehyde, 35% HEMA in water
       2. 35% HEMA in water

II Treatment agents that undergo setting or polymerization reactions
   A   Conventional glass ionomer cements
   B   Resin-reinforced glass ionomers/compomers
   C   Adhesive resin primers
   D   Adhesive resin bonding systems

III Use of mouthguards

IV Iontophoresis

V   Lasers

In covering the topic of in-office treatments for dentine hypersensitivity, the underlying assumption is that the hypersensitivity is due to hyperconductive dentinal tubules that permit hydrodynamic stimuli to activate pulpal nerves. All in-office treatments are designed to decrease the hydraulic conductance of dentine by partial or complete tubule occlusion (Brännström *et al.* 1979, Pashley 1986).

In-office treatments for hypersensitive dentine can be divided into two broad categories: treatments using applications of varnishes, precipitants, or primers that do not polymerize; or the use of cements or resins that undergo setting or polymerization reactions (see Box 30.1). Included in the first category are varnishes, oxalate-containing products, fluoride-containing products and products containing hydroxyethyl methacrylate (HEMA). Glass ionomer cements (GICs), resin-reinforced glass ionomers, adhesive primers and adhesive resin systems are included in the second category.

The clinical use of these agents will depend on the degree of sensitivity, the number of teeth involved, the amount of tooth structure lost and the amount of treatment time that would be required (which would determine the cost of the treatment). For a single quadrant of moderately sensitive teeth with little loss of tooth structure, the first therapy to try might be the use of an oxalate solution or a HEMA-containing primer. If this simple single treatment does not produce an immediate reduction in sensitivity (measured with an explorer or reduced air flow), then the treatment should be repeated. If the second treatment is without effect, the treated surface should be lightly abraded with pumice and rubber cup to remove residual material and a second, more complex treatment tried such as the use of a GIC or other adhesive material.

A review of the literature provided a good deal of evidence for the efficacy of many in-office treatments for dentine sensitivity. Where there was conflicting evidence, both observations are included. Only blinded studies that included control groups have been included in this review (unless otherwise noted). This review was not meant to be exhaustive, but only exemplary of the types of studies that have been done with the various products.

Treatment agents that do not polymerize

Varnishes, precipitants

The use of 5% sodium fluoride (NaF) in a thick varnish as a dentine desensitizer has been reported by Clark *et al.* (1985). The varnish does temporarily occlude dentinal tubules (Figure 30.2) but the material is readily lost over time. The varnish was found to be effective for the relief of dentine hypersensitivity. Hansen (1992) reported an interesting cross-over study, where patients with dentine hypersensitivity were treated first with the fluoride varnish and if that failed, with a light-cured glass ionomer. Treatment with the fluoride varnish produced 22% failures within 1 week, and a 1-year cumulative success rate of 44%. With the glass ionomer 2% of the treatments failed within the first week and the 1-year success rate was 79%. This is a good example of escalating therapy. If the simple therapy did not work, a more complex but more effective therapy was carried out.

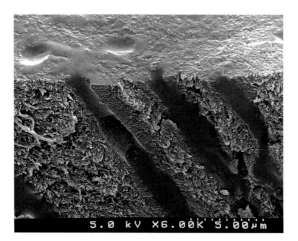

Figure 30.2

Secondary electron image of dentine surface treated with a 5% sodium fluoride varnish. The smear layer had been polished off using 0.04 μm aluminum oxide to simulate the clinical condition of open tubules. After treating with varnish, the specimen was soaked in water for 72 hours and then subjected to tooth brushing. Note the depressions in the residual film of varnish over the tubules and the 'varnish tags' extending 10–12 μm into the open tubules. (Courtesy of Dr Marcos Vargas, University of Iowa, IA, USA.)

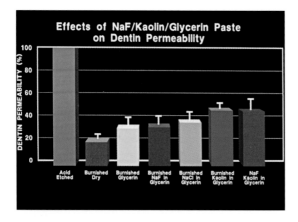

Figure 30.3

Bar graph of the effects of burnishing sodium fluoride (NaF), sodium chloride (NaCl), kaolin alone or in combination, wet versus dry, on reducing dentine permeability in vitro (from Pashley et al. 1987).

A number of treatments for hypersensitive cervical dentine are based upon occlusion of open dentinal tubules. For instance, burnishing sensitive root surfaces with a paste made up of 33% NaF, 33% kaolin and 33% glycerine has been used for over 50 years. The only clinical trial that used blinded conditions and placebo controls was done by Tarbet et al. (1979). They burnished the paste into affected dentine (or enamel in controls) with an orangewood stick for 30 s. When sensitivity was scored with cold air at 15 min and at 3, 7, 10 and 14 days after treatment, there was a significant ($P < 0.001$) immediate desensitizing effect of the treatment. The effect was lost between the seventh and tenth day of evaluation. However, the placebo paste burnished on enamel was also effective at reducing sensitivity when tested immediately, but not at the longer time periods. It was unclear whether the desensitizing result was due to the presence of NaF, kaolin or burnishing, as none of these variables were tested separately. In a simple in-vitro study, dentine permeability was measured on disks of dentine before and after burnishing with 33% NaF in glycerin or 33% sodium chloride (NaCl) in glycerin or 33% kaolin in glycerin, or burnishing the dentine with glycerin alone or burnishing dry dentine. The most effective treatment was dry burnishing ($P < 0.05$), followed by burnishing with glycerin and the other ingredients (Figure 30.3). None of the wet burnishing treatments were significantly different from each other, although all of them reduced dentine permeability following 2 min of burnishing with an orangewood stick (Pashley et al. 1987).

The clinical evidence for the efficacy of oxalate-containing solutions is mixed. Muzzin and Johnson (1989) conducted a clinical trial over 1–4 weeks using cold water as a stimulus. That study revealed that potassium oxalate was effective immediately after treatment and after 4 weeks, but not at 1 or 2 weeks. The significance level in this study ($P = 0.005$) may have been overly rigorous. Cold water was used rather than air blasts or tactile stimuli. However, another more recent clinical trial failed to objectively demonstrate the efficacy of a similar oxalate dentine desensitizer, or of an adhesive primer, although the patient's subjective impression was that both systems were effective (Gillam et al. 1997). Using a Yeaple probe, Gillam et al. (1997)

found an oxalate solution was effective at 5 min and 1 month, but not at 2 months. Air blasts failed to show any efficacy, but they may produce too severe a stimulus. In-vitro studies have confirmed that oxalates tend to solubilize over time (Pashley, unpublished observations), which may explain why they lost their effect at the 2-month evaluation period. Another clinical study by Russell et al. (1997) indicated that an oxalate solution was only marginally effective.

Imai and Akimoto (1990) demonstrated the effectiveness of a two-step procedure in which the dentine was first saturated with 5% disodium phosphate solution followed by a sequential application of 10% calcium chloride. This produced a precipitate of calcium phosphate in the tubules and on the dentine surface. The same report provided preliminary evidence of its clinical efficacy. Thirty-eight patients complaining of hypersensitive cervical dentine had their sensitivity scored with an air blast before and immediately after the sequential application of the phosphate and calcium solutions; 84% of the patients had immediate relief from hypersensitivity. No recalls were done and no statistical analyses were provided.

The precipitation of calcium phosphate that is of a particle size small enough to enter dentinal tubules depends upon the concentration of the reactants, and especially on their pH (Tung et al. 1993). This sequential, two–step approach to occluding tubules with calcium phosphate has been expanded by the work of Ishikawa et al. (1994) and Suge et al. (1995a, 1995b). That group has recently added small amounts of NaF to the solutions to promote conversion of dicalcium phosphate to apatitic crystals (Figure 30.4). No clinical trials have yet been published by this group to support the efficacy of these techniques. In a very carefully done clinical trial, Yates et al. (1998) found no effect of a sequential, two-step application of calcium chloride and potassium phosphate solutions. That is, the placebo effect was so large that they could not determine whether the decrease in hypersensitivity was due to the active agent rather than the water placebo. It is possible that testing hypersensitivity provides sufficient irritation to the pulp to initiate a series of biological responses that lead to decreases in dentine hypersensitivity.

Calcium hydroxide paste has long been used to treat hypersensitive dentine. A clinical trial by Green et al. in 1977 obtained significant desensitization to thermal stimuli (using a Peltier device) and mechanical stimulation following a 5-min treatment with calcium hydroxide paste. The desensitizing effect lasted for the 3-month

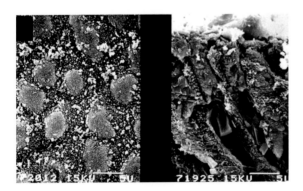
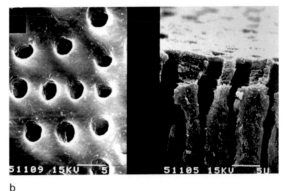

a   b

Figure 30.4

Secondary electron image of dentine surface following sequential topical treatment with acidic solutions of calcium phosphate followed by its neutralization by a basic solution (from Ishikawa et al. 1994).

a Appearance of dentine after treatment viewed from above (left) or from the side of a fractured specimen.
b Appearance of control dentine treated with water.

study. Similar results were reported, more recently by Kono *et al.* (1996).

The use of HEMA-containing primers is gaining popularity. However, few controlled clinical trials have been done to demonstrate their efficacy. Using a HEMA primer versus water-treated controls, Felton *et al.* (1991) measured the sensitivity of the facial surfaces of full crown preparations to tactile, air blast and osmotic stimuli. The primer, composed of 5% glutaraldehyde and 35% HEMA in water, was very effective in reducing dentine sensitivity both in the presence or absence of the smear layer ($P < 0.01$). The sensitivity evaluation was measured only once, 14 days after crown preparation. Similar significant results were obtained by Dondi dall'Orologio and Malferrari (1993) in a comparison of the desensitizing effects of 5% glutaraldehyde-35% HEMA primer with an aluminum nitrate/glycine (pH 2.5) conditioner. These authors evaluated the degree of hypersensitivity of cervical roots with air blasts and a dental explorer. The reductions in sensitivity ($P < 0.05$ compared with untreated control teeth) lasted for the entire 6-month trial. However, this excellent result could not be confirmed by Quarnstrom *et al.* (1998). Davidson and Suzuki (1997) reported a controlled clinical trial of the efficacy of the 5% glutaraldehyde-35% HEMA primer in reducing cervical dentine hypersensitivity. Four groups were used in the study and sensitivity was scored with explorer and air blasts immediately after treatment at 1 and 2 weeks and at 1, 3, 6 and 12 months. Group 1 teeth were treated with the complete primer, but no surface conditioning; group 2 teeth received pretreatment surface conditioning with EDTA prior to primer application; group 3 teeth received the same treatment as group 2 teeth plus application of an adhesive resin; group 4 teeth were treated with water. The teeth in groups 2 and 3 exhibited statistically significant reductions in sensitivity immediately after treatment ($P < 0.02$ and 0.03, respectively). In approximately 50% of the teeth, the sensitivity gradually returned, while 50% exhibited sustained relief of sensitivity. In a similar clinical study, Inoue *et al.* (1996) had a 79% success rate for their 8-week trial. In an interesting study by Schüpbach *et al.* (1997), buccal cusps of human molars were flattened in vivo and treated with EDTA, water, 5% glutaraldehyde or 35% HEMA in water, or the combination of 5% glutaralde-

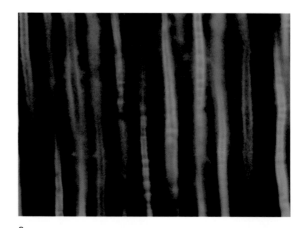

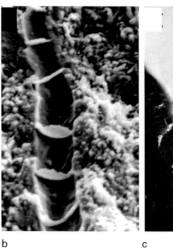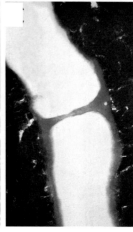

Figure 30.5

Appearance of dentinal tubules following treatment in vivo with a primer (5% glutaraldehyde, 35% HEMA in water). These septa were not observed in untreated control teeth or teeth treated with 35% HEMA alone. (from Schüpbach *et al.* 1997).

a Confocal microscopic appearance.
b Secondary electron image.
c Transmission electron micrograph.

hyde and 35% HEMA in water, and then the teeth were extracted and observed by confocal microscopy and SEM. Transluminal partitions or septa were observed (Figure 30.5) to span the lumens of dentinal tubules of teeth treated with the 5% glutaraldehyde-35% HEMA primer, but not with the other treatments. The authors speculated that the primer may have caused a precipitation of plasma proteins within dentinal fluid, causing the septa seen by both microscopic techniques. In an in-vitro study of the effects of primers used in adhesive dentistry on the permeability of dentine, Tagami *et al.* (1994) reported that most of the primers, including 5% glutaraldehyde-35% HEMA, reduced permeability if the tubules contained bovine serum, but not if they contained buffer. They also mixed adhesive primers with serum or buffer in test tubules and showed the precipitation reactions in the former, but not in the latter. Bergenholtz *et al.* (1993) treated the dentine of monkey incisors with 5% glutaraldehyde-35% HEMA primer and found that it reduced the outward movement of albumin, in vivo. No controlled studies of the treatment of hypersensitive dentine have been done using glutaraldehyde-free solutions of HEMA.

Treatment agents that undergo setting or polymerization reactions

Conventional glass ionomer cements

One of the first clinical evaluations of the use of glass ionomers for the treatment of hypersensitive dentine in cervical abrasion lesions was reported by Low (1981). The cervical lesions were etched with 50% citric acid for 30–45 s, then rinsed and dried prior to placement of the glass ionomer cement. Although the method of evaluating sensitivity was not described and no controls were used, the author reported complete loss of hypersensitivity in 89.7% of all patients.

Resin-reinforced glass ionomers

Hansen (1992) obtained a 1-year success rate of 79% using a resin-reinforced glass ionomer to treat hypersensitive dentine. This study was discussed above in the section on varnishes

because the comparison was with a fluoride varnish. These materials should be successful in treating hypersensitive dentine if they cover the affected area.

Adhesive resin primers

Theoretically, the use of adhesive primers to occlude the open tubules of hypersensitive dentine looks very attractive, because they have very thin residual film thicknesses. The use of adhesive resin primer products has been shown to decrease dentine permeability in-vitro (Simpson *et al.* 1993). The first clinical trial of the use of primers was done by Ianzano *et al.* (1993). In a small pilot study, they treated seven patients with 42 teeth sensitive to air blasts and explorer. Using a no-etch, moist-bonding technique, six to eight coats of primer were applied in unanesthetized patients. After evaporating the acetone, the treated surfaces were light-cured for 20 s. Sensitivity was scored before and immediately after treatment. The patients were asked about their sensitivity by telephone 1 month after treatment. They returned for a clinical evaluation at 9 months. About one-half of the patients had less sensitivity immediately after treatment. At 9 months, six of the seven patients were free of pain (P <0.001). There were no untreated control teeth used in the study. In another small clinical trial, Cagidiaco *et al.* (1996) covered dentine exposed during preparations for laminate veneers with one of two primer products. Postoperative sensitivity was evaluated immediately and 4 days later, compared with untreated controls, using an air blast. Both primers eliminated dentine sensitivity in this short study. The dentine was acid-etched prior to application of one of the primers. However, a full clinical trial of the use of the acid-etched primer product, done by a different group, could not demonstrate efficacy at reducing dentine hypersensitivity (Anderson and Powell 1994). One problem with resins that produce thin films is that atmospheric oxygen may diffuse into the thin films and interfere with free radical polymerization reactions (Erickson, 1989). After light-curing, unprotected resin films less than 20 µm thick may remain unpolymerized (Figure 30.6) and would be quickly lost. If thin films of resins are to be used

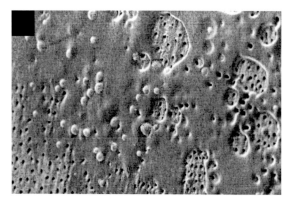

a

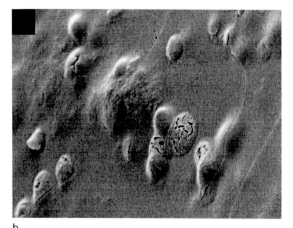

b

Figure 30.6

Secondary electron image of dentine surfaces following treatment with an adhesive primer. Although the test was done in vitro, the pulp chamber was filled with fluid under 30 cm H_2O pressure to simulate in-vivo conditions. (Courtesy of Dr Stephan Paul, University of Zurich, Switzerland.)

a The surface was light-cured for 20 s.
b The surface was light-cured for 60 s.

to treat dentine hypersensitivity, there is a need to develop polymerization initiators and reactions that are insensitive to oxygen. Thicker resin films are created using a more recently developed primer system in which the primer and adhesive components are mixed together into a single bottle. Russell *et al.* (1997) reported some success in using this system to treat cervical hypersensitive dentine.

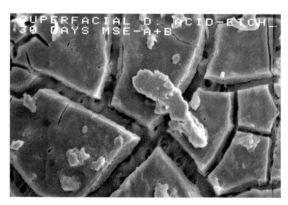

Figure 30.7

Secondary electron image of dentine following treatment with a suspension of an acidic polymer and oxalic acid. The cracks in the surface are drying artifacts (from Zhang *et al.* 1998).

An alternative resin desensitizer has been introduced recently. It is a two-bottle system; equal volumes of primers A and B are mixed and gently rubbed on the hypersensitive dentine for 30 s, followed by air-drying. The system contains oxalic acid and an emulsion of polymethylmethacrylate copolymerized with *p*-styrenesulfonic acid. The treated surface becomes covered with a layer of polymer about 5–10 µm thick (Figure 30.7) and some primitive resin tags are formed within open tubules (Nakabayashi *et al.* 1995). This treatment lowers dentine permeability in vitro (Zhang *et al.* 1998) and has been shown to be effective at reducing hypersensitive dentine in vivo (Nakabayashi *et al.* 1995, Suggs *et al.* 1996).

The long-term effectiveness of this resin product may be limited by the inability of the resin tags to bond to the walls of the peritubular dentine matrix lining most dentinal tubules. Only if the peritubular dentine is removed by acid-etching to expose the collagen fibrils of the surrounding intertubular dentine matrix can liquid resin infiltrate into the demineralized matrix and hybridize with it (Nakabayashi and Pashley, 1998). However, such acid-etching may open up previously insensitive tubules, making the treatment more difficult.

Adhesive resin bonding systems

A number of studies have been done on the use of resin bonding systems to treat dentine hypersensitivity. Dayton *et al.* (1974) evaluated the use of four first-generation dental adhesives. In a clinical study, these four adhesive systems were compared to a varnish used to treat dentine hypersensitivity. Sensitivity was evaluated with thermal stimuli (Peltier device), osmotic (1 mole/l sucrose) and scratch tests, before and immediately after treatment, and at 7 and 28 days following treatment. Two of the resin bonding adhesive treatments produced significant (P <0.001) reductions in thermal sensitivity compared with untreated controls or pretreatment sensitivity values. The reductions lasted for the duration of the 28-day study. All adhesives reduced sensitivity to tactile and osmotic stimuli. The putative desensitizing varnish was ineffective in reducing hypersensitivity.

Brännström and his colleagues were among the first to provide high resolution SEM of hypersensitive dentine treated with resins (Brännström *et al.* 1979, Nordenvall and Brännström 1980). They demonstrated that one adhesive system was effective (P <0.001) in reducing dentine hypersensitivity of exposed buccal cusp tips in premolars scheduled for extraction for orthodontic reasons (Nordenvall *et al.* 1984).

Jensen and Doering (1987) used a light-cured system to treat root surface hypersensitivity; the treatment was successful in eliminating sensitivity to air blasts and explorer in 89% of patients with extreme sensitivity, and in 97% of moderately sensitive teeth immediately after treatment. Even after 6 months, the treatments gave 75% and 94% reductions in dentine hypersensitivity, respectively.

In a 6-week study, Javid *et al.* (1987) evaluated a single application of cyanoacrylate to hypersensitive root surfaces, and found a significant (P <0.01) immediate reduction in sensitivity to air blasts that slowly returned toward pretreatment values (40% loss of effect) over the subsequent 6 weeks.

Several Japanese papers reported that the use of resin adhesives reduced radicular hypersensitivity (Suda *et al.* 1990, Yoshimine *et al.* 1991, Yoshiyama *et al.* 1991). Although they obtained good results, the investigators did not utilize statistical analyses or untreated control groups.

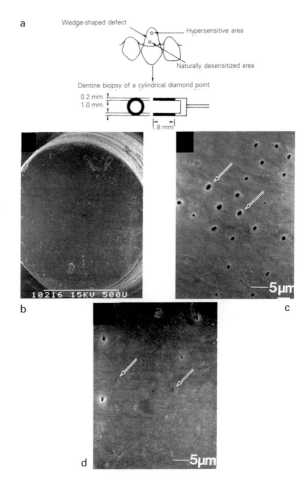

Figure 30.8

Obtaining biopsies (from Yoshiyama *et al.* 1989).

a Use of a hollow cylindrical diamond bur to obtain biopsies.
b Dentine biopsies.
c Hypersensitive dentine.
d Control, insensitive dentine.

An important morphological study was conducted by Yoshiyama *et al.* (1992) using a hard tissue biopsy technique to evaluate the long-term effects of resin treatment for hypersensitive dentine. Using a hollow cylindrical diamond bur (Figure 30.8), the authors biopsied several regions from resin-treated root surfaces 6 months after treatment. Treated regions that exhibited a recurrence of hypersensitivity were identified and biopsied, as were adjacent treated regions that remained insensitive to air blasts. In the regions exhibiting recurrence of hypersensitivity, 60% of the tubules were patent and free of resin tags. In contrast, in regions where the treatment had remained effective, over 75% of the tubules were occluded. However, in all the treated teeth, no resin coating remained on the surface, indicating that resin desensitization is due to the presence of resin tags in the tubules (Yoshiyama et al. 1993).

The use of fluoride-containing adhesive resins has been tried as a treatment for hypersensitive dentine. Orchardson et al. (1993) used multiple applications (twice weekly for 4 weeks) of a fluoride-containing, light-cured resin following pretreatment of the teeth with a paste containing fine (0.8 µm) quartz particles. They reported no consistent changes in treatment teeth compared to the controls over the 4-week study. Several patients had some desensitization, which returned when the resin became detached. The use of the pretreatment paste may have occluded the tubules with smear layer debris, thereby preventing resin penetration. Better clinical success was achieved by Tavares et al. (1994) using another fluoride-containing adhesive resin. Although these authors cleaned the surfaces with a rubber prophy cup, they acid-etched the adjacent cervical enamel with phosphoric acid. When rinsing the enamel, it is likely that the adjacent dentine was inadvertently lightly etched as well (Erickson et al. 1992). They used a primer, followed by the fluoride-containing resin. In group A, sufficient loss of tooth structure permitted placement of a layer of resin composite over the adhesive. In group B, less tooth structure was lost, so no resin composite was placed over the adhesive resin layer. Sensitivity was scored with cold (0°C) water before, immediately after treatment and at 3, 6 and 12 months. Control teeth remained sensitive. The results revealed highly significant reductions (P <0.0001) in cervical sensitivity to cold water in the resin-treated teeth at all time periods through 6 months, with group A showing lower sensitivity than group B. By 12 months, the treatment effect was no longer statistically significant due to a rise in the sensitivity of the control groups and a fall in the

efficacy of the treatment groups. Resin retention was excellent in group A (nearly 100%), but by 6 months, half of the teeth in group B had lost the resin layer. Yet, fewer than 20% of the subjects in group B reported increased sensitivity levels. The authors suggested that resin tags may have remained in the tubules even after loss of surface resin. There is no evidence in favor of the use of fluoride-containing adhesive resins over fluoride-free resins, as these studies did not include the use of such controls.

In a less well-controlled study, Calamia et al. (1996) scored sensitivity to air blast and explorer prior to and immediately after placement of an adhesive system. Postcard replies were used to assess the patients' subjective sensitivity at 1 and 7 days, but they were objectively evaluated on recall, at 1 and 6 months. Immediately after treatment, all resin bonded teeth showed much less sensitivity compared with control teeth (no statistical analyses were done). After 7 days, 29 of 31 treated teeth were less sensitive than controls. After 6 months, 19 of 21 teeth available at recall showed decreased sensitivity when tested.

Using a recently marketed adhesive system, Russell et al. (1997) reported moderate success in desensitizing cervical hypersensitive dentine, using cool water from a three-way dental syringe as a stimulus. They rescored sensitivity at 1 week and 1 month and reported that 76% of the adhesive-treated patients experienced improvements in their symptoms over the 1-month study.

In a recent, well-controlled study, Ide et al. (1998) evaluated the desensitizing effects of another adhesive system. They evaluated sensitivity with both restricted and unrestricted air stimuli, a Yeaple probe and with cold (10°C) water. Subjective response was recorded on a visual analog scale (VAS) and the short form of the McGill pain questionnaire prior to and 1 week after treatment. Control teeth had bonding agent applied to the middle third of the enamel on the sensitive control teeth. Their results indicated that the resin treatment of sensitive root surfaces produced a significant (P <0.02–0.05) reduction in tactile sensitivity, subjective sensitivity (McGill questionnaire) and sensitivity to both air stimuli, but not to cold water. The authors were so impressed with the effectiveness of the resin treatment that they suggested that it be regarded as the gold standard both for assessing techniques for estimating cervical sensitivity, and for investigating the efficacy of professionally applied topical desensitizing agents. It is important to point out that they did not acid-etch the dentine surface prior to application of the resin, as pilot experiments had shown that this treatment increased dentine sensitivity.

Other materials that have good potential for treating dentine hypersensitivity are the self-etching/self-priming bonding systems. They are usually two-bottle systems where one drop of primer A is mixed with a drop of primer B and the mixture is painted on the sensitive surface for 30 s, followed by gentle air-drying to remove volatile solvent. The surface is then covered with a thin layer of adhesive and light-cured for 20 s. Re-evaluation of the resin-covered surface should only be done with air or cold water, as the use of an explorer may tear the resin and re-expose tubules. Adhesive systems that utilize a separate acid-etching step may open up some tubules that are not covered by the second resin application step, leaving some tubules open and sensitive. The self-etching adhesive systems use an acidic methacrylate monomer dissolved in HEMA that both etches and primes the surface so that the subsequently applied adhesive is more likely to cover the primed surface and occlude all tubules. The disadvantage of the adhesive systems is that their polymerization is inhibited by atmospheric oxygen to a depth of $10-15\ \mu m$. If they are over-thinned with an air stream during placement, the resin films may not cure even though adequate light irradiation is done. This is normally not a problem in conservative dental treatment where these thin adhesive layers are covered with resin composites that exclude atmospheric oxygen and provide additional free radicals for polymerization. Although the latest generation of adhesive bonding systems are hydrophilic and provide better bonds in wet environments, the wetness should be water, not blood or protein-rich crevicular fluid which may lower bond strengths (Xie et al. 1993).

In summary, the effectiveness of adhesive resins in reducing dentine sensitivity has improved as bonding techniques and formulations have improved (Nakabayashi and Pashley, 1998). These materials are somewhat technique-sensitive and care must be taken to avoid creating a rough ledge of resin in the gingival crevice. Few well-controlled long-term studies have been performed, but most clinical trials have shown good short-term success.

Use of mouthguards

A number of clinical trials have shown the efficacy of 5% potassium nitrate (KNO_3) dentifrices at reducing dentinal hypersensitivity (Nagata et al. 1994). The dentifrices must be used twice daily for 2–4 weeks before any significant effect is seen. A 3% KNO_3/silica/NaF mouthrinse was also shown to be effective at reducing dentinal hypersensitivity after 6 weeks of treatment (Gillam et al. 1996), indicating that liquids may be as effective as pastes. The use of a mouthguard-type appliance to deliver potassium nitrate desensitizing agent was first reported by Reinhart et al. (1990). They had only partial success in that they obtained a significant reduction in sensitivity only after 2 weeks of treatment, but not at 1, 3 or 4 weeks of treatment with 10% KNO_3 gel. The lack of effectiveness of 10% KNO_3 may have been due to the short daily treatment time of 5 min. Had the patients used the gel for many hours each day or overnight, the results may have been different. They used glycerin to give the KNO_3 a gel-like consistency. These solutions are very hygroscopic and hypertonic. Had the KNO_3 been made up as an aqueous solution that was subsequently gelled, the results might have been better. In an interesting case report by Jerome (1995), a patient with severe bruxism had developed dentinal hypersensitivity in almost all of his teeth as a result of loss of enamel and much dentine. To make the patient more comfortable, a vacuum-formed mouthguard appliance was made and the patient was instructed to place small amounts of a desensitizing dentifrice containing 5% KNO_3 in the mouthguard as required for pain relief. The patient wore the mouthguard for almost 24 hours each day. Within 1 week, the patient could drink room temperature liquids without wearing the appliance, a feat that had been impossible prior to treatment. Many clinicians who are bleaching patients' teeth with the 'mouthguard' technique report that the sensitivity that sometimes develops after a few days of bleaching can be successfully treated with 5% KNO_3 toothpaste or gel in the same tray (Haywood, 1996). These treatments are usually done overnight. No controlled clinical trials have been done to confirm the efficacy of this technique, but it is something that should be considered for patients who have multiple sensitive teeth that do not respond to conventional treatments. Controlled clinical trials should be done to test the efficacy of potassium nitrate gels or pastes when used overnight.

Iontophoresis

The in-office use of iontophoresis of NaF to treat hypersensitive dentine has been advocated by Gangarosa (1983, 1994) and others (Kerns et al. 1989, Christiansen 1998). It is a technique-sensitive method that requires the purchase of an apparatus. Reports of lack of efficacy (Brough et al. 1985) may be due to inadvertent passage of current through adjacent gingival tissue rather than through cervical dentine. However, clinicians skilled in iontophoresis are strong advocates of its use for this purpose.

Lasers

Another in-office treatment for hypersensitive dentine is the use of lasers. Although there are a number of anecdotal reports of the efficacy of lasers for treating hypersensitive dentine, only two clinical trials have been published. Renton-Harper and Midda (1992) evaluated an Nd:YAG laser to treat patients with cervical sensitivity to cold air. The authors used the reduced air flow stimulus developed by Orchardson and Collins (1987). Treated roots were lasered for 2 min at 10 pulses/s at increasing power levels until the patient detected the laser energy or until a maximum of 100 mJ was reached. Although they included sensitive control teeth in the study, the treatment was not blinded to the clinician or the patient, although assessment of sensitivity on recalls was blinded. Treated teeth were less sensitive to air ($P = 0.05$) immediately after treatment and at 3, 7 and 14 day recalls. The second study was less well controlled and reported desensitization by a very low power helium-neon laser that was used for aiming the Nd:YAG laser (Gelskey et al. 1993), as well as by the Nd:YAG laser. These laser treatments were all done at power levels below that required to char dentine. The presumed mechanism of action is the coagulation and precipitation of plasma proteins in dentinal fluid as was demonstrated in vitro by Goodis et al. (1994). However, it is also possible for the thermal energy to alter intradental nerve activity (Orchardson et al. 1998). The clinical results obtained in the use of lasers to treat hypersensitive dentine do not seem to justify their very high purchase price. It is extremely difficult to produce uniform laser treatment of irregularly shaped cervical regions using a hand-held light-guide, especially if the laser operates in a pulsing mode.

Conclusion

It is clear that there are a number of in-office treatments available for hypersensitive cervical dentine. The use of restorative materials is more effective than the use of topical agents, but they require the loss of some tooth structure and they require more treatment time. Self-etching, self-priming resin adhesives are the simplest resin systems to use, but there have been no published clinical trials of their efficacy for that application.

Clinicians are urged to become familiar with these in-office products so that they can develop escalating in-office treatment approaches that are effective for mild, moderate and severe cases of hypersensitive dentine.

Acknowledgments

The author is grateful to Shirley Johnston for outstanding secretarial support. This work was supported, in part, by grant DE 06427 from the National Institute of Dental and Craniofacial Research, USA.

References

Anderson MH, Powell LV (1994) Desensitization of exposed dentine using a dentin bonding system. *J Dent Res* **73** (Special issue):297 (abstract 1559).

Bergenholtz G, Jontell M, Tuttle A, Knutsson G (1993) Inhibition of serum albumin flux across exposed dentine following conditioning with Gluma primer, glutaraldehyde or potassium oxalates. *J Dent* **21**:220–7.

Brough KM, Anderson DM, Love J, Overman PR (1985). The effectiveness of iontophoresis in reducing dentin hypersensitivity. *J Am Dent Assoc* **111**:761–5.

Brännström M, Johnson G, Nordenvall K-J (1979) Transmission and control of dentinal pain: Resin impregnation for the desensitization of dentin. *J Am Dent Assoc* **99**:612–18.

Cagidiaco MC, Ferrari M, Garberoglio R, Davidson CL (1996) Dentin contamination protection after mechanical preparation for veneering. *Am J Dent* **9**:57–60.

Calamia JR, Styner DL, Rattet AH (1996) Effect of Amalgambond on cervical sensitivity. *Am J Dent* **8**:283–4.

Chabanski MB, Gillam DG, Bulman JS, Newman HN (1996) Prevalence of cervical dentine sensitivity in a population of patients referred to a specialist periodontology department. *J Clin Periodontol* **23**:989–92.

Christiansen GJ (1998) Desensitization of cervical tooth structure. *J Am Dent Assoc* **129**:765–6.

Clark DC, Hanley HA, Geoghegan S, Vinet D (1985) The effectiveness of a fluoride varnish and a desensitizing toothpaste in treating dentinal hypersensitivity. *J Periodont Res* **20**:212–19.

Davidson DF, Suzuki M (1997) The Gluma bonding system: a clinical evaluation of its various components for the treatment of hypersensitive root dentin. *J Can Dent Assoc* **63**:38–41.

Dayton RE, DeMarco TJ, Swedlow D (1974) Treatment of hypersensitive root surfaces with dental adhesive materials. *J Periodontol* **45**:873–8.

Dondi dall'Orologio G, Malferrari S (1993) Desensitizing effects of Gluma and Gluma 2000 on hypersensitive dentin. *Am J Dent* **6**:283–6.

Erickson RL (1989) Mechanism and clinical implication of bond formation for two dentin bonding agents. *Am J Dent* **2**:117–23.

Erickson RL, Glasspoole EA, Pashley DH (1992) Dentin permeability increases from rinsing enamel etchant. *J Dent Res* **71** (Special issue): abstract 151.

Felton DA, Bergenholtz G, Kanoy BE (1991) Evaluation of the desensitizing effect of Gluma dentin bond on teeth prepared for complete coverage restorations. *Int J Prosthodontics* **4**:292–8.

Gangarosa LP (1983) *Iontophoresis in Dental Practice.* Quintessence: Chicago.

Gangarosa LP (1994) Current strategies for dentist applied treatments in the management of hypersensitive dentine. *Arch Oral Biol* **39** (Suppl):S101–S106.

Gelskey SC, White JM, Pruthi VK (1993) The effectiveness of the Nd:YAG laser in the treatment of dentinal hypersensitivity. *J Can Dent Assoc* **59**:377–86.

Gillam DG, Bulman JS, Jackson RJ, Newman HN (1996) Efficacy of a potassium nitrate mouthwash in alleviating cervical dentine sensitivity (CDS). *J Clin Periodontol* **23**:993–7.

Gillam DG, Coventry JF, Manning RH et al (1997) Comparison of two desensitizing agents for the treatment of cervical dentine sensitivity. *Endodontics Dent Trauma* **13**:36–9.

Goodis HE, White JM, Marshall SJ et al (1994) Measurement of fluid flow through laser-treated dentine. *Arch Oral Biol* **39** (Suppl):S128.

Green BL, Green ML, McFall WT (1977) Calcium hydroxide and potassium nitrate as desensitizing agents for hypersensitive root surfaces. *J Periodontol* **48**: 667–72.

Hansen EK (1992) Dentin hypersensitivity treated with a fluoride-containing varnish or a light-cured glass-ionomer liner. *Scand J Dent Res* **100**:305–9.

Haywood VB (1996) Bleaching tetracycline-stained teeth. *Esthetic Dent Update* **7**: 25–6.

Hirvonen TJ, Närhi MVO, Hakumäki MOK (1984) The excitability of dog pulp nerves in relation to the condition of dentine surface. *J Endodontics* **10**:294–8.

Ianzano JA, Gwinnet AJ, Westbay G (1993) Polymeric sealing of dentinal tubules to control sensitivity: preliminary observations. *Periodont Clin Invest* **15**:13–16.

Ide M, Morel AD, Wilson RH, Ashley FP (1998) The role of a dentine-bonding agent in reducing cervical dentine sensitivity. *J Clin Periodontol* **25**:286–90.

Imai Y, Akimoto T (1990) A new method of treatment for dentin hypersensitivity by precipitation of calcium phosphate in situ. *Dent Mat J* **9**:167–72.

Inoue M, Yoshikawa K, Okamoto A et al (1996) Clinical evaluation of Gluma 3 primer to dentin hypersensitivity. *Jap J Cons Dent* **39**:768–76.

Ishikawa K, Suge T, Yoshiyama M et al (1994) Occlusion of dentinal tubules with calcium phosphate using acidic calcium phosphate solution followed by neutralization. *J Dent Res* **73**:1197–204.

Javid B, Barkholder BA, Bhinda SV (1987) Cyanoacrylate – a new treatment for hypersensitive dentin and cementum. *J Am Dent Assoc* **114**:486–8.

Jensen ME, Doering JV (1987) A comparative study of two clinical techniques for treatment of root surface hypersensitivity. *Gen Dent* **35**: 128–32.

Jerome CE (1995) Acute care for unusual cases of dentinal hypersensitivity. *Quint Int* **26**:715–16.

Kerns D, McQuade M, Scheidt M (1989) Effectiveness of sodium fluoride on tooth hypersensitivity with and without iontophoresis. *J Periodontol* **60**:386–9.

Kono Y, Suzuki H, Hirayama S et al (1996). The effect of calcium hydroxide on dentin hypersensitivity. *Jap J Cons Dent* **39**:189–95.

Kuroiwa M, Kodoka T, Kuroiwa M, Abe M (1994) Dentin hypersensitivity. Occlusion of dentinal tubules by brushing with and without an abrasive dentifrice. *J Periodontol* **65**:291–6.

Low T (1981) The treatment of hypersensitive cervical abrasion cavities using ASPA cement. *J Oral Rehabil* **8**:81–9.

Matthews WG, Showman CD, Pashley DH (1993) Air blast-induced evaporative water loss from human dentine, *in vitro*. *Arch Oral Biol* **38**:517–23.

Muzzin KB, Johnson R (1989) Effects of potassium oxalate on dentin hypersensitivity *in vivo*. *J Periodontol* **60**:151–8.

Nagata T, Ishida H, Shinohara H et al (1994) Clinical evaluation of a potassium nitrate dentifrice for the treatment of dentinal hypersensitivity. *J Clin Periodontol* **21**:217–21.

Nakabayashi N, Pashley DH (1998) *Hybridization of Dental Hard Tissues*. Quintessence: Chicago.

Nakabayashi N, Fujii B, Horiuchi H et al (1995) Occlusion of dentinal tubules with reactive polymer emulsion. *Jap J Cons Dent* **38**:1538–48.

Nordenvall K-J, Brännström M (1980) *In vivo* resin impregnation of dentinal tubules. *J Prosthet Dent* **44**:630–7.

Nordenvall K-J, Malmgren B, Brännström M (1984) Desensitization of dentin by resin impregnation: a clinical and light-microscopic investigation. *J Dent Child* **5**:274–6.

Orchardson R, Collins WJN (1987) Thresholds of hypersensitive teeth to 2 forms of controlled stimulation. *J Clin Periodontol* **14**: 68–73.

Orchardson R, Collins WJN, Gilmour WH (1993) Pilot clinical study of a fluoride resin and conditioning paste for desensitizing dentine. *J Clin Periodontol* **20**:509–13.

Orchardson R, Peacock JM, Whitters CJ (1998) Effects of pulsed Nd:YAG laser radiation on action potential conduction in nerve fibers inside teeth, *in vitro*. *J Dent* **26**:421–6.

Pashley DH (1986) Dentin permeability, dentin sensitivity, and treatment through tubule occlusion. *J Endodontics* **12**:465–74.

Pashley DH, Leibach JG, Horner JA (1987) The effects of burnishing NaF/kaolin/glycerin paste on dentin permeability. *J Periodontol* **58**:19–23.

Pashley DH, Matthews WG, Zhang Y, Johnson M (1996) Fluid shifts across human dentin *in vitro* in response to hydrodynamic stimuli. *Arch Oral Biol* **41**:1065–72.

Quarnstrom F, Collier N, McDade E et al (1998) A randomized clinical trial of agents to reduce dentin sensitivity after crown cementation. *Gen Dent* **46**:68–74.

Reinhart TC, Killoy WJ, Love J et al (1990) The effectiveness of a patient-applied tooth desensitizing gel: a pilot study. *J Clin Periodontol* **17**:123–7.

Renton-Harper P, Midda M (1992) Nd:YAG laser treatment of dentinal hypersensitivity. *Br Dent J* **172**:13–16.

Russell CM, Dickinson GL, Downey MC et al (1997) One-Step versus Protect in the treatment of dentinal hypersensitivity. *J Dent Res* **77** (Special issue):199 (abstract 748).

Schüpbach P, Lutz F, Finger WJ (1997) Closing of dentinal tubules by Gluma desensitizer. *Eur J Oral Sci* **105**:414–21.

Simpson ME, Ciarlone AE, Pashley DH (1993) Effects of dentin primers on dentin permeability. *J Dent Res* **72** (Special issue):127 (abstract 185).

Suda R, Andoh Y, Shionome M et al (1990) Clinical evaluation of the sedative effect of HEMA solution on the hypersensitivity of dentin. *Dent Mat J* **9**:163–6.

Suge T, Ishikawa K, Kawasaki A et al (1995a). Duration of dentinal tubule occlusion formed by calcium phosphate precipitation method: *in vitro* evaluation using synthetic saliva. *J Dent Res* **74**:1709–14.

Suge T, Ishikawa K, Kawasaki A et al (1995b) Effects of fluoride on the calcium phosphate precipitation method for dentinal tubule occlusion. *J Dent Res* **74**:1079–85.

Suggs AK, Cox CF, Cox LK et al (1996) Colloidal MSE for differential diagnosis and treatment of dentin hypersensitivity. In: Shimono M, Maeda T, Suda H, Takahashi K, eds, *Dentin/Pulp Complex*, 245–7. Quintessence: Tokyo.

Tagami J, Nakajima M, Hosoda H (1994) Influence of dentine primers on the flow of bovine serum through dentine. *Arch Oral Biol* **39** (Suppl):146.

Tarbet WJ, Silverman G, Stolman JM, Fratacangelo PA (1979) An evaluation of two methods for the quantitation of dentinal hypersensitivity. *J Am Dent Assoc* **98**:914–18.

Tavares M, DePaola PF, Soparker P (1994) Using a fluoride-releasing resin to reduce cervical sensitivity. *J Am Dent Assoc* **125**:1337–42.

Trowbridge HO, Silver DR (1990) A review of current approaches to in-office management of tooth hypersensitivity. *Dent Clin North Am* **34**:561–81.

Tung MS, Bowen HJ, Derkson GD, Pashley DH (1993) Effects of calcium phosphate solutions on dentine permeability. *J Endodontics* **19**:383–7.

Xie J, Powers JM, McGuckin RS (1993) *In vitro* bond strength of two adhesives to enamel and dentin surfaces under normal and contaminated conditions. *Dent Mat J* **9**:295–99.

Yates R, Owens J, Jackson R et al (1998) A split-mouth placebo-controlled study to determine the effect of amorphous calcium phosphate in the treatment of dentine hypersensitivity. *J Clin Periodontol* **25**:687–92.

Yoshimine Y, Akamine A, Tani Y et al (1991) Clinical evaluation of a light-cured, transparent resin (Palfique-clear®) in treatment of root surface hypersensitivity. *Jap J Cons Dent* **34**: 657–62.

Yoshiyama M, Masada J, Uchida A, Ishida H (1989) Scanning electron microscopic characterization of sensitive vs. insensitive human radicular dentin. *J Dent Res* **68**:1498–502.

Yoshiyama M, Ozaki K, Noiri Y et al (1991) Treatment of dentin hypersensitivity – effect of a light-curing resin liner on tubule occlusion. *Jap J Cons Dent* **34**:76–81.

Yoshiyama M, Ozaki K, Ebisu S (1992) Morphological characterization of hypersensitive human radicular dentin and the effect of a light-curing resin liner on tubule occlusion. *Proc Finn Dent Soc* **88** (Suppl 1):337–44.

Yoshiyama M, Suge T, Kawasaki A et al (1993) Mechanisms of dentin hypersensitivity – ultrastructural characterization of both success and failure cases after topical application of a resin liner. *Jap J Cons Dent* **36**:200–5.

Zhang Y, Agee K, Pashley DH, Pashley EL (1998) The effects of Pain-Free® desensitizer on dentine permeability and tubule occlusion over time, in vitro. *J Clin Periodontol* **25**:884–91.

Index